Feeding Behavior: Neuroendocrine Control and Behavior

Feeding Behavior: Neuroendocrine Control and Behavior

Editor: John Preston

STATES
ACADEMIC PRESS
www.statesacademicpress.com

www.statesacademicpress.com

STATES
ACADEMIC PRESS

Cataloging-in-Publication Data

Feeding behavior : neuroendocrine control and behavior / edited by John Preston.
p. cm.
Includes bibliographical references and index.
ISBN 978-1-63989-785-8
1. Neuroendocrinology. 2. Psychoneuroendocrinology. 3. Neurophysiology.
4. Neuropsychology. I. Preston, John.
QP356.4 .F44 2023
612.8--dc23

States Academic Press,
109 South 5th Street,
Brooklyn, NY 11249, USA

ISBN 978-1-63989-785-8 (Hardback)

Contents

Preface

Neuroendocrinology is a discipline of biology that investigates the relationship between the nervous system and endocrine system. It studies the regulation of the hormonal activity of the body by the brain. The hypothalamus is a part of the brain that controls feeding behavior (food intake) and energy balance. Feeding behavior refers to any action of an animal that is directed towards the procurement of nutrients. Deregulation of feeding behavior, which results in weight loss or gain, has been linked to either high-grade or low-grade hypothalamic inflammation. Neuroendocrine systems are involved in the integration of hunger and satiety signals and the regulation of energy homeostasis. These hold the possibility of new treatment options for feeding disorders and diseases. This book unravels the recent studies on neuroendocrine control and behavior with respect to feeding behavior. It presents researches and studies performed by experts across the globe. Those in search of information to further their knowledge will be greatly assisted by this book.

Significant researches are present in this book. Intensive efforts have been employed by authors to make this book an outstanding discourse. This book contains the enlightening chapters which have been written on the basis of significant researches done by the experts.

Finally, I would also like to thank all the members involved in this book for being a team and meeting all the deadlines for the submission of their respective works. I would also like to thank my friends and family for being supportive in my efforts.

Editor

Preface

1

Lipid Processing in the Brain: A Key Regulator of Systemic Metabolism

Kimberley D. Bruce[1], Andrea Zsombok[2] and Robert H. Eckel[1]*

[1] University of Colorado School of Medicine, Division of Endocrinology, Metabolism and Diabetes, Aurora, CO, USA,
[2] Department of Physiology, School of Medicine, Tulane University, New Orleans, LA, USA

***Correspondence:**
Kimberley D. Bruce
kimberley.bruce@ucdenver.edu

Metabolic disorders, particularly aberrations in lipid homeostasis, such as obesity, type 2 diabetes mellitus, and hypertriglyceridemia often manifest together as the metabolic syndrome (MetS). Despite major advances in our understanding of the pathogenesis of these disorders, the prevalence of the MetS continues to rise. It is becoming increasingly apparent that intermediary metabolism within the central nervous system is a major contributor to the regulation of systemic metabolism. In particular, lipid metabolism within the brain is tightly regulated to maintain neuronal structure and function and may signal nutrient status to modulate metabolism in key peripheral tissues such as the liver. There is now a growing body of evidence to suggest that fatty acid (FA) sensing in hypothalamic neurons *via* accumulation of FAs or FA metabolites may signal nutritional sufficiency and may decrease hepatic glucose production, lipogenesis, and VLDL-TG secretion. In addition, recent studies have highlighted the existence of liver-related neurons that have the potential to direct such signals through parasympathetic and sympathetic nervous system activity. However, to date whether these liver-related neurons are FA sensitive remain to be determined. The findings discussed in this review underscore the importance of the autonomic nervous system in the regulation of systemic metabolism and highlight the need for further research to determine the key features of FA neurons, which may serve as novel therapeutic targets for the treatment of metabolic disorders.

Keywords: lipid metabolism, brain, liver, energy homeostasis, hypothalamus

INTRODUCTION

Metabolic disorders, particularly aberrations in lipid homeostasis, such as obesity, type 2 diabetes mellitus (T2D), non-alcoholic fatty liver disease, and hypertriglyceridemia, often manifest together as the metabolic syndrome (MetS) (1). Despite major advances in our understanding of the pathogenesis of these disorders, the prevalence of the MetS continues to rise (2). Since MetS constitutes an increased risk to cardiovascular morbidity and mortality (3), a more detailed understanding of the common causes, and integration between these disorders of energy homeostasis, is necessary to identify novel therapeutic targets and interventions that may halt the development of severe metabolic disease.

It is becoming increasingly apparent that the central nervous system (CNS) is a major contributor to the regulation of systemic metabolism and lipid balance. In the CNS, the nutritional status of the body is constantly being surveyed and assessed by key energy-sensing regions of the brain, such as the hypothalamus. Key nuclei within the hypothalamus, such as the ventromedial nucleus (VMH), arcuate nucleus (ARC), dorsomedial hypothalamic nucleus (DMH), and the paraventricular nucleus

(PVN), integrate signals to elicit peripheral responses, such as changes in feeding behavior, fuel mobilization, energy utilization, and energy storage (4). These nuclei detect both nutrients and nutritionally regulated endocrine factors, such as insulin (5), ghrelin (6), melanocortin (MC) (7), and leptin (8), in order to regulate feeding and energy balance. Here, in this review, we will focus on the mechanisms involved in lipid sensing in the brain and its emerging influence on systemic metabolism.

HOW DO LIPIDS ENTER THE BRAIN?

Lipids and lipid intermediates are essential components of the structure and function of the brain. In fact, the brain has the second highest lipid content behind adipose tissue, and brain lipids constitute 50% of the brain dry weight (9). However, unlike adipose tissue, which largely stores FAs as triglycerides for subsequent utilization and mobilization to other metabolic tissues, the brain is thought to mainly utilize acylated lipids to generate phospholipids for cell membranes (9). The FA composition of the brain is unique and is rich in long-chain polyunsaturated fatty acids (LC-PUFAs), particularly arachidonic acid (AA), eicosapentaenoic acid, and docosahexaenoic acid (DHA). Although some FAs can be synthesized *de novo*, essential FAs must be transported into the brain from the systemic circulation. And contrary to previously held theories, recent data suggest that this is a dynamic process, with up to 8% of LC-PUFAs actively being turned over daily and being replaced by plasma-derived FAs (10). Indeed, a number of studies have shown that FAs are able to cross the blood–brain barrier (BBB) and enter neurons. For example, radiolabeled FAs that are injected into the carotid artery of rats can be traced to neuronal cells (10). In addition, brain perfusion studies in rats have shown that radiolabeled palmitate is readily incorporated into cerebral phospholipids and neutral lipids and has a similar rate of uptake when delivered *via* whole rat plasma or a synthetic saline containing physiological levels of albumin. This suggests that FAs cross the BBB and that albumin may be important in this process (11). Even though these studies convincingly demonstrate FA uptake, they do not address the mechanism of transport.

How FAs enter the brain remains an unanswered fundamental question. Although we cannot rule out the possibility that FAs could passively diffuse across the BBB, several studies highlight the role of FA transporters in this process. The membrane localized FA transport proteins (FATP1 and FATP4) appear to be the predominant FA transport proteins expressed in the BBB based on human and mouse expression studies, whereas the FA translocase/CD36 plays a prominent role in the transport of FAs across human brain microvessel endothelial cells (12). Furthermore, cytosolic-localized fatty acid-binding protein 5 has an important function in FA transport across cultured brain microvascular cells (13). Although still under active investigation, is it plausible that some transporters may also exhibit specificity toward particular FAs. For example, the major facilitator superfamily d 2 a, which is exclusively expressed in the endothelium of the BBB, has been shown to selectively transport DHA in the form of the partially hydrolyzed phospholipid, lysophosphatidylcholine, otherwise known as lysolecithin (14).

NEURONAL UPTAKE OF LIPIDS AND FAs

Neuronal uptake of FAs remains an important yet poorly understood process. However, it is possible that once FAs have traversed the BBB, FA transporters may also play a key role in facilitating FA uptake into neurons. For example, dissociated neurons from the VMH express both FATP1 and CD36 (15). Specifically, important studies using fura-2 calcium imaging and fluorometric imaging plate reader membrane potential dye, in addition to pharmacological manipulations have shown that while neurons of the VMH and ARC respond to oleic acid (OA, C18:1 n-9) (15, 16), this response is lost when CD36 is depleted in the VMH using an adeno-associated viral (AAV) vector expressing CD36 short hairpin RNA (17). Since CD38 is an established gustatory lipid sensor, it is also plausible that other lipid sensors involved in the chemoreception of long-chain fatty acids (LCFAs)/omega-3 fatty acids (ω-3 FAs), such as GPR120, are also involved in neuronal lipid sensing. However, although GPR120 is functionally active in immortalized hypothalamic neurons and mediates the anti-inflammatory actions of the ω-3 FA, DHA (18), its role in neuronal lipid sensing *in vivo* has not been determined. In addition, FABP3, which is localized in neurons, facilitates brain AA but not palmitic acid (C16:0) uptake and trafficking into specific brain lipid pools (19).

It is also becoming more widely accepted that neurons may receive metabolic support from glial cells in a variety of forms. The "astrocyte–neuron lactate shuttle" has been postulated, whereby astrocytes metabolize glucose to release lactate, which is then taken up by the neuronally expressed monocarboxylate transporter, providing a supplemental energy source for neurons (20). Moreover, lipid metabolism in astrocytes plays a key role in FA sensing, since FA oxidation is thought to occur predominantly in the astrocyte rather than the neuron. When the levels of FAs are increased, as in the case of a high-fat diet (HFD), astrocyte-mediated lipid oxidation results in elevated ketone levels in the brain. Conversely, changes in ketone abundance within energy-sensing regions of the hypothalamus are able to modify energy homeostasis. Specifically, reduced ketone production within the VMH and ARC signals a decrease in HFD intake, and ketone production can override glucose and FA sensing in VMH neurons (21, 22). Astrocytes may play a key role in the regulation of energy balance by sensing LCFAs as metabolic signals. For example, hypothalamic but not cortical astrocytes have a high capacity for the oxidation of LCFAs (23), and this flux may be AMP-activated protein kinase (AMPK) dependent. Both neurons of the VMH and astrocytes have been shown to express many of the FA transporters, including FATP1, FATP4, and CD36. Most recently, the fatty acid bind protein 7 (FABP7) was shown to be important for astrocyte–neuron lipid homeostasis. Mice lacking FABP7 develop neuropsychiatric disorders such as schizophrenia, which may at least in part be due to aberrant dendritic spine morphology, and decreased spine density compared to WT mice (24). Moreover, transplantation of WT astrocytes into FABP7 KO mice partially attenuated cognitive impairments (24). Once transported into the cell, LCFAs are esterified by acyl-CoA-binding protein (ACBP), a protein that is ubiquitously expressed in tissues with high lipid turnover. Interestingly, ACBP is expressed in the hypothalamus and may play a role in the LCFA sensing by hypothalamic astrocytes (25).

Astrocytes are also critical for the regulation of cholesterol homeostasis in the neuron. Cholesterol is an essential component of neuronal physiology during both development and adulthood and is independently tightly regulated in the brain, largely due to the existence of the BBB (26). Cholesterol depletion in neurons impairs vital functions, including synaptic vesicle exocytosis, neuronal activity, and neurotransmission and results in synaptic loss and neurodegeneration (27, 28). Clinically, deficits in cholesterol homeostasis in the CNS manifest as severe primary neurological disorders such as Neimann–Pick C disease and Parkinson's disease (26). It is thought that astrocytes are a major site of lipoprotein synthesis and assembly in the brain (29). Of particular relevance is apolipoprotein E (ApoE), a 39-kDa protein that is highly expressed in the brain, surpassed only by hepatic ApoE production (30).

Apolipoprotein E-containing lipoproteins have been extensively studied and are known to have several major functions. For example, ApoE-containing high-density lipoprotein (HDL)-like lipoproteins are secreted by astrocytes and are taken up into neurons *via* low-density lipoprotein receptors. This transfer of key lipids and cholesterol facilitates axonal extension and neuronal survival and requires the presence of sphingomyelin in the ApoE-containing lipoprotein particle (31, 32). ApoE does not only play a major role in glia-neuronal lipid metabolism but also acts as a ligand for multiple receptors in neurons, which interact with a number of downstream physiological processes (33). In particular, a number of recent studies have shown that brain ApoE is an important regulator of peripheral energy homeostasis. In rats, intracerebroventricular (ICV) ApoE injections significantly decreased food intake, whereas infusion of ApoE antiserum stimulated feeding, therefore suggesting that ApoE may be important satiety factor in the hypothalamus (34). In support, exogenous ApoE treatment has been shown to activate phosphatidylinositol-3-kinase (PI3K)/Akt signaling, and PI3K inhibition by LY294002 attenuates both ApoE-induced signaling and satiation (35).

Apolipoprotein E has three major isoforms (ApoE2, ApoE3, and ApoE4), which have varying effects on lipid homeostasis and neuronal function. While both ApoE2 and ApoE3 preferentially associate with phospholipid rich HDL-like particles, ApoE4 prefers large triglyceride-rich VLDL particles (36). Interestingly, ApoE4 has been repeatedly implicated in the pathogenesis of Alzheimer's disease (AD) and may bind to the Aβ peptide leading to impair Aβ clearance (37). Current hypothesis suggests that the proteolytic cleavage products of ApoE4 may have a central role in AD pathology, since AD patients have markedly increased levels of these cleavage products compared to controls (38).

These findings suggest that lipoprotein metabolism in the CNS may be key to lipid homeostasis and nutrient sensing; however, to date, the molecular mechanisms underlying these processes remain largely unknown. Nonetheless, we have recently shown that lipoprotein lipase (LPL), the rate-limiting enzyme in the hydrolysis of lipoprotein-derived FAs, may facilitate the uptake of FAs into dissociated hypothalamic neurons (39). Moreover, mice with a specific neuronal LPL deficiency exhibit a defect in nutrient sensing and become hyperphagic, relatively inactive and obsessed compared to WT control mice (40). Interestingly, these mice are also polyunsaturated fatty acid (PUFA) deficient in the hypothalamus (40), and in the hippocampus, where LPL deficiency is also associated with alterations in learning and memory and synaptic function (41). In further support, a specific deletion of LPL in the hippocampus also leads to increased weight gain and decreased activity *via* a ceramide-dependent pathway (42). We have also shown that while mice lacking pan-neuronal LPL develop obesity, this obesity is not exacerbated on an HF diet, or rescued by a PUFA enriched diet, further highlighting the importance of LPL in lipid sensing and body weight regulation (43). These data highlight the potential role of LPL as a mechanistic link between brain lipid uptake, neuronal lipoprotein metabolism, and nutrient sensing; however, the precise role of LPL in lipid sensing in both neurons and glia requires further investigation.

HYPOTHALAMIC FA METABOLISM

The evidence for facilitated FA uptake into neurons is limited, which may be due to the long-held view that neurons do not derive much of their energy supply from lipids. However, neurons do express many molecular components of lipid catabolism pathways, suggesting that lipid utilization is a critical process to neuronal function. For example, neurons of the VMH express enzymes involved in the intracellular metabolism of FAs, including long-chain acyl-CoA synthase (ACS), carnitine palmitoyltransferase-1a and 1c (CPT-1a and 1c), and uncoupling protein-2 (UCP2), and enzymes involved in *de novo* lipogenesis, such as fatty acid synthase (FAS) (15). In addition, the nuclear receptor peroxisome proliferator-activated receptor (PPARγ), a key factor in lipid metabolism that can be activated by endogenous lipid ligands to promote adipogenesis and insulin sensitivity, is predominantly expressed in neurons of the hypothalamus (44), including the ARC.

Activation of these intracellular metabolic pathways in hypothalamic cells in response to FAs provides further support of the role of lipid metabolism and sensing in hypothalamic neurons. For example, UCP2, which increases proton leak from the respiratory electron transport chain, may act as a metabolic switch from glucose metabolism to mitochondrial FA oxidation in hypothalamic NPY/AgRP neurons during fasting (45). Interestingly, UCP2 likely mediates the actions of ghrelin, which is increased upon fasting, on the activation of NPY/AgRP neurons. While ghrelin increases palmitate-induced mitochondrial respiration, this is not observed in UCP2−/− mice. Moreover, NPY/AgRP neurons of UCP2−/− mice do not show the ghrelin-induced increase in mitochondrial biogenesis (45). In normal circumstances, increased FA oxidation increases reactive oxygen species (ROS), which are then scavenged by UCP2 *via* enhanced proton leak. However, in UCP2−/− mice, these ROS levels remain increased, supporting the hypothesis that ghrelin-triggered ROS production promotes UCP2 activity and mRNA expression to further promote ROS scavenging (45). These studies also suggest that ROS may be involved in neuronal lipid metabolism and activation. In further support, suppression of ROS activates NPY/AgRP neurons to promote feeding, whereas activation of ROS activates proopiomelanocortin (POMC) neurons to reduce feeding. Although further studies are warranted, it is likely that neuronal ROS accumulation may intrinsically link neuronal substrate metabolism to feeding behavior and systemic energy balance (46).

AMP-activated protein kinase may also act as a cellular energy sensor within neurons to link neuronal lipid metabolism to systemic lipid metabolism and energy balance. AMPK is widely expressed in the ARC, PVN, and VMH of the hypothalamus and is able to sense intracellular energy status by the AMP/ATP ratio and the level of adipokines (e.g., leptin and ghrelin) [see Ref. (47) for a comprehensive review]. Activated AMPK responds to the cellular energy status and can switch cellular metabolism toward catabolic processes that produce ATP and away from anabolic processes that consume ATP (48). In response to glucose, hypothalamic AMPK activity is inhibited leading to the activation of acetyl-CoA carboxylase (ACC) and the generation of malonyl-CoA from glucose-derived acetyl-CoA, with downstream effects on food intake (described in more detail below) (49). Similar to peripheral tissues, malonyl-CoA is thought to inhibit CPT-1a and LCFA oxidation in the brain (49). Specifically, glucose inhibits palmitate oxidation *via* AMPK in hypothalamic neurons (23). Hypothalamic AMPK may also regulate downstream lipid metabolism through brown adipose tissue (BAT) thermogenesis. A number of recent studies have suggested that hypothalamic AMPK is involved in the autonomic regulation of BAT thermogenesis, specifically the SNS. For example, central administration of 3,3′,5′-triiodothyronine (T_3) within the VMH stimulates a thermogenic response associated with decreased AMPK activity in the VMH and elevated sympathetic firing in BAT (50). Whether this effect is observed following neuronal glucose (or lipid) sensing remains to be seen. Nonetheless, this interesting topic has recently been reviewed in detail (51).

AMP-activated protein kinase also plays a key role in the hypothalamic response to leptin in the context of high-fat feeding. While leptin results in reduced food intake and reduced hypothalamic AMPK activity, these effects were not observed in diet-induced obese mice (52). Hypothalamic phospho-AMPK is also modulated by the FA composition of the diet and is dependent on brain region and metabolic status (53). Interestingly, AMPK regulates the activity of a number of enzymes involved in the synthesis of complex lipids that are critical for optimal brain function and metabolism. For example, long-term AMPK stimulation blunted FA-mediated induction of serine palmitoyl transferase and the synthesis of ceramides *de novo* and has thus been shown to protect against fatty acid-mediated apoptosis in the astrocyte (54). Similarly, AMPK is highly expressed in neurons due to their high-energy demands and can promote neuronal survival during periods of glucose deprivation (55). Recently, neuronal AMPK has also been implicated in the pathogenesis of AD. AMPK activity can reduce sphingomyelin levels, inhibit Aβ generation, and reduce amyloid precursor protein (APP) distribution in lipid rafts, whereas deletion of AMPKα2 increases sphingomyelin and APP distribution in lipid rafts (56).

There is growing evidence to suggest that the accumulation of FA metabolites may signal nutrient status and thus may be critical to central lipid sensing, and the modulation of systemic metabolism. For example, upon entry into the neuron, LCFAs are esterified to LCFA-CoA by ACS. It is thought that this accumulation of FA derived LCFA-CoA triggers a lipid-sensing mechanism to inhibit hepatic glucose production (HGP) and to maintain systemic glucose homeostasis (57). In support, direct inhibition of ACS in the hypothalamus disrupts the accumulation of hypothalamic LCFA-CoA, and in turn disrupts the inhibitory effect on hepatic gluconeogenesis, resulting in dysregulated glucose production (58).

In metabolic tissues, intracellular LCFA-CoAs enter the mitochondria *via* CPT-1, where they are then subject to FA β-oxidation. Importantly, the liver isoform of CPT-1, CPT-1a, is prevalent in the hypothalamus, and inhibition of hypothalamic CPT-1a causes an increase in intracellular LCFA-CoA, which triggers a satiation signal, leading to reduced systemic glucose production and food intake (59). However, the neurocircuitry is complex since the role of CPT-1a may vary between hypothalamic nuclei. For example, VMH-selective overexpression of CPT-1a causes over feeding, a phenotype which can be reversed with the CPT-1 specific inhibitor etomoxir (60). In support, long-term overexpression of permanently activated CPT-1a using a viral AAV vector injected into the VMH of rats, leads to hyperghrelinemia, increased food intake, increased body weight, hyperglycemia, and insulin resistance (61). In contrast, CPT-1a expression in the ARC does not have the same effect on the central regulation of feeding (60). Interestingly, the brain also expresses a neuron-specific isoform of CPT-1, CPT-1c, which is found in the endoplasmic reticulum (ER) of key energy-sensing nuclei of the hypothalamus (ARC) and has also been repeatedly implicated in the modulation of systemic metabolism (62–64). Specifically, CPT-1c KO mice have reduced body weight and food intake compared to control mice (62, 63). CPT-1c does not have a typical acyltransferase activity, and thus its precise molecular function is less well understood. Nonetheless, data from recent studies suggest that the orexigenic action of ghrelin is associated with increased hypothalamic (C18:0) ceramide levels, an effect that is blunted in CPT-1c KO mice (65). While the mechanism linking increased ceramide levels to energy balance remain an active area of research, recent studies have demonstrated that ceramides induce hypothalamic lipotoxicity and ER stress, which leads to sympathetic inhibition, reduced BAT thermogenesis, weight gain, and hepatic steatosis (66). In addition, recent metabolomic analysis of the brains of CPT-1c KO mice shows reduced levels of oxidized glutathione, suggesting that CPT-1c may play a role in neuronal oxidative metabolism (67). In addition, these mice show suppressed endocannabinoid levels, which offers an alternative yet consistent mechanism to account for the suppressed food intake observed in CPT-1c KO mice (67). In addition, to their established role in appetite modulation, endogenous endocannabinoids may serve as functional neuromodulatory lipids, derived from neuronal phospholipids, which once secreted undergo lipid catabolism within glial cells. A detailed description of endocannabinoid signaling is beyond the scope of this manuscript but has been previously reviewed in depth (68).

CPT-1 has been suggested to act downstream of malonyl-CoA in the hypothalamic control of feeding (60). This is particularly pertinent to FA metabolism in hypothalamic neurons since CPT-1 activity is inhibited by malonyl-CoA (69), and thus elevated malonyl-CoA leads to an accumulation of LCFA-CoA (70), which has been previously referred to as a satiety signal. Indeed, manipulation of the key enzymes involved in malonyl-CoA metabolism, including ACC, FAS, and malonyl-CoA decarboxylase (MCD), have all been shown to have major effects on food intake and peripheral metabolism (71). For example, ACC, which catalyzes the carboxylation of acetyl-CoA to malonyl-CoA, is expressed in the ARC of the hypothalamus, where it is increased following central leptin treatment resulting in elevated malonyl-CoA and reduced food intake (72). Similarly, inhibition of FAS activity by central administration of the pharmacological FAS inhibitor C75 has been shown to reduce food intake (73) and to elevate malonyl-CoA levels (74). MCD, which is important for malonyl-CoA degradation, is also important for regulating lipid intermediates and systemic metabolism. Overexpression of MCD in the mediobasal hypothalamus (MBH) chronically reduces malonyl-CoA levels and causes rapid increases in food intake and weight gain (75). In addition, MBH expression depleted both malonyl-CoA and LCFA-CoA and was sufficient to induce hepatic insulin resistance in the presence of hyperlipidemia (75). These studies begin to highlight the importance of hypothalamic sensing of circulating lipids in the maintenance of hepatic metabolism and systemic glucose homeostasis. However, the physiological and molecular mechanisms that integrate the brain–liver axis remain unresolved and an active area of investigation.

HYPOTHALAMIC LIPID SENSING AND HEPATIC METABOLISM

Early studies by Obici and colleagues, where OA was administered into the brain *via* ICV injection, were among the first to demonstrate the profound central effects of LCFAs on peripheral metabolism. Interestingly, the short chain FA octanoic acid (C8) did not have the same effect. Moreover, these studies showed that central OA administration could lower plasma insulin and glucose levels under basal physiological conditions. To determine the mode of blood glucose reduction, pancreatic euglycemic clamps were performed during ICV infusion of OA. ICV OA administration leads to a marked decline in glucose production compared to basal levels (59). However, when clamps were performed in the presence of ICV OA and sulfonylurea, a potent inhibitor of neuronal K_{ATP} channels, the profound effect of central OA on HGP was blunted, suggesting that OA acutely enhances hepatic insulin action *via* the activation of K_{ATP} channels in the hypothalamus (59). Further studies support this notion and have shown that pharmacological activation of K_{ATP} channels in the hypothalamus (*via* hypothalamic diazoxide administration) suppresses HGP (76). These observations, taken together with the findings from CPT-1 inhibition studies, strongly suggest that the accumulation of LCFA-CoAs is able to suppress HGP (70). Recent studies have suggested that this system may actually be even more complex and have shown that the effect of LCFAs on hepatic metabolism may be FA specific. For example, while bilateral infusion of OA into the MBH results in a significant reduction in HGP, palmitic acid (PA, C16:0) has a lesser effect, and linoleic acid has no effect compared to vehicle control (LA, C18:2 n-6) (77). These data suggest that mono-unsaturated fatty acids are a more potent suppressor than saturated fatty acids or PUFAs; however, the mechanisms underlying these differential effects of FAs on hepatic glucose metabolism remain to be determined.

In addition to the central regulation of HGP, hypothalamic nutrient sensing may also be a key regulator of hepatic lipid homeostasis. The liver maintains lipid homeostasis through tightly coordinated synthesis and secretion of triglyceride-rich lipoproteins (VLDL-TG), lipogenesis, and FA oxidation. Interestingly, infusion of the orexigenic neuropeptide Y directly into the third ventricle of the hypothalamus has been shown to increase hepatic VLDL-TG secretion, which may be part of the physiological response to fasting when lipids become the main energy source and NPY neurons in the ARC of the hypothalamus are activated (78). Thus, VLDL-TG secretion may be a response by the autonomic nervous system (ANS) to mobilize lipids during a period of relative nutrient deficiency. In addition, sympathetic denervation prevented the increase in the VLDL-TG secretion in the fasted state, whereas total denervation, or parasympathetic denervation did not, suggesting that the central regulation of hepatic lipid mobilization during fasting may be largely mediated through the sympathetic nervous system (78). In further support, sympathetic hepatic denervation also prevented the stimulatory effect of NPY on VLDL-TG secretion (78). This is in contrast to glucose sensing in the MBH (79), and glycine in the dorsal vagal complex (DVC) (80), which is thought to signal sufficient nutrient status and inhibit VLDL-TG secretion, possibly through the parasympathetic nervous system.

In addition to NPY, a number of studies have also shown that MC expressing neurons of the hypothalamus may also regulate hepatic lipogenesis and TG metabolism. Central administration of MTII, a synthetic MC3/4 receptor agonist, has been shown to reduce hepatic lipogenic gene expression in mice (81) and decrease hepatic TG content in rats (82), suggesting that increased MC signaling can inhibit hepatic VLDL-TG production. In support of this notion, central administration of an MC3/4 receptor antagonist, markedly increased liver TG content in rats, strongly suggesting that hepatic lipogenesis was increased (7).

Melanin-concentrating hormone (MCH) is also involved in the neuronal circuits that modify autonomic outflow to the liver and white adipose tissue. MCH-deficient mice are hyperphagic and lean when fed a normal diet (83), are resistant to age associated insulin resistance (84), and when fed an HFD they are resistant to obesity and hepatic steatosis (85). Recent key studies have also shown that genetic activation of MCH specifically in the LH triggers hepatic lipid accumulation and lipoprotein uptake (86).

This neurocircuitry is relevant to the pathogenesis of obesity, since numerous models of obesity and diabetes are characterized by elevated NPY. In a recent study, ICV administration of NPY or a selective NPY Y1 receptor agonist was shown to robustly elevate key genes involved in MUFA synthesis, such as stearol-CoA desatrate-1, and PL remodeling, such as ribosylation factor-1 (ARF-1) and lipin-1 (87). Importantly, these effects were attenuated following sympathetic denervation of the liver, supporting a model in which central NPY modifies hepatic PL and VLDL *via* the sympathetic signaling to the liver (87). Although these findings suggest that central lipid sensing may be implicated in the regulation of hepatic lipid homeostasis (see **Figure 1**), the direct mechanisms remain elusive. Nonetheless, a number of recent studies highlight the role of central FAs in hepatic lipid homeostasis. For example, central administration of PA resulted in impaired leptin signaling and pro-inflammatory response in the MBH and PVN (88). Furthermore, this was coupled with blunted leptin-induced changes in hepatic gluconeogenesis, glucose transportation, and lipogenesis (88). In a recent report, Yue and colleagues have shown that infusion of OA directly into the MBH activates a PKC-δ to K_{ATP} channel axis, which suppresses VLDL-TG secretion in rats (89). Moreover, this signaling requires DVC and hepatic innervation, highlighting a novel MBD-DVC neurocircuitry that mediates MBH FA sensing and hepatic lipid homeostasis (89). These findings are one step closer to the development of novel therapies that lower VLDL-TG secretion and restore lipid homeostasis in metabolic disorders; however, there is considerably more to learn regarding differential function of other hypothalamic neurons and their role in the autonomic regulation of hepatic metabolism.

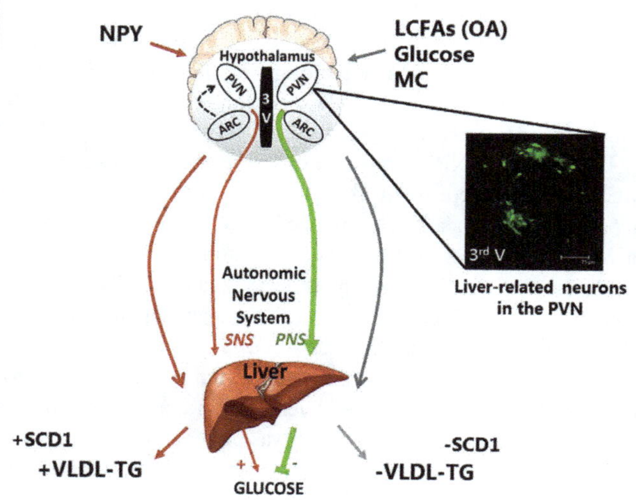

FIGURE 1 | Schematic representation of the neuronal regulation of hepatic carbohydrate and lipid metabolism. Neurons of discrete hypothalamic nuclei including the paraventricular nucleus (PVN) and arcuate nucleus (ARC) within the mediobasal hypothalamus respond to neuronal inputs to regulate hepatic glucose and very low density lipoprotein (VLDL-TG) metabolism. The accumulation or application of long-chain fatty acids (LCFAs), such as oleic acid (OA), glucose, and melanocortin (MC) signaling act through the autonomic nervous system to signal nutritional plenty a reduced requirement for energy substrate mobilization, by inhibiting VLDL-TG secretion and hepatic glucose production (HGP). This is at least in part due to reduced stearol-CoA desatrate-1 (SCD1) expression. In contrast, hypothalamic NPY is indicative of hunger and nutritional deficiency and can increase energy substrate mobilization *via* an increase in VLDL-TG and SCD1 expression and HGP. The features of these fatty acid and nutritionally sensitive neurons are unclear; however, pseudorabies virus-152 labeling supports the notion that liver-related neurons in the PVN exist and may be involved in this autonomic regulation of hepatic metabolism.

LIVER-RELATED NEURONS IN THE HYPOTHALAMUS

Recent findings support the existence of liver-related neurons in key hypothalamic nuclei; therefore, we can speculate that these liver-related neurons are the link between central lipid sensing and hepatic lipid metabolism. The control of hepatic functions by the ANS is well known. In general, beside the abovementioned examples, sympathetic stimulation of the liver enhances endogenous glucose production and glycogenolysis, while the parasympathetic nerves are responsible for inhibiting glucose production and promoting glucose storage (90–92). Preganglionic neurons are located in the spinal cord and brainstem, respectively, and transmit the information through the sympathetic and parasympathetic nerves. These autonomic motor neurons receive information from preautonomic neurons, which are located in higher brain areas and crucial for integration of brain signals (93, 94). Therefore, identifying the location of liver-related neurons and determining their cellular and molecular properties would be crucial to the understanding of brain–liver circuit.

Within the hypothalamus, the ARC, VMH, DMH, LH, and PVN are well recognized for their involvement in the regulation of a variety of metabolic functions of the body, and in particular the control of hepatic metabolism (95–101). Electrical and chemical stimulation have been feasible methods to establish direct connections between the hypothalamus and sympathetic neurons in the spinal cord or parasympathetic neurons in the brainstem and to demonstrate the importance of the autonomic control in hepatic functions (98, 102–105). On the other hand, establishing the location of premotor inputs to the sympathetic and parasympathetic motor neurons has been more challenging. Anterograde and retrograde tracers in combination with histochemical studies provided valuable information on the connections between the brain and liver (106), and the development of retrograde viral tracers opened new avenues to dissect the brain–liver pathway. Currently, transsynaptic neurotropic viruses are very valuable tools for identification of synaptic connections and neural networks. Among the neurotropic viruses, pseudorabies viruses (PRVs) are often used for circuit analysis and revealing organization of the nervous system (107–110). PRVs, such as PRV-152, an attenuated viral strain driving the expression of EGFP, are reliable and effective transsynaptic tracers, and numerous publications reported consistent organ-specific labeling of neurons (111–115). The spread of PRV-152 is strictly retrograde across synapses, and the virus is not capable of assembling in axons or glia; therefore, labeling of neurons not specific to the liver is unlikely, as has been shown (110, 116–118).

Polysynaptic neural connections between the brain and liver were identified in rodents using PRVs (118–120). PRV labeling was observed in the spinal cord of rats 3 days following inoculation, whereas at this time point no labeling was detected in parasympathetic nuclei (119). Labeled neurons in the dorsal motor nucleus of the vagus (DMV) were observed 4–5 days after inoculation of the liver. At this time point, liver-related neurons were also detected in the brainstem including the ventrolateral medulla, NTS, raphe pallidus, and few neurons were identified in the hypothalamic PVN and LH (119). Longer survival time provided labeling of liver-related neurons in nuclei connected to the PVN including the medial preoptic area, anterior hypothalamic area, and ARC. PRV-labeled cells were also present in the VMH, suprachiasmatic nuclei, central amygdala, and bed nucleus of stria terminalis (119). This study demonstrated that PRV provides reliable identification of polysynaptic sympathetic and parasympathetic pathways to the liver (113, 115, 118, 120).

Despite the identification of liver-related neurons in the CNS, labeling with PRV does not distinguish between sympathetic and parasympathetic liver-related neurons in higher brain areas. In order to identify sympathetic- or parasympathetic liver-related hypothalamic neurons in rats, PRV inoculation was combined with hepatic sympathectomy or parasympathectomy (121, 122). Following sympathetic denervation of the liver, parasympathetic liver-related neurons were identified in the brainstem DMV and nucleus ambiguus (122). Medium length survival time (~4 days) resulted in labeling of additional brainstem areas (e.g., NTS, area postrema) and hypothalamic nuclei including PVN, LH, DMH, ARC, and others (122). Retrograde labeling following parasympathectomy identified pre-sympathetic liver-related neurons in the PVN, medial preoptic area, anterior hypothalamic area, DMH, ARC, VMH, and SCN (121). These studies revealed that preautonomic PVN neurons project either to sympathetic or parasympathetic division, and the segregation of the neurons exists in other hypothalamic areas including LH and SCN suggesting functional specialization of preautonomic neurons controlling liver function. The segregation of the autonomic divisions was also supported by the observation that stimulation of PVN resulted in hyperglycemia largely due to sympathetic activation of the liver (121). On the other hand, we have to note, that viral injection into peripheral organs causes infection of nerve terminals innervating both vascular and non-vascular tissues (123). PRV injected into the liver is taken up by nerve endings near hepatocytes and sinusoidal cells, and we cannot distinguish between neurons innervating liver function or hepatic vasculature at the injection site. Therefore, it is likely that the PRV-labeled pre-sympathetic neurons contribute to both vasomotor and non-vasomotor sympathetic innervation of the liver.

Our current knowledge regarding the role and cellular properties of liver-related hypothalamic neurons is somewhat limited. Earlier studies suggested that the VMH is involved in the sympathetic control of the liver, whereas the LH plays role in the parasympathetic control of the liver (91, 124, 125). The PVN was also shown as an important, integrative center for the regulation of sympathetic and parasympathetic pathways to the liver (121, 126–128). Hypothalamic action of metabolic signals including insulin, leptin, and FAs has been shown to control glucose homeostasis (58, 59, 76, 129–133); however, the cellular properties, the phenotype, or the involved neural circuits underlying the central control of hepatic functions are less defined.

Hypothalamic nuclei are heterogeneous containing different types of neurons, which are able to control multiple organ systems; therefore, identification of pathway-related neurons is crucial. Our laboratory used the retrograde PRV tracing technique, discussed above, to identify liver-related neurons in the PVN and to reveal synaptic properties of liver-related neurons in control and hyperglycemic conditions (113). The studies determined that liver-related neurons receive transient receptor potential vanilloid type 1 (TRPV1) containing inputs. TRPV1 is a non-selective cation channel and has been linked to the development and progression of type 1 diabetes mellitus and T2D (134), and recent reviews have discussed its role in diabetes mellitus and obesity in further detail (135, 136). The TRPV1-dependent excitation of liver-related PVN neurons was diminished in a hyperglycemic, insulin-deficient mouse model. Both *in vivo* and *in vitro* insulin replacement restored the TRPV1-dependent excitatory neurotransmission *via* PI3-kinase, PKC, and/or TRPV1 trafficking (113). Similarly, TRPV1 was shown to play role in the regulation of excitatory neurotransmission to motor neurons in the DMV and stomach-related neurons in the PVN (137, 138). Furthermore, potential interaction between leptin signaling and TRPV1 has been proposed in the brainstem (114). In addition, there is limited information about the neurochemical phenotype of liver-related neurons. A study by Stanley and coworkers identified liver-related hypothalamic neurons using PRV and showed that a subpopulation of liver-related neurons co-localized with oxytocin and CRH in the mouse PVN (118). In the LH, a subset of MCH and orexin neurons was shown to be liver related. In the ARC, a subpopulation of POMC neurons but not NPY-expressing neurons were labeled with PRV, indicating that they are part of the brain–liver pathway (118).

Despite the scientific advances in our understanding of liver-related neurons, their precise role in the autonomic regulation of hepatic lipid metabolism remains to be determined. Although there is clear evidence that increased sympathetic outflow to the liver may increase VLDL-TG production, resulting in increased systemic FA availability, it remains to be determined whether the liver-related neurons of the hypothalamus are indeed FA sensitive, or indeed whether the FA-sensing neurons of the hypothalamus are liver related. It is plausible to suggest that liver-related neurons that direct hepatic triglyceride metabolism may express key lipid processing factors involved in lipid transport, e.g., CD36, FATP1 and/or TG metabolism, e.g., LPL. However, a more detailed understanding of these fundamental autonomic processes is needed in order to identify novel therapeutic targets that may halt the development of lipid-related disorders.

SUMMARY, IMPLICATIONS, AND INTERVENTIONS

The findings summarized in this review highlight the role of central lipid sensing in the regulation of systemic metabolism, including food intake, body weight, and hepatic glucose and lipid metabolism. Since increased HGP is a key factor in the development of glucose intolerance, understanding the neuronal mechanisms that drive the central regulation of HGP may be key to the development of novel therapeutic strategies that prevent hyperglycemia and the development of type 2 diabetes. In addition, our increased understanding of the hypothalamic control of TG metabolism highlights the potential utility of specifically modulating sympathetic nervous system activity toward the liver reduces VLDL-TG secretion and combat hypertriglyceridemia (139). The clinical relevance of this strategy is highlighted by a recent north European human cohort, in which elevated sympathetic nervous system activity was associated with features of the MetS, such as elevated circulated VLDL-TG (140). While current interventions for hypertriglyceridemia are aimed at reducing circulating FAs by increasing FA uptake from the plasma, an alternative approach to effectively lower TG could be though decreasing VLDL-TG production by the liver. This is the case with GLP-1 receptor agonists, which have been shown to decrease both hepatic lipogenesis (141) and VLDL-TG production (142). Based on the literature outlined in this review, interventions targeting specific liver-related or FA-sensitive neurons in of the hypothalamus could have a similar impact on systemic metabolism, and we recommend that the identification of the features of these neuronal populations should be the subject of intensive research focus.

AUTHOR CONTRIBUTIONS

KB, AZ, and RE wrote and edited the manuscript.

FUNDING

This work was in part supported by the grant awarded to AZ (NIH R01 DK099598) with RE as a consultant and to RE (NIH R01 DK089309).

REFERENCES

Eckel RH, Grundy SM, Zimmet PZ. The metabolic syndrome. *Lancet* (2005) 365:1415–28. doi:10.1016/S0140-6736(05)66378-7

Aguilar M, Bhuket T, Torres S, Liu B, Wong RJ. Prevalence of the metabolic syndrome in the United States, 2003-2012. *JAMA* (2015) 313:1973–4. doi:10.1001/jama.2015.4260

Isomaa B, Almgren P, Tuomi T, Forsen B, Lahti K, Nissen M, et al. Cardiovascular morbidity and mortality associated with the metabolic syndrome. *Diabetes Care* (2001) 24:683–9. doi:10.2337/diacare.24.4.683

Morton GJ, Cummings DE, Baskin DG, Barsh GS, Schwartz MW. Central nervous system control of food intake and body weight. *Nature* (2006) 443:289–95. doi:10.1038/nature05026

Koch L, Wunderlich FT, Seibler J, Konner AC, Hampel B, Irlenbusch S, et al. Central insulin action regulates peripheral glucose and fat metabolism in mice. *J Clin Invest* (2008) 118:2132–47. doi:10.1172/JCI31073

Theander-Carrillo C, Wiedmer P, Cettour-Rose P, Nogueiras R, Perez-Tilve D, Pfluger P, et al. Ghrelin action in the brain controls adipocyte metabolism. *J Clin Invest* (2006) 116:1983–93. doi:10.1172/JCI25811

Nogueiras R, Wiedmer P, Perez-Tilve D, Veyrat-Durebex C, Keogh JM, Sutton GM, et al. The central melanocortin system directly controls peripheral lipid metabolism. *J Clin Invest* (2007) 117:3475–88. doi:10.1172/JCI31743

Asilmaz E, Cohen P, Miyazaki M, Dobrzyn P, Ueki K, Fayzikhodjaeva G, et al. Site and mechanism of leptin action in a rodent form of con- genital lipodystrophy. *J Clin Invest* (2004) 113:414–24. doi:10.1172/ JCI200419511

Hamilton JA, Hillard CJ, Spector AA, Watkins PA. Brain uptake and utilization of fatty acids, lipids and lipoproteins: application to neuro- logical disorders. *J Mol Neurosci* (2007) 33:2–11. doi:10.1007/s12031- 007-0060-1

Rapoport SI, Chang MC, Spector AA. Delivery and turnover of plasma-derived essential PUFAs in mammalian brain. *J Lipid Res* (2001) 42:678–85.

Smith QR, Nagura H. Fatty acid uptake and incorporation in brain: studies with the perfusion model. *J Mol Neurosci* (2001) 16:167–72; discussion 215–21. doi:10.1385/JMN:16:2-3:167

Woods SC, Porte D Jr, Bobbioni E, Ionescu E, Sauter JF, Rohner-Jeanrenaud F, et al. Insulin: its relationship to the central nervous system and to the control of food intake and body weight. *Am J Clin Nutr* (1985) 42:1063–71.

Mitchell RW, On NH, Del Bigio MR, Miller DW, Hatch GM. Fatty acid transport protein expression in human brain and potential role in fatty acid transport across human brain microvessel endothelial cells. *J Neurochem* (2011) 117:735–46. doi:10.1111/j.1471-4159.2011.07245.x

Nguyen LN, Ma D, Shui G, Wong P, Cazenave-Gassiot A, Zhang X, et al. Mfsd2a is a transporter for the essential omega-3 fatty acid docosahexaenoic acid. *Nature* (2014) 509:503–6. doi:10.1038/nature13241

Le Foll C, Irani BG, Magnan C, Dunn-Meynell AA, Levin BE. Characteristics and mechanisms of hypothalamic neuronal fatty acid sensing. *Am J Physiol Regul Integr Comp Physiol* (2009) 297:R655–64. doi:10.1152/ ajpregu.00223.2009

Le Foll C, Irani BG, Magnan C, Dunn-Meynell A, Levin BE. Effects of maternal genotype and diet on offspring glucose and fatty acid-sensing ventromedial hypothalamic nucleus neurons. *Am J Physiol Regul Integr Comp Physiol* (2009) 297:R1351–7. doi:10.1152/ajpregu.00370.2009

Le Foll C, Dunn-Meynell A, Musatov S, Magnan C, Levin BE. FAT/CD36: a major regulator of neuronal fatty acid sensing and energy homeostasis in rats and mice. *Diabetes* (2013) 62:2709–16. doi:10.2337/db12-1689

Wellhauser L, Belsham DD. Activation of the omega-3 fatty acid receptor GPR120 mediates anti-inflammatory actions in immortalized hypotha- lamic neurons. *J Neuroinflammation* (2014) 11:60. doi:10.1186/1742- 2094-11-60

Murphy EJ, Owada Y, Kitanaka N, Kondo H, Glatz JF. Brain arachidonic acid incorporation is decreased in heart fatty acid binding protein gene-ablated mice. *Biochemistry* (2005) 44:6350–60. doi:10.1021/bi047292r

Pellerin L, Bouzier-Sore AK, Aubert A, Serres S, Merle M, Costalat R, et al. Activity-dependent regulation of energy metabolism by astrocytes: an update. *Glia* (2007) 55:1251–62. doi:10.1002/glia.20528

Le Foll C, Dunn-Meynell AA, Miziorko HM, Levin BE. Regulation of hypothalamic neuronal sensing and food intake by ketone bodies and fatty acids. *Diabetes* (2014) 63:1259–69. doi:10.2337/db13-1090

Le Foll C, Dunn-Meynell AA, Miziorko HM, Levin BE. Role of VMH ketone bodies in adjusting caloric intake to increased dietary fat content in DIO and DR rats. *Am J Physiol Regul Integr Comp Physiol* (2015) 308:R872–8. doi:10.1152/ajpregu.00015.2015

Taib B, Bouyakdan K, Hryhorczuk C, Rodaros D, Fulton S, Alquier T. Glucose regulates hypothalamic long-chain fatty acid metabolism via AMP-activated kinase (AMPK) in neurons and astrocytes. *J Biol Chem* (2013) 288:37216–29. doi:10.1074/jbc.M113.506238

Ebrahimi M, Yamamoto Y, Sharifi K, Kida H, Kagawa Y, Yasumoto Y, et al. Astrocyte-expressed FABP7 regulates dendritic morphology and excitatory synaptic function of cortical neurons. *Glia* (2016) 64:48–62. doi:10.1002/ glia.22902

Bouyakdan K, Taib B, Budry L, Zhao S, Rodaros D, Neess D, et al. A novel role for central ACBP/DBI as a regulator of long-chain fatty acid metabolism in astrocytes. *J Neurochem* (2015) 133:253–65. doi:10.1111/jnc.13035

Zhang J, Liu Q. Cholesterol metabolism and homeostasis in the brain. *Protein Cell* (2015) 6:254–64. doi:10.1007/s13238-014-0131-3

Linetti A, Fratangeli A, Taverna E, Valnegri P, Francolini M, Cappello V, et al. Cholesterol reduction impairs exocytosis of synaptic vesicles. *J Cell Sci* (2010) 123:595–605. doi:10.1242/jcs.060681

Liu Q, Trotter J, Zhang J, Peters MM, Cheng H, Bao J, et al. Neuronal LRP1 knockout in adult mice leads to impaired brain lipid metabolism and progressive, age-dependent synapse loss and neurodegeneration. *J Neurosci* (2010) 30:17068–78. doi:10.1523/JNEUROSCI.4067-10.2010

Wang H, Eckel RH. What are lipoproteins doing in the brain? *Trends Endocrinol Metab* (2014) 25:8–14. doi:10.1016/j.tem.2013.10.003

Linton MF, Gish R, Hubl ST, Butler E, Esquivel C, Bry WI, et al. Phenotypes of apolipoprotein B and apolipoprotein E after liver transplantation. *J Clin Invest* (1991) 88:270–81. doi:10.1172/JCI115288

Matsuo M, Campenot RB, Vance DE, Ueda K, Vance JE. Involvement of low-density lipoprotein receptor-related protein and ABCG1 in stimulation of axonal extension by apoE-containing lipoproteins. *Biochim Biophys Acta* (2011) 1811:31–8. doi:10.1016/j.bbalip.2010.10.004

Hayashi H. Lipid metabolism and glial lipoproteins in the central nervous system. *Biol Pharm Bull* (2011) 34:453–61. doi:10.1248/bpb.34.453

Beffert U, Stolt PC, Herz J. Functions of lipoprotein receptors in neurons. *J Lipid Res* (2004) 45:403–9. doi:10.1194/jlr.R300017-JLR200

Shen L, Tso P, Woods SC, Clegg DJ, Barber KL, Carey K, et al. Brain apolipoprotein E: an important regulator of food intake in rats. *Diabetes* (2008) 57:2092–8. doi:10.2337/db08-0291

Shen L, Wang DQ, Tso P, Jandacek RJ, Woods SC, Liu M. Apolipoprotein E reduces food intake via PI3K/Akt signaling pathway in the hypothalamus. *Physiol Behav* (2011) 105:124–8. doi:10.1016/j.physbeh.2011.04.018

Huang Y, Mahley RW. Apolipoprotein E: structure and function in lipid metabolism, neurobiology, and Alzheimer's diseases. *Neurobiol Dis* (2014) 72 Pt A:3–12. doi:10.1016/j.nbd.2014.08.025

Castellano JM, Kim J, Stewart FR, Jiang H, DeMattos RB, Patterson BW, et al. Human apoE isoforms differentially regulate brain amyloid-beta peptide clearance. *Sci Transl Med* (2011) 3:89ra57. doi:10.1126/scitranslmed.3002156

Jones PB, Adams KW, Rozkalne A, Spires-Jones TL, Hshieh TT, Hashimoto T, et al. Apolipoprotein E: isoform specific differences in tertiary structure and interaction with amyloid-beta in human Alzheimer brain. *PLoS One* (2011) 6:e14586. doi:10.1371/journal.pone.0014586

Libby AE, Wang H, Mittal R, Sungelo M, Potma E, Eckel RH. Lipoprotein lipase is an important modulator of lipid uptake and storage in hypothalamic neurons. *Biochem Biophys Res Commun* (2015) 465:287–92. doi:10.1016/j.bbrc.2015.08.026

Wang H, Astarita G, Taussig MD, Bharadwaj KG, DiPatrizio NV, Nave KA, et al. Deficiency of lipoprotein lipase in neurons modifies the regula- tion of energy balance and leads to obesity. *Cell Metab* (2011) 13:105–13. doi:10.1016/j.cmet.2010.12.006

Yu T, Taussig MD, DiPatrizio NV, Astarita G, Piomelli D, Bergman BC, et al. Deficiency of lipoprotein lipase in neurons decreases AMPA receptor phosphorylation and leads to neurobehavioral abnormalities in mice. *PLoS One* (2015) 10:e0135113. doi:10.1371/journal.pone.0135113

Picard A, Rouch C, Kassis N, Moulle VS, Croizier S, Denis RG, et al. Hippocampal lipoprotein lipase regulates energy balance in rodents. *Mol Metab* (2014) 3:167–76. doi:10.1016/j.molmet.2013.11.002

Wang H, Taussig MD, DiPatrizio NV, Bruce K, Piomelli D, Eckel RH. Obesity development in neuron-specific lipoprotein lipase deficient mice is not responsive to increased dietary fat content or change in fat composition. *Metabolism* (2016) 65:987–97. doi:10.1016/j.metabol.2016.01.015

Sarruf DA, Yu F, Nguyen HT, Williams DL, Printz RL, Niswender KD, et al. Expression of peroxisome proliferator-activated receptor-gamma in key neuronal subsets regulating glucose metabolism and energy homeostasis. *Endocrinology* (2009) 150:707–12. doi:10.1210/en.2008-0899

Andrews ZB, Liu ZW, Walllingford N, Erion DM, Borok E, Friedman JM, et al. UCP2 mediates ghrelin's action on NPY/AgRP neurons by lowering free radicals. *Nature* (2008) 454:846–51. doi:10.1038/nature07181

Diano S, Liu ZW, Jeong JK, Dietrich MO, Ruan HB, Kim E, et al. Peroxisome proliferation-associated control of reactive oxygen species sets melanocortin tone and feeding in diet-induced obesity. *Nat Med* (2011) 17:1121–7. doi:10.1038/nm.2421

Lopez M, Nogueiras R, Tena-Sempere M, Dieguez C. Hypothalamic AMPK: a canonical regulator of whole-body energy balance. *Nat Rev Endocrinol* (2016) 12:421–32. doi:10.1038/nrendo.2016.67

Hardie DG. AMP-activated/SNF1 protein kinases: conserved guardians of cellular energy. *Nat Rev Mol Cell Biol* (2007) 8:774–85. doi:10.1038/nrm2249

Wolfgang MJ, Cha SH, Sidhaye A, Chohnan S, Cline G, Shulman GI, et al. Regulation of hypothalamic malonyl-CoA by central glucose and leptin. *Proc Natl Acad Sci U S A* (2007) 104:19285–90. doi:10.1073/pnas.0709778104

Lopez M, Varela L, Vazquez MJ, Rodriguez-Cuenca S, Gonzalez CR, Velagapudi VR, et al. Hypothalamic AMPK and fatty acid metabolism mediate thyroid regulation of energy balance. *Nat Med* (2010) 16:1001–8. doi:10.1038/nm.2207

Lopez M. EJE PRIZE 2017: hypothalamic AMPK: a golden target against obesity? *Eur J Endocrinol* (2017). doi:10.1530/EJE-16-0927

Martin TL, Alquier T, Asakura K, Furukawa N, Preitner F, Kahn BB. Diet-induced obesity alters AMP kinase activity in hypothalamus and skeletal muscle. *J Biol Chem* (2006) 281:18933–41. doi:10.1074/jbc.M512831200

Gomez-Pinilla F, Ying Z. Differential effects of exercise and dietary docosahexaenoic acid on molecular systems associated with control of allostasis in the hypothalamus and hippocampus. *Neuroscience* (2010) 168:130–7. doi:10.1016/j.neuroscience.2010.02.070

Blazquez C, Geelen MJ, Velasco G, Guzman M. The AMP-activated protein kinase prevents ceramide synthesis de novo and apoptosis in astrocytes. *FEBS Lett* (2001) 489:149–53. doi:10.1016/S0014-5793(01)02089-0

Culmsee C, Monnig J, Kemp BE, Mattson MP. AMP-activated protein kinase is highly expressed in neurons in the developing rat brain and promotes neuronal survival following glucose deprivation. *J Mol Neurosci* (2001) 17:45–58. doi:10.1385/JMN:17:1:45

Won JS, Im YB, Kim J, Singh AK, Singh I. Involvement of AMP-activated-protein-kinase (AMPK) in neuronal amyloidogenesis. *Biochem Biophys Res Commun* (2010) 399:487–91. doi:10.1016/j.bbrc.2010.07.081

Yue JT, Lam TK. Lipid sensing and insulin resistance in the brain. *Cell Metab* (2012) 15:646–55. doi:10.1016/j.cmet.2012.01.013

Lam TK, Pocai A, Gutierrez-Juarez R, Obici S, Bryan J, Aguilar-Bryan L, et al. Hypothalamic sensing of circulating fatty acids is required for glucose homeostasis. *Nat Med* (2005) 11:320–7. doi:10.1038/nm1201

Obici S, Feng Z, Karkanias G, Baskin DG, Rossetti L. Decreasing hypothalamic insulin receptors causes hyperphagia and insulin resistance in rats. *Nat Neurosci* (2002) 5:566–72. doi:10.1038/nn0602-861

Gao S, Serra D, Keung W, Hegardt FG, Lopaschuk GD. Important role of ventromedial hypothalamic carnitine palmitoyltransferase-1a in the control of food intake. *Am J Physiol Endocrinol Metab* (2013) 305:E336–47. doi:10.1152/ajpendo.00168.2013

Mera P, Mir JF, Fabrias G, Casas J, Costa AS, Malandrino MI, et al. Long- term increased carnitine palmitoyltransferase 1A expression in ventro- medial hypothalamus causes hyperphagia and alters the hypothalamic lipidomic profile. *PLoS One* (2014) 9:e97195. doi:10.1371/journal.pone. 0097195

Wolfgang MJ, Kurama T, Dai Y, Suwa A, Asaumi M, Matsumoto S, et al. The brain-specific carnitine palmitoyltransferase-1c regulates energy homeostasis. *Proc Natl Acad Sci U S A* (2006) 103:7282–7. doi:10.1073/pnas.0602205103

Wolfgang MJ, Cha SH, Millington DS, Cline G, Shulman GI, Suwa A, et al. Brain-specific carnitine palmitoyl-transferase-1c: role in CNS fatty acid metabolism, food intake, and body weight. *J Neurochem* (2008) 105:1550–9. doi:10.1111/j.1471-4159.2008.05255.x

Lane MD, Wolfgang M, Cha SH, Dai Y. Regulation of food intake and energy expenditure by hypothalamic malonyl-CoA. *Int J Obes* (2008) 32 Suppl 4:S49–54. doi:10.1038/ijo.2008.123

Ramirez S, Martins L, Jacas J, Carrasco P, Pozo M, Clotet J, et al. Hypothalamic ceramide levels regulated by CPT1C mediate the orexigenic effect of ghrelin. *Diabetes* (2013) 62:2329–37. doi:10.2337/db12-1451

Contreras C, Gonzalez-Garcia I, Martinez-Sanchez N, Seoane-Collazo P, Jacas J, Morgan DA, et al. Central ceramide-induced hypothalamic lipotoxicity and ER stress regulate energy balance. *Cell Rep* (2014) 9:366–77. doi:10.1016/j.celrep.2014.08.057

Lee J, Wolfgang MJ. Metabolomic profiling reveals a role for CPT1c in neuronal oxidative metabolism. *BMC Biochem* (2012) 13:23. doi:10.1186/1471-2091-13-23

Pazos MR, Nunez E, Benito C, Tolon RM, Romero J. Functional neuroanatomy of the endocannabinoid system. *Pharmacol Biochem Behav* (2005) 81:239–47. doi:10.1016/j.pbb.2005.01.030

McGarry JD, Mannaerts GP, Foster DW. A possible role for malonyl-CoA in the regulation of hepatic fatty acid oxidation and ketogenesis. *J Clin Invest* (1977) 60:265–70. doi:10.1172/JCI108764

Caspi L, Wang PY, Lam TK. A balance of lipid-sensing mechanisms in the brain and liver. *Cell Metab* (2007) 6:99–104. doi:10.1016/j.cmet.2007. 07.005

Gao S, Moran TH, Lopaschuk GD, Butler AA. Hypothalamic malonyl-CoA and the control of food intake. *Physiol Behav* (2013) 122:17–24. doi:10.1016/j.physbeh.2013.07.014

Gao S, Kinzig KP, Aja S, Scott KA, Keung W, Kelly S, et al. Leptin activates hypothalamic acetyl-CoA carboxylase to inhibit food intake. *Proc Natl Acad Sci U S A* (2007) 104:17358–63. doi:10.1073/pnas.0708385104

Loftus TM, Jaworsky DE, Frehywot GL, Townsend CA, Ronnett GV, Lane MD, et al. Reduced food intake and body weight in mice treated with fatty acid synthase inhibitors. *Science* (2000) 288:2379–81. doi:10.1126/science.288.5475.2379

Andersson U, Filipsson K, Abbott CR, Woods A, Smith K, Bloom SR, et al. AMP-activated protein kinase plays a role in the control of food intake. *J Biol Chem* (2004) 279:12005–8. doi:10.1074/jbc.C300557200

He W, Lam TK, Obici S, Rossetti L. Molecular disruption of hypothalamic nutrient sensing induces obesity. *Nat Neurosci* (2006) 9:227–33. doi:10.1038/nn1626

Pocai A, Lam TK, Gutierrez-Juarez R, Obici S, Schwartz GJ, Bryan J, et al. Hypothalamic K(ATP) channels control hepatic glucose production. *Nature* (2005) 434:1026–31. doi:10.1038/nature03439

Ross RA, Rossetti L, Lam TK, Schwartz GJ. Differential effects of hypothalamic long-chain fatty acid infusions on suppression of hepatic glucose production. *Am J Physiol Endocrinol Metab* (2010) 299:E633–9. doi:10.1152/ajpendo.00190.2010

Bruinstroop E, Pei L, Ackermans MT, Foppen E, Borgers AJ, Kwakkel J, et al. Hypothalamic neuropeptide Y (NPY) controls hepatic VLDL-triglyceride secretion in rats via the sympathetic nervous system. *Diabetes* (2012) 61:1043–50. doi:10.2337/db11-1142

Lam TK, Gutierrez-Juarez R, Pocai A, Bhanot S, Tso P, Schwartz GJ, et al. Brain glucose metabolism controls the hepatic secretion of triglyceride-rich lipoproteins. *Nat Med* (2007) 13:171–80. doi:10.1038/nm1540

Yue JT, Mighiu PI, Naples M, Adeli K, Lam TK. Glycine normalizes hepatic triglyceride-rich VLDL secretion by triggering the CNS in high-fat fed rats. *Circ Res* (2012) 110:1345–54. doi:10.1161/CIRCRESAHA.112. 268276

Leckstrom A, Lew PS, Poritsanos NJ, Mizuno TM. Central melanocortin receptor agonist reduces hepatic lipogenic gene expression in streptozotocin-induced diabetic mice. *Life Sci* (2011) 88:664–9. doi:10.1016/j.lfs.2011.01.026

Wiedmer P, Chaudhary N, Rath M, Yi CX, Ananthakrishnan G, Nogueiras R, et al. The HPA axis modulates the CNS melanocortin control of liver triacylglyceride metabolism. *Physiol Behav* (2012) 105:791–9. doi:10.1016/j.physbeh.2011.10.019

Shimada M, Tritos NA, Lowell BB, Flier JS, Maratos-Flier E. Mice lacking melanin-concentrating hormone are hypophagic and lean. *Nature* (1998) 396:670–4. doi:10.1038/25341

Jeon JY, Bradley RL, Kokkotou EG, Marino FE, Wang X, Pissios P, et al. MCH-/- mice are resistant to aging-associated increases in body weight and insulin resistance. *Diabetes* (2006) 55:428–34. doi:10.2337/diabetes.55.02.06.db05-0203

Wang Y, Ziogas DC, Biddinger S, Kokkotou E. You deserve what you eat: lessons learned from the study of the melanin-concentrating hormone (MCH)-deficient mice. *Gut* (2010) 59:1625–34. doi:10.1136/gut.2010.210526

Imbernon M, Beiroa D, Vazquez MJ, Morgan DA, Veyrat-Durebex C, Porteiro B, et al. Central melanin-concentrating hormone influences liver and adipose metabolism via specific hypothalamic nuclei and efferent autonomic/JNK1 pathways. *Gastroenterology* (2013) 144:636.e–49.e. doi:10.1053/j.gastro.2012.10.051

Rojas JM, Bruinstroop E, Printz RL, Alijagic-Boers A, Foppen E, Turney MK, et al. Central nervous system neuropeptide Y regulates mediators of hepatic phospholipid remodeling and very low-density lipoprotein triglyceride secretion via sympathetic innervation. *Mol Metab* (2015) 4:210–21. doi:10.1016/j.molmet.2015.01.004

Cheng L, Yu Y, Szabo A, Wu Y, Wang H, Camer D, et al. Palmitic acid induces central leptin resistance and impairs hepatic glucose and lipid metabolism in male mice. *J Nutr Biochem* (2015) 26:541–8. doi:10.1016/j.jnutbio.2014.12.011

Yue JT, Abraham MA, LaPierre MP, Mighiu PI, Light PE, Filippi BM, et al. A fatty acid-dependent hypothalamic-DVC neurocircuitry that regulates hepatic secretion of triglyceride-rich lipoproteins. *Nat Commun* (2015) 6:5970. doi:10.1038/ncomms6970

Nonogaki K. New insights into sympathetic regulation of glucose and fat metabolism. *Diabetologia* (2000) 43:533–49. doi:10.1007/s001250051341

Shimazu T. Innervation of the liver and glucoregulation: roles of the hypothalamus and autonomic nerves. *Nutrition* (1996) 12:65–6. doi:10.1016/S0899-9007(96)90348-2

Uyama N, Geerts A, Reynaert H. Neural connections between the hypothalamus and the liver. *Anat Rec A Discov Mol Cell Evol Biol* (2004) 280:808–20. doi:10.1002/ar.a.20086

Saper CB, Loewy AD, Swanson LW, Cowan WM. Direct hypothalamo-autonomic connections. *Brain Res* (1976) 117:305–12. doi:10.1016/0006-8993(76)90738-1

Swanson LW, Sawchenko PE. Paraventricular nucleus: a site for the integration of neuroendocrine and autonomic mechanisms. *Neuroendocrinology* (1980) 31:410–7. doi:10.1159/000123111

Sandoval DA, Obici S, Seeley RJ. Targeting the CNS to treat type 2 diabetes. *Nat Rev Drug Discov* (2009) 8:386–98. doi:10.1038/nrd2874

Schwartz MW, Seeley RJ, Tschop MH, Woods SC, Morton GJ, Myers MG, et al. Cooperation between brain and islet in glucose homeostasis and diabe- tes. *Nature* (2013) 503:59–66. doi:10.1038/nature12709

Kalsbeek A, Bruinstroop E, Yi CX, Klieverik LP, La Fleur SE, Fliers E. Hypothalamic control of energy metabolism via the autonomic nervous system. *Ann N Y Acad Sci* (2010) 1212:114–29. doi:10.1111/j.1749-6632.2010.05800.x

Yi CX, la Fleur SE, Fliers E, Kalsbeek A. The role of the autonomic nervous liver innervation in the control of energy metabolism. *Biochim Biophys Acta* (2010) 1802:416–31. doi:10.1016/j.bbadis.2010.01.006

O'Hare JD, Zsombok A. Brain-liver connections: role of the preauto- nomic PVN neurons. *Am J Physiol Endocrinol Metab* (2016) 310:E183–9. doi:10.1152/ajpendo.00302.2015

Bruinstroop E, Fliers E, Kalsbeek A. Hypothalamic control of hepatic lipid metabolism via the autonomic nervous system. *Best Pract Res Clin Endocrinol Metab* (2014) 28:673–84. doi:10.1016/j.beem.2014.05.001

Puschel GP. Control of hepatocyte metabolism by sympathetic and parasympathetic hepatic nerves. *Anat Rec A Discov Mol Cell Evol Biol* (2004) 280:854–67. doi:10.1002/ar.a.20091

Lawrence D, Pittman QJ. Interaction between descending paraventricular neurons and vagal motor neurons. *Brain Res* (1985) 332:158–60. doi:10.1016/0006-8993(85)90399-3

Rogers RC, Nelson DO. Neurons of the vagal division of the solitary nucleus activated by the paraventricular nucleus of the hypothalamus. *J Auton Nerv Syst* (1984) 10:193–7. doi:10.1016/0165-1838(84)90057-2

Yamashita H, Inenaga K, Koizumi K. Possible projections from regions of paraventricular and supraoptic nuclei to the spinal cord: electrophysiological studies. *Brain Res* (1984) 296:373–8. doi:10.1016/0006-8993(84)90077-5

Cailotto C, La Fleur SE, Van Heijningen C, Wortel J, Kalsbeek A, Feenstra M, et al. The suprachiasmatic nucleus controls the daily variation of plasma glucose via the autonomic output to the liver: are the clock genes involved? *Eur J Neurosci* (2005) 22:2531–40. doi:10.1111/j.1460-9568. 2005.04439.x

Rogers RC, Hermann GE. Central connections of the hepatic branch of the vagus nerve: a horseradish peroxidase histochemical study. *J Auton Nerv Syst* (1983) 7:165–74. doi:10.1016/0165-1838(83)90044-9

Banfield BW, Kaufman JD, Randall JA, Pickard GE. Development of pseudorabies virus strains expressing red fluorescent proteins: new tools for multisynaptic labeling applications. *J Virol* (2003) 77:10106–12. doi:10.1128/JVI.77.18.10106-10112.2003

Boldogkoi Z, Reichart A, Toth IE, Sik A, Erdelyi F, Medveczky I, et al. Construction of recombinant pseudorabies viruses optimized for labeling and neurochemical characterization of neural circuitry. *Brain Res Mol Brain Res* (2002) 109:105–18. doi:10.1016/S0169-328X(02)00546-6

Card JP. Exploring brain circuitry with neurotropic viruses: new horizons in neuroanatomy. *Anat Rec* (1998) 253:176–85. doi:10.1002/ (SICI)1097-0185(199812)253:6<176::AID-AR6>3.0.CO;2-W

Card JP, Enquist LW. Transneuronal circuit analysis with pseudorabies viruses. *Curr Protoc Neurosci* (2014) 68:1.5.1–39; editorial board, Jacqueline N. Crawley … [et al.]. doi:10.1002/0471142301.ns0105s68

Cano G, Card JP, Sved AF. Dual viral transneuronal tracing of central autonomic circuits involved in the innervation of the two kidneys in rat. *J Comp Neurol* (2004) 471:462–81. doi:10.1002/cne.20040

Williams KW, Zsombok A, Smith BN. Rapid inhibition of neurons in the dor- sal motor nucleus of the vagus by leptin. *Endocrinology* (2007) 148:1868–81. doi:10.1210/en.2006-1098

Gao H, Miyata K, Bhaskaran MD, Derbenev AV, Zsombok A. Transient receptor potential vanilloid type 1-dependent regulation of liver-related neurons in the paraventricular nucleus of the hypothalamus diminished in the type 1 diabetic mouse. *Diabetes* (2012) 61:1381–90. doi:10.2337/db11-0820

Zsombok A, Jiang Y, Gao H, Anwar IJ, Rezai-Zadeh K, Enix CL, et al. Regulation of leptin receptor-expressing neurons in the brainstem by TRPV1. *Physiol Rep* (2014) 2:e12160. doi:10.14814/phy2.12160

Anwar IJ, Miyata K, Zsombok A. Brain stem as target site for the metabolic side effects of olanzapine. *J Neurophysiology* (2016) 115:1389–98. doi:10.1152/jn.00387.2015

Aston-Jones G, Card JP. Use of pseudorabies virus to delineate multisynaptic circuits in brain: opportunities and limitations. *J Neurosci Methods* (2000) 103:51–61. doi:10.1016/S0165-0270(00)00295-8

Ch'ng TH, Spear PG, Struyf F, Enquist LW. Glycoprotein D-independent spread of pseudorabies virus infection in cultured peripheral nervous system neurons in a compartmented system. *J Virol* (2007) 81:10742–57. doi:10.1128/JVI.00981-07

Stanley S, Pinto S, Segal J, Perez CA, Viale A, DeFalco J, et al. Identification of neuronal subpopulations that project from hypothalamus to both liver and adipose tissue polysynaptically. *Proc Natl Acad Sci U S A* (2010) 107:7024–9. doi:10.1073/pnas.1002790107

la Fleur SE, Kalsbeek A, Wortel J, Buijs RM. Polysynaptic neural pathways between the hypothalamus, including the suprachiasmatic nucleus, and the liver. *Brain Res* (2000) 871:50–6. doi:10.1016/S0006-8993(00)02423-9

Zsombok A, Gao H, Miyata K, Issa A, Derbenev AV. Immunohistochemical localization of transient receptor potential vanilloid type 1 and insulin receptor substrate 2 and their co-localization with liver-related neurons in the hypothalamus and brainstem. *Brain Res* (2011) 1398:30–9. doi:10.1016/j.brainres.2011.04.048

Kalsbeek A, La Fleur S, Van Heijningen C, Buijs RM. Suprachiasmatic GABAergic inputs to the paraventricular nucleus control plasma glucose concentrations in the rat via sympathetic innervation of the liver. *J Neurosci* (2004) 24:7604–13. doi:10.1523/JNEUROSCI.5328-03.2004

Buijs RM, la Fleur SE, Wortel J, Van Heyningen C, Zuiddam L, Mettenleiter TC, et al. The suprachiasmatic nucleus balances sympathetic and parasympathetic output to peripheral organs through separate preautonomic neurons. *J Comp Neurol* (2003) 464:36–48. doi:10.1002/cne.10765

Cano G, Sved AF, Rinaman L, Rabin BS, Card JP. Characterization of the central nervous system innervation of the rat spleen using viral transneuronal tracing. *J Comp Neurol* (2001) 439:1–18. doi:10.1002/cne.1331

Shimazu T. Neuronal regulation of hepatic glucose metabolism in mammals. *Diabetes Metab Rev* (1987) 3:185–206. doi:10.1002/dmr.5610030109

Shimazu T, Fukuda A, Ban T. Reciprocal influences of the ventromedial and lateral hypothalamic nuclei on blood glucose level and liver glycogen content. *Nature* (1966) 210:1178–9. doi:10.1038/2101178a0

Yi CX, Sun N, Ackermans MT, Alkemade A, Foppen E, Shi J, et al. Pituitary adenylate cyclase-activating polypeptide stimulates glucose production via the hepatic sympathetic innervation in rats. *Diabetes* (2010) 59:1591–600. doi:10.2337/db09-1398

van den Hoek AM, van Heijningen C, Schroder-van der Elst JP, Ouwens DM, Havekes LM, Romijn JA, et al. Intracerebroventricular administration of neuropeptide Y induces hepatic insulin resistance via sympathetic innervation. *Diabetes* (2008) 57:2304–10. doi:10.2337/db07-1658

Klieverik LP, Janssen SF, van Riel A, Foppen E, Bisschop PH, Serlie MJ, et al. Thyroid hormone modulates glucose production via a sympathetic pathway from the hypothalamic paraventricular nucleus to the liver. *Proc Natl Acad Sci U S A* (2009) 106:5966–71. doi:10.1073/pnas.0805355106

Lam TK, Gutierrez-Juarez R, Pocai A, Rossetti L. Regulation of blood glucose by hypothalamic pyruvate metabolism. *Science* (2005) 309:943–7. doi:10.1126/science.1112085

Lam TK, Schwartz GJ, Rossetti L. Hypothalamic sensing of fatty acids. *Nat Neurosci* (2005) 8:579–84. doi:10.1038/nn1456

Obici S, Zhang BB, Karkanias G, Rossetti L. Hypothalamic insulin signaling is required for inhibition of glucose production. *Nat Med* (2002) 8:1376–82. doi:10.1038/nm1202-798

Pocai A, Morgan K, Buettner C, Gutierrez-Juarez R, Obici S, Rossetti L. Central leptin acutely reverses diet-induced hepatic insulin resistance. *Diabetes* (2005) 54:3182–9. doi:10.2337/diabetes.54.11.3182

Pocai A, Obici S, Schwartz GJ, Rossetti L. A brain-liver circuit regulates glucose homeostasis. *Cell Metab* (2005) 1:53–61. doi:10.1016/j.cmet.2004.11.001

Razavi R, Chan Y, Afifiyan FN, Liu XJ, Wan X, Yantha J, et al. TRPV1+ sensory neurons control beta cell stress and islet inflammation in autoimmune diabetes. *Cell* (2006) 127:1123–35. doi:10.1016/j.cell.2006.10.038

Zsombok A, Derbenev AV. TRP channels as therapeutic targets in diabetes and obesity. *Pharmaceuticals (Basel)* (2016) 9:E50. doi:10.3390/ph9030050

Derbenev AV, Zsombok A. Potential therapeutic value of TRPV1 and TRPA1 in diabetes mellitus and obesity. *Semin Immunopathol* (2016) 38:397–406. doi:10.1007/s00281-015-0529-x

Zsombok A, Bhaskaran MD, Gao H, Derbenev AV, Smith BN. Functional plasticity of central TRPV1 receptors in brainstem dorsal vagal complex circuits of streptozotocin-treated hyperglycemic mice. *J Neurosci* (2011) 31:14024–31. doi:10.1523/JNEUROSCI.2081-11.2011

Boychuk CR, Zsombok A, Tasker JG, Smith BN. Rapid glucocorticoid-induced activation of TRP and CB1 receptors causes biphasic modulation of glutamate release in gastric-related hypothalamic preautonomic neurons. *Front Neurosci* (2013) 7:3. doi:10.3389/fnins.2013.00003

Geerling JJ, Boon MR, Kooijman S, Parlevliet ET, Havekes LM, Romijn JA, et al. Sympathetic nervous system control of triglyceride metabolism: novel concepts derived from recent studies. *J Lipid Res* (2014) 55:180–9. doi:10.1194/jlr.R045013

Licht CM, Vreeburg SA, van Reedt Dortland AK, Giltay EJ, Hoogendijk WJ, DeRijk RH, et al. Increased sympathetic and decreased parasympathetic activity rather than changes in hypothalamic-pituitary-adrenal axis activity is associated with metabolic abnormalities. *J Clin Endocrinol Metab* (2010) 95:2458–66. doi:10.1210/jc.2009-2801

Nogueiras R, Perez-Tilve D, Veyrat-Durebex C, Morgan DA, Varela L, Haynes WG, et al. Direct control of peripheral lipid deposition by CNS GLP-1 receptor signaling is mediated by the sympathetic nervous system and blunted in diet-induced obesity. *J Neurosci* (2009) 29:5916–25. doi:10.1523/JNEUROSCI.5977-08.2009

Parlevliet ET, Wang Y, Geerling JJ, Schroder-Van der Elst JP, Picha K, O'Neil K, et al. GLP-1 receptor activation inhibits VLDL production and reverses hepatic steatosis by decreasing hepatic lipogenesis in high-fat-fed APOE*3-Leiden mice. *PLoS One* (2012) 7:e49152. doi:10.1371/journal.pone.0049152

2

Dopamine Adaptations as a Common Pathway for Neurocognitive Impairment in Diabetes and Obesity: A Neuropsychological Perspective

Dana M. Small[1,2]*

[1] *The John B Pierce Laboratory, New Haven, CT, USA,* [2] *Department of Psychiatry, Yale University School of Medicine, New Haven, CT, USA*

Correspondence:
Dana M. Small
dana.small@yale.edu

Evidence accumulates linking obesity and diabetes with cognitive dysfunction. At present the mechanism(s) underlying these associations and the relative contribution of diet, adiposity, and metabolic dysfunction are unknown. In this perspective key gaps in knowledge are outlined and an initial sketch of a neuropsychological profile is developed that points toward a critical role for dopamine (DA) adaptations in neurocognitive impairment secondary to diabetes and obesity. The precise mechanisms by which diet, metabolic dysfunction, and adiposity influence the DA system to impact cognition remains unclear and is an important direction for future research.

Keywords: dementia, diabetes, obesity, dopamine, cognition, executive function, memory, associative learning

NEUROCOGNITIVE IMPAIRMENTS IN TYPE 2 DIABETES (T2D)

T2D is associated with cognitive decline, brain dysfunction, and dementia (Biessels et al., 2014; Koekkoek et al., 2015; Stoeckel et al., 2016). One recent study estimated that the combined overall relative risk for dementia is 73% higher in people with, compared to without T2D, indicating that between 1 in 10 and 1 in 15 incidences of dementia may be attributable to T2D (Biessels et al., 2014). Although glucose intolerance is diagnostic of T2D, a recent systematic review of 86 papers examining T2D and cognition only reported a weak association between glycaemia, and cognition (Geijselaers et al., 2015) and there is even less evidence for an association with other measures of peripheral glucose regulation and cognitive function (e.g., insulin concentration, insulin action, insulin resistance) (Geijselaers et al., 2015). Thus, although T2D is by definition associated with altered glucose metabolism, it is not clear that altered glucose metabolism contributes to cognitive change. The mechanism behind the link between cognitive dysfunction and T2D is therefore not clear.

NEUROCOGNITIVE DEFICITS MAY ARISE FROM CHRONIC CONDITIONS ASSOCIATED WITH T2D

The majority of human studies linking T2D to cognitive decline are performed in older individuals with long-standing diagnoses of diabetes (Stoeckel et al., 2016). This poses a problem for interpreting the pathophysiology of the link between T2D and cognition because individuals with chronic T2D exhibit a number of pathologies associated with cognitive decline such as damage to the blood brain barrier (BBB), neuroinflammation (Banks et al., 2012; Steculorum et al., 2014), cerebral atrophy, and small vessel disease (Biessels and Reijmer, 2014; Akrivos et al., 2015; Ramos-Rodriguez et al., 2016; Stranahan et al., 2016). The co-occurrence of these pathologies that are secondary to diabetes has led to controversy over whether it is T2D (Biessels and Reagan, 2015) or complications arising from T2D that leads to cognitive decline (De Felice and Ferreira, 2014). To rule-out confounds associated with the secondary complications of T2D it will be informative to study cognition in populations free from other chronic conditions and in populations prior to the onset of T2D. For example, it would be informative to characterize neurocognition in youth before and after the onset of prediabetes, since this population will be free from other chronic conditions that could influence cognitive function.

IT IS UNKNOWN IF NEUROCOGNITIVE DEFICITS ARE ASSOCIATED WITH T2D OR ADIPOSITY OR BOTH

Perhaps the most important limitation of the current literature is the failure to disentangle effects of metabolic dysfunction on cognition from those of adiposity and diet. Obesity has been associated with altered brain structure and function in animal models and in metabolically and neurologically healthy adults and children (Elias et al., 2003; Reinert et al., 2013; Hsu and Kanoski, 2014; Yau et al., 2014; Bocarsly et al., 2015), while diets high in saturated fat and cholesterol are correlated with compromised cognitive flexibility and processing speed in pre-pubertal children after adjusting for age, sex, socioeconomic status, IQ, VO_{2max}, and BMI (Khan et al., 2015b). Consumption of a high fat diet (HFD) can also negatively impact brain and brain function well-before obesity onset. For example, in animal models hypothalamic insulin resistance is observed following acute exposure to HFD before changes in adiposity occur (Clegg et al., 2011) and impaired performance on hippocampal-dependent tasks is observed after only 72-h access to a HFD when animals have actually lost weight, presumably due to neophobia (Kanoski and Davidson, 2010). These findings suggest that obesity can impact cognition independently from metabolic disease and that diet can impact metabolic function and cognition independently of obesity.

To date, studies have rarely taken obesity and diet into account when examining the relationship between T2D and cognition. For example, patients with T2D exhibit reduced activity in the default mode network (Musen et al., 2012), which has been associated with a wide range of neurological conditions and cognitive impairments (Browndyke et al., 2017; Contreras et al., 2017; Jockwitz et al., 2017; von Rhein et al., 2017) but BMI, which was higher in T2D, was not accounted for. Similarly, the putative confound of glucose intolerance is often not considered when examining the relationship between obesity and cognition. For example, a prospective study examining the impact of obesity on cognition excluded participants for many medical conditions likely to influence cognition, including stroke, dementia, myocardial infarction, and atrial fibrillation but NOT diabetes (Gunstad et al., 2010). They did however, include "glucose intolerance" in their mixed model regression analyses and found that this variable was related to cognitive impairments that also correlated with their adiposity measures (waist-hip ratio). In another study deficits in executive function and declarative memory were observed in 38 middle-aged adults with insulin resistance but without T2D compared to 54 age, gender, education but NOT BMI matched controls. Since the insulin resistance group had significantly higher BMI these deficits may be equally attributable to BMI (Bruehl et al., 2010).

Failure to account for confounds between diet, obesity, and metabolic dysfunction also pervade the animal literature. Rats prone to develop diabetes upon HFD are often used as a model of T2D (Levin and Routh, 1996). These models have been associated with deficits on the water maze (Li et al., 2002; Stranahan et al., 2008b), object recognition test (Stranahan et al., 2008a), contextual cue conditioning (Grillo et al., 2011), and discrimination and reversal learning (Kanoski et al., 2007, 2010). HFD has also been shown to increase inflammatory cytokines and impair neuroplasticity and learning and memory in the hippocampus (Erion et al., 2014). The extent to which adiposity or insulin resistance contributed to these observations is not known. However, impaired cognition is also observed with the streptozotocin (STX)-induced diabetic model, which impairs insulin production without increasing adiposity or requiring a high fat diet, indicating that metabolic dysfunction alone is sufficient to impair cognitive function (Stranahan et al., 2008a).

Importantly, when more than one variable is measured interactions between adiposity, diet, and impaired glucose tolerance are revealed. In obese humans without T2D, insulin sensitivity mediates the relationship between working memory-related activation in the right parietal cortex and BMI (Gonzales et al., 2010), while brain insulin action is selectively impaired in the prefrontal cortex in overweight and obese, but not diabetic adults compared to their lean counterparts (Kullmann et al., 2015), highlighting interactions between adiposity and glucose tolerance on brain function.

In summary, the relative contribution of diet, impaired glucose tolerance, and adiposity to neurocognitive impairment is largely unexplored and unknown.

CHARACTERIZATION OF GLYCEMIA

Another factor clouding the association between T2D and cognitive impairment is the use of a variety of methods to characterize glycemia, each of which reflect different, and sometimes independent, aspects of glucose metabolism (Geijselaers et al., 2015). Insulin sensitivity can be measured using a variety of techniques. HbA_{1c}, which reflects the mean glucose concentration over a period of 8–12 weeks is the most frequently used measure. Fasting blood glucose concentrations are also frequently measured, which reflect nocturnal hepatic gluconeogenesis that is influenced by hepatic insulin sensitivity, but a recent review found that studies often fail to report whether measurements are taken at the same time of day (Geijselaers et al., 2015). Other measures include post-prandial glucose concentrations, reflecting insulin secretory responses and HOMA-IR to measure insulin resistance. HbA_{1c} shows the strongest association to insulin resistance, followed by post-prandial measures. Fasting glucose, by contrast, seems to be unrelated to cognitive performance (Geijselaers et al., 2015). Interestingly, one study found that insulin resistance was related to declarative memory whereas HbA_{1c} was associated with executive dysfunction (Bruehl et al., 2010), hinting at the possibility that the different measures are associated with distinct pathophysiological effects on the brain and highlighting the need for more comprehensive measures of glucose metabolism.

NEUROCOGNITIVE IMPAIRMENTS MAY BE RELATED TO CENTRAL RATHER THAN (OR IN ADDITION TO) PERIPHERAL IMPAIRMENTS IN GLUCOSE TOLERANCE

Insulin receptors are widely distributed in the brain, with the highest concentrations in the olfactory bulb, hypothalamus, cerebral cortex, cerebellum, and hippocampus (Havrankova et al., 1978; van Houten et al., 1979). Brain-specific deletion of the insulin receptor in mice results in glycogen synthase kinase 2 beta activation resulting in hyperphosphorylation of tau protein, a hallmark of early Alzheimer's Disease (AD) (Schubert et al., 2004). There is also evidence from animal studies that disrupted central insulin and insulin-like growth factor-1 (IGF-1) signaling may lead to disrupted neurotransmitter (e.g., dopamine) and astroglial cell function, brain endothelial cell function involved in formation and regulation of BBB, mitochondrial metabolism and oxidative stress, clearance of Aβ and/or amyloid fibrils, cholesterol synthesis in the brain (important for myelination and membrane function), glucose and lipid metabolism in select regions of the brain, and regulation of central energy balance, which could relate to both metabolic and neurocognitive dysfunction (Brüning et al., 2000; Convit et al., 2003; Schubert et al., 2004; Suzuki et al., 2010; Kleinridders et al., 2014; Stouffer et al., 2015). While these data suggest a likely role for central insulin resistance in impaired neurocognitive function, it is important to note that central insulin resistance has a complicated relationship with peripheral glycemic control (Ketterer et al., 2011). Central insulin resistance is thought to result from a combination of impaired insulin receptor signaling and decreases in the transport of insulin across the BBB (Banks et al., 2012), which can occur secondary to peripheral glucose intolerance (Niswender et al., 2003). Conversely, central insulin signaling contributes to peripheral glucose regulation (Brüning et al., 2000; Heni et al., 2014) to create a dynamic brain-gut axis regulating glucose metabolism. Importantly, however, central insulin resistance can occur independently from peripheral impairments in glucose tolerance. Post-mortem studies of brain tissue from patients with AD but not T2D, reveal disrupted brain insulin signaling (De Felice and Ferreira, 2014; Yarchoan and Arnold, 2014). Accordingly, treatment with intranasal insulin, which results in direct insulin transport from the nasal cavity to the CNS via intraneuronal and extraneuronal pathways (Reger and Craft, 2006), improves cognition in patients with (Reger et al., 2008; Craft et al., 2012) and without (Hallschmid et al., 2007, 2008) dementia. These findings underscore the importance of concurrent measures of peripheral and central insulin resistance.

One promising avenue for future research is in using intranasal insulin in combination with neuroimaging methodologies and neuropsychological testing to assess the role of central insulin resistance in neurocognition (Tschritter et al., 2006; Ketterer et al., 2011; Grichisch et al., 2012; Kullmann et al., 2013, 2015; Heni et al., 2014, 2016). For example, intranasal insulin decreases the blood oxygen dependent (BOLD) response in the hypothalamus and PFC increases BOLD response in the striatum (Schilling et al., 2014) and insular cortex (Heni et al., 2012) and increases brain energy levels (Jauch-Chara et al., 2012). Critically, these effects are blunted in obesity (Tschritter et al., 2006) with evidence that hypothalamic insulin resistance is driven by visceral fat and frontal insulin resistance by peripheral insulin sensitivity (Kullmann et al., 2015). Collectively, these findings indicate a complex relationship between peripheral glucose control and central insulin resistance and they raise the possibility that central insulin resistance contributes to cognitive impairment in concert with, or independently from peripheral impaired glucose tolerance.

NEUROCOGNITIVE DEFICITS MAY BE DOMAIN-SPECIFIC AND DIFFERENTIALLY INFLUENCED BY DIET, ADIPOSITY, AND METABOLIC DYSFUNCTION

Although obesity and T2D are occasionally associated with global measures of brain atrophy (Enzinger et al., 2005; Gunstad et al., 2010; Raji et al., 2010; Brooks et al., 2013) and cognitive decline (Liang et al., 2014), many studies suggest that executive function is the domain most affected in both adults (Gunstad et al., 2007; Sabia et al., 2009; Fitzpatrick et al., 2013) (Volkow et al., 2009) and children (Convit et al., 2003; Reinert et al., 2013; Liang et al., 2014). For example, negative correlations are observed between BMI and performance on tasks of executive function but not episodic verbal memory (Volkow et al., 2009) with BMI negatively, and executive performance positively, correlated with baseline prefrontal glucose metabolism. Similarly, a recent meta-analysis of 21 studies concluded that obesity is associated with impairments in decision-making, planning and problem solving with less evidence for associations with verbal fluency and learning and memory (Fitzpatrick et al., 2013). Correspondingly, structural changes (Enzinger et al., 2005; Pannacciulli et al., 2006; Raji et al., 2010; Fotuhi et al., 2012; Bocarsly et al., 2015) and reduced brain connectivity (Musen et al., 2012) are observed in the parietal and prefrontal cortex (PFC), which are critical for executive function.

There is also strong evidence from animal work that HFD produces hippocampal insulin resistance (Biessels and Reagan, 2015) and damage (Hsu and Kanoski, 2014), resulting in impaired hippocampal-dependent cognitive functions (Kanoski and Davidson, 2011). Likewise, hippocampal atrophy is observed in obese humans (Raji et al., 2010) and altered hippocampal white matter connectivity is found in T2D (van Bussel et al., 2016). However, there are inconsistent findings with respect to alterations in hippocampal-dependent episodic memory tasks (Fitzpatrick et al., 2013). For example, significant deficits in working memory and in reinforcement learning are observed in the absence of episodic learning and memory impairment, in obese vs. healthy weight adults that are matched for age, gender, education, and IQ (Coppin et al., 2014). In contrast, impaired episodic memory and decreased hippocampal volume is observed as a function of glucose tolerance (Convit et al., 2003) and intranasal insulin increases the functional connectivity between the hippocampus and PFC in people with T2D (Zhang et al., 2015). Other studies report hippocampal-dependent impairments as a function of saturated fat intake (Francis and Stevenson, 2011) and central, but not whole body adiposity (Khan et al., 2015a). Collectively these data suggest that episodic memory may be affected by diet and metabolic dysfunction while being unrelated to BMI and whole body obesity.

This emerging neuropsychological profile provides an important insight into the pathophysiological mechanism that gives rise to neurocognitive impairment in obesity and T2D. Brain functions associated with diabetes and obesity tend to rely upon DA signaling (**Figure 1**). For example, the dopaminergic fronto-striatal loop plays a well-known role in working memory, cognitive flexibility, reinforcement learning, and incentive motivation (Frank and Fossella, 2011). It is also critical for response inhibition, the failure of which is associated with addictive like behaviors including overeating (Lokken et al., 2009; Maayan et al., 2011; Lee et al., 2013; Guo et al., 2014; Zhao et al., 2016). Finally, a role for DA in memory via a projection from the ventral tegmental area to the hippocampus has been described (Shohamy and Adcock, 2010). As reviewed above, these DA-dependent cognitive processes are altered in obesity/T2D, raising the possibility that a common pathway by which diet, adiposity and metabolic dysfunction might coalesce to impact cognition is by producing alterations in the

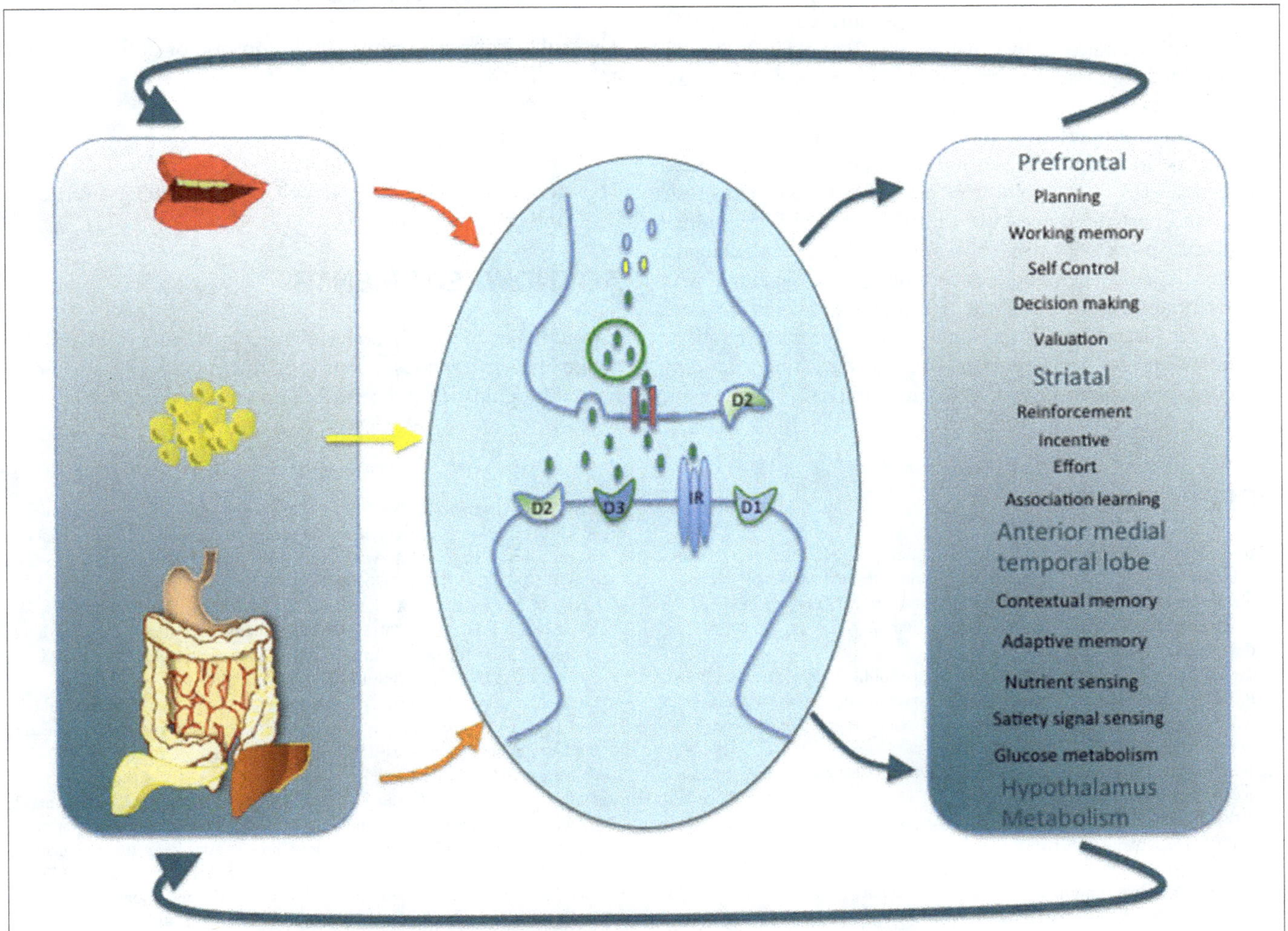

FIGURE 1 | This cartoon depicts alterations in DA signaling as a common link by which diet, adiposity, and metabolic dysfunction might impact cognition, motivation, and energy balance. A variety of mechanisms at the cellular and molecular level could support this association by regulating pre and post-synaptic DA receptor expression, DA synthesis, release, and reuptake. Alterations at any level may in turn have a wide impact on brain function and provide a parsimonious explanation for a number of dysfunctions associated with obesity and T2D.

DA system (**Figure 1**). Interestingly, although DA adaptations are considered integral in the development of compulsive behaviors and alterations in reward sensitivity they are not typically considered as a potential mechanism behind other neurocognitive complications in T2D and obesity.

There are consistent findings in the animal literature that HFD, and adiposity alter DA signaling at the cellular, and molecular levels (Anderzhanova et al., 2007; Johnson and Kenny, 2010; van de Giessen et al., 2012, 2013; Sharma and Fulton, 2013; Tellez et al., 2013; Cansell et al., 2014; Adams et al., 2015; Woods et al., 2016), as well as mounting evidence for altered DA signaling in human obesity, especially reflected in changes in DA receptor density, (Wang et al., 2001, 2011; Dunn et al., 2010; Steele et al., 2010; Eisenstein et al., 2013, 2015; Guo et al., 2014; Cosgrove et al., 2015; Horstmann et al., 2015; Karlsson et al., 2015; Caravaggio et al., 2015b; Dang et al., 2016; Gaiser et al., 2016). Additionally, there is evidence that central and peripheral insulin resistance might impact DA function. Central insulin signaling, acting through the downstream modulator Akt, is a potent modulator of DA transporter (DAT) activity, which fine-tunes DA signaling at the synapse (Kleinridders et al., 2015), demonstrating a pathway by which central IR could influence the DA system. Insulin administration also suppresses DA release by clearing DA from the synapse and concomitantly reducing the rewarding properties of food (Figlewicz and Sipols, 2010). Likewise, peripheral insulin sensitivity is associated with reduced endogenous DA levels (Murzi et al., 1996; Caravaggio et al., 2015a) and peripheral glycemia with PFC-striatal-hippocampal functional connectivity (Page et al., 2013). Thus, diet, adiposity, and insulin resistance could each impact DA signaling with the potential for additive effects and interactions. Future work aiming to disambiguate the unique and interacting effects will therefore be an important step toward understanding neurocognitive impairment in T2D and obesity.

SUMMARY

In summary, a consensus is emerging that obesity and diabetes are accompanied by cognitive impairments and brain dysfunction and that at least some of these effects are secondary to their onset. Multiple mechanisms have been proposed to underlie these associations but at present it is unclear which mechanism, or mechanisms, are critical. Also unclear is whether diet, obesity and metabolic dysfunction have distinct and/or converging pathways to neurocognitive impairment. However, work emerges to suggest that all three factors may influence DA signaling, which is provocative since the cognitive impairments that characterize diabetes and obesity uniformly rely upon the integrity of the DA system. It is therefore proposed that adaptations in DA signaling secondary to diet, adiposity and metabolic dysfunction underlie much of the neurocognitive impairment observed in diabetes and obesity.

AUTHOR CONTRIBUTIONS

The author confirms being the sole contributor of this work and approved it for publication.

FUNDING

This work was supported by NIH NCI R01CA180030 awarded to DMS and Ivan de Araujo.

ACKNOWLEDGMENTS

I would like to thank Sonia Caprio and Hubert Priessl for comments on previous versions of this manuscript and Serge Luquet for guidance and contribution on the figure.

REFERENCES

Adams, W. K., Sussman, J. L., Kaur, S., D'Souza, A. M., Kieffer, T. J., and Winstanley, C. A. (2015). Long-term, calorie-restricted intake of a high-fat diet in rats reduces impulse control and ventral striatal D2 receptor signalling - two markers of addiction vulnerability. *Eur. J. Neurosci.* 42, 3095–3104. doi: 10.1111/ejn.13117

Akrivos, J., Ravona-Springer, R., Schmeidler, J., LeRoith, D., Heymann, A., Preiss, R., et al. (2015). Glycemic control, inflammation, and cognitive function in older patients with type 2 diabetes. *Int. J. Geriatr. Psychiatry* 30, 1093–1100. doi: 10.1002/gps.4267

Anderzhanova, E., Covasa, M., and Hajnal, A. (2007). Altered basal and stimulated accumbens dopamine release in obese OLETF rats as a function of age and diabetic status. *Am. J. Physiol. Regul. Integr. Comp. Physiol.* 293, R603–R611. doi: 10.1152/ajpregu.00301.2007

Banks, W. A., Owen, J. B., and Erickson, M. A. (2012). Insulin in the brain: there and back again. *Pharmacol. Ther.* 136, 82–93. doi: 10.1016/j.pharmthera.2012.07.006

Biessels, G. J., and Reagan, L. P. (2015). Hippocampal insulin resistance and cognitive dysfunction. *Nat. Rev. Neurosci.* 16, 660–671. doi: 10.1038/nrn4019

Biessels, G. J., and Reijmer, Y. D. (2014). Brain changes underlying cognitive dysfunction in diabetes: what can we learn from MRI? *Diabetes* 63, 2244–2252. doi: 10.2337/db14-0348

Biessels, G. J., Strachan, M. W., Visseren, F. L., Kappelle, L. J., and Whitmer, R. A. (2014). Dementia and cognitive decline in type 2 diabetes and prediabetic stages: towards targeted interventions. *Lancet. Diabetes Endocrinol.* 2, 246–255. doi: 10.1016/s2213-8587(13)70088-3

Bocarsly, M. E., Fasolino, M., Kane, G. A., LaMarca, E. A., Kirschen, G. W., Karatsoreos, I. N., et al. (2015). Obesity diminishes synaptic markers, alters microglial morphology, and impairs cognitive function. *Proc. Natl. Acad. Sci. U.S.A.* 112, 15731–15736. doi: 10.1073/pnas.1511593112

Brooks, S. J., Benedict, C., Burgos, J., Kempton, M. J., Kullberg, J., Nordenskjold, R., et al. (2013). Late-life obesity is associated with smaller global and regional gray matter volumes: a voxel-based morphometric study. *Int. J. Obes.* 37, 230–236. doi: 10.1038/ijo.2012.13

Browndyke, J. N., Berger, M., Harshbarger, T. B., Smith, P. J., White, W., Bisanar, T. L., et al. (2017). Resting-state functional connectivity and cognition After major cardiac surgery in older adults without preoperative cognitive impairment: preliminary findings. *J. Am. Geriatr. Soc.* 65, e6–e12. doi: 10.1111/jgs.14534

Bruehl, H., Sweat, V., Hassenstab, J., Polyakov, V., and Convit, A. (2010). Cognitive impairment in nondiabetic middle-aged and older adults is associated with insulin resistance. *J. Clin. Exp. Neuropsychol.* 32, 487–493. doi: 10.1080/13803390903224928

Brüning, J. C., Gautam, D., Burks, D. J., Gillette, J., Schubert, M., Orban, P. C., et al. (2000). Role of brain insulin receptor in control of body weight and reproduction. *Science* 289, 2122–2125. doi: 10.1126/science.289.5487.2122

Cansell, C., Castel, J., Denis, R. G., Rouch, C., Delbes, A. S., Martinez, S., et al. (2014). Dietary triglycerides act on mesolimbic structures to regulate the rewarding and motivational aspects of feeding. *Mol. Psychiatry* 19, 1095–1105. doi: 10.1038/mp.2014.31

Caravaggio, F., Borlido, C., Hahn, M., Feng, Z., Fervaha, G., Gerretsen, P., et al. (2015a). Reduced insulin sensitivity is related to less endogenous dopamine at D-2/3 receptors in the ventral striatum of healthy nonobese humans. *Int. J. Neuropsychopharmacol.* 18:pyv014. doi: 10.1093/ijnp/pyv014

Caravaggio, F., Raitsin, S., Gerretsen, P., Nakajima, S., Wilson, A., and Graff-Guerrero, A. (2015b). Ventral striatum binding of a dopamine D2/3 receptor agonist but not antagonist predicts normal body mass index. *Biol. Psychiatry* 77, 196–202. doi: 10.1016/j.biopsych.2013.02.017

Clegg, D. J., Gotoh, K., Kemp, C., Wortman, M. D., Benoit, S. C., Brown, L. M., et al. (2011). Consumption of a high-fat diet induces central insulin resistance independent of adiposity. *Physiol. Behav.* 103, 10–16. doi: 10.1016/j.physbeh.2011.01.010

Contreras, J. A., Goni, J., Risacher, S. L., Amico, E., Yoder, K., Dzemidzic, M., et al. (2017). Cognitive complaints in older adults at risk for Alzheimer's disease are associated with altered resting-state networks. *Alzheimer's Dement.* 6, 40–49. doi: 10.1016/j.dadm.2016.12.004

Convit, A., Wolf, O. T., Tarshish, C., and de Leon, M. J. (2003). Reduced glucose tolerance is associated with poor memory performance and hippocampal atrophy among normal elderly. *Proc. Natl. Acad. Sci. U.S.A.* 100, 2019–2022. doi: 10.1073/pnas.0336073100

Coppin, G., Nolan-Poupart, S., Jones-Gotman, M., and Small, D. M. (2014). Working memory and reward association learning impairments in obesity. *Neuropsychologia* 65, 146–155. doi: 10.1016/j.neuropsychologia.2014.10.004

Cosgrove, K. P., Veldhuizen, M. G., Sandiego, C. M., Morris, E. D., and Small, D. M. (2015). Opposing relationships of BMI with BOLD and dopamine D2/3 receptor binding potential in the dorsal striatum. *Synapse* 69, 195–202. doi: 10.1002/syn.21809

Craft, S., Baker, L. D., Montine, T. J., Minoshima, S., Watson, G. S., Claxton, A., et al. (2012). Intranasal insulin therapy for Alzheimer disease and amnestic mild cognitive impairment: a pilot clinical trial. *Arch. Neurol.* 69, 29–38. doi: 10.1001/archneurol.2011.233

Dang, L. C., Samanez-Larkin, G. R., Castrellon, J. J., Perkins, S. F., Cowan, R. L., and Zald, D. H. (2016). Associations between dopamine D2 receptor availability and BMI depend on age. *Neuroimage* 138, 176–183. doi: 10.1016/j.neuroimage.2016.05.044

De Felice, F. G., and Ferreira, S. T. (2014). Inflammation, Defective insulin signaling, and mitochondrial dysfunction as common molecular denominators connecting Type 2 diabetes to Alzheimer disease. *Diabetes* 63, 2262–2272. doi: 10.2337/db13-1954

Dunn, J. P., Cowan, R. L., Volkow, N. D., Feurer, I. D., Li, R., Williams, D. B., et al. (2010). Decreased dopamine type 2 receptor availability after bariatric surgery: preliminary findings. *Brain Res.* 1350, 123–130. doi: 10.1016/j.brainres.2010.03.064

Eisenstein, S. A., Antenor-Dorsey, J. A., Gredysa, D. M., Koller, J. M., Bihun, E. C., Ranck, S. A., et al. (2013). A comparison of D2 receptor specific binding in obese and normal-weight individuals using PET with (N-[(11)C]methyl)benperidol. *Synapse* 67, 748–756. doi: 10.1002/syn.21680

Eisenstein, S. A., Bischoff, A. N., Gredysa, D. M., Antenor-Dorsey, J. A., Koller, J. M., Al-Lozi, A., et al. (2015). Emotional eating phenotype is associated with central dopamine D2 receptor binding independent of body mass index. *Sci. Rep.* 5:11283. doi: 10.1038/srep11283

Elias, M. F., Elias, P. K., Sullivan, L. M., Wolf, P. A., and D'Agostino, R. B. (2003). Lower cognitive function in the presence of obesity and hypertension: the Framingham heart study. *Int. J. Obes. Relat. Metab. Disord.* 27, 260–268. doi: 10.1038/sj.ijo.802225

Enzinger, C., Fazekas, F., Matthews, P. M., Ropele, S., Schmidt, H., Smith, S., et al. (2005). Risk factors for progression of brain atrophy in aging - Six-year follow-up of normal subjects. *Neurology* 64, 1704–1711. doi: 10.1212/01.WNL.0000161871.83614.BB

Erion, J. R., Wosiski-Kuhn, M., Dey, A., Hao, S., Davis, C. L., Pollock, N. K., et al. (2014). Obesity elicits interleukin 1-mediated deficits in hippocampal synaptic plasticity. *J. Neurosci.* 34, 2618–2631. doi: 10.1523/JNEUROSCI.4200-13.2014

Figlewicz, D. P., and Sipols, A. J. (2010). Energy regulatory signals and food reward. *Pharmacol. Biochem. Behav.* 97, 15–24. doi: 10.1016/j.pbb.2010.03.002

Fitzpatrick, S., Gilbert, S., and Serpell, L. (2013). Systematic review: are overweight and obese individuals impaired on behavioural tasks of executive functioning? *Neuropsychol. Rev.* 23, 138–156. doi: 10.1007/s11065-013-9224-7

Fotuhi, M., Do, D., and Jack, C. (2012). Modifiable factors that alter the size of the hippocampus with ageing. *Nat. Rev. Neurol.* 8, 189–202. doi: 10.1038/nrneurol.2012.27

Francis, H. M., and Stevenson, R. J. (2011). Higher reported saturated fat and refined sugar intake is associated with reduced hippocampal-dependent memory and sensitivity to interoceptive signals. *Behav. Neurosci.* 125, 943–955. doi: 10.1037/a0025998

Frank, M. J., and Fossella, J. A. (2011). Neurogenetics and pharmacology of learning, motivation, and cognition. *Neuropsychopharmacology* 36, 133–152. doi: 10.1038/npp.2010.96

Gaiser, E. C., Gallezot, J. D., Worhunsky, P. D., Jastreboff, A. M., Pittman, B., Kantrovitz, L., et al. (2016). Elevated dopamine D2/3 receptor availability in obese individuals: a PET imaging study with [11C](+)PHNO. *Neuropsychopharmacology* 41, 3042–3050. doi: 10.1038/npp.2016.115

Geijselaers, S. L., Sep, S. J., Stehouwer, C. D., and Biessels, G. J. (2015). Glucose regulation, cognition, and brain MRI in type 2 diabetes: a systematic review. *Lancet. Diabetes Endocrinol.* 3, 75–89. doi: 10.1016/s2213-8587(14)70148-2

Gonzales, M. M., Tarumi, T., Miles, S. C., Tanaka, H., Shah, F., and Haley, A. P. (2010). Insulin sensitivity as a mediator of the relationship between BMI and working memory-related brain activation. *Obesity* 18, 2131–2137. doi: 10.1038/oby.2010.183

Grichisch, Y., Çavusoglu, M., Preissl, H., Uludag, K., Hallschmid, M., Birbaumer, N., et al. (2012). Differential effects of intranasal insulin and caffeine on cerebral blood flow. *Hum. Brain Mapp.* 33, 280–287. doi: 10.1002/hbm.21216

Grillo, C. A., Piroli, G. G., Junor, L., Wilson, S. P., Mott, D. D., Wilson, M. A., et al. (2011). Obesity/hyperleptinemic phenotype impairs structural and functional plasticity in the rat hippocampus. *Physiol. Behav.* 105, 138–144. doi: 10.1016/j.physbeh.2011.02.028

Gunstad, J., Lhotsky, A., Wendell, C. R., Ferrucci, L., and Zonderman, A. B. (2010). Longitudinal examination of obesity and cognitive function: results from the Baltimore longitudinal study of aging. *Neuroepidemiology* 34, 222–229. doi: 10.1159/000297742

Gunstad, J., Paul, R. H., Cohen, R. A., Tate, D. F., Spitznagel, M. B., and Gordon, E. (2007). Elevated body mass index is associated with executive dysfunction in otherwise healthy adults. *Compr. Psychiatry* 48, 57–61. doi: 10.1016/j.comppsych.2006.05.001

Guo, J., Simmons, W. K., Herscovitch, P., Martin, A., and Hall, K. D. (2014). Striatal dopamine D2-like receptor correlation patterns with human obesity and opportunistic eating behavior. *Mol. Psychiatry* 19, 1078–1084. doi: 10.1038/mp.2014.102

Hallschmid, M., Benedict, C., Born, J., and Kern, W. (2007). Targeting metabolic and cognitive pathways of the CNS by intranasal insulin administration. *Expert Opin. Drug Deliv.* 4, 319–322. doi: 10.1517/17425247.4.4.319

Hallschmid, M., Benedict, C., Schultes, B., Born, J., and Kern, W. (2008). Obese men respond to cognitive but not to catabolic brain insulin signaling. *Int. J. Obes.* 32, 275–282. doi: 10.1038/sj.ijo.0803722

Havrankova, J., Roth, J., and Brownstein, M. (1978). Insulin receptors are widely distributed in the central nervous system of the rat. *Nature* 272, 827–829. doi: 10.1038/272827a0

Heni, M., Kullmann, S., Ahlqvist, E., Wagner, R., Machicao, F., Staiger, H., et al. (2016). Interaction between the obesity-risk gene *FTO* and the dopamine D2 receptor gene *ANKK1/TaqIA* on insulin sensitivity. *Diabetologia* 59, 2622–2631. doi: 10.1007/s00125-016-4095-0

Heni, M., Kullmann, S., Ketterer, C., Guthoff, M., Linder, K., Wagner, R., et al. (2012). Nasal insulin changes peripheral insulin sensitivity simultaneously with altered activity in homeostatic and reward-related human brain regions. *Diabetologia* 55, 1773–1782. doi: 10.1007/s00125-012-2528-y

Heni, M., Wagner, R., Kullmann, S., Veit, R., Mat Husin, H., Linder, K., et al. (2014). Central insulin administration improves whole-body insulin sensitivity via hypothalamus and parasympathetic outputs in men. *Diabetes* 63, 4083–4088. doi: 10.2337/db14-0477

Horstmann, A., Fenske, W. K., and Hankir, M. K. (2015). Argument for a non-linear relationship between severity of human obesity and dopaminergic tone. *Obes. Rev.* 16, 821–830. doi: 10.1111/obr.12303

Hsu, T. M., and Kanoski, S. E. (2014). Blood-brain barrier disruption: mechanistic links between Western diet consumption and dementia. *Front. Aging Neurosci.* 6:88. doi: 10.3389/fnagi.2014.00088

Jauch-Chara, K., Friedrich, A., Rezmer, M., Melchert, U. H., Scholand-Engler G. H., Hallschmid, M., et al. (2012). Intranasal insulin suppresses food intake via enhancement of brain energy levels in humans. *Diabetes* 61, 2261–2268. doi: 10.2337/db12-0025

Jockwitz, C., Caspers, S., Lux, S., Eickhoff, S. B., Jütten, K., Lenzen, S., et al. (2017). Influence of age and cognitive performance on resting-state brain networks of older adults in a population-based cohort. *Cortex* 89, 28–44. doi: 10.1016/j.cortex.2017.01.008

Johnson, P. M., and Kenny, P. J. (2010). Dopamine D2 receptors in addiction-like reward dysfunction and compulsive eating in obese rats. *Nat. Neurosci.* 13, 635–641. doi: 10.1038/nn.2519

Kanoski, S. E., and Davidson, T. L. (2010). Different patterns of memory impairments accompany short- and longer-term maintenance on a high-energy diet. *J. Exp. Psychol. Anim. Behav. Process.* 36, 313–319. doi: 10.1037/a0017228

Kanoski, S. E., and Davidson, T. L. (2011). Western diet consumption and cognitive impairment: links to hippocampal dysfunction and obesity. *Physiol. Behav.* 103, 59–68. doi: 10.1016/j.physbeh.2010.12.003

Kanoski, S. E., Meisel, R. L., Mullins, A. J., and Davidson, T. L. (2007). The effects of energy-rich diets on discrimination reversal learning and on BDNF in the hippocampus and prefrontal cortex of the rat. *Behav. Brain Res.* 182, 57–66. doi: 10.1016/j.bbr.2007.05.004

Kanoski, S. E., Zhang, Y., Zheng, W., and Davidson, T. L. (2010). The effects of a high-energy diet on hippocampal function and blood-brain barrier integrity in the rat. *J. Alzheimer's Dis. JAD* 21, 207–219. doi: 10.3233/JAD-2010-091414

Karlsson, H. K., Tuominen, L., Tuulari, J. J., Hirvonen, J., Parkkola, R., Helin, S., et al. (2015). Obesity is associated with decreased mu-opioid but unaltered dopamine D2 receptor availability in the brain. *J. Neurosci.* 35, 3959–3965. doi: 10.1523/JNEUROSCI.4744-14.2015

Ketterer, C., Tschritter, O., Preissl, H., Heni, M., Haring, H. U., and Fritsche, A. (2011). Insulin sensitivity of the human brain. *Diabetes Res. Clin. Pract.* 93, S47–S51. doi: 10.1016/s0168-8227(11)70013-4

Khan, N. A., Baym, C. L., Monti, J. M., Raine, L. B., Drollette, E. S., Scudder, M. R., et al. (2015a). Central adiposity is negatively associated with hippocampal-dependent relational memory among overweight and obese children. *J. Pediatr.* 166, 302–308. doi: 10.1016/j.jpeds.2014.10.008

Khan, N. A., Raine, L. B., Drollette, E. S., Scudder, M. R., and Hillman, C. H. (2015b). The relation of saturated fats and dietary cholesterol to childhood cognitive flexibility. *Appetite* 93, 51–56. doi: 10.1016/j.appet.2015.04.012

Kleinridders, A., Cai, W., Cappellucci, L., Ghazarian, A., Collins, W. R., Vienberg, S. G., et al. (2015). Insulin resistance in brain alters dopamine turnover and causes behavioral disorders. *Proc. Natl. Acad. Sci. U.S.A.* 112, 3463–3468. doi: 10.1073/pnas.1500877112

Kleinridders, A., Ferris, H. A., Cai, W., and Kahn, C. R. (2014). Insulin action in brain regulates systemic metabolism and brain function. *Diabetes* 63, 2232–2243. doi: 10.2337/db14-0568

Koekkoek, P. S., Kappelle, L. J., van den Berg, E., Rutten, G. E. H. M., and Biessels, G. J. (2015). Cognitive function in patients with diabetes mellitus: guidance for daily care. *Lancet Neurol.* 14, 329–340. doi: 10.1016/S1474-4422(14)70249-2

Kullmann, S., Frank, S., Heni, M., Ketterer, C., Veit, R., Haring, H. U., et al. (2013). Intranasal insulin modulates intrinsic reward and prefrontal circuitry of the human brain in lean women. *Neuroendocrinology* 97, 176–182. doi: 10.1159/000341406

Kullmann, S., Heni, M., Veit, R., Scheffler, K., Machann, J., Haring, H. U., et al. (2015). Selective insulin resistance in homeostatic and cognitive control brain areas in overweight and obese adults. *Diabetes Care* 38, 1044–1050. doi: 10.2337/dc14-2319

Lee, Y., Chong, M. F., Liu, J. C., Libedinsky, C., Gooley, J. J., Chen, S., et al. (2013). Dietary disinhibition modulates neural valuation of food in the fed and fasted states. *Am. J. Clin. Nutr.* 97, 919–925. doi: 10.3945/ajcn.112.053801

Levin, B. E., and Routh, V. H. (1996). Role of the brain in energy balance and obesity. *Am. J. Physiol.* 271, R491–R500.

Li, X. L., Aou, S., Oomura, Y., Hori, N., Fukunaga, K., and Hori, T. (2002). Impairment of long-term potentiation and spatial memory in leptin receptor-deficient rodents. *Neuroscience* 113, 607–615. doi: 10.1016/S0306-4522(02)00162-8

Liang, J., Matheson, B. E., Kaye, W. H., and Boutelle, K. N. (2014). Neurocognitive correlates of obesity and obesity-related behaviors in children and adolescents. *Int. J. Obes.* 38, 494–506. doi: 10.1038/ijo.2013.142

Lokken, K. L., Boeka, A. G., Austin, H. M., Gunstad, J., and Harmon, C. M. (2009). Evidence of executive dysfunction in extremely obese adolescents: a pilot study. *Surg. Obes. Relat. Dis.* 5, 547–552. doi: 10.1016/j.soard.2009.05.008

Maayan, L., Hoogendoorn, C., Sweat, V., and Convit, A. (2011). Disinhibited eating in obese adolescents is associated with orbitofrontal volume reductions and executive dysfunction. *Obesity* 19, 1382–1387. doi: 10.1038/oby.2011.15

Murzi, E., Contreras, Q., Teneud, L., Valecillos, B., Parada, M. A., DeParada, M. P., et al. (1996). Diabetes decreases limbic extracellular dopamine in rats. *Neurosci. Lett.* 202, 141–144. doi: 10.1016/0304-3940(95)12232-X

Musen, G., Jacobson, A. M., Bolo, N. R., Simonson, D. C., Shenton, M. E., McCartney, R. L., et al. (2012). Resting-state brain functional connectivity is altered in type 2 diabetes. *Diabetes* 61, 2375–2379. doi: 10.2337/db11-1669

Niswender, K. D., Morrison, C. D., Clegg, D. J., Olson, R., Baskin, D. G., Myers, M. G., et al. (2003). Insulin activation of phosphatidylinositol 3-kinase in the hypothalamic arcuate nucleus - A key mediator of insulin-induced anorexia. *Diabetes* 52, 227–231. doi: 10.2337/diabetes.52.2.227

Page, K. A., Chan, O., Arora, J., Belfort-Deaguiar, R., Dzuira, J., Roehmholdt, B., et al. (2013). Effects of fructose vs glucose on regional cerebral blood flow in brain regions involved with appetite and reward pathways. *JAMA* 309, 63–70. doi: 10.1001/jama.2012.116975

Pannacciulli, N., Del Parigi, A., Chen, K., Le, D. S., Reiman, E. M., and Tataranni, P. A. (2006). Brain abnormalities in human obesity: a voxel-based morphometric study. *Neuroimage* 31, 1419–1425. doi: 10.1016/j.neuroimage.2006.01.047

Raji, C. A., Ho, A. J., Parikshak, N. N., Becker, J. T., Lopez, O. L., Kuller, L. H., et al. (2010). Brain structure and obesity. *Hum. Brain Mapp.* 31, 353–364. doi: 10.1002/hbm.20870

Ramos-Rodriguez, J. J., Infante-Garcia, C., Galindo-Gonzalez, L., Garcia-Molina, Y., Lechuga-Sancho, A., and Garcia-Alloza, M. (2016). Increased spontaneous central bleeding and cognition impairment in APP/PS1 mice with poorly controlled diabetes mellitus. *Mol. Neurobiol.* 53, 2685–2697. doi: 10.1007/s12035-015-9311-2

Reger, M. A., and Craft, S. (2006). Intranasal insulin administration: a method for dissociating central and peripheral effects of insulin. *Drugs Today* 42, 729–739. doi: 10.1358/dot.2006.42.11.1007675

Reger, M. A., Watson, G. S., Green, P. S., Wilkinson, C. W., Baker, L. D., Cholerton, B., et al. (2008). Intranasal insulin improves cognition and modulates beta-amyloid in early AD. *Neurology* 70, 440–448. doi: 10.1212/01.WNL.0000265401.62434.36

Reinert, K. R., Po'e, E. K., and Barkin, S. L. (2013). The relationship between executive function and obesity in children and adolescents: a systematic literature review. *J. Obes.* 2013:820956. doi: 10.1155/2013/820956

Sabia, S., Kivimaki, M., Shipley, M. J., Marmot, M. G., and Singh-Manoux, A. (2009). Body mass index over the adult life course and cognition in late midlife: the Whitehall II Cohort study. *Am. J. Clin. Nutr.* 89, 601–607. doi: 10.3945/ajcn.2008.26482

Schilling, T. M., Ferreira de Sá, D. S., Westerhausen, R., Strelzyk, F., Larra, M. F., Hallschmid, M., et al. (2014). Intranasal insulin increases regional cerebral blood flow in the insular cortex in men independently of cortisol manipulation. *Hum. Brain Mapp.* 35, 1944–1956. doi: 10.1002/hbm.22304

Schubert, M., Gautam, D., Surjo, D., Ueki, K., Baudler, S., Schubert, D., et al. (2004). Role for neuronal insulin resistance in neurodegenerative diseases. *Proc. Natl. Acad. Sci. U.S.A.* 101, 3100–3105. doi: 10.1073/pnas.0308724101

Sharma, S., and Fulton, S. (2013). Diet-induced obesity promotes depressive-like behaviour that is associated with neural adaptations in brain reward circuitry. *Int. J. Obes.* 37, 382–389. doi: 10.1038/ijo.2012.48

Shohamy, D., and Adcock, R. A. (2010). Dopamine and adaptive memory. *Trends Cogn. Sci.* 14, 464–472. doi: 10.1016/j.tics.2010.08.002

Steculorum, S. M., Solas, M., and Brüning, J. C. (2014). The paradox of neuronal insulin action and resistance in the development of aging-associated diseases. *Alzheimers Dement.* 10, S3–S11. doi: 10.1016/j.jalz.2013.12.008

Steele, K. E., Prokopowicz, G. P., Schweitzer, M. A., Magunsuon, T. H., Lidor, A. O., Kuwabawa, H., et al. (2010). Alterations of central dopamine receptors before and after gastric bypass surgery. *Obes. Surg.* 20, 369–374. doi: 10.1007/s11695-009-0015-4

Stoeckel, L. E., Arvanitakis, Z., Gandy, S., Small, D. M., Kahn, C. R., Pascual-Leone, A., et al. (2016). "White Paper" meeting summary and catalyst for future inquiry: complex mechanisms linking neurocognitive dysfunction to insulin resistance and other metabolic dysfunction. *F1000Res.* 5:353. doi: 10.12688/f1000research.8300.1

Stouffer, M. A., Woods, C. A., Patel, J. C., Lee, C. R., Witkovsky, P., Bao, L., et al. (2015). Insulin enhances striatal dopamine release by activating cholinergic interneurons and thereby signals reward. *Nat. Commun.* 6:8543. doi: 10.1038/ncomms9543

Stranahan, A. M., Arumugam, T. V., Cutler, R. G., Lee, K., Egan, J. M., and Mattson, M. P. (2008a). Diabetes impairs hippocampal function through glucocorticoid-mediated effects on new and mature neurons. *Nat. Neurosci.* 11, 309–317. doi: 10.1038/nn2055

Stranahan, A. M., Hao, S., Dey, A., Yu, X., and Baban, B. (2016). Blood-brain barrier breakdown promotes macrophage infiltration and cognitive impairment in leptin receptor-deficient mice. *J. Cereb. Blood Flow Metab.* 36, 2108–2121. doi: 10.1177/0271678X16642233

Stranahan, A. M., Norman, E. D., Lee, K., Cutler, R. G., Telljohann, R. S., Egan, J. M., et al. (2008b). Diet-induced insulin resistance impairs hippocampal synaptic plasticity and cognition in middle-aged rats. *Hippocampus* 18, 1085–1088. doi: 10.1002/hipo.20470

Suzuki, R., Lee, K., Jing, E., Biddinger, S. B., McDonald, J. G., Montine, T. J., et al. (2010). Diabetes and insulin in regulation of brain cholesterol metabolism. *Cell Metab.* 12, 567–579. doi: 10.1016/j.cmet.2010.11.006

Tellez, L. A., Medina, S., Han, W., Ferreira, J. G., Licona-Limón, P., Ren, X., et al. (2013). A gut lipid messenger links excess dietary fat to dopamine deficiency. *Science* 341, 800–802. doi: 10.1126/science.1239275

Tschritter, O., Porubska, K., Preissl, H., Fritsche, A., and Haring, H. U. (2006). Cerebrocortical insulin resistance is related to visceral obesity and age, but is not independently correlated with leptin, adiponectin or the saturated long-chain fatty acids palmitate and stearate. *Diabetes* 55, A403–A404.

van Bussel, F. C., Backes, W. H., Hofman, P. A., van Boxtel, M. P., Schram, M. T., Stehouwer, C. D., et al. (2016). Altered hippocampal white matter connectivity in Type 2 diabetes mellitus and memory decrements. *J. Neuroendocrinol.* 28:12366. doi: 10.1111/jne.12366

van de Giessen, E., la Fleur, S. E., de Bruin, K., van den Brink, W., and Booij, J. (2012). Free-choice and no-choice high-fat diets affect striatal dopamine D2/3 receptor availability, caloric intake, and adiposity. *Obesity* 20, 1738–1740. doi: 10.1038/oby.2012.17

van de Giessen, E., la Fleur, S. E., Eggels, L., de Bruin, K., van den Brink, W., and Booij, J. (2013). High fat/carbohydrate ratio but not total energy intake induces lower striatal dopamine D2/3 receptor availability in diet-induced obesity. *Int. J. Obes.* 37, 754–757. doi: 10.1038/ijo.2012.128

van Houten, M., Posner, B. I., Kopriwa, B. M., and Brawer, J. R. (1979). Insulin-binding sites in the rat brain: *in vivo* localization to the circumventricular organs by quantitative radioautography. *Endocrinology* 105, 666–673. doi: 10.1210/endo-105-3-666

Volkow, N. D., Wang, G. J., Telang, F., Fowler, J. S., Goldstein, R. Z., Alia-Klein, N., et al. (2009). Inverse association between BMI and prefrontal metabolic activity in healthy adults. *Obesity* 17, 60–65. doi: 10.1038/oby.2008.469

von Rhein, D., Beckmann, C. F., Franke, B., Oosterlaan, J., Heslenfeld, D. J., Hoekstra, P. J., et al. (2017). Network-level assessment of reward-related activation in patients with ADHD and healthy individuals. *Hum. Brain Mapp.* doi: 10.1002/hbm.23522. [Epub ahead of print].

Wang, G. J., Geliebter, A., Volkow, N. D., Telang, F. W., Logan, J., Jayne, M. C., et al. (2011). Enhanced striatal dopamine release during food stimulation in binge eating disorder. *Obesity* 19, 1601–1608. doi: 10.1038/oby.2011.27

Wang, G. J., Volkow, N. D., Logan, J., Pappas, N. R., Wong, C. T., Zhu, W., et al. (2001). Brain dopamine and obesity. *Lancet* 357, 354–357. doi: 10.1016/S0140-6736(00)03643-6

Woods, C. A., Guttman, Z. R., Huang, D., Kolaric, R. A., Rabinowitsch, A. I., Jones, K. T., et al. (2016). Insulin receptor activation in the nucleus accumbens reflects nutritive value of a recently ingested meal. *Physiol. Behav.* 159, 52–63. doi: 10.1016/j.physbeh.2016.03.013

Yarchoan, M., and Arnold, S. E. (2014). Repurposing diabetes drugs for brain insulin resistance in Alzheimer Disease. *Diabetes* 63, 2253–2261. doi: 10.2337/db14-0287

Yau, P. L., Kang, E. H., Javier, D. C., and Convit, A. (2014). Preliminary evidence of cognitive and brain abnormalities in uncomplicated adolescent obesity. *Obesity* 22, 1865–1871. doi: 10.1002/oby.20801

Zhang, H., Hao, Y., Manor, B., Novak, P., Milberg, W., Zhang, J., et al. (2015). Intranasal insulin enhanced resting-state functional connectivity of hippocampal regions in type 2 diabetes. *Diabetes* 64, 1025–1034. doi: 10.2337/db14-1000

Zhao, J., Li, M., Zhang, Y., Song, H., von Deneen, K. M., Shi, Y., et al. (2016). Intrinsic brain subsystem associated with dietary restraint, disinhibition and hunger: an fMRI study. *Brain Imaging Behav.* doi: 10.1007/s11682-015-9491-4. [Epub ahead of print].

3

Food Seeking in a Risky Environment: A Method for Evaluating Risk and Reward Value in Food Seeking and Consumption in Mice

Sarah H. Lockie, Clare V. McAuley, Sasha Rawlinson, Natalie Guiney and Zane B. Andrews *

Monash Biomedicine Discovery Institute and Department of Physiology, Monash University, Clayton, VIC, Australia

***Correspondence:**
Zane B. Andrews
zane.andrews@monash.edu

Most studies that measure food intake in mice do so in the home cage environment. This necessarily means that mice do not engage in food seeking before consumption, a behavior that is ubiquitous in free-living animals. We modified and validated several commonly used anxiety tests to include a palatable food reward within the anxiogenic zone. This allowed us to assess risk-taking behavior in food seeking in mice in response to different metabolic stimuli. We modified the open field test and the light/dark box by placing palatable peanut butter chips within a designated food zone inside the anxiogenic zone of each apparatus. We then assessed parameters of the interaction with the food reward. Fasted mice or mice treated with ghrelin showed increased consumption and increased time spent in the food zone immediately around the food reward compared to *ad libitum* fed mice or mice treated with saline. However, fasted mice treated with IP glucose before exposure to the behavioral arena showed reduced time in the food zone compared to fasted controls, indicating that acute metabolic signals can modify the assessment of safety in food seeking in a risky environment. The tests described in this study will be useful in assessing risk processing and incentive salience of food reward, which are intrinsic components of food acquisition outside of the laboratory environment, in a range of genetic and pharmacological models.

Keywords: behavior, food seeking, open field test, light dark box test, reward, risk

INTRODUCTION

In a free-living situation, organisms always face a trade off in procurement of food. They must evaluate the risk of obtaining food in an unsafe environment, against the reward value of the food itself once obtained. This calculation must necessarily be dynamic and quickly recalculated when changes to either the environment or the nutritional needs of the organism occur. This flexible value attached to the food reward can be termed the "incentive salience" of the reward. The incentive salience (i.e., the importance) of the food is heavily influenced by physiological state (Lockie and Andrews, 2013). Studies of feeding behavior in laboratory animals, generally focused on mice, do not tend to take this balance into account, with most relying on a simple measurement of food consumed in the safe home cage environment. This largely removes the food-seeking behavioral component of food consumption, which is ubiquitous in animals outside of those kept as pets. Even humans in the current "obesigenic" environment must engage in food seeking behavior with some inherent risk, such as driving to the grocery store or restaurants. Studies that measure only food intake in a cage may miss deficits in the complete feeding behavioral spectrum, as they are not equipped to measure them. We have set out to address this issue by establishing and optimizing a set of simple and cost-effective behavioral tasks, using traditional behavioral equipment, designed to evaluate the incentive salience of a food reward in a risky environment.

Previous models of risk have approached this idea differently, using an operant conditioning paradigm and either a variable reward schedule or choice between a small, safe reward, and a large, "risky" reward—where "risky" is defined as an intermittent reward schedule for that lever (Leblond et al., 2011). This falls short of modeling "risk" as loss of a potential reward does not result in punishment or loss of personal resources. This task was redesigned to include a possible foot shock delivered along with the food reward (Simon and Setlow, 2012). These variations are informative regarding decision making in reward seeking, but fall short of modeling environmental risk *per se* as the animal can choose to avoid the risky lever entirely. Current mouse risk/reward paradigms do not incorporate the intrinsic risk associated with reward or food seeking in natural environments, such as injury and predation risk (Anselme, 2015). Others have previously used a modified light/dark box task with food included in the light zone (Teegarden and Bale, 2007; Cottone et al., 2012; Liu et al., 2016) as a measure of food seeking in a risky environment, and in this paper we seek to expand, validate and standardize this idea. Considering the light/dark box, like most common tests of unconditioned anxiety, relies upon the evolutionarily conserved fear of predation (Crawley, 2006), we supposed that this could be exploited to model ecologically relevant risk processing in food-seeking behavior in mice.

We have modified several standard behavioral tests of anxiety-like behavior to include a food reward element in the anxiogenic zone. We have experimentally validated these tests in a number of paradigms designed to alter the motivational state of the animal and/or the incentive salience of the reward. We fasted mice for 16 h or administered exogenous ghrelin, as both interventions are well-known to enhance food consumption, food seeking, and lever pressing in operant conditioning tasks (Tang-Christensen et al., 2004; Overduin et al., 2012; Skibicka et al., 2012). To examine the tests' sensitivity to acute metabolic state, we also included a group that had been fasted for 16 h and then administered IP glucose. Previous studies have shown that glucose can inhibit feeding in fasted mice, and that blood glucose levels can influence reported hunger levels in humans (Mayer, 1953; Bady et al., 2006), so we hypothesized that these mice should behave like fed mice.

METHODS

Animals

C57black/6 male mice were obtained from Monash Animal Services at 8 weeks of age. For modified light/dark box and open field they were housed in pairs at 22°C in a 12:12 light/dark cycle. They were fed standard laboratory chow (Specialty Feeds, Glen Forrest, WA). Palatable food rewards were Reece's peanut butter chips (The Hersey Company, Hershey, PA, USA), referred to throughout as PB chips. All mice were exposed to the PB chips three times in the home cage before the test day to avoid neophobia and to familiarize mice with the taste and caloric content of the chips. All experiments were performed in the last 4 h of the light phase. For fasting experiments, food was removed at 1 h after the onset of the dark on the previous day and testing was conducted in the last 4 h of the light cycle on the test day. Food was returned immediately upon completion of the behavioral task.

Drugs

Ghrelin (Rat, SC1356, lot number HF40076B, PolyPeptide group, Strasbourg, France) was administered at 0.3 mg/kg, in saline, and injected IP at 10 ml/kg. This dose was previously determined by dose response to be the lowest to reliably increase feeding in a 2 h window (Lockie et al., 2015). Ghrelin or saline vehicle were given 5 min before mice were placed in the apparatus. Glucose was given at 2.25 g/kg in 10 ml/kg of distilled water, not saline, to limit hypertonicity of the injection. Control mice for glucose injections received saline, not distilled water, avoid hypotonicity of the injection. Glucose was given 10 min before mice were placed in the apparatus.

Behavioral Tasks

Modified Open Field

The open field arena consisted of a circular area with a larger than normal diameter of 800 mm to increase the open field and enhance anxiety. PB chips were placed in an equilateral triangle within the center zone of the open field, with each PB chip being 280 mm from the external wall. PB chips of known weight were secured to the floor of the arena with Blu-Tack (Bostic). All other parameters were as per usual open field protocols, as follows. After injections, each mouse was placed in the same area of the perimeter of the open field and allowed to explore the space without interruption for 10 min. The trial was filmed for later analysis. After 10 min, the mouse was removed from the arena and placed back in the home cage with *ad libitum* access to food and water. The PB chips were removed and weighed and the apparatus cleaned with mild soap and water and allowed to dry.

Modified Light/Dark Box

The light dark box apparatus consisted of a two-chambered box, with a large, white zone (480 × 300 mm) and a smaller black zone (150 × 300 mm). Both zones were open to the light at the top. A single, previously weighed PB chip was secured in the center of the center of light zone with Blu-Tack, 240 mm from the entry to the dark zone. Mice were injected, then placed in the dark side of the apparatus. They were allowed 10 min to explore the apparatus undisturbed, and trials were taped for later analysis.

Modified Elevated Plus Maze

The elevated plus maze apparatus was a standard mouse plus maze with two open and two closed arms, with each arm being 50

× 300 mm, and a center zone 50 × 50 mm. Each open arm was baited with a PB chip 150 mm from the center zone, which was fixed to the arm with Blu-Tack. Mice were placed in the center zone facing the same open arm each time. They were allowed to explore the apparatus for 6 min and trials were filmed for later analysis.

Video Analysis

All behavior tests were filmed and video analysis was done later using CleverSys TopScan software. Zoning for software analysis included a "food zone," which was the area immediately surrounding the PB chip. For images of sample arenas, see Supplementary Figure 2. The food zone was always 78 mm in diameter, with the PB chip at the center of the zone. Mice were tracked from the center of the body and time in food zone was defined as center of the body within the 78 mm zone. Individual bouts were defined as the mouse entering and then leaving the zone, with the length of the bout being defined as the amount of time the mouse was continuously tracked within that zone. Latency was defined as time to approach one of the PB chips after introduction into the arena. For the reward-baited open field, approach of any one of the three pellets was considered the initial entry into the food zone.

Validation Parameters and Statistics

We were aiming to see data variation consistent with our results from standard versions of open field, elevated plus maze, and light/dark box, typically needing around 15/group to achieve an alpha of <0.05 for an effect size of ~ 0.8. We required the tests to be similarly sensitive to the non-modified open field, light dark box, and elevated plus maze. We intend to use these tests to screen genetically modified mice, and so we require a large to very large effect size to minimize animal numbers used in these tests, meaning values of Cohen's d-values of 0.8–1.2. Accepting an α of 0.05 and a β of 0.8, we need a sample size in the range of 10–21 mice/group, calculated using G*power (Faul et al., 2007). All statistics were performed using Graphpad prism software. Independent measures t-tests were used to compare results, with an alpha level of <0.05 being considered significant.

RESULTS

Validation of Tests Comparing Fasted and Ad Lib Fed Mice

We started with three common tests of "anxiety" in mice, the open field, the light/dark box, and the elevated plus maze. We used fasted mice to validate the concept, as fasting is a well-established method to induce motivated responding and food intake (Toth and Gardiner, 2000). We considered a number of aspects of experimental design that might impact upon test performance. To this end, we performed our tests close to the end of the light cycle, when mice are naturally becoming more alert and hungry. We considered the distance between the safe zone and the food reward, which we felt needed to carefully balance the anxiogenic nature of the open zone, with the motivational pull of the PB chip reward. We found that in general, we needed group sizes of 12–15 mice to see significant results for time spent in the food zone and amount of PB chip consumed in the experiments we performed. **Figure 1** shows the results of the three tests. Mice fasted for 18 h spent significantly more time in the food zone (**Figures 1A,E**) and ate significantly more of the PB chip (**Figures 1D,H**) in both the open field and the light dark box tests. We did not see any differences in latency to approach to food zone (**Figures 1B,F**) or number of bouts in the foods zone (**Figures 1C,G**) for either test. In the elevated plus maze, we did not see any differences in time spent in the food zone, which was overall very low, or in any other parameter (**Figures 1I–K**). Variability of results was particularly high for this test. We concluded that the elevated plus maze was a less suitable test for these modifications than the open field and light dark box, so did not pursue this test further. We then set out to validate our modified open field and light dark box test in additional experimental conditions of modified metabolic and motivational states.

Ghrelin Treatment Increases PB Chip Consumption and Time in Food Zone

Similarly to fasting, ghrelin has been well-described to increase both food consumption and motivated responding in operant tasks (Dickson et al., 2011). We administered ghrelin or saline to fed mice and repeated the baited open field and light/dark box as for the fasted mice. In both the light dark box (**Figure 2A**) and the open field (**Figure 2E**), we saw a significant increase in time spent in the food zone in the ghrelin-treated mice. This was supported by increased consumption of the PB chip in ghrelin treated mice (**Figures 2D,H**), in line with the well-known orexigenic actions of ghrelin. We did not see differences in latency to approach the food zone (**Figures 2B,F**) or number of bouts in the food zone (**Figures 2C,G**) in either test, suggesting that there were no differences in baseline anxiety-like behavior in ghrelin and vehicle-treated mice. Interestingly, we saw significant increase in locomotor activity in ghrelin-treated mice in the light/dark box only (Supplementary Figure 1C), which was not seen in the open field test.

Glucose Pretreatment Reduces PB Consumption and Food Zone Time in Fasted Mice

In order to validate that energy status was driving the motivated behavior in the anxiogenic environment, we wondered if acutely mitigating the energy deficit in fasted mice with IP administration of glucose would reduce interest in the PB chip. We found that, indeed, giving glucose to fasted mice 10 min before testing significantly reduced the amount of time fasted mice spent in the food zone in both the light/dark box (**Figure 3A**) and the open field (**Figure 3E**). Additionally, it significantly reduced the amount of PB chip consumed in both tests (**Figures 3D,H**). Again, no differences were noted in either latency to approach (**Figures 3B,F**) or number of bouts in the food zone (**Figures 3C,G**).

Generally, we did not see differences in time spent in the anxiogenic (center of the open field or light side of the light dark box) or anxiolytic zones (perimeter zone of the open field or

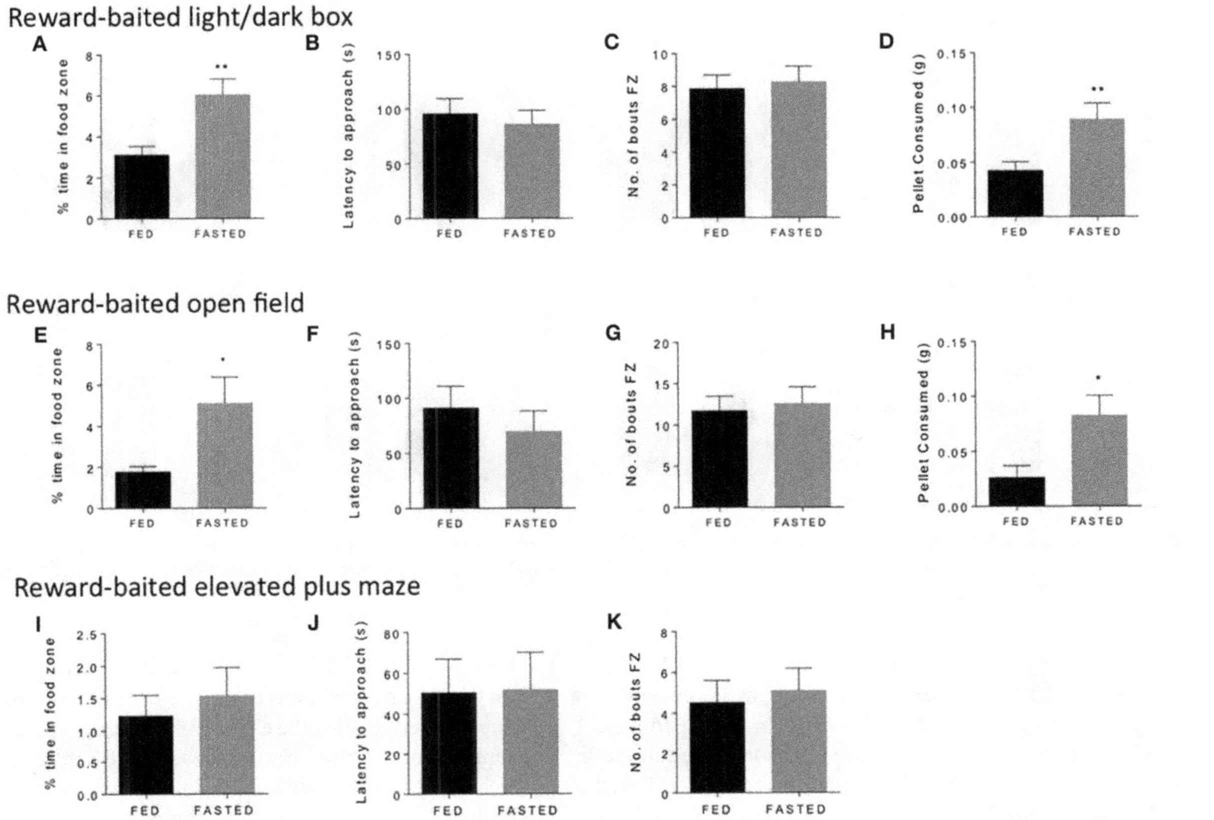

FIGURE 1 | Fasting increases time in food zone and consumption of peanut butter chip reward. Comparison of *ad libitum* fed and 18 h fasted mice in the reward-baited light/dark box **(A–D)**, $n = 18$; reward-baited open field test **(E–H)**, $n = 12$; and reward-baited elevated plus maze, **(I–K)**, $n = 20$–25. FZ, food zone; $^{*}p < 0.05$, $^{**}p < 0.01$, independent measures t-test.

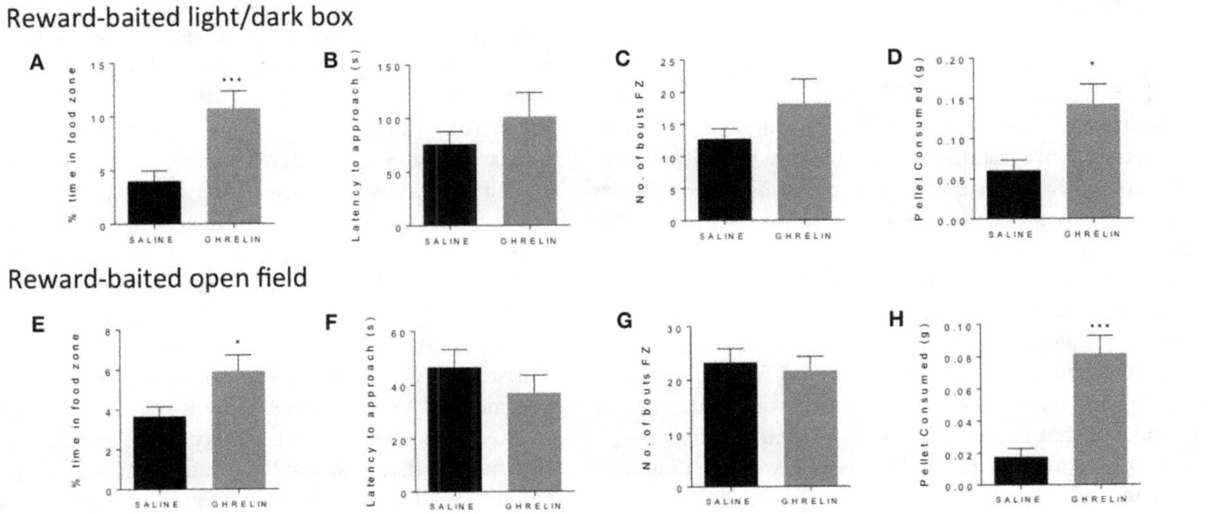

FIGURE 2 | Ghrelin treatment increases time in food zone and consumption of peanut butter chip reward. Comparison of saline treated and ghrelin treated mice in the reward-baited light/dark **(A–D)**, $n = 8$; and reward-baited open field test **(E–H)**, $n = 16$–18. FZ, food zone; $^{*}p < 0.05$, $^{***}p < 0.001$, independent measures t-test.

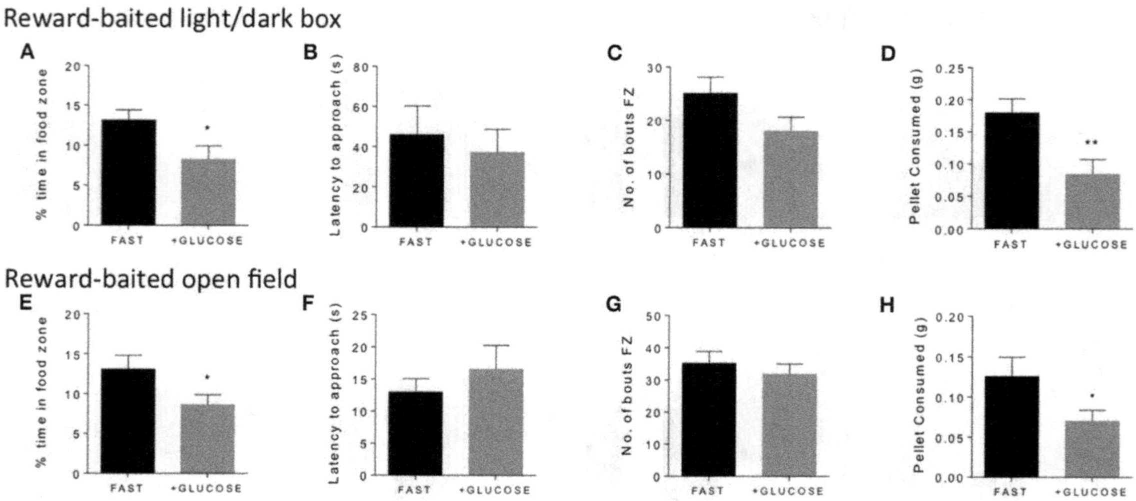

FIGURE 3 | Glucose treatment in fasted mice decreases time in food zone and consumption of peanut butter chip reward. Comparison of 18 h fasted, saline treated, and 18 h fasted, glucose treated mice in the reward-baited light/dark **(A–D)**, $n = 15$–16; and reward-baited open field test **(E–H)**, $n = 12$–14. FZ, food zone; $^{*}p < 0.05$, $^{**}p < 0.01$, independent measures t-test.

dark side of the light/dark box; Supplementary Figure 1). The exceptions to this were decreased time spent in the perimeter zone for fasted mice compared to fed mice in the open field (Supplementary Figure 1K) and increased time in the perimeter zone for fasted mice treated with glucose compared to fasted mice treated with saline (Supplementary Figure 1Q). Both these results reflect the increased time the fasted group spent in the food zone, and do not represent a true anxiety based result. With the exception of the already mentioned ghrelin-treated group we did not see alterations in locomotor activity between groups (Supplementary Figure 1).

DISCUSSION

Food consumption in laboratory rodents is almost exclusively measured in the context of *ad libitum* feeding in a home-cage environment. This fails to adequately model the reality of food seeking in a natural environment where attainment of food necessarily involves risk taking. We designed a series of experiments in which the mouse understands the value of the reward, but not the risk required to obtain the reward. To validate these tests, we manipulated the metabolic state to influence the decision to commit to food seeking in the novel, anxiogenic environment. We specifically set out to address a hole in the current battery of tests used to assess feeding and food reward, and attempted to design tests that would incorporate ecologically relevant risk processing, as currently available tests do this poorly (Anselme, 2015). To this end, we have described and validated two tests, which have innate perceived risk to the mouse, are sensitive to metabolic state, and are repeatable. These two tests are the reward-baited open field, the reward-baited light/dark box, which have the additional advantage of being cheap, time-effective and using standardized equipment readily available to most labs. We attempted to modify the elevated plus maze in a similar manner, by baiting the open arms with PB chips, but this test proved difficult to validate. It showed high variability within groups and low levels of investigation/consumption of the BP chips. We concluded the elevated plus maze apparatus was not appropriate for this modification to assess risk in food seeking.

We found no differences in time spent in the light zone of the light/dark box or center zone of the open field for any experimental condition, which demonstrates that mice explore the novel anxiogenic space similarly, regardless of metabolic state. This is an important parameter to measure to preclude the possibility that the experimental variable being tested influences anxiety state. Increases in anxiety will alter perceived risk and may confound assessment of the motivational/rewarding aspects of interaction with the PB chip. In two experiments, we report a difference in time spent in the perimeter zone of the open field, with the more metabolically replete (ad lib fed or glucose-treated) mice showing increased time in this space. This is reflective of the increased time the fasted mice spend in the food zone, and indicates greater motivation for the food reward rather than an altered anxiety state (Lockie and Andrews, 2013).

Locomotor activity was similar between all groups except for ghrelin-treated mice in the light/dark box. Ghrelin has previously been shown to increase locomotor activity in the absence of food (Jerlhag et al., 2006), although others have demonstrated that it has the opposite effect in the presence of food (Tang-Christensen et al., 2004). We might have expected, given the presence and increased consumption of the PB chip in this group, to have reduced locomotor activity in the ghrelin treated mice. We suggest that this result is due to an interaction between ghrelin signaling and the novelty and anxiogenic nature of the arena, as ghrelin has been shown to reduce anxiety in the face of stress (Spencer et al., 2012).

The results were most uniform in the ghrelin-treated experiment, and least uniform in the fasted mice treated with glucose, which likely reflects the greater innate physiological variability of the interventions. Ghrelin targets key neuronal populations that influence food seeking and motivation. Hypothalamic AgRP neurons are highly ghrelin sensitive and are active during fasting. Artificial activation of these neurons results in increased motivation to obtain food, increased consumption of food (Aponte et al., 2011; Krashes et al., 2011) and increased risk taking behavior around food acquisition (Jikomes et al., 2016).

One criticism of the current models of risk/reward decision making in mice is that the organism's survival is not endangered by bad choices, because at worst "bad" choices lead to loss of reward, not punishment (Anselme, 2015). Negative consequences, or at least concrete fear of them, is required to generate real awareness of risk within the organism, as is clearly demonstrated in food seeking and foraging choices undertaken in the wild (Holmes, 1984; Anderson, 1986). This can be done by punishment intrinsic to experimental procedure, or fear of natural consequences, like starvation, or predation. We used a larger than normal open field to exploit and exacerbate the natural fear of predation in open spaces (Holmes, 1984; Anderson, 1986), which underlies the traditional open field and light/dark box tests (Crawley, 2006), and force the mouse to make a calculated decision about the value of a known palatable food reward situated in the anxiogenic zone. This value ascribed to the PB chip following this assessment by the mouse can be termed the incentive salience of the reward, and should be sensitive to the metabolic state of the mouse. If this was the case, we would expect the lure of the PB chip to be greater in those mice experiencing metabolic need, and that these mice would make "riskier" choices about approaching and consuming the PB chip. Indeed, we demonstrated that hunger or exogenous ghrelin increased time spent eating and total amount consumed of the chip, while fasted mice injected with glucose immediately prior to the test behaved like fed mice. This indicates that the metabolic state of the mouse, while in the test situation, greatly influences its behavioral choices. Others have demonstrated that manipulation of AgRP neurons is capable of directing similar behavioral choices, driving food consumption in the presence of foot shocks (Jikomes et al., 2016) or directing more risky foraging behavior (Padilla et al., 2016). While we did not directly assess the role of AgRP neurons in our experiments, given that they are active in the fasted state (Yang et al., 2011), are targeted by ghrelin (Nakazato et al., 2001), and are glucose sensitive (Claret et al., 2007), we propose AgRP neurons are likely involved in mediating these behavioral changes.

Importantly, we do not see differences in other measures of exploratory or anxiety-like behavior such as time spent in anxiogenic zone or latency to approach PB chip. This demonstrates that we are not impacting these behaviors by altering metabolic state, but having a focused effect on consumptive behavior. Several times we saw a significant difference in time spent in the non-anxiogenic zone (open field perimeter zone or dark zone in light dark box), with the non-metabolically challenged mice showing increased time in this space. This is likely to be the reciprocal of the decreased time spent in the food zone during these tests. This indicates that mice are spending a similar amount of time exploring the anxiogenic zone, but without a pressing metabolic need to be in the food zone they prefer to spend time in the non-anxiogenic zone. This reflects the preference mice have for safer spaces when there is no incentive to leave them.

If we understand hunger, or high ghrelin, as a signal of food resource scarcity, the risk of starvation becomes more salient to the mouse than the risk of predation. In the fed state, there is no resource pressure as food has been constantly available. Fasting or administering ghrelin creates perceived resource pressure on the food supply, and amplifies the perceived consequences of forgoing the PB chip out of fear. Therefore these mice are more likely to spend time in the unsafe zone consuming a known high-energy food source, as the cost of forgoing this opportunity is greater than the fear of predation. Fed mice are much more conservative in their risk/reward calculation because they have no immediate metabolic pressure to contend with. We used highly palatable PB chips, however some experiments may require use of standard chow or other less well-liked food rewards to avoid ceiling effects on food exploration and consumption.

Others have used modified light/dark box to assess food consumption in an aversive environment (Teegarden and Bale, 2007; Cottone et al., 2012; Liu et al., 2016). Each of these previous uses of the modified light dark box comprise of a food reward placed in the light compartment and then investigated both time spent in the light compartment and time spent consuming food. An increased amount of time spent in the light compartment has universally been described as "risk-taking behavior," however what consumption of the food under those circumstances means is more controversial. Cottone describes it as "compulsive-like eating" based on the premise that food intake is usually suppressed when a rat faces adverse circumstances like exposure in an open arena. However, arguing against "compulsive" eating is the fact that ad lib fed mice do not consume much of the PB chip, compared to fasted or ghrelin-treated mice. We feel that rather than representing "compulsivity" in fasted and ghrelin-treated mice, food consumption in an aversive environment is rather a logical response to a metabolic need, which is more pressing than the risky environment of the open arena. This paper offers a standardized and validated protocol for use of a reward-baited light/dark box, in addition to a reward-baited open field test. Using both tests in conjunction provides comprehensive assessment of risk vs. reward seeking in mice.

Food seeking in the modern human situation rarely has this perceived level of risk associated with it, none the less it is not risk free. Aside from the basic risks associated with driving or walking to the grocery store, there are social risks around food selection and consumption, which can make eating psychologically taxing. Perhaps the point here though, is not that we are modeling the human situation, but rather that we are trying to better model the natural food seeking-obtaining-consuming cycle of wild animals, which necessarily contains motivational, reward, and risk-taking elements. We propose that this test battery will be a useful addition to standard food intake measurements, and standard behavior tests to assess deficits in global processing of food attainment in genetic and other mouse models.

AUTHOR CONTRIBUTIONS

ZBA, designed research and drafted manuscript. SHL, designed research, performed research, analyzed data, and drafted manuscript. CM, performed research and analyzed data. SR, performed research and analyzed data. NG, Performed research and analyzed data.

FUNDING

This work was supported by fellowships from the Australian National Health and Medical Research Council to ZBA (1084344) and SHL (1072364).

REFERENCES

Anderson, P. K. (1986). Foraging range in mice and voles: the role of risk. *Can. J. Zool.* 64, 2645–2653. doi: 10.1139/z86-384

Anselme, P. (2015). Does reward unpredictability reflect risk? *Behav. Brain Res.* 280, 119–127. doi: 10.1016/j.bbr.2014.12.003

Aponte, Y., Atasoy, D., and Sternson, S. M. (2011). AGRP neurons are sufficient to orchestrate feeding behavior rapidly and without training. *Nat. Neurosci.* 14, 351–355. doi: 10.1038/nn.2739

Bady, I., Marty, N., Dallaporta, M., Emery, M., Gyger, J., Tarussio, D., et al. (2006). Evidence from glut2-null mice that glucose is a critical physiological regulator of feeding. *Diabetes* 55, 988–995. doi: 10.2337/diabetes.55.04.06.db05-1386

Claret, M., Smith, M. A., Batterham, R. L., Selman, C., Choudhury, A. I., Fryer, L. G., et al. (2007). AMPK is essential for energy homeostasis regulation and glucose sensing by POMC and AgRP neurons. *J. Clin. Invest.* 117, 2325–2336. doi: 10.1172/JCI31516

Cottone, P., Wang, X., Park, J. W., Valenza, M., Blasio, A., Kwak, J., et al. (2012). Antagonism of sigma-1 receptors blocks compulsive-like eating. *Neuropsychopharmacology* 37, 2593–2604. doi: 10.1038/npp.2012.89

Crawley, J. N. (2006). *What's Wrong with My Mouse?: Behavioral Phenotyping of Transgenic and Knockout Mice.* Hoboken, NJ: John Wiley and Sons, Inc.

Dickson, S. L., Egecioglu, E., Landgren, S., Skibicka, K. P., Engel, J. A., and Jerlhag, E. (2011). The role of the central ghrelin system in reward from food and chemical drugs. *Mol. Cell. Endocrinol.* 340, 80–87. doi: 10.1016/j.mce.2011.02.017

Faul, F., Erdfelder, E., Lang, A. G., and Buchner, A. (2007). G*Power 3: a flexible statistical power analysis program for the social, behavioral, and biomedical sciences. *Behav. Res. Methods* 39, 175–191. doi: 10.3758/BF03193146

Holmes, W. G. (1984). Predation risk and foraging behavior of the hoary marmot in Alaska. *Behav. Ecol. Sociobiol.* 15, 923–301. doi: 10.1007/BF00292992

Jerlhag, E., Egecioglu, E., Dickson, S. L., Andersson, M., Svensson, L., and Engel, J. A. (2006). Ghrelin stimulates locomotor activity and accumbal dopamine-overflow via central cholinergic systems in mice: implications for its involvement in brain reward. *Addict. Biol.* 11, 45–54. doi: 10.1111/j.1369-1600.2006.00002.x

Jikomes, N., Ramesh, R. N., Mandelblat-Cerf, Y., and Andermann, M. L. (2016). Preemptive stimulation of AgRP neurons in fed mice enables conditioned food seeking under threat. *Curr. Biol.* 26, 2500–2507. doi: 10.1016/j.cub.2016.07.019

Krashes, M. J., Koda, S., Ye, C. P., Rogan, S. C., Adarns, A. C., Cusher, D. S., et al. (2011). Rapid, reversible activation of AgRP neurons drives feeding behavior in mice. *J. Clin. Invest.* 121, 1424–1428. doi: 10.1172/JCI46229

Leblond, M., Fan, D., Brynildsen, J. K., and Yin, H. H. (2011). Motivational state and reward content determine choice behavior under risk in mice. *PLoS ONE* 6:e25342. doi: 10.1371/journal.pone.0025342

Liu, S., Globa, A. K., Mills, F., Naef, L., Qiao, M., Bamji, S. X., et al. (2016). Consumption of palatable food primes food approach behavior by rapidly increasing synaptic density in the VTA. *Proc. Natl. Acad. Sci. U.S.A.* 113, 2520–2525. doi: 10.1073/pnas.1515724113

Lockie, S. H., and Andrews, Z. B. (2013). The hormonal signature of energy deficit: increasing the value of food reward. *Mol. Metab.* 2, 329–336. doi: 10.1016/j.molmet.2013.08.003

Lockie, S. H., Dinan, T., Lawrence, A. J., Spencer, S. J., and Andrews, Z. B. (2015). Diet-induced obesity causes ghrelin resistance in reward processing tasks. *Psychoneuroendocrinology* 62, 114–120. doi: 10.1016/j.psyneuen.2015.08.004

Mayer, J. (1953). Glucostatic mechanism of regulation of food intake. *N.Engl. J. Med.* 249, 13–16. doi: 10.1056/NEJM195307022490104

Nakazato, M., Murakami, N., Date, Y., Kojima, M., Matsuo, H., Kangawa, K., et al. (2001). A role for ghrelin in the central regulation of feeding. *Nature* 409, 194–198. doi: 10.1038/35051587

Overduin, J., Figlewicz, D. P., Bennett-Jay, J., Kittleson, S., and Cummings, D. E. (2012). Ghrelin increases the motivation to eat, but does not alter food palatability. *Am. J. Physiol. Regul. Integr. Comp. Physiol.* 303, R259–R269. doi: 10.1152/ajpregu.00488.2011

Padilla, S. L., Qiu, J., Soden, M. E., Sanz, E., Nestor, C. C., Barker, F. D., et al. (2016). Agouti-related peptide neural circuits mediate adaptive behaviors in the starved state. *Nat. Neurosci.* 19, 734–741. doi: 10.1038/nn.4274

Simon, N. W., and Setlow, B. (2012). Modeling risky decision making in rodents. *Methods Mol. Biol.* 829, 165–175. doi: 10.1007/978-1-61779-458-2_10

Skibicka, K. P., Hansson, C., Egecioglu, E., and Dickson, S. L. (2012). Role of ghrelin in food reward: impact of ghrelin on sucrose self-administration and mesolimbic dopamine and acetylcholine receptor gene expression. *Addict. Biol.* 17, 95–107. doi: 10.1111/j.1369-1600.2010.00294.x

Spencer, S. J., Xu, L., Clarke, M. A., Lemus, M., Reichenbach, A., Geenen, B., et al. (2012). Ghrelin regulates the hypothalamic-pituitary-adrenal axis and restricts anxiety after acute stress. *Biol. Psychiatry* 72, 457–465. doi: 10.1016/j.biopsych.2012.03.010

Tang-Christensen, M., Vrang, N., Ortmann, S., Bidlingmaier, M., Horvath, T. L., and Tschöp, M. (2004). Central administration of ghrelin and Agouti-related protein (83-132) increases food intake and decreases spontaneous locomotor activity in rats. *Endocrinology* 145, 4645–4652. doi: 10.1210/en.2004-0529

Teegarden, S. L., and Bale, T. L. (2007). Decreases in dietary preference produce increased emotionality and risk for dietary relapse. *Biol. Psychiatry* 61, 1021–1029. doi: 10.1016/j.biopsych.2006.09.032

Toth, L. A., and Gardiner, T. W. (2000). Food and water restriction protocols: physiological and behavioral considerations. *Contemp. Top. Lab. Anim. Sci.* 39, 9–17.

Yang, Y. L., Atasoy, D., Su, H. H., and Sternson, S. M. (2011). Hunger states switch a flip-flop memory circuit via a synaptic AMPK-dependent positive feedback loop. *Cell* 146, 991–1002. doi: 10.1016/j.cell.2011.07.039

4

Combination of Selective Immunoassays and Mass Spectrometry to Characterize Preproghrelin-Derived Peptides in Mouse Tissues

Rim Hassouna [1,2†], Dominique Grouselle [1†], Giovanni Chiappetta [3], Joanna Lipecka [1], Oriane Fiquet [1], Catherine Tomasetto [4], Joëlle Vinh [3], Jacques Epelbaum [1,5] and Virginie Tolle [1]*

[1] Centre de Psychiatrie et Neurosciences, UMR-S 894 Institut National de la Santé et de la Recherche Médicale, Université Paris Descartes, Sorbonne Paris Cité, Paris, France, [2] Department of Pediatrics, Naomi Berrie Diabetes Center, Columbia University Medical Center, New York, NY, USA, [3] ESPCI Paris, PSL Research University, Spectrométrie de Masse Biologique et Protéomique (SMPB), CNRS USR 3149, Paris, France, [4] UMR-7104 Centre Nationnal de la Recherche Scientifique/U596, Institut National de la Santé et de la Recherche Médicale, Institut de génétique et de biologie moléculaire et cellulaire, Université de Strasbourg, Illkirch, France, [5] UMR 7179 Centre Nationnal de la Recherche Scientifique, MNHN, Adaptive Mechanism and Evolution (MECADEV), Brunoy, France

***Correspondence:**
Virginie Tolle
virginie.tolle@inserm.fr

† These authors have contributed equally to this work.

Preproghrelin is a prohormone producing several preproghrelin-derived peptides with structural and functional heterogeneity: acyl ghrelin (AG), desacyl ghrelin (DAG), and obestatin. The absence of selective and reliable assays to measure these peptides simultaneously in biological samples has been a limitation to assess their real proportions in tissues and plasma in physiological and pathological conditions. We aimed at reliably measure the ratio between the different preproghrelin-derived peptides in murine tissues using selective immunoassays combined with a highly sensitive mass spectrometry method. AG-, DAG-, and obestatin-immunopositive fractions from the gastrointestinal tract of adult wild-type and ghrelin-deficient mice were processed for analysis by mass spectrometry (MS) with a Triple Quadrupole mass spectrometer. We found that DAG was predominant in mouse plasma, however it only represented 50% of total ghrelin (AG+DAG) production in the stomach and duodenum. Obestatin plasma levels accounted for about 30% of all circulating preproghrelin-derived peptides, however, it represented <1% of total preproghrelin-derived peptides production (AG+DAG+Obestatin) in the stomach. Assays were validated in ghrelin-deficient mice since neither ghrelin nor obestatin immunoreactivities were detected in their stomach, duodenum nor plasma. MS analyses confirmed that obestatin-immunoreactivity in stomach corresponded to the C-terminal amidated form of the peptide but not to des(1–10)-obestatin, nor to obestatin-Gly. In conclusion, specificity of ghrelin and obestatin immunoreactivities in gastrointestinal tissues using selective immunoassays was validated by MS. Obestatin was less abundant than AG or DAG in these tissues. Whether this is due to inefficient processing rate of preproghrelin into mature obestatin in gastrointestinal mouse tissues remains elusive.

Keywords: acyl ghrelin, desacyl ghrelin, obestatin, immunoreactivity, mass spectrometry

INTRODUCTION

Preproghrelin is a complex prohormone that, upon post-translational processing, leads to the production of several derived peptides with structural and functional heterogeneity. Ghrelin is a 28 amino acid peptide originating from the stomach (Kojima et al., 1999; Hosoda et al., 2000; Tomasetto et al., 2000) and identified as the endogenous ligand of the Growth Hormone Secretagogue Receptor (GHS-R; Howard et al., 1996). The addition of an acyl-group by the Ghrelin-O-Acyl-Transferase (GOAT; Yang et al., 2008), enables ghrelin (Acyl-ghrelin, AG) to stimulate GH secretion and appetite (Tolle et al., 2001, 2002). Another endogenous form of ghrelin is desacyl ghrelin (DAG) reported as the most abundant form in plasma (Hosoda et al., 2000). Its specific roles are to regulate glucose, lipid, and bone metabolism (Delhanty et al., 2013). Obestatin is a 23 amino acid amidated peptide derived from the same precursor as ghrelin. Originally isolated as the endogenous ligand for the GPR39 and described as an anorexigenic factor in rodents (McKee et al., 1997; Zhang et al., 2005), its physiological relevance has since been questioned (Zhang et al., 2005; Bresciani et al., 2006; Lauwers et al., 2006; Seoane et al., 2006; Yamamoto et al., 2007). Both DAG and obestatin interact pharmacologically with AG to modulate food intake, GH secretion or glucose metabolism through yet unidentified receptors (Hassouna et al., 2012; Delhanty et al., 2013; Gargantini et al., 2013). Previous studies found equimolar ratios of plasma AG and obestatin levels in the rat (Zhang et al., 2005; Zizzari et al., 2007), consistent with both peptides being processed from the same prohormone. However, evidence that tissue specific splicing variant encoding obestatin but not ghrelin exist in humans suggests that obestatin could also be produced independently of ghrelin (Seim et al., 2009).

With regard to the literature, many issues remain to be addressed concerning obestatin: its main source of production in the body and its abundance relative to ghrelin as well as its molecular form and way of processing. Obestatin was initially extracted from rat stomach and found in rat plasma (Zhang et al., 2005). In addition, obestatin immunoreactivity was detected in a number of human tissues using immunohistochemistry (Grönberg et al., 2008) and in cultured pancreatic islets *in vitro* (Granata et al., 2008). However, other studies failed to detect significant amounts of obestatin in rat plasma or stomach using radioimmunoassay (RIA) coupled to High Performance Liquid Chromatography (HPLC; Bang et al., 2007; Mondal et al., 2008).

The absence of selective and reliable assays to measure all three preproghrelin-derived peptides (AG, DAG, and obestatin) simultaneously in biological samples is an obstacle to further characterization of their specific physiological and pathophysiological functions. In this study, we developed selective immunoassays combined to a highly sensitive targeted mass spectrometry method in order to reliably measure and characterize the ratios of the different preproghrelin-derived peptides in mice. Preproghrelin gene deficient mice that do not produce AG or DAG (Hassouna et al., 2014) were used as negative controls to further validate the immunoreactivity and mass spectrometry assays.

MATERIALS AND METHODS

Animals

Dissections were performed on 7–12 weeks old preproghrelin deficient (*ghrl−/−*) mice and wild type (*ghrl+/+*) littermates backcrossed on the C57BL/6J genetic background as previously reported (Hassouna et al., 2014). Mice were housed in a room under controlled illumination (0700–1900 h) and temperature (22–24°C) and had free access to food and water. Offsprings were genotyped by PCR amplification of tail DNA. All experiments were carried out in accordance with the European Communities Council Directive (86/609/EEC) and were approved by the Animal Experimentation Committee of Paris Descartes University (agreement number 03422.02).

Peptides

Peptides used as standards in liquid chromatography (LC) were provided by NeoMPS (Strasbourg, France): rat/mouse acyl ghrelin (AG) and desacyl ghrelin (DAG), rat/mouse amidated obestatin (obestatin-NH_2), Des(1–10)-obestatin and obestatin-Gly (Sequences presented in Table S1 and Figure S1).

Dissection, Extraction, and Purification of Tissue Samples

Gastric epithelia, 1 cm proximal duodenum, small intestine and colon were collected and the tissues were extracted in 2N acetic acid during 10 min at 90°C, sonicated and frozen at −80°C for 24 h. The homogenate was centrifuged 20 min at 12,000 g at 4°C. Supernatants were lyophilized and further dissolved in phosphate assay buffer. Extracts were first filtered on a 10 kDa filter (Amicon Ultra, Millipore, Molsheim, France) then purified using SepPak C18 columns (Waters, Saint-Quentin-en-Yvelines, France). Briefly, the supernatants were loaded onto a SepPak C18 cartridge pre-equilibrated in 0.1% trifluoroacetic acid (TFA). The samples were desalted with aqueous TFA 0.1% and eluted with an acetonitrile gradient (10–100%).

Plasma Collection and Processing

Blood samples were collected from trunk blood on EDTA (1 mg/ml) and PHMB (0.4 mM final), a serine protease inhibitor and centrifuged at 1,000 g during 10 min at 4°C. Plasma were immediately acidified with HCl (0.1 M final) and stored at −80°C.

Hormone Assays

Immunoreactivities were measured in plasma, whole tissue and SepPak fractions (10–70 and 100%) with selective sandwich immunoassays for AG, DAG (SPIbio Bertin pharma, A05118 for the acyl form and A05117 for the desacyl form, Montigny-le-Bretonneux, France) and competitive assay for obestatin (Phoenix Pharmaceuticals, Burlingame, USA). Immunoreactive fractions were further analyzed by Mass Spectrometry (MS).

Mass Spectrometry

Mass Spectrometry (MS) analyses were performed in the Selected Reaction Monitoring (SRM) mode using a high pressure nanoLC (U3000 RSLC, Thermo Fisher Scientific) coupled to a triple quadrupole (QqQ) mass spectrometer (TSQ Vantage^{TM}, Thermo

Fisher Scientific, San Jose, CA, USA) in nano-ESI mode. Briefly, peptides were loaded and desalted on a C18 cartridge (C18 PepMap, 3 mm, 100 A°, 75 mm i.d., 2 cm length) using a loading buffer containing 0.05% aq TFA/acetonitrile 98:2 (v/v) at 10 μL/min. Peptides were then separated on a C18 analytical column (C18 PepMap, 2 mm, 100 A°, 75 mm i.d., 15 cm length) with a 60 min gradient from 99% A [0.1% aq formic acid/acetonitrile 98:2 (v/v)] to 50% B [0.1% aq formic acid/acetonitrile 10:90 (v/v)] at 300 nL/min. Standard was injected before each series of experiments. Blank runs were interposed until necessary to avoid peptide carry-over effects. QqQ parameters were set as follows: first and third quadrupole widths set at 0.7, scan time 200 ms/transition and total dwell time 3 s (method performed in unscheduled mode). The transitions for AG (retention time 29.1 min) were 553.1 (precursor MH_6^{6+}) → 513.3 (y_4); 641.4 (y_5); 712.4;(y_6); 809.5 (y_7) 906.5(y_8). The transitions for DAG (retention time 20.0 min) were 532.1 (precursor MH_6^{6+}) → 513.3 (y_4); 641.4 (y_5); 712.4; (y_6); 809.5 (y_7); 906.5(y_8). The transitions for obestatin-NH_2 (retention time 38.3 min) were 630.8 (precursor MH_5^{5+}) → 262.1(b_2); 416.2 (y_4); 553.3 (y_5); 681.4;(y_6); 972.5 (y_8). The transitions for obestatin-Gly (retention time 33.4 min) were 858.8 (precursor MH_3^{3+}) → 262.1 (b_2); 333.2 (b_3); 473.2 (y_5); 610.3 (y_6) 1029.5(y_9). The transitions for des(1–10)-obestatin (retention time 17.9 min) were 476.9 (precursor MH_3^{3+}) → 201.1 (b_2); 553.2 (y_5); 681.3;(y_6); 809.5 (y_7); 972.5(y_8) (Supplementary Table S1).

RESULTS

Preproghrelin-Derived Peptides Immunoreactivities in the Gastrointestinal Tract and Plasma

In adult mice, stomach is known to be the major source of ghrelin, however the main source of obestatin remains elusive. Accordingly, since ghrelin gene is widely expressed throughout the gastro-intestinal (GI) tract, we thus measured all preproghrelin-derived peptides in the different portions of the GI tract (stomach, duodenum, intestine, and colon) in mice using selective antibodies (Figure S1). Amongst all preproghrelin-derived peptides, AG and DAG were the most abundant forms found in stomach. In this tissue, AG represented 50%, DAG 50%, and obestatin <1% of all preproghrelin-derived peptides. Although their proportions varied in the different sections of the GI tract, ghrelin (AG and DAG) remained predominant compared to obestatin. In duodenum, AG represented 34%, DAG 38%, and obestatin 29% of all preproghrelin-derived peptides. Differences in proportions of obestatin relative to ghrelin may partly be due to the utilization of different techniques to detect specific immunoreactivities and revelation procedures (sandwich enzymoimmunoassays for ghrelin vs. competitive radioimmunoassay for obestatin). Whereas, AG and DAG levels were gradually decreasing from caudal to distal region of the GI tract, obestatin concentrations were slightly higher in the duodenum than in the stomach (**Table 1**). Both the intestine and colon produced small amounts of all three peptides (data not shown).

Previous studies using competition assays indicated that DAG accounts for 80–90% of total circulating ghrelin (Hosoda et al., 2000). In the present study, DAG accounted for nearly 80% of total circulating ghrelin (i.e., AG+DAG) and 60% of total circulating preproghrelin-derived peptides (i.e., AG+DAG+Obestatin; **Table 1**). Obestatin plasma levels represented about 30% of all circulating preproghrelin-derived peptides, which is much higher than its proportion in gastrointestinal tissues (**Table 1**).

Mass Spectrometry (MS) Analysis of Preproghrelin-Derived Peptides in *ghrl*+/+ and *ghrl*−/− mice

Selected Reaction Monitoring (SRM) method was set up using synthetic peptides AG, DAG, Obestatin-NH_2, Des(1–10)-Obestatin and Obestatin-Gly. The SRM method selected the best five transitions obtained by testing all the theoretic "y" and "b" ion fragments from MH_3^{3+} to MH_6^{6+} precursors (**Figure 1**).

TABLE 1 | Tissue content or concentrations, percentage and molar ratio of preproghrelin-derived peptides immunoreactivities in the stomach, duodenum, and plasma of *ghrl*+/+ mice (n = 6–10).

	Acyl ghrelin (AG)	Desacyl ghrelin (DAG)	Obestatin	AG/TG	DAG/TG	Obestatin/TG
STOMACH						
Tissue content (pmol/tissue)	184 ± 9	197 ± 19	0.65 ± 0.02		Molar ratio	
% of total preproghrelin-derived peptides	49 ± 3%	51 ± 3%	0.17 ± 0.01%	1/2	1/2	1/616
DUODENUM						
Tissue content (pmol/tissue)	1.32 ± 0.39	1.39 ± 0.42	1.00 ± 0.52		Molar ratio	
% of total preproghrelin-derived peptides	34 ± 6%	38 ± 10%	29 ± 12%	1/2	1/2	1/2.5
PLASMA						
Concentration (pmol/L)	103 ± 29	370 ± 44	210 ± 79		Molar ratio	
% of total preproghrelin-derived peptides	16 ± 4%	57 ± 5%	27 ± 8%	1/5	1/1.2	1/1.7

AG, Acyl ghrelin; DAG, Desacyl ghrelin; TG, Total Ghrelin (AG+DAG). Limits of detection are 0.03 pmol for AG and DAG and 0.08 pmol for obestatin. Data are expressed as Mean ± SEM, molar ratio or as percentages of total preproghrelin-derived peptides (AG+DAG+obestatin).

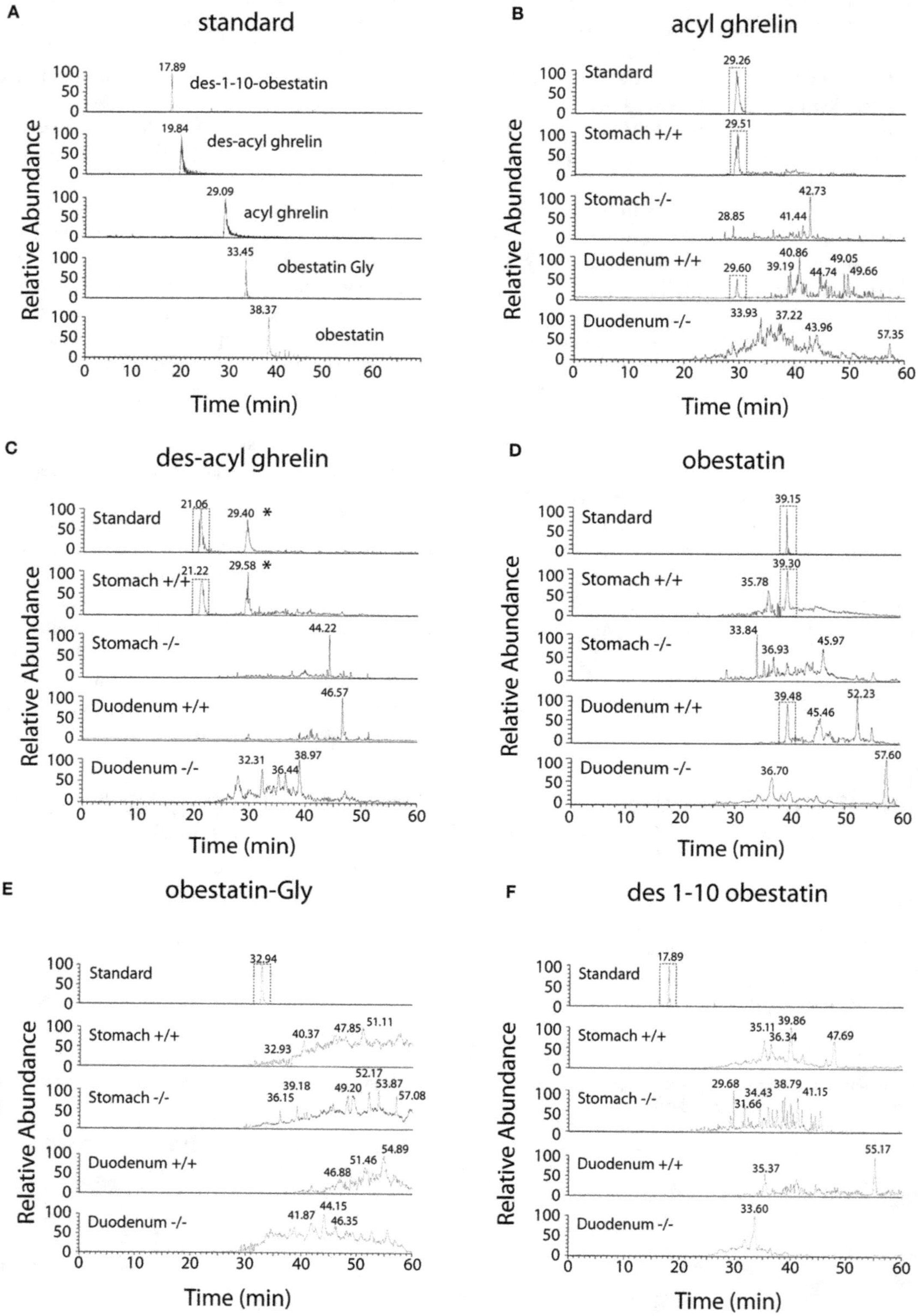

FIGURE 1 | Chromatographic profiles of SRM analyses related to preproghrelin-derived peptides in the stomach and duodenum from 60% chromatographic fractions in *ghrl+/+* and *ghrl−/−* mice. SRM analyses of the synthetic peptide (standard) and tissue samples obtained from the fraction eluted with 60% acetonitrile: **(A)** standard, **(B)** acyl ghrelin, **(C)** des-acyl ghrelin, **(D)** obestatin, **(E)** obestatin-Gly, **(F)** des(1–10)-obestatin. Acyl ghrelin and obestatin-NH_2 were present in both the stomach and duodenum of *ghrl+/+* mice but absent in the tissues of *ghrl−/−* mice. Des-acyl ghrelin was present in the stomach but not in the duodenum of *ghrl+/+* mice and absent in the tissues of *ghrl−/−* mice. The star (*) denotes a peak in ghrelin chromatogram that is related to the "in source" neutral loss of the acyl group of acyl ghrelin converted partially acyl ghrelin to desacyl ghrelin after LC separation. Obestatin-Gly and des(1–10)-obestatin were absent in both the stomach and duodenum of *ghrl+/+* and *ghrl−/−* mice. See experimental section for SRM method design.

The detection limits for AG and DAG was 10–50 fmol and for obestatin-NH_2 and its derivatives 1–5 fmol.

As preproghrelin-derived peptides are highly concentrated in stomach and duodenum, purified SepPak fractions from these tissue protein extracts from both *ghrl+/+* and *ghrl−/−* mice were used for mass spectrometry. Preproghrelin-derived peptides immunoreactivities were retrieved in stomach and duodenum of *ghrl+/+* mice but not in the same tissues in *ghrl−/−* mice (**Table 2** and data not shown). The residual immunoreactivity for obestatin found in two out of six *ghrl−/−* mice was unspecific, since it did not correspond to the correct specific masses in MS experiments (See below). To decrease the dynamic range and the complexity of the whole protein extract, samples were first depleted to conserve only peptides below 10 kDa. The resulting mixtures were further submitted to solid phase extraction on C18 stationary phase to remove hydrophilic species. According to standard synthetic peptides properties, the endogenous peptides of interest were expected to be eluted using 10–70% acetonitrile. The fractions were submitted to stepwise elution with successive 10% increments of acetonitrile. Immunoreactivity of each preproghrelin-derived peptides (AG, DAG, and Obestatin) was measured in each eluted fraction. In *ghrl+/+* mice, 30, 40, and 60% acetonitrile-containing fractions presented the most intense immunoreactivity and were further analyzed by SRM LC-MS. The matched fractions obtained from *ghrl−/−* mice contained no immunoreactivity for all three preproghrelin-derived peptides and were also analyzed in SRM LC-MS.

Ghrelin and obestatin were detected by mass spectrometry in both *ghrl+/+* mice stomach and duodenum, only in 60% acetonitrile fractions (**Table 3**). Thus LC-MS profiles of SRM analyses related to preproghrelin-derived peptides in stomach and duodenum were restricted to 60% acetonitrile fractions from *ghrl+/+* and *ghrl−/−* mice (**Figure 1**). The antibody used in the obestatin immunoassay may detect other forms of obestatin, such as a truncated peptide, des(1–10)-obestatin, and a modified form of obestatin with additional glycine at the C-terminal position, obestatin-Gly. Thus, the presence of des(1–10)-obestatin and obestatin-Gly was also assayed by SRM in order to evaluate a possible antibody cross-reactivity. To develop a specific and sensitive detection method for the peptides of interest, a mix of AG, DAG, obestatin, Des(1–10)-obestatin and obestatin-Gly standards (100 fmol of each) was used to calibrate the SRM method before each analysis. Blanks were run to assure the absence of contaminations from standards before the analysis of samples. Comparison between the chromatographic profiles of SRM analyses related to the fractions eluted at 60% ACN of the stomach and duodenum tissues were compared between *ghrl+/+* and *ghrl−/−* mice (**Figures 1B–F**). As further described below, only native obestatin-NH2 was present in the extracts analyzed (**Table 3**).

The three preproghrelin-derived peptides were present in stomach LC fractions of *ghrl+/+* mice. In duodenum LC fractions of *ghrl+/+* mice, AG, and obestatin were present while DAG was absent. As shown on **Table 3**, and **Figure 1**, SRM analyses further confirmed that obestatin-immunoreactivity in stomach and duodenum corresponded to the amidated (**Figure 1D**) form of the peptide but not to obestatin-Gly (**Figure 1E**) nor Des(1–10)-obestatin (**Figure 1F**). No MS signal for any preproghrelin-derived peptides was detected in stomach or duodenum of *ghrl−/−* mice. This further validated the specificity of the spectrometric signal detected (**Figures 1B–F**). In stomach and duodenum extracts from *ghrl+/+* and *ghrl−/−* mice, extracted ion chromatograms related to DAG transitions (**Figure 1C**) presented two peaks instead of one, respectively associated to DAG retention time (21 min) and AG retention time (29 min). The "in source" neutral loss of the acyl group of AG converted partially AG to DAG after LC separation, so that DAG SRM signature can also be detected at AG retention time. On the opposite, when DAG and AG standards are analyzed separately (**Figure 1A**) no signals are detected at DAG retention time with AG transitions.

TABLE 2 | Preproghrelin-derived peptides immunoreactivities in the stomach and duodenum of *ghrl+/+* and *ghrl−/−* mice.

	Ghrl+/+ (n = 6)		*Ghrl−/−* (n = 6)	
	Stomach (pg)	Duodenum (pg)	Stomach (pg)	Duodenum (pg)
Acyl ghrelin	606,100 ± 30,826	4,350 ± 1,301	UN	UN
Desacyl ghrelin	649,767 ± 64,027	4,587 ± 1,385	UN	UN
Total ghrelin	1,255,867 ± 67,509	8,937 ± 2,312	UN	UN
Obestatin	1,632 ± 57	2,600 ± 1,293	UN	710 ± 328*

*Acyl ghrelin, desacyl ghrelin, and obestatin immunoreactivities measured using selective assays are detected in the stomach and duodenum of ghrl+/+ mice (n = 6) but are undetectable in ghrl−/− mice (n = 6). Limits of detection are 10 pg for AG and DAG and 200 pg for obestatin. Data are expressed as Mean ± SEM. UN: Under detection limit. *Immunoreactivity is unspecific.*

DISCUSSION

Using a combination of selective immunoassays and highly sensitive mass spectrometry, we validate the presence of a specific immunoreactivity signal for amidated obestatin in protein extracts from stomach and duodenum and further characterize the ratio of the different preproghrelin-derived peptides in mouse gastrointestinal tract. Specific presence of each preproghrelin-derived peptide was validated by the lack of signal in preproghrelin deficient mice using both immunodetection and MS.

Until now, very few studies characterized all preproghrelin-derived peptides in murine tissues. This can be explained by the lack of sensitive and specific methods to simultaneously detect the three preproghrelin-derived peptides in a given biological sample. Moreover, their relative proportions in tissues and plasma remained unclear. Previous studies using competitive immunoassays reported equimolar ratios of acyl ghrelin and obestatin in rat plasma (Zhang et al., 2005; Zizzari et al., 2007) consistent with a model previewing both peptides obtained by the processing of the same prohormone, while ratios of 2:1–4:1 were reported in humans (Germain et al., 2009, 2010). The reason for such discrepancy is unclear but this could evoke alternative

TABLE 3 | SRM detection of preproghrelin-derived peptides in the different chromatographic fractions (30, 40, and 60% Acetonitrile) in the stomach and duodenum of *ghrl+/+* mice.

Tissue	LC Fraction (%age acetonitrile)	Acyl ghrelin	Desacyl ghrelin	Obestatin-NH2	Obestatin-Gly	des(1–10) -obestatin
Stomach	30	–	+	–	–	–
	40	+	–	–	–	–
	60	+	+	+	–	–
Duodenum	30	–	–	–	–	–
	40	–	–	–	–	–
	60	+	–	+	–	–

Acyl ghrelin and obestatin-NH_2 were detected in the stomach and duodenum whereas, desacyl ghrelin was only detected in the stomach LC fractions of ghrl+/+ mice. MS-MS analyses further confirmed that obestatin-immunoreactivity in tissues is specific to the amidated peptide but not to obestatin-Gly nor des(1–10)-obestatin.

splicing and/or different processing mechanism in rodents and humans. Although one study demonstrated that obestatin is produced in gastrointestinal tract in humans (Grönberg et al., 2008), two other studies failed to identify significant amounts of obestatin in rat plasma or stomach by RIA coupled to HPLC (Bang et al., 2007; Mondal et al., 2008) in contrast with the original data from Zhang and collaborators in the rat (Zhang et al., 2005). Moreover, in the study by Mondal et al., the ratio of obestatin/ghrelin in gastric fundus of rats was 0.004%, which is far less than what is expected in plasma.

These inconsistent results raise many interrogations regarding the exact obestatin site of production, the abundance of the peptide, and the specificity of the signal measured, as well as specific differences between humans and rodents. To gain more knowledge on obestatin, we explored its presence in different murine tissues, including the gastrointestinal tract using immunological detection in association with MS analyses in order to identify the positive immune signals. Our data confirm that both forms of ghrelin as well as obestatin are produced in majority in the gastrointestinal tract in mice.

We show that in stomach, DAG represents 50% of total ghrelin production while in plasma, it accounts for about 60% of total preproghrelin-derived peptides and nearly 80% of total ghrelin. The latter result is in accordance with previous studies using competitive immunoassays which demonstrated that DAG accounts for 80–90% of total circulating ghrelin (Hosoda et al., 2000). Moreover, we find that while plasma obestatin levels represent about 30% of all circulating preproghrelin-derived peptides, obestatin is 500–1,000 times less abundant than total ghrelin in stomach.

Although we find equimolar concentrations of total ghrelin and obestatin in mouse plasma, the amount of obestatin in tissues is negligible compared to those of ghrelin. Several hypotheses may explain this observation. First of all, conditions of sampling, processing and storage may be inadequate to preserve immunoreactive obestatin. Furthermore, a low processing rate of obestatin from preproghrelin in the stomach cannot be excluded. Finally, the existence of different transcripts arising from the preproghrelin gene in a tissue-specific manner (Seim et al., 2009), including a human transcript that encodes obestatin but not ghrelin, also suggests that obestatin transcripts may be produced independently of ghrelin.

The specificity of the immunoreactive detection for all three preproghrelin-derived peptides in both stomach and duodenum was assessed by MS and further validated by the absence of signal in preproghrelin deficient mice (Hassouna et al., 2014). Residual immunoreactivity for obestatin was detected in duodenum of two out of six preproghrelin deficient mice. This is the result of an artifact as no MS signal confirmed that it was actually obestatin. Furthermore, we also confirmed by MS that the immunoreactivity detected in tissues was specific of the amidated form of obestatin. No MS signal for all preproghrelin-derived peptides was present in stomach or duodenum of *ghrl−/−* mice, confirming specificity of the assay.

In this study, we used a very sensitive mass spectrometer system. Indeed detection limits is estimated to be 10–50 fmol for AG and DAG and 1–5 fmol for Obestatin-NH_2 and its derivatives, allowing to detect very small amounts of the peptides. The specificity was verified by determining the transitions for each peptide and analyzing ions fragments. In the original study by Zhang et al. (2005), obestatin was extracted from rat stomach but its relative abundance as compared to ghrelin was not discussed. As far as we know, this is the first attempt to identify and quantify these peptides in mouse tissues and to validate the existence of a mature form of obestatin (Obestatin-NH2) in mouse gastrointestinal tract.

In conclusion, both forms of ghrelin and obestatin can be detected with very selective immunoassays coupled with MS in gastrointestinal tract in mice. In this tissue, obestatin appears to be far less abundant than AG or DAG. This could be the result of either a lower processing rate of proghrelin into mature obestatin in gastrointestinal tissues or degradation of the peptide during the different extraction/purification procedures. Whether the main source of obestatin production and/or processing is outside the gastrointestinal tract has to be further investigated.

AUTHOR CONTRIBUTIONS

RH: contributed to the conception and design of the work, performed experiments and analyses of data, participated to manuscript redaction. DG: contributed to reagents/materials/analysis tools, performed experiments, and analyses of data, participated to manuscript redaction. GC: contributed to the acquisition and analyses of MS data and participated to manuscript redaction. JL: contributed to the experiments and acquisition of data. OF: contributed to the experiments. CT: contributed to reagents/materials/analysis tools and revised the manuscript. JV: contributed to reagents/materials/analysis tools and revised the manuscript. JE: contributed to the conception of the work and revised the manuscript. VT: contributed to the conception and design of the work, analyses, and interpretation of data, manuscript redaction.

FUNDING

This work was supported by an Agence Nationale de la Recherche (ANR) Jeunes Chercheuses Jeunes Chercheurs ANR-12-JSV1-0013-01 grant to VT, University Paris Descartes Sorbonne Paris Cité, Institut National de la Santé et de la Recherche Médicale (INSERM) and Ecole Supérieure de Physique et de Chimie Industrielles (ESPCI) Paris.

ACKNOWLEDGMENTS

We would like to thank Dr. Philippe Zizzari for his contribution in preparing the manuscript. We are grateful to Alice Cougnon and Chloé Got and the Plateau d'Exploration Fonctionnelle du Petit Animal in the Center for Psychiatry and Neurosciences for the care of the animals. We are grateful to Bertin Pharma (Montigny-le-Bretonneaux, France) for providing the AG and DAG assays.

REFERENCES

Bang, A. S., Soule, S. G., Yandle, T. G., Richards, A. M., and Pemberton, C. J. (2007). Characterisation of proghrelin peptides in mammalian tissue and plasma. *J. Endocrinol.* 192, 313–323. doi: 10.1677/JOE-06-0021

Bresciani, E., Rapetti, D., Dona, F., Bulgarelli, I., Tamiazzo, L., Locatelli, V., et al. (2006). Obestatin inhibits feeding but does not modulate GH and corticosterone secretion in the rat. *J. Endocrinol. Invest.* 29, RC16–RC18. doi: 10.1007/BF03344175

Delhanty, P. J., Neggers, S. J., and van der Lely, A. J. (2013). Des-acyl ghrelin: a metabolically active peptide. *Endocr. Dev.* 25, 112–121. doi: 10.1159/000346059

Gargantini, E., Grande, C., Trovato, L., Ghigo, E., and Granata, R. (2013). The role of obestatin in glucose and lipid metabolism. *Horm. Metab. Res.* 45, 1002–1008. doi: 10.1055/s-0033-1351325

Germain, N., Galusca, B., Grouselle, D., Frere, D., Billard, S., Epelbaum, J., et al. (2010). Ghrelin and obestatin circadian levels differentiate bingeing-purging from restrictive anorexia nervosa. *J. Clin. Endocrinol. Metab.* 95, 3057–3062. doi: 10.1210/jc.2009-2196

Germain, N., Galusca, B., Grouselle, D., Frere, D., Tolle, V., Zizzari, P., et al. (2009). Ghrelin/obestatin ratio in two populations with low bodyweight: constitutional thinness and anorexia nervosa. *Psychoneuroendocrinology* 34, 413–419. doi: 10.1016/j.psyneuen.2008.10.001

Granata, R., Settanni, F., Gallo, D., Trovato, L., Biancone, L., Cantaluppi, V., et al. (2008). Obestatin promotes survival of pancreatic beta-cells and human islets and induces expression of genes involved in the regulation of beta-cell mass and function. *Diabetes* 57, 967–979. doi: 10.2337/db07-1104

Grönberg, M., Tsolakis, A. V., Magnusson, L., Janson, E. T., and Saras, J. (2008). Distribution of obestatin and ghrelin in human tissues: immunoreactive cells in the gastrointestinal tract, pancreas, and mammary glands. *J. Histochem. Cytochem.* 56, 793–801. doi: 10.1369/jhc.2008.951145

Hassouna, R., Zizzari, P., Tomasetto, C., Veldhuis, J. D., Fiquet, O., Labarthe, A., et al. (2014). An early reduction in GH peak amplitude in preproghrelin-deficient male mice has a minor impact on linear growth. *Endocrinology* 155, 3561–3571. doi: 10.1210/en.2014-1126

Hassouna, R., Zizzari, P., Viltart, O., Yang, S. K., Gardette, R., Videau, C., et al. (2012). A natural variant of obestatin, Q90L, inhibits ghrelin's action on food intake and GH secretion and targets NPY and GHRH neurons in mice. *PLoS ONE* 7:e51135. doi: 10.1371/journal.pone.0051135

Hosoda, H., Kojima, M., Matsuo, H., and Kangawa, K. (2000). Ghrelin and des-acyl ghrelin: two major forms of rat ghrelin peptide in gastrointestinal tissue. *Biochem. Biophys. Res. Commun.* 279, 909–913. doi: 10.1006/bbrc.2000.4039

Howard, A. D., Feighner, S. D., Cully, D. F., Arena, J. P., Liberator, P. A., Rosenblum, C. I., et al. (1996). A receptor in pituitary and hypothalamus that functions in growth hormone release. *Science* 273, 974–977. doi: 10.1126/science.273.5277.974

Kojima, M., Hosoda, H., Date, Y., Nakazato, M., Matsuo, H., and Kangawa, K. (1999). Ghrelin is a growth-hormone-releasing acylated peptide from stomach. *Nature* 402, 656–660. doi: 10.1038/45230

Lauwers, E., Landuyt, B., Arckens, L., Schoofs, L., and Luyten, W. (2006). Obestatin does not activate orphan G protein-coupled receptor GPR39. *Biochem. Biophys. Res. Commun.* 351, 21–25. doi: 10.1016/j.bbrc.2006.09.141

McKee, K. K., Tan, C. P., Palyha, O. C., Liu, J., Feighner, S. D., Hreniuk, D. L., et al. (1997). Cloning and characterization of two human G protein-coupled receptor genes (GPR38 and GPR39) related to the growth hormone secretagogue and neurotensin receptors. *Genomics* 46, 426–434. doi: 10.1006/geno.1997.5069

Mondal, M. S., Toshinai, K., Ueno, H., Koshinaka, K., and Nakazato, M. (2008). Characterization of obestatin in rat and human stomach and plasma, and its lack of acute effect on feeding behavior in rodents. *J. Endocrinol.* 198, 339–346. doi: 10.1677/JOE-08-0082

Seim, I., Herington, A. C., and Chopin, L. K. (2009). New insights into the molecular complexity of the ghrelin gene locus. *Cytokine Growth Factor Rev.* 20, 297–304. doi: 10.1016/j.cytogfr.2009.07.006

Seoane, L. M., Al-Massadi, O., Pazos, Y., Pagotto, U., and Casanueva, F. F. (2006). Central obestatin administration does not modify either spontaneous or ghrelin-induced food intake in rats. *J. Endocrinol. Invest.* 29, RC13–RC15. doi: 10.1007/BF03344174

Tolle, V., Bassant, M.-H., Zizzari, P., Poindessous-Jazat, F., Tomasetto, C., Epelbaum, J., et al. (2002). Ultradian rhythmicity of ghrelin secretion in relation with GH, feeding behavior, and sleep-wake patterns in rats. *Endocrinology* 143, 1353–1361. doi: 10.1210/endo.143.4.8712

Tolle, V., Zizzari, P., Tomasetto, C., Rio, M. C., Epelbaum, J., and Bluet-Pajot, M. T. (2001). *In vivo* and *in vitro* effects of ghrelin/motilin-related peptide on growth hormone secretion in the rat. *Neuroendocrinology* 73, 54–61. doi: 10.1159/000054620

Tomasetto, C., Karam, S. M., Ribieras, S., Masson, R., Lefèbvre, O., Staub, A., et al. (2000). Identification and characterization of a novel gastric peptide hormone: the motilin-related peptide. *Gastroenterology* 119, 395–405. doi: 10.1053/gast.2000.9371

Yamamoto, I., Numao, M., Sakaguchi, Y., Tsushima, N., and Tanaka, M. (2007). Molecular characterization of sequence and expression of chicken GPR39. *Gen. Comp. Endocrinol.* 151, 128–134. doi: 10.1016/j.ygcen.2006.12.002

Yang, J., Brown, M. S., Liang, G., Grishin, N. V., and Goldstein, J. L. (2008). Identification of the acyltransferase that octanoylates ghrelin, an appetite-stimulating peptide hormone. *Cell* 132, 387–396. doi: 10.1016/j.cell.2008.01.017

Zhang, J. V., Ren, P.-G., Avsian-Kretchmer, O., Luo, C.-W., Rauch, R., Klein, C., et al. (2005). Obestatin, a peptide encoded by the ghrelin gene, opposes ghrelin's effects on food intake. *Science* 310, 996–999. doi: 10.1126/science.1117255

Zizzari, P., Longchamps, R., Epelbaum, J., and Bluet-Pajot, M. T. (2007). Obestatin partially affects ghrelin stimulation of food intake and growth hormone secretion in rodents. *Endocrinology* 148, 1648–1653. doi: 10.1210/en.2006-1231

5

Hunger and Satiety Gauge Reward Sensitivity

Ryan Michael Cassidy and Qingchun Tong*

Brown Foundation of the Institute of Molecular Medicine for the Prevention of Human Diseases of McGovern Medical School, Neuroscience Program MD Anderson Cancer Center and UTHealth Graduate School of Biological Sciences, The University of Texas Health Science Center at Houston, Houston, TX, USA

***Correspondence:**
Ryan Michael Cassidy
ryan.m.cassidy@uth.tmc.edu

Many of the neurocircuits and hormones known to underlie the sensations of hunger and satiety also substantially alter the activity of the dopaminergic reward system. Much interest lies in the ways that hunger, satiety, and reward tie together, as the epidemic of obesity seems tied to the recent development and mass availability of highly palatable foods. In this review, we will first discuss the basic neurocircuitry of the midbrain and basal forebrain reward system. We will elaborate how several important mediators of hunger—the agouti-related protein neurons of the arcuate nucleus, the lateral hypothalamic nucleus, and ghrelin—enhance the sensitivity of the dopaminergic reward system. Then, we will elaborate how mediators of satiety—the nucleus tractus solitarius, pro-opiomelanocortin neurons of the arcuate nucleus, and its peripheral hormonal influences such as leptin—reduce the reward system sensitivity. We hope to provide a template by which future research may identify the ways in which highly rewarding foods bypass this balanced system to produce excessive food consumption.

Keywords: hunger, satiety, obesity, hypothalamus, reward, superstimulus, dopamine

INTRODUCTION

In evolutionary psychology, a supernormal stimulus or "superstimulus" is some evolutionarily novel concentration of engaging characteristics, which produces a stronger response than the natural one (1). As Pinker described it, strawberry cheesecake is a superstimulus as compared to a Neolithic human diet; it overloads the senses and drives caloric overconsumption, combining the "sweet taste of ripe fruit, the creamy mouth feel of fats and oils from nuts and meat, and the coolness of fresh water" (2). The debate is ongoing as to what exactly differentiates a superstimulus from a regular one or whether it is truly maladaptive to create them or seek them out (1). Nevertheless, an important concept for neuroscience emerges from this discussion; certain systems governing the reaction to rewarding stimulus can be overloaded and their negative feedback component overridden. This hypothesis provides explanation for the panoply of excessive behaviors we cope with as a society,

Abbreviations: AgRP, agouti-related protein; Arc, arcuate nucleus of the hypothalamus; CCK, cholecystokinin; D1R, D2R, dopamine receptors; GHS1R, growth hormone secretagogue 1 receptor (ghrelin receptor); GLP1/GLP1R, glucagon-like peptide 1/receptor; LepR, leptin receptor; LH, lateral hypothalamic area; LTD, long-term depression; LTP, long-term potentiation; MC3R, MC4R, melanocortin receptors; MCH/MCH1R, melanin concentrating hormone/receptor; MSH, melanocyte-stimulating hormone (natural MCR agonist); MSN, medium spiny neuron; MTII, melanotan II (non-selective MCR agonist); NAc, nucleus accumbens; NAcc, nucleus accumbens core; NAcSh, nucleus accumbens shell; NTS, nucleus tractus solitarius; O1R, O2R, orexin receptors; POMC, pro-opiomelanocortin; PPG, preproglucagon; PVH, paraventricular hypothalamic nucleus; VTA, ventral tegmental area.

often conceptualized as "behavioral addictions": drug addiction, internet addiction, porn addiction, food addiction, and so on (3). Even physical activity in some individuals meets the criteria for behavioral addiction, demonstrating the complex nature of this phenomenon (4). It is necessary to provide biological evidence for the existence of the balanced system which these superstimuli overload.

The neurocircuitry and endocrinology underlying hunger and satiety may represent the best studied system in this regard. It clearly produces a physiological balance in certain conditions with regular stimulus, such as a laboratory mouse fed rodent chow its whole life producing a normal weight, and is dysregulated in other conditions that contain superstimuli, such as when that mouse is fed a high-fat, high-carbohydrate diet producing obesity. The signals encoding hunger and satiety alter the brain's dopaminergic reward system in a multitude of ways. In this review, we will discuss the mechanisms by which these signals, primarily hypothalamic neurocircuits and neuropeptides in combination with peripheral hormones, modulate midbrain dopaminergic activity to alter reward salience and value. By laying out this evidence, we provide a substrate for future research to examine how superstimulus foods, such as cheesecake or high-fat/high-carbohydrate chow, drive so-called hedonic feeding and produce obesity.

The relationship of the midbrain dopaminergic reward system and hypothalamic neurocircuits governing hunger and satiety, hereafter referred to as the *reward system* and *hunger system*, is ancient. The patterned expression of genes necessary to produce segmentation of the brain at the mesencephalon (midbrain) and diencephalon (hypothalamus) occurred very early in chordate evolution (5, 6). Both dopamine neuronal receptors and hypothalamic feeding-related peptides and their associated receptors are present in most vertebrates and have similar functions across taxa (7–9). Given this intimate association, it is not surprising that they share a fundamental interdependence. For example, dopamine-deficient mice stop feeding a few weeks after birth; administration of L-DOPA reverses this phenotype and restores normal growth (10). Conversely, knockout of orexin, a hypothalamic neuropeptide associated with hunger, reduces dopamine response to cocaine (11). They also produce cross-sensitization or desensitization; food-restricted, hungry mice have enhanced response and reinforcement to amphetamine or cocaine (drugs which flood the brain with dopamine), and satiety signals such as leptin reduce the drive to seek self-administration of these drugs (12, 13). As will be discussed below, hypothalamic and endocrine components of the hunger system alter the activity of the reward system. To demonstrate this, we will first present a brief overview of the neurocircuitry of the reward system. Then, we will chart the various ways the hunger system interacts with the reward system.

NEUROCIRCUITRY OF THE REWARD SYSTEM

The Ventral Tegmental Area (VTA)

The VTA and substantia nigra pars compacta (SNc) are immediately caudal to the posterior hypothalamus, brace the third ventricle, and contain the major source of dopaminergic outflow to the rest of the brain. The SNc is best known for its role in the nigrostriatal pathway regulating the dorsal striatum in movement, and the VTA for mediating salience, motivation, and reward and aversion-related learning (14, 15). Salience refers to the attention paid to the stimulus; an increase in salience means the stimulus, if identified, will be more likely to draw the organism's attention. The value of the stimulus, whether it is rewarding or aversive, refers to whether a stimulus induces behavior to acquire it or avoid it, respectively (15). Rewarding stimuli produce a positive valence when acquired and a negative valence when unable to be acquired; the converse is true with aversive stimuli (15).

The VTA dopaminergic neurons are the primary mediators of the behavioral response to a rewarding or aversive stimulus (16). They are not uniform in their activity or projection targets, and thus activation of one neuron may produce substantially different behavioral output than another. This is why studies evaluating the rewarding nature of dopamine often focus on the VTA to nucleus accumbens (NAc) projections specifically; this will be discussed below. However, much effort has been spent elucidating the ways in which local VTA dopaminergic neurons encode reward across brain regions by alteration in firing pattern, increase or decrease in action potential frequency, and projection target. The literature is incomplete on this topic, but discussion of some of these mechanisms sets the stage for further discussion of how the hunger system interfaces with the VTA dopaminergic neurons. For example, *in vivo* recording of the VTA during a conditioned place preference task suggests that one subset of dopaminergic neurons exhibits phasic activation in response to reward-related cues or reward consumption; another exhibits phasic inhibition in response to aversive stimulus or the absence of reward consumption after a reward cue (17). Tonic activation of dopaminergic neurons can produce the opposite effect of phasic activity on the same target and will decrease reward consumption (18). Thus, a given projection target receives either increased or decreased dopamine input dependent on the valence of the reward. Furthermore, dopaminergic neurons vary in their projection targets; the VTA's projections are heterogeneous. Dependent on the projection target, an increase in dopamine outflow produces either rewarding or aversive responses (14, 19). As has been well-established, VTA projections to the NAc core (NAcc) and NAc shell (NAcSh) increase dopamine release in response to a rewarding stimulus and induce goal-direct behavior to acquire and consume it (14). Conversely, VTA dopaminergic neurons projecting to the medial prefrontal cortex are activated in response to an aversive stimulus and produce aversive behaviors (19). However, even within the same target, dopaminergic activation can code both types of behaviors; VTA dopaminergic projections to the lateral portion of the NAcSh are activated in response to both rewarding and aversive stimulus (19).

The VTA also possesses neurons releasing the classic neurotransmitters glutamate and GABA. The function of these glutamatergic and GABAergic neurons is less well-known, but recent evidence indicates they also participate in valence-related responses. VTA glutamatergic projections to the lateral habenula

(LHb) play a significant role in encoding aversive learning (20). VTA glutamatergic projections to the NAcSh act in concert with the dopaminergic projections to produce reward-mediated behavior (14). Finally, VTA GABAergic neurons projecting to the LHb appear to inhibit this area to enhance positive valence responses (21). Recent analysis has identified that some VTA neurons corelease glutamate and dopamine—it is as yet unknown whether this occurs at the same synapse or at separate synaptic targets (14). Further research is needed to fully evaluate how the classic fast-acting neurotransmitters coordinate with dopaminergic neurons to produce the full suite of valence-related behaviors and alter future learned responses.

The NAc

The NAc is part of the ventral striatum and extended amygdala in the basal forebrain, and it mediates much of the motivated behavior produced in response to VTA dopaminergic outflow after sensation of a rewarding stimulus. Many components of the hunger system act here as well as in the VTA to alter the responsiveness to rewarding stimulus; thus, some description of its components and basic activity follows. The NAc is divided into a medial shell (NAcSh) and lateral core (NAcc). Self-administration of cocaine into the NAcSh is highly rewarding and rapidly produces cue-responsiveness with locomotor sensitization to anticipation of the drug (22–24). Self-administration of cocaine into the NAcc, however, is not reinforcing (22). Phasic activity of VTA dopaminergic projections to the NAcc instead responds to risk and prediction error in response to reward presentation (22, 24, 25). Thus, a basic paradigm can be constructed, where the NAcc responds to the salience, availability, and risk of acquiring the reward to produce motivation to pursue it, and the NAcSh responds to the positive valence of the reward acquisition, learns the cues which associate with the reward, and enhances the future salience of those cues. Interestingly, if dopamine is depleted in the NAc but reward acquisition is low effort, rats will still take the reward; however, if it requires high effort, rats will choose less effort-requiring behaviors (26). Thus, the level of dopamine in the NAc may provide a rough proxy for the amount of motivation an animal has to ignore risk and effort costs of acquiring a reward.

Both the shell and the core are inhibitory on all downstream targets; the vast majority of neurons are the GABAergic medium spiny neurons (MSNs). These are divided by receptor profile. There are D1R-MSNs, possessing excitatory D1R-like dopamine receptors (D1R and D5R), and D2R-MSNs, possessing inhibitory D2R-like dopamine receptors (D2R, D3R, and D4R). A significant minority express both receptor subtypes (27). The projection fields of the NAcSh and NAcc are wide and differ from each other in several important respects for their mediation of behavior. The NAcSh densely projects to the ventromedial ventral pallidum, lateral hypothalamic area (LH), and lateral preoptic area, whereas the NAcc projects to the dorsolateral ventral pallidum, subthalamic nucleus, and substantia nigra pars reticulata (22). The NAcSh shares significant reciprocal connections with feeding-related areas of the hypothalamus, whereas the NAcc primarily interacts with the basal ganglia. Thus, the NAcSh responds more to signals from the hunger system than the NAcc and will feature more prominently in this discussion.

HUNGER NEUROCIRCUITS SELECT FOR INCREASED REWARD SYSTEM ACTIVITY IN THE PRESENCE OF FOOD

There are numerous and dense interconnections between the hypothalamic nuclei, VTA, and NAc, and a wealth of neuropeptide and neurocircuit data exists to support the powerful influence of the several hypothalamic nuclei and their specific neuronal subtypes on the reward system. The interaction is complex and dynamic, depending upon both the availability of food and the endocrine manipulation of the system, as will be discussed later. A summary of the major hunger and satiety neurocircuits influencing the reward system is shown in **Figure 1**.

Arcuate Nucleus

The arcuate nucleus of the hypothalamus (Arc) sits adjacent to the third ventricle immediately ventral to the paraventricular hypothalamic nucleus (PVH). These two nuclei share the distinction of integrating central nervous system (CNS) input into the hypothalamic–pituitary axis and are the major source of the "releasing hormones," which are secreted into the hypophyseal portal veins to alter anterior pituitary production of various hormones. Thus, the Arc possesses a multitude of neuronal populations defined by their neuropeptide content, such as gonadotropin-releasing hormone neurons, growth hormone releasing hormone neurons, kisspeptin neurons, tuberoinfundibular dopamine (TIDA) neurons regulating prolactin release, somatostatin neurons, and so on. Many of these neurons alter feeding behavior, but their interaction with the dopaminergic reward system is poorly understood at this point in time (28). Thus, our discussion will focus on the agouti-related protein (AgRP)/neuropeptide Y (NPY) neurons that govern hunger and TIDA neurons role in feeding behavior. The pro-opiomelanocortin (POMC) neurons that govern satiety will be discussed later.

AgRP/NPY-Expressing Neurons

The AgRP/NPY-expressing neurons are found solely within the Arc (29). NPY acts on NPY receptors (Y1, Y2, Y4, and Y5 which are G_iPCRs) (30). AgRP is an inverse agonist of melanocortin receptors (MCRs; MC3R and MC4R, which are G_sPCRs and MAPK pathway activators) (31–35). Perhaps because of this, these neurons share with POMC neurons the same set of connections with hypothalamic and extrahypothalamic nuclei (29, 36). Thus, AgRP neurons are strong inhibitors of their downstream targets *via* GABA release, inverse agonism of MC-Rs, and NPYR-Gi activity. These neurons respond to a wide array of peripheral and central signals of energy balance, such as leptin, ghrelin, low glucose concentration, and gustatory sensation, and are activated during fasting (37–41). Surprisingly, given this role, knockout of AgRP by itself or in combination with NPY does not produce any obvious phenotype either in *ad libitum* or starvation feeding conditions—only in old age do they demonstrate slightly reduced body weight and adiposity due to increased metabolic

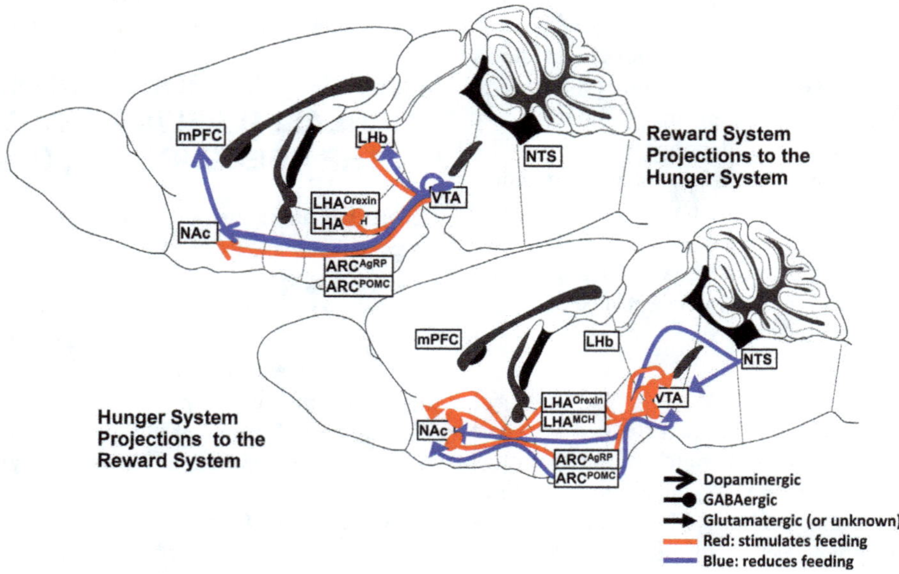

FIGURE 1 | Hunger and satiety neurocircuits interface with the midbrain–basal forebrain reward pathway.

rate (42, 43). Furthermore, neonatal destruction of the AgRP/NPY neurons has minimal effect on feeding; only adult ablation of these neurons prevents feeding behavior and leads mice in this condition to starve to death (44–46). Interestingly, several AgRP/NPY neuronal projections are not formed until a week postnatal in mice, such as to the PVH; there are many opportunities for developmental compensation to alter the neonatal AgRP/NPY ablation phenotype, which deserve further study to understand the homeostasis of feeding behavior (47). Much recent effort has been spent on understanding the acute dynamics of AgRP/NPY neuronal activity in hunger and reward.

Optogenetic stimulation produces food seeking and food consuming behaviors, with enhanced risk-taking and reduced anxiety (48–51). Their activity is aversive, as mice avoid the side of a chamber associated with their optogenetic activation (52). AgRP neurons select for food consumption; when activated, they reduce motivation to engage in other behaviors such as social interactions or drinking water when thirsty (51). Sustained AgRP neuronal activity is not necessary to produce feeding, and *in vivo* recording demonstrates that these neurons stop firing in the presence of food cues (53). Further optogenetic evidence demonstrates that a brief period of activation, prior to presentation with any food stimulus, will produce subsequent feeding, enhanced motivation to work for food, and selection for calorie dense foods (54). As strength of AgRP signal increases, there is a first-order kinetic increase in length of feeding and motivation to work which saturates (54). Stimulating AgRP projections to the PVH, bed nucleus of the stria terminalis, or LH are all individually sufficient to produce this effect (54). However, AgRP neurons also synapse on the VTA and regulate the reward system through this connection. AgRP projections to the VTA inhibit dopaminergic and glutamatergic release in the NAc and reduce the development of long-term potentiation (LTP) (55). It can be argued that AgRP neurons in the Arc reduce activity of the reward system while activating the hunger system, priming it to respond to food and not other stimuli; once food is spotted, cessation of AgRP neuronal activity releases the brakes on the reward system to enhance dopaminergic outflow. The increase in dopamine in the NAc likely increases the willingness to work for food and take risks to acquire it.

TIDA Neurons

The dopaminergic neurons of the Arc regulate the release of prolactin from the anterior pituitary. A subset of TIDA neurons appear to be functionally distinct from governing prolactin; these corelease GABA and dopamine, and deletion of prolactin receptor within this subpopulation has no effect on prolactin secretion regulation (56). A recent study demonstrated that optogenetic stimulation of these neurons produces feeding behavior independent of their stimulation of prolactin release, and inhibition of these neurons reduces body weight (57). Activation of these neurons, which are ghrelin sensitive, inhibited POMC neurons and excited AgRP/NPY neurons. While these are not considered part of the dopaminergic reward system, their role in detecting the intersection of hunger and reward is relevant to this discussion as any manipulation altering whole-brain dopamine systems (such as dopamine reuptake inhibitors such as cocaine) will alter the activity of these neurons and may subtly alter the phenotype.

The Lateral Hypothalamus

One of the major downstream targets of AgRP neurons is the LH. This was classically understood as both a hunger center and reward hot spot from early lesion and electrical stimulation studies. The LH has extensive projections divided by multiple subpopulations of neurons that express various neuropeptides as well as solely fast-acting neurotransmitter neurons (58). Many of these fast-acting projections play a role in mediating hunger and reward. LH glutamatergic projections to the LHb prevent consumption of a conditioned reward of sucrose and has negative valence (59). Inhibition of this same projection has positive valence and induces sucrose consumption. Conversely, LH GABAergic projections appear to mediate consumption; activation of LH GABAergic neurons produces consumption regardless of the target's food value, such as ethanol, water, saccharin, sucrose, or wood (60). The projection targets of the LH GABAergic neurons may relate to different aspects of this behavior. For example, LH GABAergic projections to the PVH produce directed food consumption (61). However, activation of the LH-VTA GABAergic projections produce non-directed gnawing and licking of immediately available objects, despite the availability of a sucrose reward distant from the mouse (62). These LH-VTA GABAergic neurons inhibit both a subpopulation of dopaminergic and GABAergic neurons within the VTA. Interestingly, the reciprocal VTA-LH projection is observed to be activated in response to reward omission; the disorganized feeding behavior from LH-VTA projection may occur because of the lack of this feedback information (62). Indeed, a recent study evaluating lateral septum inhibitory influence on the LH found that one subset of LH GABAergic neurons are activated during food approach and another during food consumption, indicating that a temporal sequence of GABAergic subpopulation activation occurs to produce successful food consumption (63).

Orexin Neurons

Another reciprocal functional relationship between LH neuronal subtypes can be found in orexin (hypocretin) and melanin-concentrating hormone (MCH) neuropeptide-expressing neurons. Orexin, as the name suggests, is an orexigenic or food consumption-inducing neuropeptide released primarily by glutamatergic neurons in the medial and dorsal portions of the LH. Orexin A and B are co-released from the same neurons and bind to their receptors O1R and O2R, potently inducing arousal *via* G_s signaling. Orexin release dramatically increases in release in the human amygdala upon waking up or during arousing positive stimuli such as laughing or talking (64). Orexinergic neurons are activated in response to learned reward cues, but not novel objects; for example, activating them can reinstate extinguished drug-seeking behavior (65). Indeed, O2R protein levels in the NAc are elevated for up to 60 days after discontinuation of repeated cocaine administration (66). They are depolarized in response to low glucose, and directly activate VTA dopaminergic neurons which project to both the medial and lateral portions of the NAcSh (67). Orexin receptors also exist within both of these subdivisions; injection of Orexin A into the medial NAcSh induces a sucrose pleasure-associated facial response, whereas injection into the lateral NAcSh induces a sucrose seeking reaction (68). O1R activation increases NMDA glutamate receptor activity, a sign of LTP formation, whereas blockade of O1R in the VTA reduces the rate of self-administration of cocaine or chocolate (11, 69). Thus, orexinergic neurons clearly enhance the seeking and acquisition of a learned reward, partially *via* activation of the dopaminergic pathway as well as potentially enhancing the reinforcing quality of those rewards.

MCH Neurons

Melanin-concentrating hormone neurons are released from the anatomically adjacent dorsolateral LH and have a complex reciprocal relationship with orexin neurons. They linked with induction of sleep and directly inhibit orexin neurons *via* the MCH receptor (MCH1R) G_i protein coupled signaling (70). Their interaction with feeding behavior is complex. Knockdown of MCH1R produces hyperphagia, hyperactivity with increased foraging behaviors; however, these mice have a baseline lower body weight than controls, gain less weight on a high-fat diet, and exhibit an increased metabolic rate (71, 72). Elevation of glucose concentration from fasting levels to fed-state levels inhibits orexin neurons and depolarizes MCH neurons. It appears that MCHergic activity appears to play a role in placing a brake on orexin-induced seeking and consuming behaviors after food is acquired (73). However, injection of MCH into the lateral ventricle increases food consumption, without producing long-term weight gain (74). It appears that MCH neurons integrate olfactory, taste, and gut sensory input about the nutritional value of food and project to the VTA, NAc, and dorsal striatum in order to enhance the rewarding value of nutritionally valuable foods (75, 76). To this end, optogenetic stimulation of MCH neurons increases dopamine levels in the striatum only when paired with active consumption of an artificial sweetener; without stimulation, only caloric foods like sucrose induce this dopamine release (76). Pairing these stimuli produced a future preference for the artificial sweetener over sucrose—opposite of the control mouse preference. As further evidence of this, ablation of MCH neurons prevented the natural spike of dopamine in the striatum after the consumption of sucrose—though, interestingly, it did not ablate preference for sweet flavor over water, indicating that other mechanisms are at play (76). Thus, MCH neuronal activity increases when olfaction, taste, and gut nutrient sensors indicate that the food under active consumption is calorically valuable; it enhances the rewarding value of food by increasing VTA dopaminergic activity in the NAc.

The pattern of MCH1R activation within the NAc is similarly complex and deserves some further discussion. These receptors are coexpressed with D1R and D2R on opioid-producing MSNs. Activation of MCH1R here induces feeding and causes a depressed phenotype on the forced swim test, implying reduced locomotor drive (77, 78). Given that MCH1R is inhibitory, it is unsurprising that MSNs have decreased membrane excitability and reduced AMPA glutamatergic receptor currents; furthermore, antagonism of MCH1R reduces cocaine self-administration or cue-induced reinstatement of cocaine seeking behavior. However, on MSNs which coexpress D1R, D2R, and MCH1R, there is a unique synergy which enhances their firing activity and activates a phosphorylation cascade known to increase NMDA receptor activation (79). Some of this response is opioid dependent, as blockade of any of the three opioid receptors in the NAcSh prevents MCH-induced facial pleasure expression in response to oral gavage of sucrose (80). It appears that MCH1R activity within the NAc may shift the reward system response to enhance immediate food consumption and learning the nutrient value of food and dampen the seeking function of the reward system.

Hunger Enhances Sensitivity to Reward

The above discussion details how several neuronal populations—AgRP/NPY neurons, LH GABAergic neurons, orexin neurons, and MCH neurons—each alter the activity of the reward system in a distinct way as part of their contribution to the sensation of hunger. AgRP neurons reduce reward system sensitivity and inhibit its function until food is detected. The food cue silences their activity, disinhibiting the VTA and NAc to produce a large increase in dopamine release. This increases both the salience and value of the food cue. A subset of LH GABAergic neurons act in concert with orexin neurons to respond to these cues and produce food-seeking behavior, enhancing VTA dopaminergic release into the NAc. Other LH GABAergic neurons act with MCH neurons to also enhance the rewarding value of food and increase learning of nutritionally valuable food-related cues, producing food consumption. Once this process begins, satiety neurocircuits begin to act in order to limit overconsumption, as will be detailed below.

SATIETY NEUROCIRCUITS DECREASE THE ACTIVITY OF THE REWARD SYSTEM

The neurocircuitry of satiety is not as well-known as that of hunger. The general paradigm appears to be as follows: peripheral signals of positive energy balance, primarily hormonal, travel to the brain to inhibit the activity of hunger-producing neurocircuits. However, three populations of neurons within the CNS, defined by their neuropeptide content, are activated by these signals and directly influence the reward system. These are the POMC neurons of the Arc, the POMC neurons of the nucleus tractus solitarius (NTS), and the preproglucagon (PPG) neurons of the NTS. The NTS neurons integrate peripheral satiety signals, such as leptin, cholecystokinin (CCK), glucagon-like peptide 1 (GLP1), and gut distention, to induce rapid satiety. The role of POMC neurons is more complex, but appears to reduce the immediate value of the food reward while maintaining future responsiveness to that same reward.

PPG Neurons in NTS

The NTS has multiple functions both related to primary routing of taste information as well as being the routing point for significant amounts of autonomic and peripheral hormonal information entering the brain. It is situated in the dorsal motor vagal nerve complex and receives the vagal sensory afferents. These afferents are activated by GLP1, CCK, and leptin. The first two are released from stomach and intestinal cells and leptin from adipocytes in response to increased nutrient availability. They all synergistically increase the activity of the GLP1 producing neurons (termed PPG, or PPG neurons) in the NTS (81, 82).

The PPG NTS neurons have a wide projection field and synapse directly onto the VTA and NAc (83). Intestinally released GLP1 does not appear to cross the blood–brain barrier (BBB), and GLP1 receptor (GLP1R) signaling in the midbrain and basal forebrain requires NTS-mediated release of GLP1 (84). Activating GLP1R decreases highly palatable food intake and produces long-term weight loss; conversely, inhibiting them increases food consumption (83). Both changes occur due to changes in meal size, not frequency, indicating their role in terminating meal consumption. GLP1R activity in the VTA reduces LTP formation on dopaminergic neuron (85). GLP1 administration significantly increases dopamine transporter expression, increasing dopamine clearance from the synapse (86). GLP1R activity in the reward system may act to place the brakes on dopaminergic response to nutrient contents in the gut and prevent excessive learning of a food reward—or any reward, given the wide applicability of the reward system pathway. Consistent with this prediction, GLP1R knockout mice exhibit enhanced reward learning on the conditioned place preference test and increased cocaine-induced locomotion—receptor agonism had the inverse effect (87, 88). Thus, the PPG NTS neurons clearly mediate a dopamine-dampening function in the reward system and use this as a mechanism to reduce the reward salience and value of food or other objects.

POMC Neurons in the NTS and the Arcuate Nucleus

The role of POMC neurons is more complex, and much effort has been expended to explore their role in satiety. POMC is a precursor polypeptide which is cleaved by prohormone convertase 1 or 2 into α-, β-, or γ-melanocyte-stimulating hormone (MSH), corticotropin, and β-endorphin (89). These neuropeptides act *via* the MCR family, the best studied of which in regard to satiety are MC3R and MC4R. Deletion of MC4R produces obesity and hyperphagia; furthermore, the most common syndromic cause of obesity, Prader–Willi, occurs in part due to reduced cleavage of POMC (90, 91). The NTS and Arc POMC neurons both drive satiety *via* their actions on their receptors, but at different time scales. Optogenetic stimulation of the POMC NTS immediately halts feeding, but long-term activation does not produce weight loss (92). Stimulation of POMC Arc neurons has no immediate effect on feeding, but over many hours reduces feeding and produces weight loss (37). Both populations of POMC neurons project to the NAc and VTA—however, evidence is lacking on what effect direct stimulation of these projections produces (36). Both GABA-expressing and glutamate-expressing neurons have been found within the POMC neurons of the arcuate nucleus; but, the effects of fast neurotransmission from these neurons are not well explored (93). Instead, this discussion will focus on the pharmacological and receptor-related data that exist on the role of MC3R and MC4R in these regions.

MCR Signaling

The pharmacological effects of MCR activation are complex and their signaling mechanisms require some discussion before elaborating on their influence on the reward system. Multiple endogenous ligands for melanocortins exist. AgRP is an inverse agonist of MC3R and MC4R. α-, β-, and γ-MSHs and adrenocorticotropin hormone are produced from POMC by alternative cleavage and have varying affinities for each MCR type. Their downstream signaling activity is significantly altered dependent on their heterodimerization with other receptors such as dopamine receptors or ghrelin receptors. MC4R can couple with G_s, G_q, or $G_{i/o}$ protein complexes dependent upon allosteric binding-related conformational changes and thus produce increases in intracellular calcium, increased cAMP signaling, or inhibit these same pathways (33). The two neuron-activating pathways, G_s and G_q, mediate distinct physiologic effects; knockout of PVH G_q, but not G_s, prevented the efficacy of MC4R agonism to prevent food intake (94). Conversely, the ghrelin receptor, when coupled with either MC3R or MC4R, selects for G_s signaling in both proteins in the PVH, for example, emphasizing that in conditions of increased hunger, MSH activity may select for activation (95). One of the most commonly used non-selective synthetic MCR agonists, melanotan II (MTII), also selects for G_s signaling (33, 95). AgRP, discussed above, is an inverse agonist of MC4R and reduces cAMP levels independent of the presence of any agonist (33–35). Hypothetically, AgRP activity may select for the G_i signaling conformation of MC4R, as it both antagonizes the ligand-binding site and binds to the allosteric site to cause a conformational change; it also induces receptor internalization and alters MC4R-mediated inhibition of L-type calcium channel activity (31–33, 96). While it has been demonstrated conclusively that intracerebroventricular infusion of the MC3R/MC4R agonist α-MSH suppresses feeding and infusion of AgRP suppresses feeding, the multiple signaling pathways invoked by each ligand as compared to MTII are important considerations while evaluating the pharmacological data for melanocortin influence on the reward system (97).

MC4R is found on D1R MSNs in the NAc. Application of α-MSH to *ex vivo* brain slices produces a decreased post-synaptic ratio of AMPA/NMDA glutamatergic receptor signaling and fewer excitatory post-synaptic currents—a sign of long-term depression (LTD) (98). These MC4R-linked D1R MSNs synapse onto LH GABAergic neurons; optogenetic activation of these prevents feeding (99). This reduction in feeding also occurs by MCR activity in the VTA; injection of MTII decreases sucrose consumption (100). Thus, MC4R activity may increase activity of these neurons to inhibit feeding, but lose their synaptic strength to prevent excessive inhibition of feeding behavior and simultaneously reduce their rewarding value. This coincides with evidence that administration of MC4R shRNA (knockdown) prevents the natural decrease in reward seeking induced by a chronic stress paradigm (98). Furthermore, blockade of NAc MC4R prevents chronic stress-elicited anhedonia, a known low-dopamine phenomenon (98).

However, in other conditions MCRs may play a role in reward-mediated learning and sensitivity to reward. After 2 h, intraventricular injection of MTII reduced the threshold for brain self-stimulation (101). Furthermore, mice with knockdown or inhibition of MC4R display reduced cocaine-induced reinforcement and reduced locomotor sensitization (102, 103). Injection of alpha-MSH into the posterior VTA increases the activity of MC4R-expressing dopaminergic neurons and induces ethanol self-administration (104). These neurons coexpress MC3R, and agonism of these neurons with γ-MSH increases motivation to work for sucrose reward in a dopamine-dependent fashion (105). Indeed, it appears that the level of glucose increase in response to food intake induces excitatory synaptic plasticity in a subpopulation of POMC neurons, which may enhance some of these downstream dopaminergic responses (106).

Thus, the multiple combinations of POMC cleavage products, the heterodimerization and allosteric-binding configurations of MCRs, and the differences in activity dependent on brain region all indicate that further evaluation of intracellular signaling pathways is needed. However, a possible synthesis may be as follows. MC4R signaling reduces ongoing feeding *via* its action on D1R MSNs in the NAc, with a naturally decaying signal because of the development of LTD. Simultaneously, in other regions and neuronal subpopulations, MC3R and MC4R enhance synaptic plasticity to encode future responses to that food reward—hence, knockdown of these receptors reduces reward consumption. The balance of melanocortin-mediated LTP and LTD in striatal neurons is important to halt ongoing food consumption, but appropriately encourage future responsiveness to rewarding food cues. One demonstration of this phenomena arises when hyperphagic MC4R knockout mice have induced second deletion of synapse-associated protein 90/post-synaptic density protein 95-associated protein 3 (SAPAP3) in the striatum (90). This double deletion both cures the compulsive grooming behavior of these mice and normalizes their weight. Deletion of SAPAP3 induces excessive LTD formation, and one may postulate that this helps reduce the excessive excitatory synapses formed in the VTA by unchecked MC3R signaling that in turn promote feeding behavior (107).

FOOD-RELATED HORMONES INFLUENCE DOPAMINERGIC ACTIVITY AND SENSITIVITY TO REWARD

The above discussion has focused on the interaction between neurons encoding hunger and satiety and the reward system. However, these are all interoceptive and are responsible for the integration of internal and external sensory information to produce unified behaviors. As is to be expected, the sensory input into this system is both neuronal (gut distention, pain, olfaction, taste, etc.) and endocrine. While the vast majority of endocrine pathways are altered in some way in response to variations in energy stores and the presence or absence of food in the gut, the best studied of these which appear to act directly on the reward system are the hunger hormone ghrelin and the satiety hormone leptin.

Ghrelin

Ghrelin is a peptide hormone first discovered as an endogenous ligand of the growth hormone secretagogue receptor (GHS1R), produced in the oxyntic glands of the stomach (108). Copies of ghrelin mRNA and ghrelin immunoreactivity are found in abundance in the antrum and fundus of the stomach and to a lesser degree in the duodenum, jejunum, ileum, and pancreas (109–111). Both peripheral and intracerebroventricular injections of ghrelin produce feeding in mice, and knockout of neuronal GHS1R prevents the development of diet-induced obesity; this places the CNS activity of ghrelin as a primary mediator of ghrelin's orexigenic effect (112, 113).

The mechanics governing ghrelin release and the neuronal response to ghrelin are complex and deserve some consideration. Ghrelin secretion occurs in ultradian pulses, peaking immediately before onset of meals and declining soon after, with the greatest rise occurring overnight preceding breakfast (114). Several neurotransmitters, hormones, and metabolic signals also affect ghrelin release; acetylcholine, CCK, gastrointestinal peptide, and low glucose concentration enhance it, whereas insulin, gastrin, somatostatin, GLP-1, and increasing glucose concentration inhibit its release (115–117). Once ghrelin is produced, it can undergo post-translational modification with fatty acid linkage (octanoylation). This appears to affect ghrelin transport across the BBB; human octanoylated ghrelin and mouse des-octanoyl ghrelin are preferentially transported into the brain, whereas mouse octanoylated ghrelin (with two amino acid differences) is preferentially transported into the blood (118). The rate of BBB transport is enhanced by elevated serum triglycerides and fasting and blunted in aging, indicating physiological state modulation of this mechanism (119). There is also some evidence suggesting that a subpopulation of ghrelin-producing neurons may exist within the hypothalamus itself, which would not be affected by BBB transport and would have entirely unique, as yet undescribed, regulation (38). Finally, GHS1R-Gq-induced calcium flux (i.e., the signal strength) is attenuated by its heterodimerization with serotonin (specifically 5-HT2C), dopamine (D1R), and melanocortin (MC3R) receptors (120). Given that GHS1R possesses one of the highest levels of basal Gq activity of any GPCR, this dimerization may be important for reducing basal signaling except in the presence of the appropriate ligands for each receptor, potentiating the signal strength of the ghrelin-GHS1R active conformation or increasing GHS1R Gq-signaling *via* dedimerization after dopamine-D1R or serotonin-5-HT2C interactions (121).

After integrating the influences of pulsivity, BBB transport, and heterodimerization considered, ghrelin induces feeding behavior by depolarizing neurons expressing GHS1R. Chief among these, AgRP/NPY neurons express GHS1R-G_q-coupled signaling; this produces feeding behavior and reduced thermogenesis (112, 122). Thus, in the absence of any food cues, ghrelin actually reduces sensitivity to reward, acting *via* AgRP/NPY neurons and inhibiting the VTA and NAc as described earlier. However, GHS1R is also found in the VTA and laterodorsal VTA, a source of midbrain acetylcholine; injecting ghrelin into either of these places increases locomotor activity, food consumption, and NAc dopamine levels (123). Indeed, ghrelin enhances the rewarding value of high fat diet in *ad libitum*-fed mice (124). If no food is consumed after VTA ghrelin injection, VTA GABAergic neurons increase activity and reduce the release of dopamine into the NAc (123). These effects occur both due to ghrelin action on the VTA cell body and by alteration of pre-synaptic activity, especially the LH as orexin-deficient mice are resistant to the effect of ghrelin (40, 124–126).

These effects may be cross-sensitive for non-food rewards such as alcohol and amphetamines. In recovering alcoholics, ghrelin injection increases craving for alcohol; coincident with this, ghrelin receptor blockade attenuates both alcohol and amphetamine-induced locomotion sensitization (127–130). However, once sensitization has occurred, blockade of ghrelin transport into the brain does not appear to alter alcohol-induced locomotor activity or expression of conditioned place preference in rats (131). Thus, ghrelin may act to enhance learning of non-food rewards, but not be necessary to express this preference (132). Notably, GHS1R is found in the hippocampus; here it may enhance dopamine-induced synaptic plasticity within the hippocampus, promoting retention of the food-related reward *via* GHS1R-D1R heterodimer interactions (133).

Ghrelin action in gaging reward sensitivity can be summarized in three ways. First, by acting on AgRP/NPY neurons, it selects for food-seeking and food-consuming behavior and ignoring of other rewards. Second, by acting on the VTA, it increases the amplitude of dopamine release once cue-mediated silencing of AgRP/NPY neurons disinhibits these regions. Third, by acting on the hippocampus, it promotes dopamine-induced synaptic plasticity and future salience of the reward cue. Given the complexity and numerous levels of signal modification in the ghrelin system, future research will undoubtedly expand upon this story.

Leptin

Leptin is a signal of positive energy balance and appears to exert a dampening effect on the reward system. Leptin is a protein hormone released by white adipose tissue in pulses, highest around midnight in humans; the amplitude of each pulse directly correlates with the total amount of adipose tissue (114, 134). Glucose, insulin, glucocorticoids, TNF-alpha, and IL-6 all increase leptin release (134). Leptin acts on its receptors (leptin receptor, LepR), which are located in the CNS, particularly the hypothalamus. It can influence neuronal activity from the blood *via* action on the circumventricular organs and vagal afferents and is also translocated across the BBB *via* the action of tanycytes (135). The Arc, ventromedial and dorsomedial hypothalamus, LH, and NTS most densely express LepRs, and leptin action can be either inhibitory or excitatory on these neurons to inhibit food consumption and induce satiety (136). LepR also exists within the VTA on the dopaminergic projections to the extended central amygdala; exciting these neurons reduces food intake (137–139). This is consistent with the central amygdala's role in mediating the stress response.

Other populations of LepR expressing dopaminergic neurons have their activity inhibited by leptin and produce a general reward-dampening effect. Direct administration of leptin into the VTA and into the Arc increases the threshold for brain self-stimulation reward and decreases food intake (140). Conversely, knockdown or inhibition of LepRs within the VTA increases dopamine release onto the NAc and enhances cocaine-conditioned place preference (13). LepR depletion within the NAc core mediates the same effect (13). Interestingly, it also prevented D2R agonism from reducing cocaine reinforcement, implying that there is some synergy between LepR inhibitory action and D2R's reduction of synaptic plasticity mechanisms (13). This may occur *via* LepR activation of the signal transducer and activator of transcription 3 signaling pathway in the VTA, which reduces both feeding behavior and motivation to exercise (141). Finally, the hyperleptinemia of diet-induced obesity is also sufficient to produce the generalized reward-dampening effects described above. Mice with diet-induced obesity have reduced drive to self-administer cocaine, express less amphetamine conditioned place preference, and are less likely to express operant response to sucrose (142, 143). These mice are demonstrated to have reduced dopamine turnover in the NAc (142, 143). Interestingly, alcohol consumption does not appear to follow this paradigm. Leptin administration significantly increased the consumption of ethanol in mice exposed to an ethanol deprivation-then-reinstatement procedure (144). High leptin levels at onset of alcohol withdrawal in humans were predictive of cravings and alcohol relapse; anti-opioid receptor drugs used to prevent relapse reduced leptin levels (145). Future research is necessary to understand how alcohol bypasses the dopaminergic reward system pathway to induce opioid release in a leptin-potentiated manner. Nevertheless, leptin clearly induces satiety by directly reducing activity of both the hunger system and the reward system, with generalizable reduction of the salience and value of both food and non-food rewards.

LIMITATIONS IN THE STUDY OF THE INTERFACE BETWEEN THE HUNGER AND REWARD SYSTEMS

The above reviewed evidence is not comprehensive, as the relationship between the hunger system and reward system is of great interest and under active research with exciting new evidence unveiled daily. Given the ancient association of these two systems and the necessity of proper balance of food consumption to sustain life, it is understandable that nearly every neuronal and endocrine system appears to alter food consumption and manipulate the reward system in some way. Furthermore, the developmental activity of these systems may differ from their adult activity, and disruptions to these systems may result in significant compensation over the developmental period. The techniques utilized to study feeding and reward behavior are also limited by the necessity of overactivation, for an extended period, a single node within the feeding system. Given the interconnected nature of these neuronal circuits within the hunger system, continuous activation of any part likely engages the other portions and produces the unified behavioral response. However, it is likely that each neuronal pathway described above does not independently induce or inhibit food or reward consumption, but instead activates a certain portion of a "reward consumption sequence." A clear example of this is how LH-VTA GABAergic activation induces gnawing and licking behaviors, but not sucrose seeking (62). The nature of this reward consumption sequence remains to be uncovered, and will likely require further molecular characterization of each of these components of the reward sequence, *in vivo* recording of their activity, and more advanced optogenetic and chemogenetic stimulation techniques to better approximate physiological activity.

CONCLUSION

The hunger system manipulates the reward system to increase the salience and value of food and enhance future response to rewarding food cues. Ghrelin and AgRP neurons prime the reward system to activate only in the presence of food cues. LH fast neurotransmitters and orexin neurons produce food-seeking paradigm in response to a learned cue. Other LH GABAergic neurons and MCH neurons increase food consumption, reducing reward seeking behavior and producing reward consuming behavior by their action on the VTA and NAc. Early satiety signals like GLP1 and CCK put the brakes on food consumption by dampening reward system activity, reducing its value. POMC neuronal activity produces a balanced synaptic plasticity to respond effectively to future food stimulus, while gradually inducing satiety. Late satiety signals like leptin dampen reward system activity generally to reduce effort for acquiring food or other rewards while in a positive energy state. A summary of these effects is presented in **Table 1**.

TABLE 1 | Hunger system activity and influence on the reward system.

	Fasting state	Food cue response	Feeding and fed state
Arcuate agouti-related protein (AgRP)/ neuropeptide Y neurons	Inhibits reward system activity	Decreased activity	Decreased activity
Lateral hypothalamic area (LH) GABAergic neurons	Unknown	Inhibit subpopulation ventral tegmental area (VTA) DA and GABAergic neurons	Inhibit different subpopulation of VTA DA and GABA neurons
LH Orexin neurons	Increase reward system sensitivity	Increase VTA DA firing	Reduced activity as glucose increases
LH melanin-concentrating hormone neurons	Inhibited in low glucose	Integrate gustatory cues, enhance nucleus accumbens (NAc) sensitivity	Activate in response to gustatory nutrient content, enhance NAc-mediated reward consumption
Nucleus tractus solitarius (NTS) preproglucagon neurons	Decreased activity	Decreased activity	Integrates cholecystokinin, leptin, glucagon-like peptide 1, gut distention to inhibit reward system
NTS pro-opiomelanocortin (POMC) neurons	Decreased activity	Decreased activity	Increase in response to gut distention, reduce feeding
Arcuate POMC neurons	Decreased activity	Decreased activity	Activated by leptin, decrease NAc sensitivity but increase VTA encoding of food cue
Ghrelin	Dual action: increases AgRP neuronal activity and increases intrinsic reward system sensitivity	Increases reward system sensitivity	Reduces after food consumption
Leptin	Decreased activity	Decreased activity	Increases with insulin activity and decreases reward system activity

With this paradigm in mind, we can return to the superstimulus concept and observe how extreme rewards may bypass this balanced relationship of hunger systems enhancing food rewards to increase food consumption, and satiety systems reducing food rewards to reduce consumption. Highly palatable foods can induce food consumption in fed mice, even with adult ablation of AgRP neurons—a disruption which typically produces starvation (146). This relies on dopaminergic tone to produce the feeding response. A natural extension of this finding is this: if the reward's learned value is high enough to stimulate a large dopamine spike upon sighting, overcoming the reward-dampening influence of satiety circuits and hormones, this triggers the feeding sequence. It can be speculated that normally, AgRP neurons *via* their aversive, inhibitory action sensitize the reward system so that when it is finally released, even an intrinsically low-value food cue produces a large spike in dopaminergic activity. This is in keeping with the old saying that "hunger is the best sauce." Thus, it may not be that there are separate hedonic and homeostatic feeding mechanisms, but instead that highly palatable foods bypass the natural inhibition of the reward system by the hunger system.

AUTHOR CONTRIBUTIONS

RC prepared and wrote the manuscript. QT revised the manuscript and provided critical input for new ideas and content to be added to the manuscript.

FUNDING

Work in the Tong lab was supported by NIH R01DK092605 and R01DK109934, UT BRAIN Initiative and CTSA UL1 TR000371, Welch Foundation (L-AU0002), Grand-in-aid from American Heart Association (15GRNT22370024), and Basic Research Award (1-15-BS-184) from American Diabetes Association; QT is the holder of Cullen Chair in Molecular Medicine at McGovern Medical School. RC is supported by the Center for Clinical and Translational Sciences at UTHealth (4TL1TR000369-10).

REFERENCES

De Block A, Du Laing B. Amusing ourselves to death? Superstimuli and the evolutionary social sciences. *Philos Psychol* (2010) 23(6):821–43. doi:10.1080/ 09515089.2010.529048

Pinker S. *How the Mind Works*. New York, NY: W.W. Norton (1997).

Longo DL, Volkow ND, Koob GF, McLellan AT. Neurobiologic advances from the brain disease model of addiction. *N Engl J Med* (2016) 374(4):363–71. doi:10.1056/NEJMra1511480

Freimuth M, Moniz S, Kim SR. Clarifying exercise addiction: differential diagnosis, co-occurring disorders, and phases of addiction. *Int J Environ Res Public Health* (2011) 8(10):4069–81. doi:10.3390/ijerph8104069

Murakami Y, Kuratani S. Brain segmentation and trigeminal projections in the lamprey; with reference to vertebrate brain evolution. *Brain Res Bull* (2008) 75(2):218–24. doi:10.1016/j.brainresbull.2007.10.057

Pani AM, Mullarkey EE, Aronowicz J, Assimacopoulos S, Grove EA, Lowe CJ. Ancient deuterostome origins of vertebrate brain signalling centres. *Nature* (2012) 483(7389):289–94. doi:10.1038/nature10838

Jackson PJ, Douglas NR, Chai B, Binkley J, Sidow A, Barsh GS, et al. Structural and molecular evolutionary analysis of agouti and agou- ti-related proteins. *Chem Biol* (2006) 13(12):1297–305. doi:10.1016/j. chembiol.2006.10.006

Västermark Å, Krishnan A, Houle ME, Fredriksson R, Cerdá-Reverter JM, Schiöth HB. Identification of distant agouti-like sequences and re-evaluation of the evolutionary history of the agouti-related peptide (AgRP). *PLoS One* (2012) 7(7):e40982. doi:10.1371/journal.pone.0040982

Callier S, Snapyan M, Crom S, Prou D, Vincent J-D, Vernier P. Evolution and cell biology of dopamine receptors in vertebrates. *Biol Cell* (2003) 95(7):489–502. doi:10.1016/S0248-4900(03)00089-3

Zhou Q-Y, Palmiter RD. Dopamine-deficient mice are severely hypoactive, adipsic, and aphagic. *Cell* (1995) 83(7):1197–209. doi:10.1016/0092-8674(95)90145-0

España RA, Oleson EB, Locke JL, Brookshire BR, Roberts DC, Jones SR. The hypocretin-orexin system regulates cocaine self-administration via actions on the mesolimbic dopamine system. *Eur J Neurosci* (2010) 31(2):336–48. doi:10.1111/j.1460-9568.2009.07065.x

Zheng D, De Vaca SC, Carr KD. Food restriction increases acquisition, persistence and drug prime-induced expression of a cocaine-conditioned place preference in rats. *Pharmacol Biochem Behav* (2012) 100(3):538–44. doi:10.1016/j.pbb.2011.10.021

Shen M, Jiang C, Liu P, Wang F, Ma L. Mesolimbic leptin signaling negatively regulates cocaine-conditioned reward. *Transl Psychiatry* (2016) 6(12):e972. doi:10.1038/tp.2016.223

Morales M, Margolis EB. Ventral tegmental area: cellular heterogeneity, connectivity and behaviour. *Nat Rev Neurosci* (2017) 18(2):73–85. doi:10.1038/ nrn.2016.165

Bromberg-Martin ES, Matsumoto M, Hikosaka O. Dopamine in motivational control: rewarding, aversive, and alerting. *Neuron* (2010) 68(5):815–34. doi:10.1016/j.neuron.2010.11.022

Bariselli S, Glangetas C, Tzanoulinou S, Bellone C. Ventral tegmental area subcircuits process rewarding and aversive experiences. *J Neurochem* (2016) 139(6):1071–80. doi:10.1111/jnc.13779

Cohen JY, Haesler S, Vong L, Lowell BB, Uchida N. Neuron-type-specific signals for reward and punishment in the ventral tegmental area. *Nature* (2012) 482(7383):85–8. doi:10.1038/nature10754

Mikhailova MA, Bass CE, Grinevich VP, Chappell AM, Deal AL, Bonin KD, et al. Optogenetically-induced tonic dopamine release from VTA-nucleus accumbens projections inhibits reward consummatory behaviors. *Neuroscience* (2016) 333:54–64. doi:10.1016/j.neuroscience.2016.07.006

Lammel S, Ion DI, Roeper J, Malenka RC. Projection-specific modulation of dopamine neuron synapses by aversive and rewarding stimuli. *Neuron* (2011) 70:855–62. doi:10.1016/j.neuron.2011.03.025

Root DH, Mejias-Aponte CA, Qi J, Morales M. Role of glutamatergic projections from ventral tegmental area to lateral habenula in aver- sive conditioning. *J Neurosci* (2014) 34(42):13906–10. doi:10.1523/ JNEUROSCI.2029-14.2014

Stamatakis AM, Jennings JH, Ung RL, Blair GA, Weinberg RJ, Neve RL, et al. A unique population of ventral tegmental area neurons inhibits the lateral habenula to promote reward. *Neuron* (2013) 80(4):1039–53. doi:10.1016/j. neuron.2013.08.023

Zahm DS. Functional-anatomical implications of the nucleus accumbens core and shell subterritories. *Ann N Y Acad Sci* (1999) 877:113–28. doi:10.1111/ j.1749-6632.1999.tb09264.x

Wheeler RA, Aragona BJ, Fuhrmann KA, Jones JL, Day JJ, Cacciapaglia F, et al. Cocaine cues drive opposing context-dependent shifts in reward processing and emotional state. *Biol Psychiatry* (2011) 69(11):1067–74. doi:10.1016/j. biopsych.2011.02.014

Saddoris MP, Cacciapaglia F, Wightman RM, Carelli RM. Differential dopamine release dynamics in the nucleus accumbens core and shell reveal complementary signals for error prediction and incentive motivation. *J Neurosci* (2015) 35(33):11572–82. doi:10.1523/JNEUROSCI.2344-15.2015

Sugam JA, Day JJ, Wightman RM, Carelli RM. Phasic nucleus accumbens dopamine encodes risk-based decision-making behavior. *Biol Psychiatry* (2012) 71(3):199–205. doi:10.1016/j.biopsych.2011.09.029

Salamone JD, Correa M, Farrar A, Mingote SM. Effort-related func- tions of nucleus accumbens dopamine and associated forebrain circuits.

Psychopharmacology (Berl) (2007) 191(3):461–82. doi:10.1007/ s00213-006-0668-9

Yager LM, Garcia AF, Wunsch AM, Ferguson SM. The ins and outs of the striatum: role in drug addiction. *Neuroscience* (2015) 301:529–41. doi:10.1016/j.neuroscience.2015.06.033

Waterson MJ, Horvath TL. Neuronal regulation of energy homeostasis: beyond the hypothalamus and feeding. *Cell Metab* (2015) 22(6):962–70. doi:10.1016/j.cmet.2015.09.026

Haskell-Luevano C, Chen P, Li C, Chang K, Smith MS, Cameron JL, et al. Characterization of the neuroanatomical distribution of agouti-related protein immunoreactivity in the rhesus monkey and the rat [1]. *Endocrinology* (1999) 140(3):1408–15. doi:10.1210/endo.140.3.6544

Colmers WF, Bleakman D. Effects of neuropeptide Y on the electrical properties of neurons. *Trends Neurosci* (1994) 17(9):373–9. doi:10.1016/ 0166-2236(94)90046-9

Tao YX. The melanocortin-4 receptor: physiology, pharmacology, and pathophysiology. *Endocr Rev* (2010) 31(4):506–43. doi:10.1210/er.2009-0037

Ollmann MM, Wilson BD, Yang YK, Kerns JA, Chen Y, Gantz I, et al. Antagonism of central melanocortin receptors in vitro and in vivo by agouti-related protein. *Science* (1997) 278(5335):135–8. doi:10.1126/ science.278.5335.135

Yang Y. Structure, function and regulation of the melanocortin receptors. *Eur J Pharmacol* (2011) 660(1):125–30. doi:10.1016/j.ejphar.2010.12.020

Tolle V, Low MJ. In vivo evidence for inverse agonism of agouti-related peptide in the central nervous system of proopiomelanocortin-deficient mice. *Diabetes* (2007) 57(1):86–94. doi:10.2337/db07-0733

Nijenhuis WA, Oosterom J, Adan RA. AgRP(83-132) acts as an inverse agonist on the human-melanocortin-4 receptor. *Mol Endocrinol* (2001) 15:164–71. doi:10.1210/me.15.1.164

Wang D, He X, Zhao Z, Feng Q, Lin R, Sun Y, et al. Whole-brain mapping of the direct inputs and axonal projections of POMC and AgRP neurons. *Front Neuroanat* (2015) 9:40. doi:10.3389/fnana.2015.00040

Aponte Y, Atasoy D, Sternson SM. AGRP neurons are sufficient to orchestrate feeding behavior rapidly and without training. *Nat Neurosci* (2011) 14(3):351–5. doi:10.1038/nn.2739

Cowley MA, Smith RG, Diano S, Tschöp M, Pronchuk N, Grove KL, et al. The distribution and mechanism of action of ghrelin in the CNS demonstrates a novel hypothalamic circuit regulating energy homeostasis. *Neuron* (2003) 37(4):649–61. doi:10.1016/S0896-6273(03)00063-1

Varela L, Horvath TL. Leptin and insulin pathways in POMC and AgRP neurons that modulate energy balance and glucose homeostasis. *EMBO Rep* (2012) 13(12):1079–86. doi:10.1038/embor.2012.174

Schaeffer M, Langlet F, Lafont C, Molino F, Hodson DJ, Roux T, et al. Rapid sensing of circulating ghrelin by hypothalamic appetite-modifying neurons. *Proc Natl Acad Sci U S A* (2013) 110(4):1512–7. doi:10.1073/ pnas.1212137110

Takahashi KA, Cone RD. Fasting induces a large, leptin-dependent increase in the intrinsic action potential frequency of orexigenic arcuate nucleus neuropeptide Y/Agouti-related protein neurons. *Endocrinology* (2005) 146(3):1043–7. doi:10.1210/en.2004-1397

Qian S, Chen H, Weingarth D, Trumbauer ME, Novi DE, Guan X, et al. Neither agouti-related protein nor neuropeptide Y is critically required for the regulation of energy homeostasis in mice. *Mol Cell Biol* (2002) 22(14):5027–35. doi:10.1128/MCB.22.14.5027-5035.2002

Wortley KE, Anderson KD, Yasenchak J, Murphy A, Valenzuela D, Diano S, et al. Agouti-related protein-deficient mice display an age-related lean phenotype. *Cell Metab* (2005) 2(6):421–7. doi:10.1016/j.cmet.2005.11.004

Luquet S, Perez FA, Hnasko TS, Palmiter RD. NPY/AgRP neurons are essential for feeding in adult mice but can be ablated in neonates. *Science* (2005) 310(5748):683–5. doi:10.1126/science.1115524

Gropp E, Shanabrough M, Borok E, Xu AW, Janoschek R, Buch T, et al. Agouti-related peptide-expressing neurons are mandatory for feeding. *Nat Neurosci* (2005) 8(10):1289–91. doi:10.1038/nn1548

Bewick GA, Gardiner JV, Dhillo WS, Kent AS, White NE, Webster Z, et al. Postembryonic ablation of AgRP neurons in mice leads to a lean, hypophagic phenotype. *FASEB J* (2005) 21(3):1–22. doi:10.1096/fj.04-3434fje

Bouret SG, Draper SJ, Simerly RB. Formation of projection pathways from the arcuate nucleus of the hypothalamus to hypothalamic regions implicated in the neural control of feeding behavior in mice. *J Neurosci* (2004) 24(11):2797–805. doi:10.1523/JNEUROSCI.5369-03.2004

Tong Q, Ye C-P, Jones JE, Elmquist JK, Lowell BB. Synaptic release of GABA by AgRP neurons is required for normal regulation of energy balance. *Nat Neurosci* (2008) 11(9):998–1000. doi:10.1038/nn.2167

Dietrich MO, Zimmer MR, Bober J, Horvath TL. Hypothalamic Agrp neurons drive stereotypic behaviors beyond feeding. *Cell* (2015) 160(6):1222–32. doi:10.1016/j.cell.2015.02.024

Nakajima K, Cui Z, Li C, Meister J, Cui Y, Fu O, et al. Gs-coupled GPCR signalling in AgRP neurons triggers sustained increase in food intake. *Nat Commun* (2016) 7:10268. doi:10.1038/ncomms10268

Burnett CJ, Li C, Webber E, Tsaousidou E, Xue SY, Brüning JC, et al. Hunger-driven motivational state competition. *Neuron* (2016) 92(1):187–201. doi:10.1016/j.neuron.2016.08.032

Betley JN, Xu S, Cao ZF, Gong R, Magnus CJ, Yu Y, et al. Neurons for hunger and thirst transmit a negative-valence teaching signal. *Nature* (2015) 521(7551):180–5. doi:10.1038/nature14416

Chen Y, Lin YC, Kuo TW, Knight ZA. Sensory detection of food rapidly modulates arcuate feeding circuits. *Cell* (2015) 160(5):829–41. doi:10.1016/j.cell.2015.01.033

Chen Y, Lin YC, Zimmerman CA, Essner RA, Knight ZA. Hunger neurons drive feeding through a sustained, positive reinforcement signal. *Elife* (2016) 5:e18640. doi:10.7554/eLife.18640

Dietrich MO, Bober J, Ferreira JG, Tellez LA, Mineur YS, Souza DO, et al. AgRP neurons regulate development of dopamine neuronal plasticity and nonfood-associated behaviors. *Nat Neurosci* (2012) 15(8):1108–10. doi:10.1038/nn.3147

Brown RSE, Kokay IC, Phillipps HR, Yip SH, Gustafson P, Wyatt A, et al. Conditional deletion of the prolactin receptor reveals functional subpopulations of dopamine neurons in the arcuate nucleus of the hypo- thalamus. *J Neurosci* (2016) 36(35): 9173–85. doi:10.1523/ JNEUROSCI.1471- 16.2016

Zhang X, van den Pol AN. Hypothalamic arcuate nucleus tyrosine hydroxylase neurons play orexigenic role in energy homeostasis. *Nat Neurosci* (2016) 19(10):1341–7. doi:10.1038/nn.4372

Stuber GD, Wise RA. Lateral hypothalamic circuits for feeding and reward. *Nat Neurosci* (2016) 19(2):198–205. doi:10.1038/nn.4220

Stamatakis AM, Van Swieten M, Basiri ML, Blair GA, Kantak P, Stuber GD. Lateral hypothalamic area glutamatergic neurons and their projections to the lateral habenula regulate feeding and reward. *J Neurosci* (2016) 36(2):302–11. doi:10.1523/JNEUROSCI.1202-15.2016

Navarro M, Olney JJ, Burnham NW, Mazzone CM, Lowery-Gionta EG, Pleil KE, et al. Lateral hypothalamus GABAergic neurons modulate consummatory behaviors regardless of the caloric content or biological relevance of the consumed stimuli. *Neuropsychopharmacology* (2016) 41(6):1505–12. doi:10.1038/npp.2015.304

Wu Z, Kim ER, Sun H, Xu Y, Mangieri LR, Li DP, et al. GABAergic projections from lateral hypothalamus to paraventricular hypothalamic nucleus promote feeding. *J Neurosci* (2015) 35(8):3312–8. doi:10.1523/ JNEUROSCI.3720-14.2015

Nieh EH, Matthews GA, Allsop SA, Presbrey KN, Leppla CA, Wichmann R, et al. Decoding neural circuits that control compulsive sucrose seeking. *Cell* (2015) 160(3):528–41. doi:10.1016/j.cell.2015.01.003

Carus-Cadavieco M, Gorbati M, Ye L, Bender F, van der Veldt S, Kosse C, et al. Gamma oscillations organize top-down signalling to hypothalamus and enable food seeking. *Nature* (2017) 542:232–6. doi:10.1038/ nature21066

Blouin AM, Fried I, Wilson CL, Staba RJ, Behnke EJ, Lam HA, et al. Human hypocretin and melanin-concentrating hormone levels are linked to emotion and social interaction. *Nat Commun* (2013) 4:1547. doi:10.1038/ ncomms2461

Harris GC, Wimmer M, Aston-Jones G. A role for lateral hypothalamic orexin neurons in reward seeking. *Nature* (2005) 437(7058):556–9. doi:10.1038/ nature04071

Zhang G-C, Mao L-M, Liu X-Y, Wang JQ. Long-lasting up-regulation of orexin receptor type 2 protein levels in the rat nucleus accumbens after chronic cocaine administration. *J Neurochem* (2007) 103(1):400–7. doi:10.1111/j.1471-4159.2007.04748.x

Sheng Z, Santiago AM, Thomas MP, Routh VH. Metabolic regulation of lat- eral hypothalamic glucose-inhibited orexin neurons may influence midbrain reward neurocircuitry. *Mol Cell Neurosci* (2014) 62:30–41. doi:10.1016/j.mcn.2014.08.001

Castro DC, Terry RA, Berridge KC. Orexin in rostral hotspot of nucleus accumbens enhances sucrose "liking" and intake but scopolamine in caudal shell shifts "liking" toward "disgust" and "fear". *Neuropsychopharmacology* (2016) 41(8):2101–11. doi:10.1038/npp.2016.10

Borgland SL, Chang SJ, Bowers MS, Thompson JL, Vittoz N, Floresco SB, et al. Orexin A/hypocretin-1 selectively promotes motivation for positive reinforcers. *J Neurosci* (2009) 29(36):11215–25. doi:10.1523/JNEUROSCI.6096-08.2009

Gao XB, Van Den Pol AN. Melanin concentrating hormone depresses synaptic activity of glutamate and GABA neurons from rat lateral hypothalamus. *J Physiol* (2001) 533(1):237–52. doi:10.1111/j.1469-7793.2001.0237b.x

Eiler WJA, Chen Y, Slieker LJ, Ardayfio PA, Statnick MA, Witkin JM. Consequences of constitutive deletion of melanin-concentrating hormone-1 receptors for feeding and foraging behaviors of mice. *Behav Brain Res* (2017) 316:271–8. doi:10.1016/j.bbr.2016.09.028

Marsh DJ, Weingarth DT, Novi DE, Chen HY, Trumbauer ME, Chen AS, et al. Melanin-concentrating hormone 1 receptor-deficient mice are lean, hyperactive, and hyperphagic and have altered metabolism. *Proc Natl Acad Sci U S A* (2002) 99(5):3240–5. doi:10.1073/pnas.052706899

Burdakov D, Gerasimenko O, Verkhratsky A. Physiological changes in glucose differentially modulate the excitability of hypothalamic melanin-concentrating hormone and orexin neurons in situ. *J Neurosci* (2005) 25(9):2429–33. doi:10.1523/JNEUROSCI.4925-04.2005

Rossi M, Choi SJ, O'Shea D, Miyoshi T, Ghatei MA, Bloom SR. Melanin-concentrating hormone acutely stimulates feeding, but chronic administration has no effect on body weight. *Endocrinology* (1997) 138(1):351–5. doi:10.1210/endo.138.1.4887

Pérez CA, Stanley SA, Wysocki RW, Havranova J, Ahrens-Nicklas R, Onyimba F, et al. Molecular annotation of integrative feeding neural circuits. *Cell Metab* (2011) 13(2):222–32. doi:10.1016/j.cmet.2010.12.013

Domingos AI, Sordillo A, Dietrich MO, Liu ZW, Tellez LA, Vaynshteyn J, et al. Hypothalamic melanin concentrating hormone neurons communicate the nutrient value of sugar. *Elife* (2013) 2:e01462. doi:10.7554/eLife.01462

Chung S, Hopf FW, Nagasaki H, Li CY, Belluzzi JD, Bonci A, et al. The melanin-concentrating hormone system modulates cocaine reward. *Proc Natl Acad Sci U S A* (2009) 106(16):6772–7. doi:10.1073/pnas.0811331106

Georgescu D, Sears RM, Hommel JD, Barrot M, Bolaños CA, Marsh DJ, et al. The hypothalamic neuropeptide melanin-concentrating hormone acts in the nucleus accumbens to modulate feeding behavior and forced-swim performance. *J Neurosci* (2005) 25(11):2933–40. doi:10.1523/JNEUROSCI.1714-04.2005

Sears RM, Liu RJ, Narayanan NS, Sharf R, Yeckel MF, Laubach M, et al. Regulation of nucleus accumbens activity by the hypothalamic neuropeptide melanin-concentrating hormone. *J Neurosci* (2010) 30(24):8263–73. doi:10.1523/JNEUROSCI.5858-09.2010

Lopez CA, Guesdon B, Baraboi E-D, Roffarello BM, Hétu M, Richard D. Involvement of the opioid system in the orexigenic and hedonic effects of melanin-concentrating hormone. *Am J Physiol Regul Integr Comp Physiol* (2011) 301(4):R1105–11. doi:10.1152/ajpregu.00076.2011

Cheung GW, Kokorovic A, Lam CK, Chari M, Lam TK. Intestinal cholecystokinin controls glucose production through a neuronal network. *Cell Metab* (2009) 10(2):99–109. doi:10.1016/j.cmet.2009.07.005

Baggio LL, Drucker DJ. Biology of Incretins: GLP-1 and GIP. *Gastroenterology* (2007) 132(6):2131–57. doi:10.1053/j.gastro.2007.03.054

Alhadeff AL, Rupprecht LE, Hayes MR. GLP-1 neurons in the nucleus of the solitary tract project directly to the ventral tegmental area and nucleus accumbens to control for food intake. *Endocrinology* (2012) 153(2):647–58. doi:10.1210/en.2011-1443

Alhadeff AL, Mergler BD, Zimmer DJ, Turner CA, Reiner DJ, Schmidt HD, et al. Endogenous glucagon-like peptide-1 receptor signaling in the nucleus tractussolitariusisrequiredforfoodintakecontrol. *Neuropsychopharmacology* (2016). doi:10.1038/npp.2016.246

Mietlicki-Baase EG, Ortinski PI, Rupprecht LE, Olivos DR, Alhadeff AL, Pierce RC, et al. The food intake-suppressive effects of glucagon-like peptide-1 receptor signaling in the ventral tegmental area are mediated by AMPA/kainate receptors. *Am J Physiol Endocrinol Metab* (2013) 305(11):E1367–74. doi:10.1152/ajpendo.00413.2013

Reddy IA, Pino JA, Weikop P, Osses N, Sørensen G, Bering T, et al. Glucagon-like peptide 1 receptor activation regulates cocaine actions and dopamine homeostasis in the lateral septum by decreasing arachidonic acid levels. *Transl Psychiatry* (2016) 6(5):e809. doi:10.1038/tp.2016.86

Harasta AE, Power JM, von Jonquieres G, Karl T, Drucker DJ, Housley GD, et al. Septal glucagon-like peptide 1 receptor expression determines suppression of cocaine-induced behavior. *Neuropsychopharmacology* (2015) 40(8):1969–78. doi:10.1038/npp.2015.47

Schmidt HD, Mietlicki-Baase EG, Ige KY, Maurer JJ, Reiner DJ, Zimmer DJ, et al. Glucagon-like peptide-1 receptor activation in the ventral tegmental area decreases the reinforcing efficacy of cocaine. *Neuropsychopharmacology* (2016) 41(7):1917–28. doi:10.1038/npp.2015.362

Benjannet S, Rondeau N, Day R, Chrétien M, Seidah NG. PC1 and PC2 are proprotein convertases capable of cleaving proopiomelanocortin at distinct pairs of basic residues. *Proc Natl Acad Sci U S A* (1991) 88(9):3564–8. doi:10.1073/PNAS.88.9.3564

Xu P, Grueter BA, Britt JK, McDaniel L, Huntington PJ, Hodge R, et al. Double deletion of melanocortin 4 receptors and SAPAP3 corrects compulsive behavior and obesity in mice. *Proc Natl Acad Sci U S A* (2013) 110(26):10759–64. doi:10.1073/pnas.1308195110

Burnett LC, LeDuc CA, Sulsona CR, Paull D, Rausch R, Eddiry S, et al. Deficiency in prohormone convertase PC1 impairs prohormone processing in Prader-Willi syndrome. *J Clin Invest* (2017) 127(1):293–305. doi:10.1172/JCI91307

Zhan C, Zhou J, Feng Q, Zhang JE, Lin S, Bao J, et al. Acute and long-term suppression of feeding behavior by POMC neurons in the brainstem and hypothalamus, respectively. *J Neurosci* (2013) 33(8):3624–32. doi:10.1523/JNEUROSCI.2742-12.2013

Hentges ST, Otero-Corchon V, Pennock RL, King CM, Low MJ. Proopiomelanocortin expression in both GABA and glutamate neurons. *J Neurosci* (2009) 29(43):13684–90. doi:10.1523/JNEUROSCI.3770-09.2009

Li YQ, Shrestha Y, Pandey M, et al. Gq/11α and Gsα mediate distinct physiological responses to central melanocortins. *J Clin Invest* (2016) 126(1):40–9. doi:10.1172/JCI76348

Rediger A, Piechowski CL, Habegger K, Grüters A, Krude H, Tschöp MH, et al. MC4R dimerization in the paraventricular nucleus and GHSR/MC3R heterodimerization in the arcuate nucleus: is there relevance for body weight regulation? *Neuroendocrinology* (2012) 95(4):277–88. doi:10.1159/000334903

Agosti F, Cordisco Gonzalez S, Martinez Damonte V, Tolosa MJ, Di Siervi N, Schioth HB, et al. Melanocortin 4 receptor constitutive activity inhibits L-type voltage-gated calcium channels in neurons. *Neuroscience* (2017) 346:102–12. doi:10.1016/j.neuroscience.2017.01.007

Pandit R, van der Zwaal EM, Luijendijk MC, Brans MA, van Rozen AJ, Oude Ophuis RJ, et al. Central melanocortins regulate the motivation for sucrose reward. *PLoS One* (2015) 10(3):e0121768. doi:10.1371/journal.pone.0121768

Lim BK, Huang KW, Grueter BA, Rothwell PE, Malenka RC. Anhedonia requires MC4R-mediated synaptic adaptations in nucleus accumbens. *Nature* (2012) 487(7406):183–9. doi:10.1038/nature11160

O'Connor EC, Kremer Y, Lefort S, Harada M, Pascoli V, Rohner C, et al. Accumbal D1R neurons projecting to lateral hypothalamus authorize feeding. *Neuron* (2015) 88(3):553–64. doi:10.1016/j.neuron.2015.09.038

Yen HH, Roseberry AG. Decreased consumption of rewarding sucrose solutions after injection of melanocortins into the ventral tegmental area of rats. *Psychopharmacology (Berl)* (2015) 232(1):285–94. doi:10.1007/s00213-014-3663-6

Cabeza de Vaca S, Kim G-YY, Carr KD. The melanocortin receptor agonist MTII augments the rewarding effect of amphetamine in ad-libitum-fed and food-restricted rats. *Psychopharmacology (Berl)* (2002) 161(1):77–85. doi:10.1007/s00213-002-0998-1

Cui H, Lutter M. The expression of MC4Rs in D1R neurons regulates food intake and locomotor sensitization to cocaine. *Genes Brain Behav* (2013) 12(6):658–65. doi:10.1111/gbb.12057

Hsu R, Taylor JR, Newton SS, Alvaro JD, Haile C, Han G, et al. Blockade of melanocortin transmission inhibits cocaine reward. *Eur J Neurosci* (2005) 21(8):2233–42. doi:10.1111/j.1460-9568.2005.04038.x

Shelkar GP, Kale AD, Singh U, Singru PS, Subhedar NK, Kokare DM. Alpha-melanocyte stimulating hormone modulates ethanol self-administration in posterior ventral tegmental area through melanocortin-4 receptors. *Addict Biol* (2015) 20(2):302–15. doi:10.1111/adb.12126

Pandit R, Omrani A, Luijendijk MC, de Vrind VA, Van Rozen AJ, Ophuis RJ, et al. Melanocortin 3 receptor signaling in midbrain dopamine neurons increases the motivation for food reward. *Neuropsychopharmacology* (2016) 41(9):2241–51. doi:10.1038/npp.2016.19

Hu J, Jiang L, Low MJ, Rui L. Glucose rapidly induces different forms of excitatory synaptic plasticity in hypothalamic POMC neurons. *PLoS One* (2014) 9(8):e105080. doi:10.1371/journal.pone.0105080

Chen M, Wan Y, Ade K, Ting J, Feng G, Calakos N. Sapap3 deletion anomalously activates short-term endocannabinoid-mediated synaptic plasticity. *J Neurosci* (2011) 31(26):9563–73. doi:10.1523/JNEUROSCI.1701- 11.2011

Kojima M, Hosoda H, Date Y, Nakazato M, Matsuo H, Kangawa K. Ghrelin is a growth-hormone-releasing acylated peptide from stomach. *Nature* (1999) 402(6762):656–60. doi:10.1038/45230

Ghelardoni S, Carnicelli V, Frascarelli S, Ronca-Testoni S, Zucchi R. Ghrelin tissue distribution: comparison between gene and protein expression. *J Endocrinol Invest* (2006) 29(2):115–21. doi:10.1007/BF03344083

Gnanapavan S. The tissue distribution of the mRNA of ghrelin and sub- types of its receptor, GHS-R, in humans. *J Clin Endocrinol Metab* (2002) 87(6):2988–2988. doi:10.1210/jc.87.6.2988

Matsui-Sakata A, Ohtani H, Sawada Y. Receptor occupancy-based analysis of the contributions of various receptors to antipsychotics-induced weight gain and diabetes mellitus. *Drug Metab Pharmacokinet* (2005) 20(5):368–78. doi:10.2133/dmpk.20.368

Shintani M, Ogawa Y, Ebihara K, Aizawa-Abe M, Miyanaga F, Takaya K, et al. Ghrelin, an endogenous growth hormone secretagogue, is a novel orexigenic peptide that antagonizes leptin action through the activation of hypotha- lamic neuropeptide Y/Y1 receptor pathway. *Diabetes* (2001) 50(2):227–32. doi:10.2337/diabetes.50.2.227

Lee JH, Lin L, Xu P, Saito K, Wei Q, Meadows HE, et al. Neuronal deletion of ghrelin receptor almost completely prevents diet-induced obesity. *Diabetes* (2016) 65(8):2169–78. doi:10.2337/db15-1587

Yildiz BO, Suchard MA, Wong M-L, Mccann SM, Licinio J. *Alterations in the Dynamics of Circulating Ghrelin, Adiponectin, and Leptin in Human Obesity.* (2004). Available from: http://www.pnas.org.ezproxyhost.library.tmc.edu/content/101/28/10434.full.pdf

Shrestha YB, Wickwire K, Giraudo SQ. Direct effects of nutrients, acetylcholine, CCK, and insulin on ghrelin release from the isolated stomachs of rats. *Peptides* (2009) 30(6):1187–91. doi:10.1016/j.peptides.2009.02.001

Sakata I, Park WM, Walker AK, Piper PK, Chuang JC, Osborne-Lawrence S, et al. Glucose-mediated control of ghrelin release from primary cultures of gastric mucosal cells Glucose-mediated control of ghrelin release from primary cultures of gastric mucosal cells. *Am J Physiol Endocrinol Metab* (2012) 302(10):E1300–10. doi:10.1152/ajpendo.00041.2012

Lippl F, Kircher F, Erdmann J, Allescher H-D, Schusdziarra V. Effect of GIP, GLP-1, insulin and gastrin on ghrelin release in the isolated rat stomach. *Regul Pept* (2004) 119(1):93–8. doi:10.1016/j.regpep.2004.01.003

Banks WA, Tschop M, Robinson SM, Heiman ML. Extent and direction of ghrelin transport across the blood-brain barrier is determined by its unique primary structure. *J Pharmacol Exp Ther* (2002) 302(2):822–7. doi:10.1124/jpet.102.034827

Banks WA, Burney BO, Robinson SM. Effects of triglycerides, obesity, and starvation on ghrelin transport across the blood-brain barrier. *Peptides* (2008) 29(11):2061–5. doi:10.1016/j.peptides.2008.07.001

Schellekens H, van Oeffelen WE, Dinan TG, Cryan JF. Promiscuous dimerization of the growth hormone secretagogue receptor (GHS-R1a) attenuates ghrelin-mediated signaling. *J Biol Chem* (2013) 288(1):181–91. doi:10.1074/jbc.M112.382473

Damian M, Mary S, Maingot M, M'Kadmi C, Gagne D, Leyris JP, et al. Ghrelin receptor conformational dynamics regulate the transition from a preassembled to an active receptor: Gq complex. *Proc Natl Acad Sci U S A* (2015) 112(5):1601–6. doi:10.1073/pnas.1414618112

Wu CS, Bongmba OYN, Yue J, Lee JH, Lin L, Saito K, et al. Suppression of GHS-R in AgRP neurons mitigates diet-induced obesity by acti- vating thermogenesis. *Int J Mol Sci* (2017) 18(4):832. doi:10.3390/ ijms18040832

Jerlhag E, Egecioglu E, Dickson SL, Douhan A, Svensson L, Engel JA. Ghrelin administration into tegmental areas stimulates locomotor activity and increases extracellular concentration of dopamine in the nucleus accumbens. *Addict Biol* (2007) 12(1):6–16. doi:10.1111/j.1369-1600.2006. 00041.x

Perello M, Sakata I, Birnbaum S, Chuang JC, Osborne-Lawrence S, Rovinsky SA, et al. Ghrelin increases the rewarding value of high-fat diet in an orexin-dependent manner. *Biol Psychiatry* (2010) 67(9):880–6. doi:10.1016/j.biopsych.2009.10.030

Olszewski PK, Li D, Grace MK, Billington CJ, Kotz CM, Levine AS. Neural basis of orexigenic effects of ghrelin acting within lateral hypothalamus. *Peptides* (2003) 24(4):597–602. doi:10.1016/S0196-9781(03)00105-0

Seoane LM, López M, Tovar S, Casanueva FF, Señarís R, Diéguez C. Agouti-related peptide, neuropeptide Y, and somatostatin-producing neurons are targets for ghrelin actions in the rat hypothalamus. *Endocrinology* (2003) 144(2):544–51. doi:10.1210/en.2002-220795

Jerlhag E, Egecioglu E, Landgren S, Salomé N, Heilig M, Moechars D, et al. Requirement of central ghrelin signaling for alcohol reward. *Proc Natl Acad Sci U S A* (2009) 106(27):11318–23. doi:10.1073/pnas.0812809106

Suchankova P, Engel JA, Jerlhag E. Sub-chronic ghrelin receptor blockade attenuates alcohol- and amphetamine-induced locomotor stimulation in mice. *Alcohol Alcohol* (2016) 51(2):121–7. doi:10.1093/alcalc/agv100

Haass-Koffler CL, Aoun EG, Swift RM, de la Monte SM, Kenna GA, Leggio L. Leptin levels are reduced by intravenous ghrelin administration and cor- related with cue-induced alcohol craving. *Transl Psychiatry* (2015) 5(9):e646. doi:10.1038/tp.2015.140

Leggio L, Zywiak WH, Fricchione SR, Edwards SM, de la Monte SM, Swift RM, et al. Intravenous ghrelin administration increases alcohol craving in alcohol-depe1ndent heavy drinkers: a preliminary investiga- tion. *Biol Psychiatry* (2014) 76(9):734–41. doi:10.1016/j.biopsych.2014. 03.019

Jerlhag E, Ivanoff L, Vater A, Engel JA. Peripherally circulating ghrelin does not mediate alcohol-induced reward and alcohol intake in rodents. *Alcohol Clin Exp Res* (2014) 38(4):959–68. doi:10.1111/acer.12337

Gomez JL, Cunningham CL, Finn DA, Young EA, Helpenstell LK, Schuette LM, et al. Differential effects of ghrelin antagonists on alco- hol drinking and reinforcement in mouse and rat models of alcohol dependence. *Neuropharmacology* (2015) 97:182–93. doi:10.1016/j.neuropharm.2015.05.026

Kern A, Mavrikaki M, Ullrich C, Albarran-Zeckler R, Brantley AF, Smith RG. Hippocampal dopamine/DRD1 signaling dependent on the ghrelin receptor. *Cell* (2015) 163(5):1176–90. doi:10.1016/j.cell.2015.10.062

Park H-KK, Ahima RS. Physiology of leptin: energy homeostasis, neuroendocrine function and metabolism. *Metabolism* (2015) 64:24–34. doi:10.1016/j.metabol.2014.08.004

Balland E, Dam J, Langlet F, Caron E, Steculorum S, Messina A, et al. Hypothalamic tanycytes are an erk-gated conduit for leptin into the brain. *Cell Metab* (2014) 19:293–301. doi:10.1016/j.cmet.2013.12.015

Schwartz MW, Seeley RJ, Campfield LA, Burn P, Baskin DG. Identification of targets of leptin action in rat hypothalamus. *J Clin Invest* (1996) 98(5):1101–6. doi:10.1172/JCI118891

Domingos AI, Vaynshteyn J, Voss HU, Ren X, Gradinaru V, Zang F, et al. Leptin regulates the reward value of nutrient. *Nat Neurosci* (2011) 14(12):1562–8. doi:10.1038/nn.2977

Hommel JD, Trinko R, Sears RM, Georgescu D, Liu ZW, Gao XB, et al. Leptin receptor signaling in midbrain dopamine neurons regulates feeding. *Neuron* (2006) 51(6):801–10. doi:10.1016/j.neuron.2006.08.023

Leshan RL, Opland DM, Louis GW, Leinninger GM, Patterson CM, Rhodes CJ, et al. Ventral tegmental area leptin receptor neurons specifically project to and regulate cocaine- and amphetamine-regulated transcript neurons of the extended central amygdala. *J Neurosci* (2010) 30(16):5713–23. doi:10.1523/JNEUROSCI.1001-10.2010

Bruijnzeel AW, Corrie LW, Rogers JA, Yamada H. Effects of insulin and leptin in the ventral tegmental area and arcuate hypothalamic nucleus on food intake and brain reward function in female rats. *Behav Brain Res* (2011) 219(2):254–64. doi:10.1016/j.bbr.2011.01.020

Fernandes MF, Matthys D, Hryhorczuk C, Sharma S, Mogra S, Alquier T, et al. Leptin suppresses the rewarding effects of running via STAT3 signaling in dopamine neurons. *Cell Metab* (2015) 22(4):741–9. doi:10.1016/j.cmet.2015.08.003

Wellman PJ, Nation JR, Davis KW. Impairment of acquisition of cocaine self-administration in rats maintained on a high-fat diet. *Pharmacol Biochem Behav* (2007) 88(1):89–93. doi:10.1016/j.pbb.2007.07.008

Davis JF, Tracy AL, Schurdak JD, Tschöp MH, Lipton JW, Clegg DJ, et al. Exposure to elevated levels of dietary fat attenuates psychostimulant reward and mesolimbic dopamine turnover in the rat. *Behav Neurosci* (2008) 122(6):1257–63. doi:10.1037/a0013111

Kiefer F, Jahn H, Wolf K, Kampf P, Knaudt K, Wiedemann K. Free-choice alcohol consumption in mice after application of the appetite regulating peptide leptin. *Alcohol Clin Exp Res* (2001) 25(5):787–9. doi:10.1111/j.1530-0277.2001.tb02280.x

Kiefer F, Jahn H, Otte C, Demiralay C, Wolf K, Wiedemann K. Increasing leptin precedes craving and relapse during pharmacological abstinence maintenance treatment of alcoholism. *J Psychiatr Res* (2005) 39(5):545–51. doi:10.1016/j.jpsychires.2004.11.005

Denis RG, Joly-Amado A, Webber E, Langlet F, Schaeffer M, Padilla SL, et al. Palatability can drive feeding independent of AgRP neurons. *Cell Metab* (2015) 22(4):646–57. doi:10.1016/j.cmet.2015.07.011

6

Central Nervous Insulin Administration before Nocturnal Sleep Decreases Breakfast Intake in Healthy Young and Elderly Subjects

*João C. P. Santiago [1, 2, 3] and Manfred Hallschmid [1, 2, 3]**

[1] Institute of Medical Psychology and Behavioral Neurobiology, University of Tübingen, Tübingen, Germany, [2] German Center for Diabetes Research, Tübingen, Germany, [3] Institute for Diabetes Research and Metabolic Diseases of the Helmholtz Center Munich at the University of Tübingen, Tübingen, Germany

***Correspondence:**
Manfred Hallschmid
manfred.hallschmid@uni-tuebingen.de

Peripheral insulin acts on the brain to regulate metabolic functions, in particular decreasing food intake and body weight. This concept has been supported by studies in humans relying on the intranasal route of administration, a method that permits the direct permeation of insulin into the CNS without substantial absorption into the blood stream. We investigated if intranasal insulin administration before nocturnal sleep, a period of reduced metabolic activity and largely absent external stimulation, affects food intake and energy turnover on the subsequent morning. Healthy participants who were either young (16 men and 16 women; mean age ± SEM, 23.68 ± 0.40 years, mean BMI ± SEM, 22.83 ± 0.33 kg/m^2) or elderly (10 men, 9 women; 70.79 ± 0.81 years, 25.27 ± 0.60 kg/m^2) were intranasally administered intranasal insulin (160 IU) or placebo before a night of regular sleep that was polysomnographically recorded. Blood was repeatedly sampled for the determination of circulating glucose, insulin, leptin and total ghrelin. In the morning, energy expenditure was assessed via indirect calorimetry and subjects were offered a large standardized breakfast buffet from which they could eat *ad libitum*. Insulin compared to placebo reduced breakfast size by around 110 kcal (1,054.43 ± 50.91 vs. 1,162.36 ± 64.69 kcal, $p = 0.0095$), in particular decreasing carbohydrate intake (502.70 ± 25.97 vs. 589.82 ± 35.03 kcal, $p = 0.0080$). This effect was not dependent on sex or age (all $p > 0.11$). Sleep architecture, blood glucose and hormonal parameters as well as energy expenditure were not or only marginally affected. Results show that intranasal insulin administered to healthy young and elderly humans before sleep exerts a delayed inhibitory effect on energy intake that is not compensated for by changes in energy expenditure. While the exact underlying mechanisms cannot be derived from our data, findings indicate a long-lasting catabolic effect of central nervous insulin delivery that extends across sleep and might be of particular relevance for potential therapeutic applications.

Keywords: intranasal insulin, food intake behavior, sleep, aging, sex distribution

INTRODUCTION

Eating behavior is tightly regulated by central nervous circuitries that receive hormonal feedback on body fat stores and nutritional status from the body periphery (Morton et al., 2014). In addition to the adipocyte-derived hormone leptin, insulin is one of the major peripheral signals that contribute to the central nervous control of ingestive behavior. Both leptin and insulin circulate in direct proportion to the size of body fat stores and reach the CNS via active, saturable transport mechanisms across the blood-brain barrier (Baura et al., 1993; Schwartz et al., 1996; William and Banks, 2001). Studies in animals (Woods et al., 1979; McGowan et al., 1992; Air et al., 2002) and humans (Benedict et al., 2008; Hallschmid et al., 2012) have conclusively shown that insulin administered directly to the brain reduces food intake, independent of its peripheral glucoregulatory action. In humans, the inhibitory effect of central nervous insulin on food intake has been mainly investigated by means of the intranasal route of peptide administration (Hallschmid et al., 2004a, 2012; Benedict et al., 2008), a non-invasive method of substance delivery to the brain that largely bypasses the blood-brain barrier (Born et al., 2002; Dhuria et al., 2010). Intranasal administration of 160 IU insulin to healthy, fasted young subjects reduced calorie intake in male, but not female participants (Benedict et al., 2008). Accordingly, intranasal insulin treatment (4×40 IU/day) for 8 weeks resulted in loss of body weight and body fat in men but not in women (Hallschmid et al., 2004a). Still, young women who intranasally received 160 IU insulin after a standardized lunch displayed an enhancement of post-prandial satiety and a reduction in the intake of palatable snacks (Hallschmid et al., 2012). Ample evidence for a distinct effect of insulin on food intake-regulatory networks has also been found in related neuroimaging studies (see Heni et al., 2015; Kullmann et al., 2016 for reviews).

Sleep has turned out to be an important factor in the maintenance of energy homeostasis and the regulation of food intake (St-Onge et al., 2016). Habitually short sleep duration is associated with increased body weight (Magee and Hale, 2012; Vgontzas et al., 2014) and a more pronounced risk of impairments in glucose homeostasis (Gangwisch et al., 2007; Cappuccio et al., 2010). Fittingly, individuals exposed to acute sleep deprivation tend to consume more food on the subsequent day (Brondel et al., 2010), to reduce their physical activity (Schmid et al., 2009) and to display a deterioration in glucoregulation (Schmid et al., 2011). It has been proposed that increased energy expenditure due to sleep loss is overcompensated by an exaggerated increase in energy intake, resulting, on the long run, in a higher risk of obesity and related metabolic impairments (Penev, 2012; Schmid et al., 2015). We have previously shown that insulin applied to the CNS before nocturnal sleep increases growth hormone concentrations during early sleep and impacts memory function on the subsequent day (Feld et al., 2016), indicating that central nervous insulin signaling is relevant for sleep-associated neuroendocrine regulation. In the present study, we investigated the effect of intranasal insulin administered before sleep on eating behavior on the subsequent morning. We assumed that the acute enhancement of brain insulin signaling during sleep, i.e., a period of reduced metabolic activity and largely absent external input, exerts a delayed but discernible attenuating effect on breakfast intake, i.e., calorie consumption immediately following the sleep period. This hypothesis was tested in a group of healthy young men and women, thereby enabling the detection of potential sex differences. Considering reports that food-cue elicited changes in brain activity in response to a meal decrease with advancing age (Cheah et al., 2013), we moreover included a group of healthy elderly participants in order to investigate if age is a relevant modulatory factor in this context.

METHODS AND MATERIALS

Participants

Thirty-two healthy young subjects (16 men and 16 women, mean age $\pm$ SEM, 23.68 $\pm$ 0.40 years) and 19 elderly participants (10 men and 9 women, 70.79 $\pm$ 0.81 years) were recruited from the community for this study. All young subjects were normal-weight (BMI, 22.83 $\pm$ 0.33 kg/m^2, $p = 0.49$ for men vs. women) while the elderly participants were normal- or mildly overweight (25.27 $\pm$ 0.60 kg/m^2, $p = 0.70$ for men vs. women; $p < 0.001$ for young vs. elderly participants). All subjects were non-smokers. The women in the young group were taking oral contraceptives (estrogen dominant, single-phase; Valette, Jenapharm, Jena, Germany), but were otherwise free of medication, as were the men. Clinical examination excluded previous illness prior to inclusion in the study. In order to restrict the burden of experimental participation for the elderly subjects, some assessments (in particular energy expenditure and continuous heart rate monitoring) were omitted and less blood parameters were determined in this group. Written informed consent was obtained from all subjects and the study conformed to the Declaration of Helsinki and was approved by the local ethics committee.

Study Design and Procedure

The experiments were conducted according to a placebo-controlled, double-blind, within-subject crossover design. All participants took part in two experimental sessions which were identical except for the intranasal administration of insulin (Actrapid®, Novo Nordisk, Bagsværd, Denmark) or placebo (vehicle). Sessions were performed in a balanced order, i.e., half of the sample received first placebo and then the active agent, with the reversed order for the other half of the sample. In addition, participants spent an adaption night in the sleep lab (i.e., including the placement of electrodes for polysomnographic recordings), with at least a 24-h delay between adaptation and the first experiment. Experimental sessions were scheduled to be apart as close to 28 days as possible, ensuring that the young women were tested during the same phase of contraceptive intake in both sessions.

Subjects were instructed not to take naps and not to engage in intense physical activities on experimental days. They were told to abstain from caffeine and to follow their usual dinner routines around 1800–1900 h. Participants arrived at the sleep lab at 2000 h. Adherence to the instructions for the experimental day was confirmed and an intravenous catheter was placed in a vein of the dominant arm. At 2120 h, participants underwent a memory test battery (see Feld et al., 2016, for details and respective results in the group of young subjects) before receiving intranasal insulin or placebo via sixteen 0.1-ml puffs (8 per nostril) in 1-min intervals, amounting to a total dose of 1.6 ml insulin (160 IU) or placebo at 2220 h. This dose was chosen in order to enable comparisons with previous studies on the role of central nervous insulin in the acute regulation of food intake (Benedict et al., 2008; Hallschmid et al., 2012). Subjects went to bed at 2300 h for 8 h of polysomnographically recorded sleep, resulting in an overnight fast of at least 12 h in all subjects. Subjects were awakened at approximately 0700 h; care was taken not to wake participants up from rapid eye movement (REM) sleep or slow wave sleep. In the young subjects, heart rate was recorded throughout the night and energy expenditure was assessed at 0710 h in the morning. At 0815 h, breakfast was offered to all subjects. Throughout the session, blood was repeatedly sampled, without disturbing the participants, from an adjacent room with a thin plastic tube attached to the catheter for the determination of relevant parameters. Venous patency was maintained with a NaCl 0.9% drip.

Assessment of Breakfast Intake

Participants were offered a standardized test buffet of approximately 4,550 kcal at 0815 h and were allowed to eat ad-libitum and undisturbed for 30 min (see **Table 1** for a list of ingredients). All ingredients were weighed before and after eating to calculate the net amount consumed. Participants were allowed to take any leftovers with them in order to prevent them from overconsumption. They were told that this breakfast was scheduled to fill the gap between cognitive tests and provide them with the possibility to follow their usual breakfast routine, so that the experimental nature of this buffet remained undisclosed. One male and three female participants of the young group and one male and two female participants of the elderly group abstained from eating breakfast and were excluded from food intake analyses. All participants rated their hunger, thirst and tiredness on visual analog scales (VAS) before breakfast.

Energy Expenditure

In the participants of the young group, energy expenditure was measured at 0710 h via indirect calorimetry using a ventilated-hood system (Deltatrac II, MBM-200 Metabolic Monitor; Datex-Engström Deutschland, Achim, Germany). Before each use, the device was calibrated with Quick Cale calibration gas to 5% CO_2 and 95% O_2. Due to technical failures, assessments were not possible in two subjects.

Blood Parameters

Blood samples for the determination of blood glucose levels and circulating concentrations of hormones were obtained before intranasal insulin administration and repeatedly throughout the night. Blood glucose was determined immediately after each blood draw (HemoCue Glucose 201 Analyzer, HemoCue AB, Ångelholm, Schweden). The remaining samples were centrifuged and serum and plasma were frozen at −80°C for later analyses.

TABLE 1 | Composition of the test breakfast buffet.

Food	Weight (g)	Energy (kcal)	Carbohydrate (g)	Fat (g)	Protein (g)
NEUTRAL					
Whole milk	750	491	36	26.3	24.8
Buns	240	275	122.4	3.4	6.3
Whole wheat bread	165	360	71	2.3	12
White bread	30	72	14.6	0.4	2.2
Butter	120	928	0.7	99.8	0.8
SWEET					
Orange juice	400	173	36	1	4
Strawberry milk	200	167	18.2	6.8	7.4
Apple	195	104	22.2	1.2	0.6
Orange	180	72	15	0.4	1.8
Banana	179	168	38.3	0.4	2
Pear	140	78	17.4	0.4	0.7
Fruit curd	125	140	19.3	3.3	7.7
Vanilla pudding	125	134	20.8	3.8	3.5
Tangerine	80	35	8.2	0	0.5
Strawberry jam	50	147	35.8	0.1	0.1
Hazelnut spread	40	218	21.6	12.8	2.8
Honey	40	123	30	0	0.1
Sugar	24	98	24	0	0
HEARTY					
Sliced cheese	100	374	0.1	29.2	25.5
Poultry sausage	40	74	0.1	4.3	8.3
Cream cheese (herbs)	40	124	1	11.6	3.2
Cervelat sausage	34	120	0.1	10.2	6.1
Cream cheese	33	87	0.6	7.8	3
Total	3,330	4,562	553.4	225.5	123.4

All values are rounded to the closest decimal.

Insulin concentrations were determined in young and elderly participants (Insulin ELISA Kit, Dako, Glostrup, Denmark). In the young participants, plasma concentrations of total ghrelin (RIA; Linco Research, St. Charles, MO; sensitivity 93 pg/ml, intra-assay and inter-assay CV, 10 and 17.8%) and serum concentrations of leptin (RIA; Linco Research, St. Charles, MO; sensitivity, 0.5 ng/ml, intra-assay and inter-assay CV, 8.3% and 6.2%) were measured at time-points of relevance throughout the night.

Polysomnography and Heart Rate

EEG was recorded continuously from electrodes (Ag-AgCl) placed at C3 and C4 according to the 10-20 System and referenced to two coupled electrodes attached at the mastoids. EEG signals were filtered between 0.16 and 35 Hz and sampled at a rate of 200 Hz using an EEG amplifier system (BrainAmp DC, BrainProducts GmbH, Munich, Germany). Additionally, eye movements and muscle tone were recorded by electrodes placed diagonally above the left and below the right eye and electrodes attached to the chin, respectively. Sleep EEG scoring was carried out independently by two experienced technicians who were blind to the assigned treatment. Sleep architecture was determined according to standard polysomnographic criteria using EEG recordings from C3 and C4, diagonal EOG and chin EMG (Rechtschaffen and Kales, 1968). For each night, total sleep time, i.e., the time between the first detection of transition from sleep stages 1 to 2 and lights on, was used to calculate relative time spent in the different sleep stages, i.e., wake, REM sleep and NonREM sleep stages 1–4. Heart rate was recorded by electrocardiography (Actiheart, CamNtech, Boerne TX USA) in the young subjects during sleep until shortly after awakening. In the elderly subjects, it was monitored before and after sleep.

Statistical Analyses

R 3.3.1 (R Core Team, 2016) was used for statistical analyses. We used *lme4* (Bates et al., 2015) to build linear mixed-effects models to compensate for missing blood values in some cases (less than four per experiment). Main effects were tested for significance using likelihood-ratio tests with Satterthwaite approximations to degrees of freedom. For the indirect calorimetry data, we used condition (placebo or insulin) and sex as fixed effects and random intercepts for subjects. For breakfast consumption, we built an initial model using condition, sex, age group (young, elderly), macronutrient (carbohydrate, fat, protein) and interactions between condition, sex and macronutrient, condition and sex, condition and age and sex and macronutrient as fixed effects, random slopes for macronutrient and random intercepts for subjects. The inclusion of a random slope takes into account individual food preferences of each subject, thus optimally capturing between-subject differences. To evaluate intake by food type (hearty, neutral, sweet), we replaced macronutrient with food type in the previous model. For the VAS we built a model with fixed effects for treatment, sex, age group and random intercepts for subjects. We used *lsmeans* (Lenth, 2016) to run *post-hoc* comparisons with multivariate t adjustment. Levene's test for homogeneity of variance was used to test for equality of variances in our factors of interest, with only sex showing a deviation ($p < 0.01$; $p \geq 0.12$ for age and treatment). For analyses of blood parameters, the fixed factors sex, condition and time were used and areas under the curve (AUC) according to the trapezoidal rule were calculated. Results are presented as means ± SEM. A $p < 0.05$ was considered significant.

RESULTS

Breakfast Intake and Hunger Ratings

Intranasal insulin administration before sleep reduced breakfast intake by 110 kcal or around 9% (**Table 2** and **Figure 1A** and **Supplementary Figure 1**). This hypophagic effect of insulin primarily concerned carbohydrate intake, whereas consumption of fat and protein was not affected [$F_{(2, 170)} = 3.23$, $p = 0.042$ for treatment × macronutrient; **Table 2**]. The insulin effect was modified neither by sex nor age (all $p > 0.11$ for interaction with treatment; **Figure 1B**) and did not specifically affect individual food types [hearty, neutral, sweet; $F_{(2, 233)} = 0.71$, $p = 0.49$ for treatment × food type]. Independent of insulin treatment, men consumed more energy than women [1,276.23 ± 86.76 vs. 913.23 ± 50.64 kcal, $F_{(1, 43)} = 17.34$, $p = 0.0001$; **Figures 1C–F**], in

TABLE 2 | Consumption from the breakfast buffet.

	All subjects			Men			Women			Young subjects			Elderly subjects		
	Insulin	Placebo	p	Insulin	Placebo	p	Insulin	Placebo	p	Insulin	Placebo	p	Insulin	Placebo	p
Overall consumption	1,054.43 ± 50.91	1,162.36 ± 64.69	0.0095	1,188.79 ± 72.29	1,363.66 ± 97.42	0.0146	893.20 ± 54.30	932.30 ± 47.87	0.0143	1,032.90 ± 60.44	1,128.64 ± 70.78	0.0285	1,092.12 ± 96.11	1,217.89 ± 127.38	0.0210
MACRO-NUTRIENTS															
Carbohydrate	502.70 ± 25.97	589.82 ± 35.03	0.0079	543.82 ± 39.02	678.63 ± 55.67	0.0075	453.36 ± 30.66	488.32 ± 27.31	0.0073	531.03 ± 28.66	587.09 ± 36.26	0.001	453.12 ± 50.91	594.32 ± 72.64	0.0090
Fat	413.85 ± 28.95	430.65 ± 30.92	0.9866	485.51 ± 41.06	516.50 ± 46.48	0.9856	327.84 ± 32.46	332.54 ± 27.67	0.9853	368.75 ± 30.92	404.93 ± 33.51	0.9922	492.76 ± 55.63	473.02 ± 60.48	0.9916
Protein	137.89 ± 8.70	141.89 ± 9.15	1	159.46 ± 13.25	168.54 ± 13.29	1	112.00 ± 7.94	111.43 ± 8.68	1	133.12 ± 10.39	136.62 ± 11.28	1	146.23 ± 16.23	150.55 ± 15.74	1

Results are means ± SEM kcal, rounded to the nearest decimal. P-values are derived from least-squares means with multivariate t adjustment.

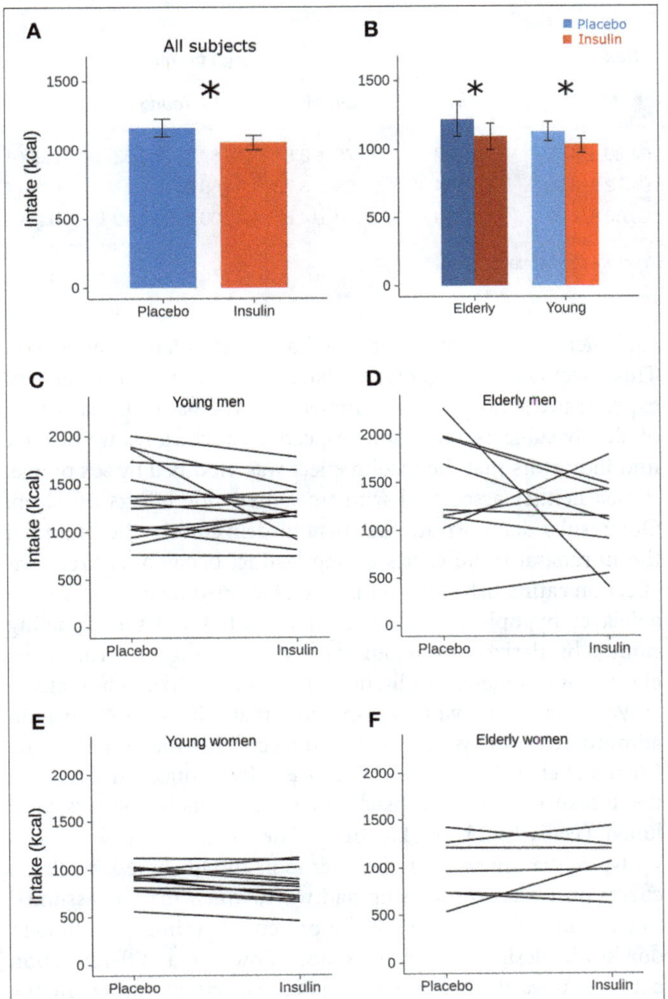

FIGURE 1 | Calorie intake. Mean (± SEM) calorie intake from the breakfast buffet assessed in the morning after intranasal administration of placebo (vehicle; blue bars) and insulin (160 IU; red bars) at 2220 h of the preceding evening in **(A)** all subjects and **(B)** according to age groups. **(C–F)** Individual calorie intake from the breakfast buffet in the placebo (left) and the insulin condition (right) in respectively, the young and elderly men and women. Individual values of both sessions are connected by lines. Note that omitting the male subjects showing the largest insulin effect yielded *p*-values for the factor condition of 0.015 and 0.079 in the groups of young and, respectively, elderly subjects. $n = 14$ young and 9 elderly men, and 14 young and 7 elderly women; *$p < 0.05$ for comparisons between conditions (least-square means with multivariate *t* adjustment).

particular fat [501.01 ± 43.50 vs. 330.25 ± 29.72 kcal, $t_{(54)} = 4.33$, $p = 0.0008$; $p > 0.05$ for carbohydrates and protein; $F_{(2,54)} = 4.13$, $p = 0.02$ for sex × macronutrient]. Men also ate more neutral-taste foods than women [248.74 ± 43.48 vs. 168.80 ± 22.92 kcal, $t_{(146)} = 5.73$, $p < 0.0001$; $p > 0.84$ for hearty and sweet foods]. Calorie intake of young and elderly participants was generally comparable [1,080.77 ± 65.85 vs. 1,156.91 ± 111.48 kcal, $F_{(1,44)} = 0.64$, $p = 0.43$; $F_{(1,55)} = 0.69$, $p = 0.41$ for sex × age; **Figures 1C–F**] and also did not differ regarding food types [$F_{(2,231)} = 0.53$, $p = 0.59$]. Age and macronutrient showed a significant interaction [$F_{(2,54)} = 4.38$, $p = 0.02$] that, however, did not yield significant age-dependent effects on macronutrient intake (all $p > 0.17$).

Overall, intranasal insulin did not alter hunger, thirst and tiredness as rated before breakfast (all $p > 0.50$), and there was no influence of sex on these values (all $p > 0.33$; **Table 3**). Elderly participants reported significantly lower hunger than their young counterparts [43.75 ± 3.81 vs. 67.56 ± 4.52%, $t_{(122)} = -4.64$, $p = 0.0001$], with no differences in thirst and tiredness (all $p > 0.19$; **Table 3**).

Energy Expenditure

Intranasal insulin administration before sleep did not affect resting energy expenditure measured in the young subjects before breakfast [1,637.96 ± 50.25 vs. 1,656.32 ± 50.87 kcal/day for insulin and placebo, respectively, $F_{(1,29)} = 0.971$, $p = 0.33$; **Figure 2**] and also did not induce sex-dependent changes [$F_{(1,28)} = 0.07$, $p = 0.80$]. Across conditions, women displayed significantly lower energy expenditure than men [1,418.63 ± 41.56 vs. 1,847.05 ± 46.24 kcal/day, $F_{(1,28)} = 49.27$, $p < 0.0001$].

Blood Parameters

In the young participants, a transient peak in plasma insulin concentration emerged 10 min after intranasal insulin administration (111.19 ± 9.38 vs. 56.67 ± 4.79 pmol/L after placebo; $p \leq 0.001$) that was followed by a slight dip in blood glucose values (4.38 ± 0.13 vs. 4.86 ± 0.06 mmol/L; $p \leq 0.01$). Neither of these changes was correlated with the intranasal insulin-induced decrease in breakfast intake in the subsequent morning ($r = -0.15$, $p = 0.54$, and $r = 0.02$, $p = 0.95$, respectively, Pearson's coefficients). During the rest of the night, respective values were comparable between conditions [$F_{(6,156)} = 0.86$, $p = 0.65$ for treatment × time; see Feld et al., 2016, for detailed results], without any statistical difference to the elderly group ($p = 0.24$ for age). Serum insulin as well as blood glucose concentrations were not affected by insulin administration in the elderly subjects (all $p > 0.58$). Across conditions, blood glucose levels were lower in elderly than young [$F_{(1,105)} = 14.49$, $p < 0.001$ for age] and in female than male individuals [$F_{(1,25)} = 10.14$, $p < 0.01$ for sex].

Plasma concentrations of total ghrelin, measured only in the group of young subjects, did not differ between conditions [17,940.26 ± 830.37 vs. 17,903.28 ± 763.61 h × pg/ml for insulin and placebo, respectively; $F_{(1,108)} = 0.01$, $p = 0.95$; $F_{(1,909)} = 0.0042$, $p = 0.95$ for time × treatment; **Figures 3A,B**]. They were generally elevated in women compared to men [20,258.09 ± 915.24 vs. 15,429.69 ± 967.39 h×pg/ml, $F_{(1,29)} = 16.31$, $p = 0.0004$]. Serum leptin concentrations in the young participants also remained unaffected by intranasal insulin [154.10 ± 23.25 vs. 156.47 ± 23.75 h × ng/ml, $F_{(1,31)} = 0.04$, $p = 0.85$; $F_{(1,406)} = 0.18$, $p = 0.67$ for time × treatment] and, as expected, were markedly higher in women compared to men [259.78 ± 27.57 vs. 50.69 ± 6.30 h × ng/ml, $F_{(1,30)} = 67.35$, $p < 0.0001$, **Figures 3C,D**].

Sleep and Heart Rate

Total sleep time for the young participants was 461.59 ± 3.37 min in the insulin and 460.70 ± 4.57 min in the placebo condition (*p*

TABLE 3 | Visual analog scale ratings obtained before breakfast.

	Overall			Sex			Age group		
	Insulin	Placebo	*p*	Female	Male	*p*	Elderly	Young	*p*
Hungry	58.96 ± 3.55	60.10 ± 3.63	1	55.84 ± 5.78	62.86 ± 4.26	0.4382	43.75 ± 3.81	67.56 ± 4.52	0.0001
Thirsty	63.00 ± 2.94	61.33 ± 3.25	0.9311	59.31 ± 4.77	64.72 ± 3.96	0.7564	54.69 ± 3.78	65.95 ± 4.17	0.1974
Tired	32.93 ± 3.17	36.98 ± 3.40	0.9837	41.14 ± 4.71	29.60 ± 4.37	0.3319	31.29 ± 4.61	36.83 ± 4.40	0.9398

Results are means ± SEM %. p values are derived from least-square means contrasts with multivariate t adjustment.

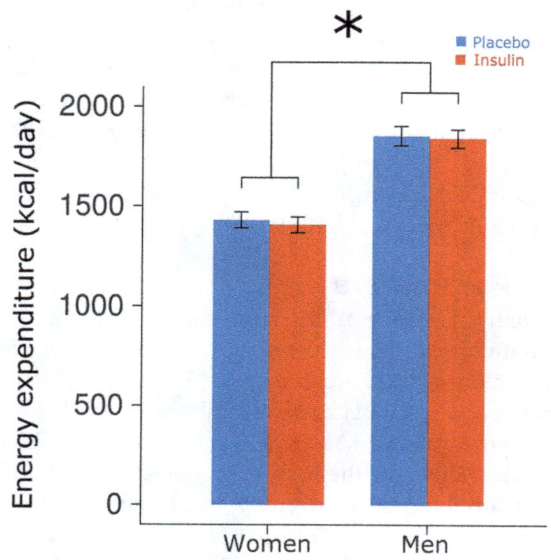

FIGURE 2 | Energy expenditure. Mean ± SEM energy expenditure measured in the young participants via indirect calorimetry in the morning after intranasal administration of placebo (vehicle; blue bars) and insulin (160 IU; red bars) at 2220 h of the preceding evening. Calorimetry was performed in the fasted state at 0710 h before breakfast. $^*p < 0.05$ for comparisons between sexes.

> 0.84). Elderly participants spent comparable amounts of time asleep (456.57 ± 11.12 vs. 458.39 ± 5.68 min, $p > 0.89$; $p > 0.57$ for group effect). Intranasal insulin compared to placebo did not alter sleep latency, whole-night sleep architecture and total sleep time (all $p > 0.29$). Heart rate measured in the young subjects throughout the night was unchanged by insulin [58.77 ± 1.59 vs. 58.98 ± 1.48 bpm, $F_{(1, 29{,}006)} = 0.08$, $p = 0.77$; **Figure 4**]. Independent of treatment, it showed a trend toward increased values in women compared to men [61.19 ± 1.96 vs. 56.63 ± 2.10 bpm; $F_{(1, 30)} = 3.72$, $p = 0.063$]. Heart rate measured in the elderly subjects before and after sleep was not modulated by intranasal insulin (all $p \geq 0.18$).

DISCUSSION

We investigated whether a single dose of intranasal insulin administered to healthy young and elderly subjects before nocturnal sleep attenuates calorie intake from a large, standardized ad-libitum breakfast buffet on the subsequent day. We found that pre-sleep insulin treatment reduced breakfast consumption by around 110 kcal, which is roughly equivalent to a large banana or half a chocolate-caramel bar. This effect emerged against the background of unaltered energy expenditure. Although the number of participants, in particular of elderly subjects, may limit respective conclusions, we did not find indicators that the insulin effect was modified by sex or age. It was neither associated with unwanted side effects on sleep. Our results demonstrate that insulin delivered to the brain via the intranasal route exerts a long-lasting, behaviorally relevant effect on eating behavior. While the exact mediators behind such a delayed hypophagic action of enhanced brain insulin signaling cannot be derived from our data, this finding underlines the efficacy of intranasal insulin in curbing food intake in humans.

We have previously shown that intranasal insulin administered to young male subjects in the fasted state (Benedict et al., 2008) acutely decreases food intake, and reduces the intake of palatable snacks in young female subjects after lunch (Hallschmid et al., 2012). The latter effect concerned post-prandial snacking in the afternoon and likely resulted from effects on reward-processing pathways, which may be assumed to have also played a role in the present experiments, although our study design clearly does not allow for a differentiation between reward- and hunger-related aspects of eating. In the former experiment (Benedict et al., 2008), the hypophagic insulin effect in the young men was observed in the late morning and around 80 min after intranasal delivery of 160 IU insulin, i.e., the same dose as applied in the present experiments. It was found during ad-libitum intake from a breakfast buffet that was comparable in composition and size to the buffet offered in the present study. Insulin administration in the morning led to a macronutrient-unspecific reduction in calorie intake of around 190 kcal in young men, which exceeded the drop in food intake of 110 kcal found in the young male subjects of the present experiments. Both effects developed against the background of well-comparable overall calorie intake (1,350 vs. 1,330 kcal in the respective placebo conditions of the former and, for the young men, the present study). In the former study (Benedict et al., 2008), young female participants did not show an insulin-induced reduction in food intake whereas pre-sleep insulin delivery reduced breakfast size in the young women of the present experiments. There are some indicators that central nervous insulin, with regard to food intake, may be less efficient in female compared to male organisms (Clegg et al., 2003, 2006). However, the women of our previous study (Benedict et al., 2008) ate around 130 kcal less than their female counterparts of the present experiments (769 vs. 895 kcal in the respective placebo conditions), so that a biasing contribution of bottom effects cannot be excluded.

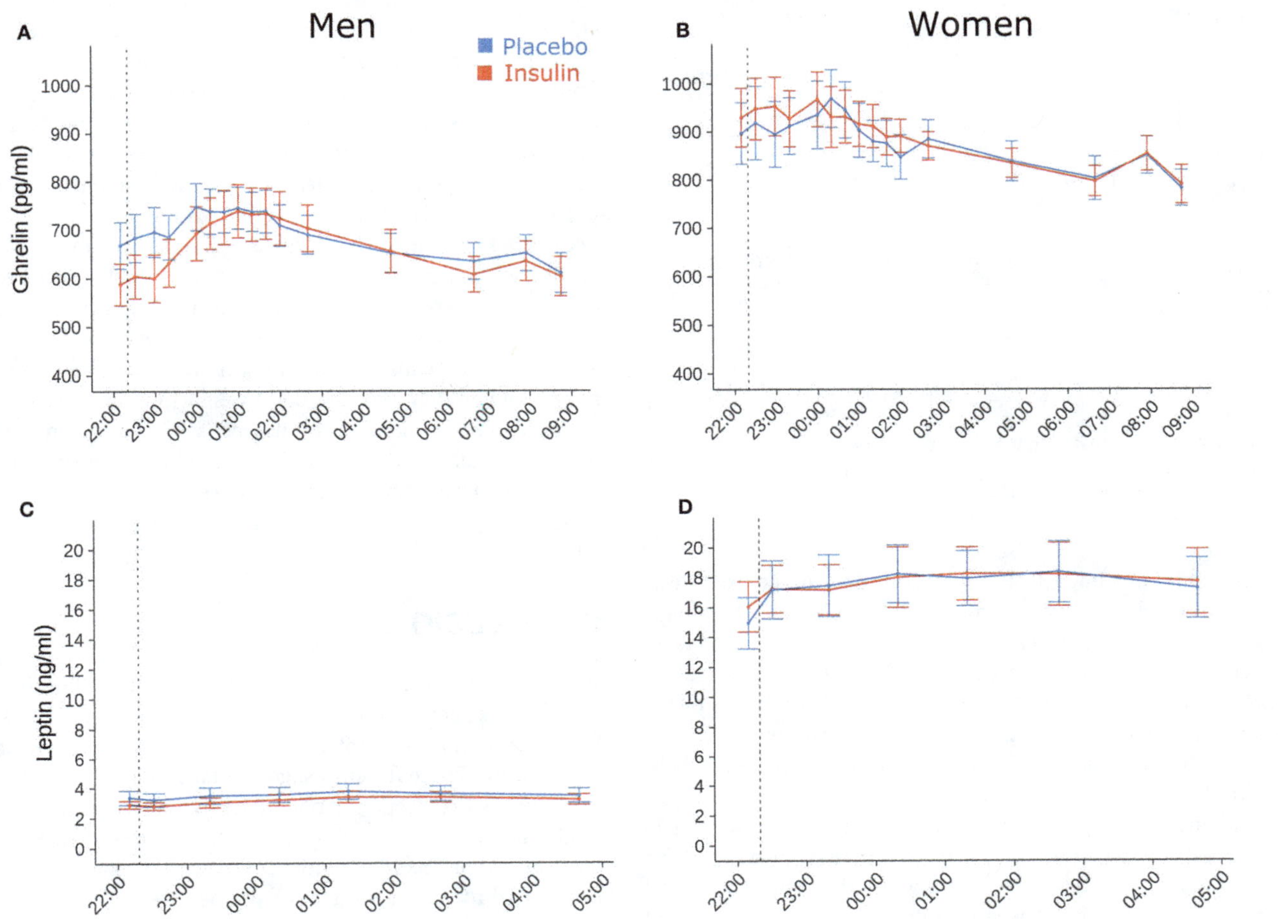

FIGURE 3 | Blood parameters. Mean ± SEM concentrations of **(A,B)** plasma total ghrelin and **(C,D)** serum leptin measured in young male (n = 16; left panels) and female participants (n = 16; right panels) who were intranasally administered insulin (160 IU; red lines) or placebo (blue lines) at 2220 h (dotted line). Note that leptin concentrations were determined only until 0440 h in the morning.

Basal energy expenditure assessed in the young subgroup before breakfast was comparable between conditions, indicating that the reduction in breakfast intake was not a compensatory effect, but yielded a net decrease in energy intake. This effect was primarily caused by a drop in the consumption of carbohydrates. This finding ties in with experiments in rats indicating that insulin administration to the CNS reduces sugar intake (Figlewicz et al., 2008) and suggests that, in accordance with the major role of peripheral insulin for blood glucose regulation, the anorexigenic effect of the hormone on the brain might focus on carbohydrates. However, the relative paucity of available data in humans (Benedict et al., 2008; Hallschmid et al., 2012; Jauch-Chara et al., 2012) and animals (Woods et al., 1979; McGowan et al., 1992; Air et al., 2002; Clegg et al., 2003, 2006) at the moment does not permit sound conclusions on macronutrient-specific effects of brain insulin on eating behavior (for review see Kullmann et al., 2016; Lee et al., 2016). Animal research has indicated that the adiposity signals insulin and leptin can directly act on the brain reward circuitry to decrease the intake of particularly palatable foods (Figlewicz et al., 2007). Although at a first glance, the insulin-induced reduction in carbohydrate intake would fit with the assumption that intranasal insulin specifically reduces the intake of highly rewarding foods (Hallschmid et al., 2012), sweet items as a food category were not differentially affected here. Considering that hunger ratings were comparable between conditions, it may be concluded that intranasal insulin did not affect hunger motivation, but rather acted via satiating factors that contribute to the termination of a meal. We did not find discernible treatment-induced changes in ghrelin and leptin, two hormones of paramount relevance for food intake control (Morton et al., 2014). A mild insulin-induced decrease in plasma glucose concentration apparently was restricted to the young participants although our study was not designed to detect respective differences between age groups. This dip in blood glucose, which was presumably due to absorption of insulin into the blood stream via the nasal mucosa (Ott et al., 2015), was statistically unrelated to the insulin-induced reduction in breakfast intake. It can be safely excluded to have affected breakfast intake because of its transient nature, and because nocturnal decreases in blood glucose levels rather increase than attenuate food intake in the morning (Schmid et al., 2008).

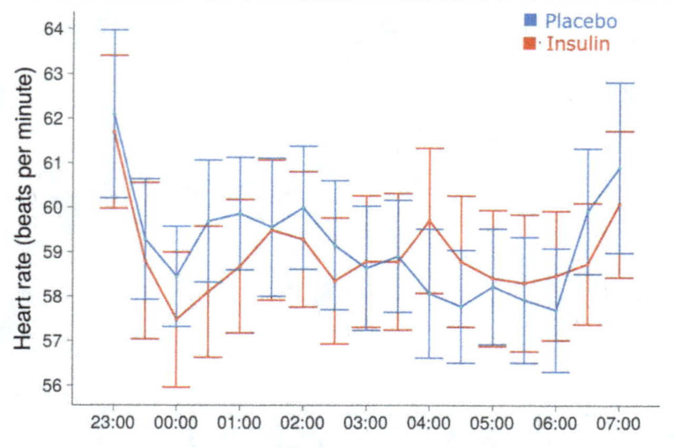

FIGURE 4 | Heart rate during the sleep period. Mean ± SEM heart rate averaged across 30-min blocks from minute-to-minute recordings. No signs of coherent treatment effects were detected (see Results).

The inhibitory impact on ad-libitum food intake exerted by intranasal insulin emerged across 10 h, which is a surprisingly long period of time when compared to respective effects in related studies (Benedict et al., 2008; Hallschmid et al., 2012; Jauch-Chara et al., 2012). Considering that degradation of the insulin molecule in the central nervous compartment can be assumed to be relatively delayed in comparison to its half-life in the circulation of 4–6 min (Duckworth et al., 1998), the enhanced brain insulin signal may in principle be still functionally active after a prolonged period of time. This assumption is supported by the finding that shifts in direct current EEG potentials triggered by intranasal insulin do not yet reach their maximum after around 90 min of recording (Hallschmid et al., 2004b). Alternatively, an indirect mediation of the observed effect might be assumed, but cannot be derived from our data inasmuch as endocrine signals like ghrelin and leptin, but also indicators of sympathovagal balance were unchanged and our study does not warrant a strict differentiation between central and peripheral mediators. Intranasal insulin exerted its anorexigenic effect across an interval of nocturnal sleep which, in itself, has turned out to be a relevant modulator of food intake (Schmid et al., 2015). Total sleep deprivation for one night leads to activity changes in brain functions that favor food intake (Greer et al., 2013), and partial sleep deprivation of 4 h for one night strongly increases breakfast intake in healthy men (Brondel et al., 2010). Since we did not observe differences in total sleep time nor in sleep architecture between conditions, insulin presumably did not exert major effects on sleep. However, sleep might have prolonged the insulin effect by reducing interfering effects of external stimuli, or increases in hunger typically developing in awake subjects across extended periods of time.

The relative reduction in pre-breakfast hunger ratings in the elderly, as compared to young participants, might be related to decreasing responses to food cues (Cheah et al., 2013) and impaired dynamics of satiety-regulating factors (Rolls et al., 1995) that emerge during aging, but was not reflected in differences in actual food intake. Young and elderly participants were also equally responsive to the anorexigenic effect of insulin. However, probably because of the relatively small number of elderly participants the effect appeared to be less robust in this group so that further studies should substantiate this finding. While decreases in central nervous insulin sensitivity have been linked to cognitive deficits and Alzheimer's disease, pathologies associated with advanced age (Freiherr et al., 2013), our results suggest that, at least in healthy individuals, age does not independently affect the role of insulin in central nervous networks that control food intake. Likewise, insulin sensitivity in the body periphery is not independently affected by biological age as long there is no increase in fat mass (Karakelides et al., 2010). Thus, the good health status of our elderly participants, as verified by clinical examination and evidenced by their merely moderately elevated body weight in comparison to our young subjects, might have ensured sufficient potency of the insulin signal. Vice versa, indicators of high cerebral insulin sensitivity have been found to be associated with successful loss of body fat during lifestyle intervention (Tschritter et al., 2012).

CONCLUSION

In sum, we demonstrate that intranasal insulin administration before nocturnal sleep elicits a reduction in breakfast intake in healthy subjects that is not compensated for by changes in energy expenditure. These findings suggest that insulin administered to the brain before sleep may potentiate the satiating effect of food intake in the next morning. The effect observed here was of moderate impact, and potential compensatory changes in eating behavior throughout the rest of the day were not investigated. In previous studies, four daily doses of intranasal insulin, one of them administered before going to bed, induced a reduction in body weight and fat in healthy participants (Hallschmid et al., 2004a), suggesting that on the long run the anorexigenic effect of (pre-sleep) intranasal insulin administration can affect body weight regulation. Thus, central nervous insulin administration regimens focusing on the sleep period may exert beneficial effects on metabolic health and might even help prevent or treat the brain insulin resistance associated with metabolic disorders (Kullmann et al., 2016).

AUTHOR CONTRIBUTIONS

JS conducted the data analyses. MH collected the data and contributed to the analyses. Both authors interpreted the data and wrote the manuscript.

FUNDING

This research was supported by grants from the Deutsche Forschungsgemeinschaft (DFG; SFB 654 "Plasticity and Sleep"), from the German Federal Ministry of Education and Research (BMBF) to the German Center for Diabetes Research (DZD e.V.; 01GI0925), and the Helmholtz Alliance ICEMED—Imaging and Curing Environmental Metabolic Diseases (ICEMED), through the Initiative and Networking Fund of the Helmholtz

Association. The funding sources had no input in the design and conduct of this study; in the collection, analysis, and interpretation of the data; or in the preparation, review, or approval of the article.

ACKNOWLEDGMENTS

We would like to thank Monika Schönauer and Matthias Thienel for major support and inspiring discussions while drafting this paper.

SUPPLEMENTARY MATERIAL

Supplementary Figure 1 | Boxplots of calorie intake from the breakfast buffet assessed in the morning after intranasal administration of placebo (vehicle; blue bars) and insulin (160 IU; red bars) at 2220 h of the preceding evening (A) according to age groups (elderly subjects, darker shades; young subjects, brighter shades) and **(B)** according to sex.

REFERENCES

Air, E. L., Benoit, S. C., Blake Smith, K. A., Clegg, D. J., and Woods, S. C. (2002). Acute third ventricular administration of insulin decreases food intake in two paradigms. *Pharmacol. Biochem. Behav.* 1, 423–429. doi: 10.1016/S0091-3057(01)00780-8

Bates, D., Mächler, M., Bolker, B., and Walker, S. (2015). Fitting linear mixed-effects models using lme4. *J. Stat. Softw.* 1, 1–48. doi: 10.18637/jss.v067.i01

Baura, G. D., Foster, D. M., Porte, D., Kahn, S. E., Bergman, R. N., Cobelli, C., et al. (1993). Saturable transport of insulin from plasma into the central nervous system of dogs *in vivo*. A mechanism for regulated insulin delivery to the brain. *J. Clin. Invest.* 4, 1824–1830. doi: 10.1172/JCI116773

Benedict, C., Kern, W., Schultes, B., Born, J., and Hallschmid, M. (2008). Differential sensitivity of men and women to anorexigenic and memory-improving effects of intranasal insulin. *J. Clin. Endocrinol. Metab.* 4, 1339–1344. doi: 10.1210/jc.2007-2606

Born, J., Lange, T., Kern, W., McGregor, G. P., Bickel, U., and Fehm, H. L. (2002). Sniffing neuropeptides: a transnasal approach to the human brain. *Nat. Neurosci.* 6, 514–516. doi: 10.1038/nn0602-849

Brondel, L., Romer, M. A., Nougues, P. M., Touyarou, P., and Davenne, D. (2010). Acute partial sleep deprivation increases food intake in healthy men. *Am. J. Clin. Nutr.* 6, 1550–1559. doi: 10.3945/ajcn.2009.28523

Cappuccio, F. P. F., D'Elia, L., Strazzullo, P., and Miller, M. A. (2010). Quantity and quality of sleep and incidence of type 2 diabetes: a systematic review and meta-analysis. *Diabetes Care* 2, 414–420. doi: 10.2337/dc09-1124

Cheah, Y. S., Lee, S., Ashoor, G., Nathan, Y., Reed, L. J., Zelaya, F. O., et al. (2013). Ageing diminishes the modulation of human brain responses to visual food cues by meal ingestion. *Int. J. Obes.* 9, 1186–1192. doi: 10.1038/ijo.2013.237

Clegg, D. J., Brown, L. M., Woods, S. C., and Benoit, S. C. (2006). Gonadal hormones determine sensitivity to central leptin and insulin. *Diabetes* 4, 978–987. doi: 10.2337/diabetes.55.04.06.db05-1339

Clegg, D. J., Riedy, C. A., Smith, K. A., Benoit, S. C., and Woods, S. C. (2003). Differential sensitivity to central leptin and insulin in male and female rats. *Diabetes* 3, 682–687. doi: 10.2337/diabetes.52.3.682

Dhuria, S. V., Hanson, L. R., and Frey, W. H. (2010). Intranasal delivery to the central nervous system: mechanisms and experimental considerations. *J. Pharm. Sci.* 4, 1654–1673. doi: 10.1002/jps.21924

Duckworth, W. C., Bennett, R. G., and Hamel, F. G. (1998). Insulin degradation: progress and potential. *Endocr. Rev.* 5, 608–624. doi: 10.1210/er.19.5.608

Feld, G. B., Wilhem, I., Benedict, C., Rüdel, B., Klameth, C., Born, J., et al. (2016). Central nervous insulin signaling in sleep-associated memory formation and neuroendocrine regulation. *Neuropsychopharmacology* 6, 1540–1550. doi: 10.1038/npp.2015.312

Figlewicz, D. P., Bennett, J. L., Aliakbari, S., Zavosh, A., and Sipols, A. J. (2008). Insulin acts at different CNS sites to decrease acute sucrose intake and sucrose self-administration in rats. *Am. J. Physiol. Regul. Integr. Comp. Physiol.* 2, R388–R394. doi: 10.1152/ajpregu.90334.2008

Figlewicz, D. P., Naleid, A. M., and Sipols, A. J. (2007). Modulation of food reward by adiposity signals. *Physiol. Behav.* 5, 473–478. doi: 10.1016/j.physbeh.2006.10.008

Freiherr, J., Hallschmid, M., Frey, W. H., Brünner, Y. F., Chapman, C. D., Hölscher, C., et al. (2013). Intranasal insulin as a treatment for alzheimer's disease: a review of basic research and clinical evidence. *CNS Drugs* 7, 505–514. doi: 10.1007/s40263-013-0076-8

Gangwisch, J. E., Heymsfield, S. B., Boden-Albala, B., Buijs, R. M., Kreier, F., Pickering, T. G., et al. (2007). Sleep duration as a risk factor for diabetes incidence in a large U.S. sample. *Sleep* 12, 1667–1673.

Greer, S. M., Goldstein, A. N., and Walker, M. P. (2013). The impact of sleep deprivation on food desire in the human brain. *Nat. Commun.* 4, 2259. doi: 10.1038/ncomms3259

Hallschmid, M., Benedict, C., Schultes, B., Fehm, H.-L., Born, J., and Kern, W. (2004a). Intranasal Insulin reduces body fat in men but not in women. *Diabetes* 11, 3024–3029. doi: 10.2337/diabetes.53.11.3024

Hallschmid, M., Higgs, S., Thienel, M., Ott, V., and Lehnert, H. (2012). Postprandial administration of intranasal insulin intensifies satiety and reduces intake of palatable snacks in women. *Diabetes* 4, 782–789. doi: 10.2337/db11-1390

Hallschmid, M., Schuttes, B., Marshall, L., Mölle, M., Kern, W., Bredthauer, J., et al. (2004b). Transcortical direct current potential shift reflects immediate signaling of systemic insulin to the human brain. *Diabetes* 9, 2202–2208. doi: 10.2337/diabetes.53.9.2202

Heni, M., Kullmann, S., Preissl, H., Fritsche, A., and Häring, H.-U. (2015). Impaired insulin action in the human brain: causes and metabolic consequences. *Nat. Rev. Endocrinol.* 12, 701–711. doi: 10.1038/nrendo.2015.173

Jauch-Chara, K., Friedrich, A., Rezmer, M., Melchert, U. H., Scholand-Engler, H. G., Hallschmid, M., et al. (2012). Intranasal insulin suppresses food intake via enhancement of brain energy levels in humans. *Diabetes* 9, 2261–2268. doi: 10.2337/db12-0025

Karakelides, H., Irving, B. A., Short, K. R., O'Brien, P., and Nair, K. S. (2010). Age, obesity, and sex effects on insulin sensitivity and skeletal muscle mitochondrial function. *Diabetes* 1, 89–97. doi: 10.2337/db09-0591

Kullmann, S., Heni, M., Hallschmid, M., Fritsche, A., Preissl, H., and Häring, H.-U. (2016). Brain insulin resistance at the crossroads of metabolic and cognitive disorders in humans. *Physiol. Rev.* 4, 1169–1209. doi: 10.1152/physrev.00032.2015

Lee, S. H., Zabolotny, J. M., Huang, H., Lee, H., and Kim, Y. B. (2016). Insulin in the nervous system and the mind: functions in metabolism, memory, and mood. *Mol. Metab.* 8, 589–601. doi: 10.1016/j.molmet.2016.06.011

Lenth, R. V. (2016). Least-squares means: the R package lsmeans. *J Stat Softw.* 1, 1–33. doi: 10.18637/jss.v069.i01

Magee, L., and Hale, L. (2012). Longitudinal associations between sleep duration and subsequent weight gain: a systematic review. *Sleep Med. Rev.* 3, 231–241. doi: 10.1016/j.smrv.2011.05.005

McGowan, M. K., Andrews, K. M., and Grossman, S. P. (1992). Chronic intrahypothalamic infusions of insulin or insulin antibodies alter body weight and food intake in the rat. *Physiol. Behav.* 4, 753–766. doi: 10.1016/0031-9384(92)90112-F

Morton, G. J., Meek, T. H., and Schwartz, M. W. (2014). Neurobiology of food intake in health and disease. *Nat. Rev. Neurosci.* 6, 367–378. doi: 10.1038/nrn3745

Ott, V., Lehnert, H., Staub, J., Wönne, K., Born, J., and Hallschmid, M. (2015). Central nervous insulin administration does not potentiate the acute glucoregulatory impact of concurrent mild hyperinsulinemia. *Diabetes* 3, 760–765. doi: 10.2337/db14-0931

Penev, P. D. (2012). Update on energy homeostasis and insufficient sleep. *J. Clin. Endocrinol Metab.* 97, 1792–1801. doi: 10.1210/jc.2012-1067

R Core Team (2016). *R: A Language and Environment for Statistical Computing.* Vienna: R Foundation for Statistical Computing.

Rechtschaffen, A., and Kales, A. (1968). *A Manual of Standardized Terminology, Techniques and Scoring System for Sleep Stages of Human Subject.* Washington, DC: US Government Printing Office; US Public Health Service.

Rolls, B. J., Dimeo, K. A., and Shide, D. J. (1995). Age-related impairments in the regulation of food intake. *Am. J. Clin. Nutr.* 5, 923–931.

Schmid, S. M., Hallschmid, M., Jauch-Chara, K., Wilms, B., Lehnert, H., Born, J., et al. (2011). Disturbed glucoregulatory response to food intake after moderate sleep restriction. *Sleep* 3, 371–377.

Schmid, S. M., Hallschmid, M., Jauch-Chara, K., Wilms, B., Benedict, C., Lehnert, H., et al. (2009). Short-term sleep loss decreases physical activity under free-living conditions but does not increase food intake under time-deprived laboratory conditions in healthy men. *Am. J. Clin. Nutr.* 6, 1476–1482. doi: 10.3945/ajcn.2009.27984

Schmid, S. M., Hallschmid, M., and Schultes, B. (2015). The metabolic burden of sleep loss. *Lancet Diabetes Endocrinol.* 1, 52–62. doi: 10.1016/S2213-8587(14)70012-9

Schmid, S. M., Jauch-Chara, K., Hallschmid, M., Oltmanns, K. M., Born, J., and Schultes, B. (2008). Short-term nocturnal hypoglycaemia increases morning food intake in healthy humans. *Diabet. Med.* 2, 232–235. doi: 10.1111/j.1464-5491.2007.02347.x

Schwartz, M. W., Peskind, E., Raskind, M., Boyko, E. J., and Porte, D. (1996). Cerebrospinal fluid leptin levels: relationship to plasma levels and to adiposity in humans. *Nat. Med.* 5, 589–593. doi: 10.1038/nm0596-589

St-Onge, M.-P., Bormes, A., and Salazar, I. (2016). The role of sleep duration on energy balance: an update. *Curr. Nutr. Rep.* 4, 278–285. doi: 10.1007/s13668-016-0178-2

Tschritter, O., Preissl, H., Hennige, A. M., Sartorius, T., Stingl, K. T., Heni, M., et al. (2012). High cerebral insulin sensitivity is associated with loss of body fat during lifestyle intervention. *Diabetologia* 1, 175–182. doi: 10.1007/s00125-011-2309-z

Vgontzas, A. N., Fernandez-Mendoza, J., Miksiewicz, T., Kritikou, I., Shaffer, M. L., Liao, D., et al. (2014). Unveiling the longitudinal association between short sleep duration and the incidence of obesity: the Penn State Cohort. *Int. J. Obes.* 6, 825–832. doi: 10.1038/ijo.2013.172

William, A., and Banks, B. S. P. (2001). Leptin transport across the blood-brain barrier: implications for the cause and treatment of obesity. *Curr. Pharm. Des.* 2, 125–133. doi: 10.2174/1381612013398310

Woods, S. C., Lotter, E. C., McKay, L. D., and Porte, D. (1979). Chronic intracerebroventricular infusion of insulin reduces food intake and body weight of baboons. *Nature* 5738, 503–505. doi: 10.1038/282503a0

7

Central Amino Acid Sensing in the Control of Feeding Behavior

*Nicholas Heeley and Clemence Blouet**

Medical Research Council Metabolic Disease Unit, Institute of Metabolic Science, University of Cambridge, Cambridge, UK

***Correspondence:**
Clemence Blouet
csb69@medschl.cam.ac.uk

Dietary protein quantity and quality greatly impact metabolic health *via* evolutionary-conserved mechanisms that ensure avoidance of amino acid imbalanced food sources, promote hyperphagia when dietary protein density is low, and conversely produce satiety when dietary protein density is high. Growing evidence supports the emerging concept of protein homeostasis in mammals, where protein intake is maintained within a tight range independently of energy intake to reach a target protein intake. The behavioral and neuroendocrine mechanisms underlying these adaptations are unclear. While peripheral factors are able to signal amino acid deficiency and abundance to the brain, the brain itself is exposed to and can detect changes in amino acid concentrations, and subsequently engages acute and chronic responses modulating feeding behavior and food preferences. In this review, we will examine the literature describing the mechanisms by which the brain senses changes in amino acids concentrations, and how these changes modulate feeding behavior.

Keywords: food intake, amino acids, protein, leucine, brain, appetite

INTRODUCTION

Over the past 20 years, a large number of studies have refined our understanding of how neuroendocrine networks detect internal energy availability and modulate behavioral circuits controlling energy intake to maintain energy homeostasis (1). Food intake is also driven by factors independent of internal energy balance. This is well illustrated by the contribution of the sensory and hedonic value of a diet to the control of energy intake independently of energy homeostasis (2). In addition, the need for specific macronutrients or nutrients can affect appetite and food choices, but the mechanisms underlying how individual macronutrients influence feeding behavior or how appetite for specific macronutrients/nutrients influences energy intake remain unclear.

Ensuring sufficient consumption of protein is essential for growth, reproduction, and species survival (3). Animals, from insects to mammals, have evolved mechanisms to ensure quantitatively and qualitatively adequate protein intake (3, 4). Detection of lack or abundance of single amino acids can have profound acute and chronic effects on feeding behavior and food preference (5, 6). In addition, within a certain range, dietary protein content is a determinant of total

---

Abbreviations: eIF2, eukaryotic initiation factor 2α; AAA, aromatic amino acids; AgRP, agouti-related peptide; APC, anterior piriform cortex; ATP, adenosine triphosphate; BBB, blood–brain barrier; BCAA, branched-chain amino acids; BCAT, branched-chain amino acid transferase; BCKDH, branched-chain ketoacid dehydrogenase; CNS, central nervous system; EAA, essential amino acids; GABA, γ-aminobutyric acid; GCN2, general control non-derepressible 2; HP, high protein; icv, intracerebroventricular; KIC, α-ketoisocaproic acid; KO, knock out; LP, low protein; MBH, mediobasal hypothalamus; mTOR, mammalian target of rapamycin; NPY, neuropeptide Y; NTS, nucleus tractus solitarii; OVN, overnight; POMC, pro-opio melanocortin; PVH, paraventricular nucleus of the hypothalamus; TCA, tricarboxylic acid; WT, wild type.

energy intake (7). Moderately low-protein diets are associated with an increase in energy intake, adjusted to match minimum requirements for nitrogen and essential amino acids (EAA) (8). Conversely, high-protein diets reduce energy intake, presumably to prevent excessive amino acid levels potentially toxic for the brain (9). This remarkable bidirectional adjustment of energy intake based on dietary protein content has been proposed to target a protein intake of 15% across multiple species from insects to humans (10) and supports the idea that protein intake is regulated by homeostatic mechanisms somewhat independent of energy intake or intake of carbohydrate and fat.

In this review, we will examine the literature exploring how the brain monitors internal amino acid availability and how this central detection modulates food intake. We will not discuss in detail the peripheral mechanisms by which amino acids are sensed and how these mechanisms may interact with the brain to control food intake (8, 11).

DIET-INDUCED CHANGES IN BRAIN AMINO ACID CONCENTRATIONS

The unique morphological and functional properties of mammalian cerebral endothelial cells that form the blood–brain barrier (BBB) allow the brain to be protected from toxins and sheltered from variations in blood composition, presumably providing the central nervous system (CNS) with an optimal chemical environment for cerebral functions. Amino acid homeostasis is particularly critical in the brain, as a number of non-EAA – L-glutamate, L-aspartate, L-cysteine, L-homocysteine, glycine, alanine, and taurine – can act directly as neurotransmitters when released at the synapse, while other amino acids, L-tyrosine and L-tryptophan, serve as precursors for neurotransmitters, the catecholamines, and serotonin, respectively. In addition, branched-chain amino acids (leucine, isoleucine, and valine – BCAA) serve as precursors for the neurotransmitter glutamate and pathologically high BCAA concentrations, as seen in Maple Syrup Disease, cause excessive glutamatergic signaling and neurological symptoms (9).

Four facilitative saturable amino acid carriers have currently been identified to be expressed on the luminal side (blood side) of the mammalian BBB, maintaining intra-cerebral levels of amino acids within a narrow range to about 10% of plasma levels (12–14). However, the idea that all amino acids are non-specifically buffered to that fraction is challenged by discoveries demonstrating selective transport of amino acids across the BBB. This was first suggested by the observation that following arterial delivery of radiolabeled amino acids in rats, brain uptake of essential neutral amino acids is 5- to 10-fold greater than that of non-EAA (15, 16). Molecular support for this observation indicates that the system L1 amino acid transporter, which carries most EAA including branched-chain (leucine, isoleucine, and valine – BCAA) and aromatic (phenylalanine, tyrosine, and tryptophan – AAA) amino acids, is the predominant amino acid transport system expressed in the brain endothelium (13, 17, 18). In addition, the luminal and abluminal (brain side) membranes of the brain endothelium are functionally distinct, as sodium-dependent amino acid transport systems are present exclusively on the abluminal membrane, providing the BBB with a mechanism to actively export amino acids against the concentration gradient (13, 19). Thus, the BBB expresses transport systems that allow selective import and exports of amino acids and active regulation of brain extracellular amino acid composition.

BCAA and AAA compete for transport through system L1, and consequently, the blood ratio of BCAA to AAA levels is a major determinant of brain extracellular and cerebrospinal amino acid composition (9). Decreased plasma BCAA levels, as seen in specific contexts including endurance training or adaptation to ketogenic diets, are associated with decreased brain BCAA levels, increased uptake of tryptophan and tyrosine into brain, and increased synthesis of serotonin and catecholamines (20, 21). Conversely, increased plasma BCAA levels are reflected in brain BCAA levels, and negatively impact brain AAA uptake and serotonin synthesis (9, 13). Such changes have been reported in contexts associated with chronic increases in BCAA levels including diabetes or maintenance on a high-protein diet (12, 22–25) but also acutely following food ingestion (26). In fact, while the plasma level of most amino acids remains relatively stable in the postprandial period, BCAA levels rapidly and transiently rise as they largely escape first-pass splanchnic metabolism (27–29), resulting in a rapid increase in brain BCAA levels (26, 30–32). This observation led to the hypothesis that circulating BCAA levels may represent a signal of postprandial protein availability that regulates various anabolic functions modulated by dietary proteins. Consistently, BCAA have been shown to mediate protein-induced transcription, insulin secretion, and protein synthesis (33–35). Likewise, brain BCAA levels may mediate protein-induced modulations of centrally controlled functions, including appetite and metabolism, as discussed below.

Only a few studies have explored the regional differences in the kinetics of brain amino acid uptake following meal ingestion. Microdialysis studies in rats demonstrated that after oral gavage of a balanced amino acid mix or ingestion of a 50% protein meal, there were consistent increases in the concentrations of BCAA in the lateral and periventricular nuclei of the hypothalamus within 20–40 min of meal consumption, while the concentrations of the majority of other amino acids remained unchanged, with the exception of methionine and tyrosine that consistently increase in these brain regions following a meal (36–38). Whether this effect is specific to these brain regions or also occurs in other areas of the brain, including other hypothalamic nuclei, remains to be determined. In contrast, regional differences in the concentration of BCAA and AAA following the ingestion of amino acid imbalanced diets have been described. In this context, while the concentration of the limiting amino acid decreases in discrete sites, including the pyriform cortex, locus coeruleus, and the nucleus of the solitary tract, hypothalamic areas are protected from this deficiency (39–41). Collectively, these data indicate that amino acid concentrations in the brain are not a simple reflection of the plasma amino acid profile but vary selectively in discrete sites under specific dietary contexts.

CENTRAL DETECTION OF ESSENTIAL AMINO ACID DEVOID OR UNBALANCED DIETS

The marked reduction in energy intake and growth of animals maintained on diets containing very low protein amounts (<8% in rats; <5% in mice) or imbalanced EAA ratios was first described over 100 years ago (42). Seminal studies from Harper and colleagues demonstrated that the anorectic response to imbalanced amino acid diets is the cause rather than the consequence of growth failure, supporting a direct role for dietary amino acids in the regulation of food intake (43–46). Analysis of the behavioral responses to the ingestion of a diet devoid in one EAA indicated that the initial rapid anorectic response is followed by the onset of a learned conditioned taste aversion and the development of a specific appetite for the limiting amino acid (5, 47–51). These two latter adaptations have been associated with chronic changes in feeding-regulating circuits and are secondary to acute neuronal amino acid sensing, as reviewed in (52).

The rapid initial aversive response to EAA-devoid diets, manifested by a decrease in meal size and an increase in inter-meal interval, occurs within 20–40 min following feeding onset and is dependent on acute amino acid interoception. This response is independent of food sensory stimuli or peripheral signals (53–55) and instead relies on direct neuronal sensing of EAA imbalance by the anterior piriform cortex (APC). This assertion is supported by the following observations: (i) APC lesions prevent rats discriminating between AA containing and AA devoid diets (56, 57), (ii) concentrations of the limiting EAA in the APC rapidly fall after the introduction of the devoid diet (41, 48), through competition at the capillary endothelial amino acid transport system (58–60), and (iii) replacement of the limiting EAA into the APC *via* microinjections rapidly increases intake of a diet deficient in that EAA (49, 57, 61, 62). Importantly, this aversive response was shown to be independent of diet palatability and novelty (63). Thus, the APC is both necessary and sufficient to produce rapid hypophagia in response to EAA imbalanced diets.

Neurophysiological and neuroanatomical evidence further indicate that local APC EAA sensing initiates the response to EAA-devoid diets and engages neurocircuits connected to hypothalamic, pontine, and hindbrain feeding-regulating networks (**Figure 1A**). Neurons in the APC have been shown to be excited by the absence of threonine or the presence of the amino alcohols, which cause tRNA uncharging (61, 64). Changes in local interneuron interactions, at least in part *via* decreased local inhibitory GABAergic tone (65), cause a change in output signal from glutamatergic APC neurons (66) – their excitatory output is potentiated when GABAergic inhibitory control is lost. Tracing studies from the APC identified the projection targets of APC EAA sensing neurons [reviewed in Ref. (52)], but the functional

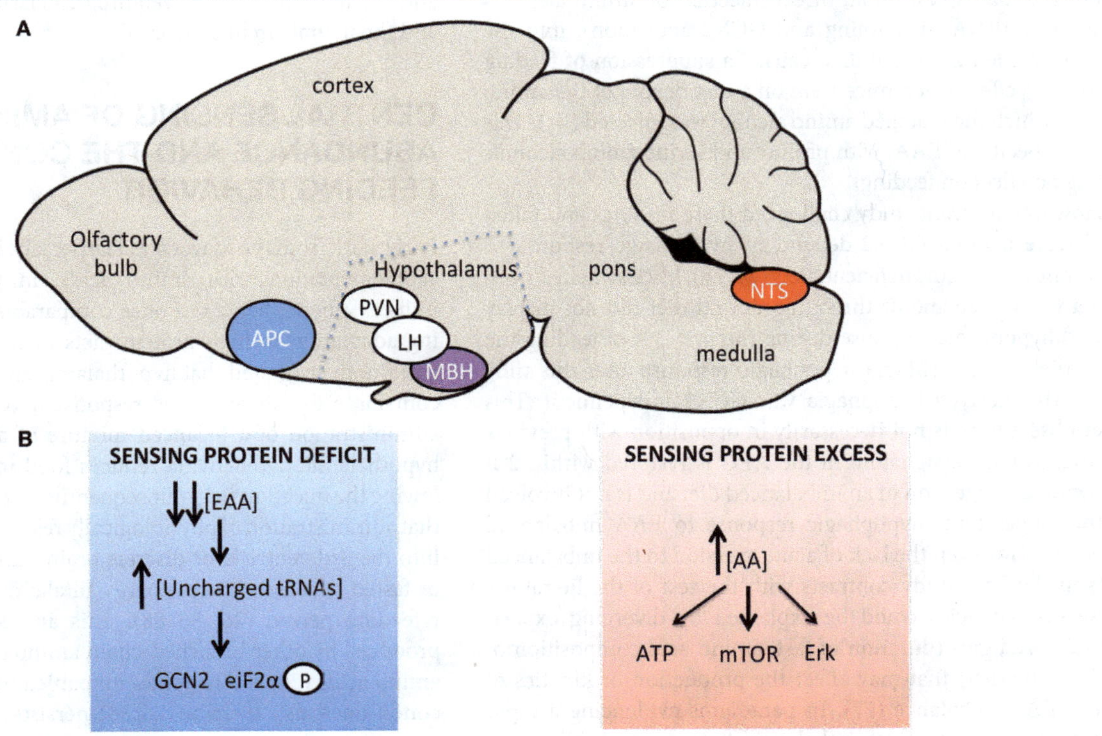

FIGURE 1 | Brain regions and signaling pathways involved in central amino acid sensing. (A) Sagittal representation of the rodent brain with amino acid sensing brain regions identified. Blue – regions sensing amino acid imbalanced diets or very low-protein diets, Red – regions sensing increases in amino acid concentrations, Purple – regions involved in sensing bidirectional changes in amino acid concentrations, White – regions involved in neurocircuitory of amino acid sensing, which are not primary sensing sites. **(B)** Signaling pathways implicated in central sensing of amino acid deficit or excess.

relevance of the targets in the acute aversion to EAA deficiency has not been directly addressed. Two hypothalamic regions have been implicated in this acute response: the VMH and the LH, both rapidly activated in response to a lysine-deficient meal according to fMRI assessments in rats (67). Norepinephrine and dopamine levels are rapidly increased in these regions under these conditions (39, 62), providing some neurochemical insights into the circuits engaged from APC EAA imbalance chemodetection. Clearly, the precise circuits engaged downstream from the APC in mammals to produce the rapid aversion to EAA imbalance remain partially characterized, and novel circuit mapping tools would prove useful to decipher these circuits.

Work by two independent groups demonstrated that the rapid detection of dietary EAA deficiency within the APC occurs *via* a GCN2-dependent mechanism in mice; this pathway is also required for rejection of for EAA imbalanced diets in drosophila (68). The GCN2 pathway is an evolutionarily conserved pathway identified in yeast to mediate the detection of amino acid deficiency (69, 70). When cellular amino acid levels fall, uncharged tRNAs accumulate in the cell, bind to GCN2 that displays kinase activity toward eiF2α (eukaryotic initiation factor 2α), causing a global suppression of translation, but increased transcription of starvation relevant transcripts (**Figure 1B**). Evidence supporting a role for this pathways in the aversion to unbalanced EAA diet was obtained using GCN2 knockout mice, in which the rapid aversion to unbalanced diets is markedly blunted (71, 72) and downstream signaling, increased eiF2α phosphorylation (73), is absent (71, 72). In addition, direct injection of amino alcohols (that cause tRNA uncharging and GCN2 activation), into the APC of rats fed a normal diet, caused a suppression of feeding but had no effect when mice were on a diet devoid of the amino acid for which the matched amino alcohol was injected (71). This effect is specific to EAA, with proline and serine amino alcohols having no effect on feeding.

However, a recent study challenged these findings and failed to observe a rapid GCN2-dependent hypophagic response to threonine and leucine deficient diets (74, 75). Mice switched from a control to a leucine or threonine-devoid diet did not display a rapid hypophagic response during the first 3 h of feeding the novel diet but did show a hypophagic response after this time point. This delayed hypophagia was GCN2 independent. This latter observation is not necessarily in opposition with previous reports, as GCN2 signaling in the APC is restored within 2 h following the ingestion of an imbalanced diet and is not involved in the longer term hypophagic response to EAA imbalanced diets (76). However, the lack of acute aversion to the imbalanced diets in the Leib study contrasts with the rest of the literature. These discrepancies could be explained by diverging experimental paradigms (duration of fast, amino acid composition of the baseline diet) that may affect the production or kinetics of central EAA imbalance (77). In paradigms evidencing a rapid aversive response to EAA imbalance diets, a rapid fall in the APC concentration of the limiting amino acid occurred in the same time course as the production of the hypophagic response, within 40 min of diet exposure (41, 48, 78), and correlated with the activation of the GCN2 pathway in the APC (71, 72). In the Leib study, plasma concentrations of the missing amino acid and APC GCN2 signaling 1 h after diet exposure were unchanged, suggesting that the EAA imbalance failed to reach the APC during early exposure to the diet in these conditions.

More recently, the mediobasal hypothalamus has been proposed to be a primary sensing site of EAA deficiency (79). After an overnight fast, a leucine devoid diet caused an increase in eIF2α phosphorylation in the MBH within 40 min of diet consumption. Adenoviral-mediated knockdown of GCN2 in the MBH blunted the anorectic response to a leucine deficient diet over an hour of diet consumption. In addition, icv L – leucinol injection increased eiF2α phosphorylation selectively in the MBH and was sufficient to inhibit feeding in WT mice, but not GCN2 KO mice. Importantly, L – leucinol did not activate eiF2α signaling in the APC, demonstrating (i) the specificity of the protocol to target the MBH alone and (ii) the sufficiency of the MBH to initiate an aversive response to a leucine deficient diet. However, in earlier studies, no changes in the concentration of the limiting amino acid were found in three hypothalamic nuclei studied (39), suggesting changes in amino acid concentrations are not uniform across the brain. While the hypothalamus is clearly involved downstream of the APC in the anorectic response to AA deficient diets (80–82), further work will be needed to explore if the MBH is required for primary sensing of EAA deficiency.

While there is controversy about the mechanism and site(s) of central amino acid sensing in this context (75, 77), the ability of central amino acid absence to regulate feeding behavior is clear, and further work will be required to clarify these mechanisms and the neural circuits involved.

CENTRAL SENSING OF AMINO ACID ABUNDANCE AND THE CONTROL OF FEEDING BEHAVIOR

Early work from the Mayer and Harper labs identified that dietary supplementation with amino acids, in particular L-leucine, induces a hypophagic response comparable to that seen following adaptation to high-protein diets in rats (83, 84). Panskeep and Booth suggested that hypothalamic amino acid sensing may contribute to this anorectic response and reported that direct administration of a balanced mixture of amino acids into the hypothalamic parenchyma reduces food intake within 1 h following the injection (85). Subsequently, several groups confirmed that administration of physiologically relevant amounts of leucine into the 3rd ventricle or discrete brain nutrient-sensing regions of fasted rodents reduces energy intake during the subsequent refeeding period (26, 86–88). This anorectic response is not produced by other branched-chain amino acids or any aromatic amino acids (26, 87), is not accompanied by the development of conditioned taste aversion (26, 86), persists for 24 h, and produces a significant decrease in body weight gain (26, 86), as summarized in **Table 1**. Brain leucine levels are increased following a meal, and brain leucine administration reduces food intake, suggesting that brain amino acid levels may constitute a signal of energy and/or protein availability detected by brain nutrient-sensing regions that modulate homeostatic feeding-regulatory circuits.

TABLE 1 | Effects of centrally administered amino acids on food intake.

Paper	Species	Conditions	Time of injection	Route	Amino Acid	Dose	Food intake
(86)	Rat	24 h fast	Before onset of dark cycle	3rd icv	Leucine	1.1 μg	↓
(88)	Rat	24 h fast	–	3rd icv	RPMI Amino Acid Mix Leucine	1 μg Leucine, and other EAA 1, 3, 10 μg	↓ ↓
(89)	Rat	6 h fast	5–6 pm (onset of dark cycle)	3rd icv	Leucine	197 ng, 787 ng, 1.6 μg	No effect of 197 ng, others lowered feeding
(26)	Rat Mouse	OVN fast 6 h fast	1 h before onset of dark cycle 1 h before onset of dark cycle	MBH MBH	Leucine Leucine Valine	56 ng 28 ng 28 ng	↓ ↓ No effect
(90)	Rat	OVN fast	1 h before onset of dark cycle	NTS	Leucine Valine	28 ng 28 ng	↓ No effect
(87, 91)	Rat Rat	24 h fast 24 h fast	2 h prior to lights off 2 h prior to lights off	3rd icv 3rd icv	Leucine Tryptophan, Methionine, Lysine, Threonine, Serine	10 ug 10 ug	↓ No effect
	Rat	No fast LP diet	2 h prior to lights off	3rd icv	Leucine	10 μg	↓
(92)	Mouse	OVN fast	After overnight fast	3rd icv	Leucine	2.2 μg	No effect
(93)	Mouse	6 h fast	1 h before onset of dark cycle	NTS	Leucine	14 ng	↓

Leucine abundance is detected in the brain through neurochemically diverse and neuroanatomically distributed networks modulating feeding behavior. This is supported by the observation that both the mediobasal hypothalamus and the nucleus of the solitary tract in the caudomedial brainstem contain leucine-sensing cells that can modulate feeding behavior in response to leucine abundance (**Figure 1A**). Although these two apparently redundant sensing sites produce similar behaviors when injected with leucine, further studies are necessary to understand how they may differently be engaged in physiological contexts. Within each of these sensing sites, the population of leucine-sensing cells is heterogeneous. In the mediobasal hypothalamus, POMC neurons but also non-POMC neurons are activated in response to local leucine administration (26). Likewise, in the NTS, leucine-sensing cells are diverse and comprise POMC neurons, catecholaminergic neurons, and maybe as yet uncharacterized cell types (90). However, this is based on the sole use of c-FOS as a marker of neuronal activation, and we know very little about the electrophysiological response of these cells to leucine. Based on c-FOS studies, only a sub-population of cells within the MBH or NTS respond to leucine (26, 90), but what makes a cell leucine-sensitive or not is an open question, and whether leucine-sensing cells share a common molecular signature remains to be determined. To date, only arcuate POMC neurons have been shown to depolarize in response to leucine bath application in slice preparations, and the underlying mechanisms remains to be characterized (26, 92) (**Figure 1B**).

The detailed analysis of the feeding response to increased leucine levels within the hypothalamus or brainstem further supports the idea that leucine sensing engages multiple behavioral output circuits to control food intake. Indeed, meal pattern analyses show that the reduction in food intake measured in food-deprived rats and mice who received brain injections of leucine results from the alteration of various components of the feeding sequence: increased first meal latency (and therefore decreased orexigenic tone), decreased meal size and decreased meal frequency. One circuit implicated in the acute reduction in meal size following hypothalamic leucine sensing involves hypothalamic POMC neurons, their melanocortinergic projections to PVH oxytocin neurons and oxytocinergic projections to the nucleus of the solitary tract in the caudomedial brainstem (26). However, pharmacological inhibition of this circuit is neither sufficient to suppress the rapid reduction in first meal latency nor entirely blunt the anorectic response to leucine, suggesting that other circuits are involved in the overall behavioral response to brain leucine detection. One possible candidate to mediate the immediate increase in first meal latency following leucine hypothalamic administration in fasted rodents is AgRP neurons. This neuronal population is critical to the development of hunger and foraging during food deprivation (94, 95). Consistent with this possibility, leucine was found to regulate AgRP expression in hypothalamic GT1-7 cells (88). However, whether leucine can rapidly affect electrical or synaptic activity of AgRP neurons is unknown, and more generally, how changes in extracellular concentrations of leucine can rapidly and more chronically affect neuronal activity remains poorly characterized.

Activation of mTORC1 has been consistently associated with brain leucine sensing in the regulation of feeding (86). mTORC1 is an evolutionary-conserved signaling pathway that couples nutrient and growth factor sensing in the control of protein synthesis, growth, cell cycle progression and other processes (96). Within 30 min following discrete injections of leucine into the rodent MBH or NTS, phosphorylation of one of the major effector of mTORC1, p70 S6 kinase 1 (S6K1), increases in the respective site (26, 90). In rats, co-administration of rapamycin, a specific mTORC1 inhibitor, blunts leucine's effect on meal size and early hypophagia, implicating activation of mTORC1 in the mechanisms underlying leucine-sensing in hypothalamic and brainstem feeding-regulating circuits. Further evidence in support for a role of mTOR in the regulation of feeding indicates that inhibition of MBH or Dorsal Vagal Complex mTOR signaling with rapamycin in fed rodents rapidly drives feeding and increases meal size

(26, 86, 90). Conversely, constitutive activation of S6K1 inhibits feeding *via* a specific decrease in meal size in both the MBH and the Dorsal Vagal Complex. These data support a role for endogenous mTOR signaling in the control of meal size and foraging behavior. Interestingly, activation of neuronal TOR signaling has also been implicated in the control of feeding in drosophila. In this invertebrate, activation of p70 S6K1 signaling in neurons that control feeding produces hypophagia in fasted larvae, whereas its down-regulation produces increased foraging and feeding in fed larvae, and these responses engage neuropeptide Y-like signaling (97). Collectively, these data indicate that mTOR in discrete nutrient-sensing neurons is an evolutionary-conserved regulator of feeding behavior.

To better characterize the neurochemical populations of the MBH in which mTOR signaling is important in the control of feeding and metabolism in mice, Smith et al. generated mice with germline deletion of S6K1 from either POMC or AgRP neurons (92). Unexpectedly, a thorough metabolic phenotyping revealed that both lines had normal food intake, feeding behavior and energy expenditure under various experimental conditions. S6K1 deletion in both POMC and AgRP neurons reduced neuronal excitability, and reduces synaptic strength in AgRP neurons, resulting in impaired POMC and AgRP tone in these mice, but these alterations are not sufficient to produce a phenotype. This latter observation is consistent with reports showing that germline loss of AgRP neurons fail to affect energy balance, which supports the idea that feeding-regulatory circuits are plastic during development (98). This raises the possibility that S6K1 loss of function is compensated for in these lines. Further investigations are required to clarify the role of S6K1 in AgRP and POMC neurons in the regulation of energy balance in adult rodents.

As mentioned above, increased mTOR signaling is not sufficient to account for decreased meal frequency following MBH or NTS leucine administration (26, 90). We hypothesized that intracellular leucine metabolism, leading to ATP production, may contribute to neuronal leucine sensing in a mechanism analogous to the pancreatic and brain glucose sensing mechanism (99–101). Leucine undergoes intracellular metabolism, producing α-ketoisocaproic acid (KIC) and isovaleryl – CoA, respectively by branched-chain amino acid transferase (BCAT) and branched-chain ketoacid dehydrogenase (BCKDH), leading to the production of TCA cycle intermediates and ATP production that could contribute to leucine sensing in the MBH. Consistently, KIC injection into the mouse MBH suppressed feeding but through a specific decrease in meal number, without affecting meal size, suggesting that this mechanism is not recruited for the acute effects of leucine on foraging and meal size (26). Moreover, injection of an activator of BCKDK, resulting in an increase in the metabolism of leucine, caused a suppression of food intake, due to specific reduction in meal number. In addition, data obtained in mice bearing a whole body deletion of BCATm, expressed in astrocytes in the CNS and peripheral tissues, suggest that long-term high BCAA levels in the brain affect dietary preferences (102). This deletion produces high brain leucine concentrations. Although energy intake does not differ between the KO and the controls, these mice have a higher preference for a low BCAA diet over a normal diet, indicating that chronic abundance of BCAA in the brain induces changes in food choices that do not require BCAA transamination.

To our knowledge, leucine is the only EAA that has been found to produce an anorectic response when administered alone (**Table 1**). Orexin/hypocretin neurons, an orexigenic neuronal population in the lateral hypothalamus, have been shown to respond specifically to non-EAA using c-FOS staining and slice electrophysiology (103). The depolarization of these neurons in response to non-EAA was mediated by System A amino acid transporters and a suppression of the hyperpolarizing activity of K_{ATP} channels. Unlike in the MBH, leucine did not activate these neurons, as assessed by c-FOS immunohistochemistry and electrophysiology. The sensing of non-EAA was shown to be mTOR independent. Whether this sensing mechanism modulates feeding behavior remains to be established.

DIETS WITH VARYING PROTEIN CONTENT: THE PROTEIN LEVERAGE HYPOTHESIS

As discussed above, a number of species avoid and develop conditioned aversion for diets very low in protein or with imbalanced EAA compositions. In contrast, marginally low-protein diets (LP, 8–10% of energy as protein in rats) with balanced EAA profiles induce a hyperphagic response restoring nitrogen and EAA intakes which, together with various metabolic adaptions, are sufficient to enable growth (87, 91, 104–108). Conversely, high-protein diets (HP, 20–70% of energy as protein) produce a sustained decrease in energy intake that is not caused by taste aversion even at very high-protein levels (109, 110). These bidirectional behavioral responses to shifts in dietary protein content are evolutionary conserved from insects to humans (111), and protein intake has been proposed to be regulated independently of energy intake (7, 112). In the following section, we will highlight the literature describing the role of brain amino acid sensing in the bidirectional regulation of energy intake in response to changes in dietary protein content.

Response to Low-Protein Diets

Rats develop hyperphagia (starting day 2) following transition to a 10% protein diet (87, 113), but little is known about the behavioral components of this response, and to our knowledge, meal pattern analysis has not been performed in this context. Plasma levels of most EAA drop in the first 24 h after shift to a LP diet, but this response is only transient (87), and consistently, brain levels of amino acids, including BCAA and AAA, are not affected by LP feeding (12, 87). However, plasma and brain levels of BCAA and AAA fail to increase in response to food ingestion in rats adapted to a LP diet (87), suggesting that the inability to detect amino acids in the postprandial period could reduce satiety and contribute to hyperphagia. Consistent with this hypothesis, icv administration of leucine produces anorexia in LP-fed rats (87). To directly test the role of brain BCAA sensing in the hyperphagic response to LP diets, Morrison et al. measured energy intake in rats fed LP diets supplemented with leucine or BCAA (87). None of these treatments suppressed the hyperphagic response to LP diets, but confirmation that they produce increases in brain BCAA levels is missing. The authors went on and treated LP-fed rats with icv chronic amino acid infusions (87). They found that icv amino acid infusions could only partially blunt LP-induced hyperphagia, suggesting that the hyperphagic response to LP diets primarily involves peripheral amino acid sensing sites. These data argue against a role for direct brain amino acid detection in LP-induced hyperphagia but are not sufficient to rule out a contribution of brain amino acid sensing is this adaptation, as a lack of dynamic changes in BCAA or leucine levels in discrete nutrient-sensing regions, typically in the postprandial period, may contribute to reduced satiety in this model.

Data from the same group implicate hepatic FGF21 production in the metabolic and feeding responses to LP diets (91, 114). FGF21 circulating levels are dramatically increased in response to LP diets in mice, rats, and humans (91), and remarkably, *Fgf21* knockout mice are protected against the metabolic effects of LP diets (114). Using *Gcn2* knockout mice, the authors provided evidence suggesting that hepatic GCN2 responds to LP diets and promotes FGF21 production and release. These data clearly implicate FGF21 signaling in the metabolic adaptations to protein restriction, but whether brain amino acid sensing contributes to these responses remains to be clarified (**Figure 1B**). Interestingly, mTOR signaling interacts with GCN2 signaling (115, 116) and bidirectionally regulates FGF21 production (117), suggesting that multiple amino acid sensing pathways may orchestrate the overall metabolic and feeding responses to LP diets.

Response to High-Protein Diets

At the other end of the spectrum, high-protein diets have been consistently shown to reduce energy intake in multiple species, from flies to humans (7, 111). When rats previously adapted to a normal-protein diet are offered a HP diet, they immediately decrease their food intake and progressively but incompletely re-increase food intake on the following days (118–121). Gut amino acid sensing and recruitment of local vagal afferents have been implicated in these responses, as reviewed in Ref. (11, 122). However, vagal afferents are not sufficient to produce the anorectic response to HP diets, as subdiaphragmatic vagotomy does not abolish the ability of a HP diet to reduce food intake (123). Brain detection of increased amino acid levels, particularly BCAA, may therefore also contribute.

Meal pattern analysis of rats exposed to a HP diet indicates that the initial important anorectic response to HP diets is mainly driven by a transient decrease in meal size, whereas after adaptation to the diet, decreased meal frequency is primarily accounting for the reduced energy intake (109). Ropelle et al. implicated activation of hypothalamic mTOR signaling in this response and found interestingly that although adaptation to a HP diet induced a chronic increase in brain leucine concentrations, hypothalamic mTOR signaling was only transiently increased (89). Thus, transient increase in hypothalamic mTOR signaling could account for the transient decrease in meal size during early exposure to HP feeding. In contrast, increase hypothalamic leucine catabolism may underlie the chronic decrease in meal frequency. However, there is currently no direct evidence to support this interpretation, and research in this field would significantly progress with the identification of a central mechanism specifically mediating the identification of protein abundance. Likewise, little is known about the neurocircuits involved in the hypophagic response to HP diets. Expression of *Pomc*-, *Npy*-, and *Agrp*-feeding neuropeptides is altered in response to a HP diet in rats (89), but these findings have been recently challenged (124), leaving open the contribution of melanocortinergic feeding circuits in the hypophagic response to increased dietary protein intake.

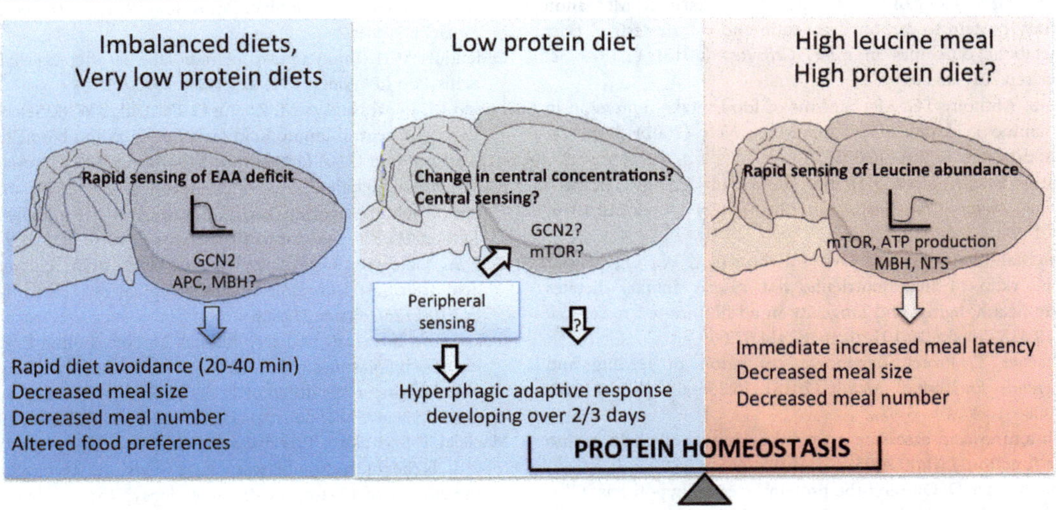

FIGURE 2 | Central detection of amino acid availability in the regulation of feeding behavior. Discrete cell populations in the brain monitor extracellular amino acid availability through a variety of mechanisms and engage downstream feeding-regulatory circuits to prevent or limit the ingestion of diets with imbalanced essential amino acid content, produce hyperphagia if dietary protein content is low and conversely reduce food intake if dietary protein content is high.

CONCLUSION

Collectively, the data reviewed here support a role for a distributed network of discrete brain regions in primary amino acid sensing in the control of multiple behavioral responses to changes in dietary amino acid intake, as summarized in **Figure 2**. Many gaps remain to be filled to complete our understanding of these processes, and a key poorly described step is the intracellular coupling of intracellular amino acid availability to neuronal electrical and synaptic activity, as highlighted in **Figure 1B**. Does this coupling rely on specific intracellular components that could perhaps represent a unique molecular signature of amino acid sensing neurons, making these cells amenable to molecular genetics? Identifying a molecular marker for amino acid sensing neurons would prove extremely useful in the characterization of neurocircuits engaged downstream from primary brain sensors to regulate feeding behavior.

Brain amino acid sensing also modulates feeding behavior on a chronic basis and in some cases affects food preferences. The neurobiological substrates supporting these chronic changes are poorly characterized, and how dietary amino acids may affect the remodeling of central circuits regulating energy balance is unknown.

Central amino acid sensing has also been implicated in the regulation of metabolism and glucose homeostasis. Studies in flies and rodents suggest that decreased protein intake accounts for the beneficial metabolic effects of caloric restriction (3, 4, 125). Further work is required to determine how central amino acid sensing processes implicated in the control of feeding behavior may also coordinate metabolic effectors of energy balance and possibly mediate the beneficial effects of caloric restriction of metabolic health and lifespan.

Lastly, although we did not discuss in depth the evidence supporting the concept of protein homeostasis, understanding how distributed peripheral and central amino acid sensors monitor amino acid quantitative and qualitative availability to adjust feeding behavior is a long-term challenge in the field. The characterization of this "homeostatic" control could help identify novel targets for the prevention or treatment of obesity, potentially uncoupling the beneficial satiety effects of protein from their deleterious consequences on metabolic health.

AUTHOR CONTRIBUTIONS

Both authors contributed to the preparation of the manuscript.

FUNDING

This work was supported by the Medical Research Council Metabolic Disease Unit [MR/M501736/1].

REFERENCES

Morton GJ, Meek TH, Schwartz MW. Neurobiology of food intake in health and disease. *Nat Rev Neurosci* (2014) 15:367–78. doi:10.1038/nrn3745

Zheng H, Lenard NR, Shin AC, Berthoud H-R. Appetite control and energy balance regulation in the modern world: reward-driven brain overrides repletion signals. *Int J Obes (Lond)* (2009) 33(Suppl 2):S8–13. doi:10.1038/ijo.2009.65

Fontana L, Partridge L. Promoting health and longevity through diet: from model organisms to humans. *Cell* (2015) 161:106–18. doi:10.1016/j.cell.2015.02.020

Solon-Biet SM, Mitchell SJ, Coogan SCP, Cogger VC, Gokarn R, McMahon AC, et al. Dietary protein to carbohydrate ratio and caloric restric- tion: comparing metabolic outcomes in mice. *Cell Rep* (2015) 11:1529–34. doi:10.1016/j.celrep.2015.05.007

Gietzen DW, Hao S, Anthony TG. Mechanisms of food intake repression in indispensable amino acid deficiency. *Annu Rev Nutr* (2007) 27:63–78. doi:10.1146/annurev.nutr.27.061406.093726

Schwartz G. Central leucine sensing in the control of energy homeostasis. *Endocrinol Metab Clin North Am* (2013) 42:81–7. doi:10.1016/j.ecl.2012.12.001

Solon-Biet SM, McMahon AC, Ballard JWO, Ruohonen K, Wu LE, Cogger VC, et al. The ratio of macronutrients, not caloric intake, dictates cardiometabolic health, aging, and longevity in ad libitum-fed mice. *Cell Metab* (2014) 19:418–30. doi:10.1016/j.cmet.2014.02.009

Morrison CD, Laeger T. Protein-dependent regulation of feeding and metabolism. *Trends Endocrinol Metab* (2015) 26:256–62. doi:10.1016/j.tem.2015.02.008

Fernstrom JD. 4th amino acid assessment workshop branched-chain amino acids and brain function. *J Nutr* (2005) 135:1539S–46S.

Simpson SJ, Raubenheimer D. Obesity: the protein leverage hypothesis. *Obes Rev* (2005) 6:133–42. doi:10.1111/j.1467-789X.2005.00178.x

Fromentin G, Darcel N, Chaumontet C, Marsset-Baglieri A, Nadkarni N, Tomé D. Peripheral and central mechanisms involved in the control of food intake by dietary amino acids and proteins. *Nutr Res Rev* (2012) 25:29–39. doi:10.1017/S0954422411000175

Colombo J, Cervantes H, Kokorovic M, Pfister U, Perritaz R. Effect of differ- ent protein diets on the distribution of amino acids in plasma, liver and brain in the rat. *Ann Nutr Metab* (1992) 36:23–33. doi:10.1159/000177695

Hawkins RA, O'Kane RL, Simpson IA, Vina JR. Structure of the blood-brain barrier and its role in the transport of amino acids. *J Nutr* (2006) 136:218S–26S.

Nishimura F, Nishihara M, Mori M, Torii K, Takahashi M. Excitability of neurons in the ventromedial nucleus in rat hypothalamic slices: modulation by amino acids at cerebrospinal fluid levels. *Brain Res* (1995) 691:217–22. doi:10.1016/0006-8993(95)00719-7

Battistin L, Grynbaum A, Lajtha A. The uptake of various amino acids by the mouse brain in vivo. *Brain Res* (1971) 29:85–99. doi:10.1016/0006-8993(71)90419-7

Oldendorf WH. Brain uptake of radiolabeled after arterial amino injection acids. *Am J Physiol* (1971) 221:1629–39.

Boado RJ, Li JY, Nagaya M, Zhang C, Pardridge WM. Selective expression of the large neutral amino acid transporter at the blood-brain barrier. *Proc Natl Acad Sci U S A* (1999) 96:12079–84. doi:10.1073/pnas.96.21.12079

Killian DM, Chikhale PJ. Predominant functional activity of the large, neutral amino acid transporter (LAT1) isoform at the cerebrovasculature. *Neurosci Lett* (2001) 306:1–4. doi:10.1016/S0304-3940(01)01810-9

Betz A, Goldstein G. Polarity of the blood-brain barrier: neutral amino acid transport into isolated brain capillaries. *Science* (1978) 202:225–7. doi:10.1126/science.211586

Blomstrand E, Perrett D, Parry-Billings M, Newsholme E. Effect of sustained exercise on plasma amino acid concentrations and on 5-hydroxytryptamine metabolism in six different brain regions in the rat. *Acta Physiol Scand* (1989) 136:473–81. doi:10.1111/j.1748-1716.1989.tb08689.x

Maciejak P, Szyndler J, Turzyńska D, Sobolewska A, Kołosowska K, Krząścik P, et al. Is the interaction between fatty acids and tryptophan responsible for the efficacy of a ketogenic diet in epilepsy? The new hypoth- esis of action. *Neuroscience* (2016) 313:130–48. doi:10.1016/j.neuroscience. 2015.11.029

Crandall E, Fernstrom J. Effect of experimental diabetes on the levels of aromatic and branched-chain amino acids in rat blood and brain. *Diabetes* (1983) 32:222–30. doi:10.2337/diabetes.32.3.222

Glanville N, Anderson G. The effect of insulin deficiency, dietary protein intake, and plasma amino acid concentrations on brain amino acid levels in rats. *Can J Physiol Pharmacol* (1985) 63:487–94. doi:10.1139/y85-084

Masiello P, Balestreri E, Bacciola D, Bergamini E. Influence of experimental diabetes on brain levels of monoamine neurotransmitters and their precursor amino acids during tryptophan loading. *Acta Diabetol Lat* (1987) 24:43–50. doi:10.1007/BF02732052

Peters JC, Harper A. Adaptation of rats to diets containing different levels of protein: effects on food intake, plasma and brain amino acid concentrations and brain neurotransmitter metabolism. *J Nutr* (1985) 115:382–98.

Blouet C, Jo Y-H, Li X, Schwartz GJ. Mediobasal hypothalamic leucine sensing regulates food intake through activation of a hypothalamus-brainstem circuit. *J Neurosci* (2009) 29:8302–11. doi:10.1523/JNEUROSCI.1668-09.2009

Brosnan JT, Brosnan ME. Branched-chain amino acids: enzyme and substrate regulation. *J Nutr* (2006) 136:207S–11S.

Nishioka M, Imaizumi A, Ando T, Tochikubo O. The overnight effect of dietary energy balance on postprandial plasma free amino acid (PFAA) profiles in Japanese adult men. *PLoS One* (2013) 8:e62929. doi:10.1371/ journal.pone.0062929

Wahren J, Felig P, Hagenfeld L. Effect of protein ingestion on splachnic and leg metabolism in normal man and in patients with diabetes mellitus. *J Clin Invest* (1976) 57:987–99. doi:10.1172/JCI108375

Glaeser BS, Maher TJ, Wurtman RJ. Changes in brain levels of acidic, basic, and neutral amino acids after consumption of single meals containing various proportions of protein. *J Neurochem* (1983) 41:1016–21. doi:10.1111/j.1471-4159.1983.tb09045.x

Kanamori K, Ross BD, Kondrat RW. Rate of glutamate synthesis from leucine in rat brain measured in vivo by 15N NMR. *J Neurochem* (1998) 70:1304–15. doi:10.1046/j.1471-4159.1998.70031304.x

Voog L, Eriksson T. Relationship between plasma and brain large neutral amino acids in rats fed diets with different compositions at different times of the day. *J Neurochem* (1992) 59:1868–74. doi:10.1111/j.1471-4159.1992.tb11022.x

Henquin J-C, Dufrane D, Nenquin M. Nutrient control of insulin secretion in isolated normal human islets. *Diabetes* (2006) 55:3470–7. doi:10.2337/db06-0868

Kimball SR, Jefferson LS. Signaling pathways and molecular mechanisms through which branched-chain amino acids mediate translational control of protein synthesis. *J Nutr* (2006) 136:227S–31S.

Nair KS, Schwartz RG, Welle S. Leucine as a regulator of whole body and skel- etal muscle protein metabolism in humans. *Am J Physiol* (1992) 263:E928–34.

Choi Y, Chang N, Anderson G. An intragastric amino acid mixture influences extracellular amino acid profiles in the lateral hypothalamic area of freely moving rats. *Can J Physiol Pharmacol* (1999) 77:827–34. doi:10.1139/y99-082

Choi YH, Fletcher PJ, Anderson GH. Extracellular amino acid profiles in the paraventricular nucleus of the rat hypothalamus are influenced by diet composition. *Brain Res* (2001) 892:320–8. doi:10.1016/S0006-8993(00)03267-4

Currie PJ, Chang N, Luo S, Anderson GH. Microdialysis as a tool to measure dietary and regional effects on the complete profile of extracel- lular amino acids in the hypothalamus of rats. *Life Sci* (1995) 57:1911–23. doi:10.1016/0024-3205(95)02178-L

Gietzen DW, Leung PMB, Rogers QR. Dietary amino acid imbalance and neurochemical changes in three hypothalamic areas. *Physiol Behav* (1989) 46:503–11. doi:10.1016/0031-9384(89)90028-0

Gietzen DW, Leung PM, Rogers QR. Norepinephrine and amino acids in prepyriform cortex of rats fed imbalanced amino acid diets. *Physiol Behav* (1986) 36:1071–80. doi:10.1016/0031-9384(86)90482-8

Koehnle TJ, Russell MC, Morin AS, Erecius LF, Gietzen DW. Diets deficient in indispensable amino acids rapidly decrease the concentration of the limiting amino acid in the anterior piriform cortex of rats. *J Nutr* (2004) 134:2365–71.

Willcock E, Hopkins F. The importance of individual amino-acids in metabolism: observations on the effect of adding tryptophane to a dietary in which zein is the sole nitrogenous constituent. *J Physiol* (1906) 35:88–102. doi:10.1113/jphysiol.1906.sp001181

Harper A, Benevenga N, Wohlhueter R. Effects of ingestion of disproportionate amounts of amino acids. *Physiol Rev* (1970) 50:428–558.

Rogers QR, Morris JG, Freedland RA. Lack of hepatic adaptation to low and high levels of dietary protein in the adult rat. *Enzyme* (1977) 55:348–56.

Rogers QR, Egan AR. Amino acid imbalance in the liquid-fed lamb. *Aust J Biol Sci* (1975) 28:169–81.

Leung PM, Rogers QR. Effect of amino acid imbalance and deficiency on dietary choice patterns of rats. *Physiol Behav* (1986) 37:747–58.

Feurté S, Tomé D, Gietzen D, Even P, Nicolaïdis S, Fromentin G. Feeding patterns and meal microstructure during development of a taste aversion to a threonine devoid diet. *Nutr Neurosci* (2002) 5:269–78. doi:10.1080/10284150290032003

Feurté S, Nicolaïdis S, Even PC, Tome D, Mahe S, Fromentin G. Rapid fall in plasma threonine followed by increased intermeal interval in response to first ingestion of a threonine-devoid diet in rats. *Appetite* (1999) 33:329–41. doi:10.1006/appe.1999.0242

Gietzen DW, Rogers QR. Nutritional homeostasis and indispensable amino acid sensing: a new solution to an old puzzle. *Trends Neurosci* (2006) 29:91–9. doi:10.1016/j.tins.2005.12.007

Mori M, Kawada T, Ono T, Torii K. Taste preference and protein nutrition and l-amino acid homeostasis in male Sprague-Dawley rats. *Physiol Behav* (1991) 49:987–95. doi:10.1016/0031-9384(91)90212-7

Torii K, Mawatari K, Yugari Y. Effect of dietary protein on the taste preference for amino acids and sodium chloride in rats. *Ann N Y Acad Sci* (1987) 510:665–8. doi:10.1080/87559129809541162

Gietzen DW, Aja SM. The brain's response to an essential amino acid-deficient diet and the circuitous route to a better meal. *Mol Neurobiol* (2012) 46:332–48. doi:10.1007/s12035-012-8283-8

Leung PMB, Larson DM, Rogers QR. Food intake and preference of olfactory bulbectomized rats fed amino acid imbalanced or deficient diets. *Physiol Behav* (1972) 9:553–7. doi:10.1016/0031-9384(72)90011-X

Markison S, Gietzen DW, Spector AC. Essential amino acid deficiency enhances long-term intake but not short-term licking of the required nutri- ent. *J Nutr* (1999) 129:1604–12.

Washburn BS, Jiang JC, Cummings SL, Dixon K, Gietzen DW. Anorectic responses to dietary amino acid imbalance: effects of vagotomy and tropisetron. *Am J Physiol* (1994) 266:R1922–7.

Leung P, Rogers Q. Importance of prepyriform cortex in food-intake response of rats to amino acids. *Am J Physiol* (1971) 221:929–35.

Beverly JL, Gietzen DW, Rogers QR. Effect of dietary limiting amino acid in prepyriform cortex on food intake. *Am J Physiol* (1990) 259:R709–15.

Tackman JM, Tews JK, Harper AE. Dietary disproportions of amino acids in the rat: effects on food intake, plasma and brain amino acids and brain serotonin. *J Nutr* (1990) 120:521–33.

Tews JK, Kim YW, Harper AE. Induction of threonine imbalance by dispensable amino acids: relation to competition for amino acid transport into brain. *J Nutr* (1979) 109:304–15.

Tews JK, Good SS, Harper AE. Transport of threonine and tryptophan by rat brain slices: relation to other amino acids at concentrations found in plasma. *J Neurochem* (1978) 31:581–9. doi:10.1111/j.1471-4159.1978.tb07828.x

Rudell JB, Rechs AJ, Kelman TJ, Ross-Inta CM, Hao S, Gietzen DW. The anterior piriform cortex is sufficient for detecting depletion of an indispensable amino acid, showing independent cortical sensory function. *J Neurosci* (2011) 31:1583–90. doi:10.1523/JNEUROSCI.4934-10.2011

Russell M, Koehnle T, Barrett J, Blevins J, Gietzen D. The rapid anorectic response to a threonine imbalanced diet is decreased by injection of threonine into the anterior piriform cortex of rats. *Nutr Neurosci* (2003) 6:247–51. doi:10.1080/1028415031000151567

Koehnle TJ, Russell MC, Gietzen DW. Rats rapidly reject diets deficient in essential amino acids. *J Nutr* (2003) 133:2331–5.

Magrum LJ, Hickman MA, Gietzen DW. Increased intracellular calcium in rat anterior piriform cortex in response to threonine after threonine deprivation. *J Neurophysiol* (1999) 81:1147–9.

Truong BG, Magrum LJ, Gietzen DW. GABA(A) and GABA(B) receptors in the anterior piriform cortex modulate feeding in rats. *Brain Res* (2002) 924:1–9. doi:10.1016/S0006-8993(01)03213-9

Blevins JE, Truong BG, Gietzen DW. NMDA receptor function within the anterior piriform cortex and lateral hypothalamus in rats on the control of intake of amino acid-deficient diets. *Brain Res* (2004) 1019:124–33. doi:10.1016/j.brainres.2004.05.089

Yokawa T, Tabuchi E, Takezawa M, Ono T, Torii K. Recognition and neural plasticity responding to deficient nutrient intake scanned by a functional

MRI in the brain of rats with l-lysine deficiency. *Obes Res* (1995) 3(Suppl 5): 685S–8S. doi:10.1002/j.1550-8528.1995.tb00486.x

Bjordal M, Arquier N, Kniazeff J, Pin JP, Leopold P. Sensing of amino acids in a dopaminergic circuitry promotes rejection of an incomplete diet in drosophila. *Cell* (2014) 156:510–21. doi:10.1016/j.cell.2013.12.024

Dong J, Qiu H, Garcia-Barrio M, Anderson J, Hinnebusch A. Uncharged tRNA activates GCN2 by displacing the protein kinase moiety from a bipartite tRNA-binding domain. *Mol Cell* (2000) 6:269–79. doi:10.1016/ S1097-2765(00)00028-9

Zhang P, McGrath BC, Reinert J, Olsen DS, Lei L, Gill S, et al. The GCN2 eIF2alpha kinase is required for adaptation to amino acid deprivation in mice. *Mol Cell Biol* (2002) 22:6681–8. doi:10.1128/MCB.22.19.6681

Hao S, Sharp J, Ross-Inta C, McDaniel B, Anthony T, Wek R, et al. Uncharged tRNA and sensing of amino acid deficiency in mammalian piriform cortex. *Science* (2005) 307:1776–8. doi:10.1002/9780470114735. hawley00624

Maurin AC, Jousse C, Averous J, Parry L, Bruhat A, Cherasse Y, et al. The GCN2 kinase biases feeding behavior to maintain amino acid homeo- stasis in omnivores. *Cell Metab* (2005) 1:273–7. doi:10.1016/j.cmet.2005. 03.004

Gietzen DW, Ross CM, Hao S, Sharp JW. Phosphorylation of eIF2a is involved in the signaling of indispensible amino acid deficiency in the anterior piriform cortex of the brain in rats. *J Nutr* (2004) 134:717–23.

Leib DE, Knight ZA. Re-examination of dietary amino acid sensing reveals a GCN2-independent mechanism. *Cell Rep* (2015) 13:1081–9. doi:10.1016/ j.celrep.2015.09.055

Leib DE, Knight ZA. Rapid sensing of dietary amino acid deficiency does not require GCN2. *Cell Rep* (2016) 16:2051–2. doi:10.1016/j.celrep.2016. 08.022

Magrum L, Teh P, Kreiter M, Hickman M, Gietzen D. Transfer ribonucleic acid charging in rat brain after consumption of amino acid-imbalanced diets. *Nutr Neurosci* (2002) 5:125–30. doi:10.1080/10284150290018982

Gietzen DW, Anthony TG, Fafournoux P, Maurin A-C, Koehnle TJ. Letter measuring the ability of mice to sense dietary essential amino acid deficiency: the importance of amino acid status and timing. *Cell Rep* (2016) 16:2049–50. doi:10.1016/j.celrep.2016.08.021

Gloaguen M, Le Floc'h N, Corrent E, Primot Y, van Milgen J. Providing a diet deficient in valine but with excess leucine results in a rapid decrease in feed intake and modifies the postprandial plasma amino acid and α-keto acid concentrations in pigs. *J Anim Sci* (2012) 90:3135–42. doi:10.2527/ jas.2011-4956

Maurin AC, Benani A, Lorsignol A, Brenachot X, Parry L, Carraro V, et al. Hypothalamic eIF2a signaling regulates food intake. *Cell Rep* (2014) 6:438–44. doi:10.1016/j.celrep.2014.01.006

Bellinger LL, Evans JF, Tillberg CM, Gietzen DW. Effects of dorsomedial hypothalamic nuclei lesions on intake of an imbalanced amino acid diet. *Am J Physiol* (1999) 277:R250–62.

Blevins JE, Dixon KD, Hernandez EJ, Barrett JA, Gietzen DW. Effects of threonine injections in the lateral hypothalamus on intake of amino acid imbalanced diets in rats. *Brain Res* (2000) 879:65–72. doi:10.1016/ S0006-8993(00)02734-7

Gietzen DW, Erecius LF, Rogers QR. Neurochemical changes after imbal- anced diets suggest a brain circuit mediating anorectic responses to amino acid deficiency in rats. *J Nutr* (1998) 128:771–81.

Krauss R, Mayer J. Influence of protein and amino acids on food intake in the rat. *Am J Physiol* (1965) 209:479–83.

Rogers Q, Tannous R, Harper A. Effects of excess leucine on growth and food selection. *J Nutr* (1967) 91:561–72.

Panskeep J, Booth D. Decreased feeding after injections of amino acids into the hypothalamus. *Nature* (1971) 233:341–2. doi:10.1038/233341a0

Cota D, Proulx K, Smith KAB, Kozma SC, Thomas G, Woods SC, et al. Hypothalamic mTOR signaling regulates food intake. *Science* (2006) 312:927–30. doi:10.1126/science.1124147

Laeger T, Reed SD, Henagan TM, Fernandez DH, Taghavi M, Addington A, et al. Leucine acts in the brain to suppress food intake but does not function as a physiological signal of low dietary protein. *Am J Physiol Regul Integr Comp Physiol* (2014) 307:R310–20. doi:10.1152/ajpregu.00116.2014

Morrison CD, Xi X, White CL, Ye J, Martin RJ. Amino acids inhibit Agrp gene expression via an mTOR-dependent mechanism. *Am J Physiol Endocrinol Metab* (2007) 70808:165–71. doi:10.1152/ajpendo.00675.2006

Ropelle ER, Pauli R, Fernandes MFA, Rocco SA, Marin RM, Morari J, et al. A central role for neuronal AMP-activated protein kinase (AMPK) and mammalian target of rapamycin (mTOR) in high-protein diet–induced weight loss. *Diabetes* (2008) 57:594–605. doi:10.2337/db07-0573.2-DG

Blouet C, Schwartz GJ. Brainstem nutrient sensing in the nucleus of the solitary tract inhibits feeding. *Cell Metab* (2012) 16:579–87. doi:10.1016/ j.cmet.2012.10.003

Laeger T, Münzberg H, Henagan TM, Hutson SM, Albarado DC, Gettys TW, et al. FGF21 is an endocrine signal of protein restriction. *J Clin Invest* (2014) 124:1–3. doi:10.1172/JCI77508

Smith M, Katsouri L, Irvine EE, Hankir MK, Pedroni SM, Voshol PJ, et al. Ribosomal S6K1 in POMC and AgRP neurons regulates glucose homeostasis but not feeding behavior in mice. *Cell Rep* (2015) 11:335–43. doi:10.1016/ j.celrep.2015.03.029

Cavanaugh AR, Schwartz GJ, Blouet C. High-fat feeding impairs nutrient sensing and gut brain integration in the caudomedial nucleus of the solitary tract in mice. *PLoS One* (2015) 10:1–12. doi:10.1371/journal.pone. 0118888

Atasoy D, Betley JN, Su HH, Sternson SM. Deconstruction of a neural circuit for hunger. *Nature* (2012) 488:172–7. doi:10.1038/nature11270

Krashes MJ, Koda S, Ye C, Rogan SC, Adams AC, Cusher DS, et al. Rapid, reversible activation of AgRP neurons drives feeding behavior in mice. *J Clin Invest* (2011) 121:2–6. doi:10.1172/JCI46229DS1

Laplante M, Sabatini DM. mTOR signaling in growth control and disease. *Cell* (2012) 149:274–93. doi:10.1016/j.cell.2012.03.017

Wu Q, Zhang Y, Xu J, Shen P. Regulation of hunger-driven behaviors by neural ribosomal S6 kinase in *Drosophila*. *Proc Natl Acad Sci U S A* (2005) 102(37):13289–94. doi:10.1073/pnas.0501914102

Luquet S, Perez F, Hnasko T, Palmiter R. NPY/AgRP neurons are essential for feeding in adult mice but can be ablated in neonates. *Science* (2005) 310:683–5. doi:10.1126/science.1115524

Kang L, Dunn-Meynell AA, Routh VH, Gaspers LD, Nagata Y, Nishimura T, et al. Glucokinase is a critical regulator of ventromedial hypothalamic neuronal glucosensing. *Diabetes* (2006) 55:412–20. doi:10.2337/diabetes.55.02.06. db05-1229

Kang L, Routh VH, Kuzhikandathil EV, Gaspers LD, Levin BE. Physiological and molecular characteristics of rat hypothalamic ventromedial nucleus glucosensing neurons. *Diabetes* (2004) 53:549–59. doi:10.2337/diabetes. 53.3.549

Ogunnowo-Bada EO, Heeley N, Brochard L, Evans ML. Brain glucose sensing, glucokinase and neural control of metabolism and islet function. *Diabetes Obes Metab* (2014) 16(Suppl 1):26–32. doi:10.1111/dom.12334

Purpera MN, Shen L, Taghavi M, Münzberg H, Martin RJ, Hutson SM, et al. Impaired branched chain amino acid metabolism alters feeding behavior and increases orexigenic neuropeptide expression in the hypothalamus. *J Endocrinol* (2012) 212:85–94. doi:10.1530/JOE-11-0270

Karnani MM, Apergis-Schoute J, Adamantidis A, Jensen LT, de Lecea L, Fugger L, et al. Activation of central orexin/hypocretin neurons by dietary amino acids. *Neuron* (2011) 72:616–29. doi:10.1016/j.neuron.2011.08.027

Du F, Higginbotham D, White B. Food intake, energy balance and serum leptin concentrations in rats fed low-protein diets. *J Nutr* (2000) 130:514–21.

Morrison CD, Reed SD, Henagan TM. Homeostatic regulation of protein intake: in search of a mechanism. *Am J Physiol Regul Integr Comp Physiol* (2012) 302:R917–28. doi:10.1152/ajpregu.00609.2011

Peng Y, Meliza L, Vavich M, Kemmerer A. Changes in food intake and nitrogen metabolism of rats while adapting to a low or high protein diet. *J Nutr* (1974) 104:1008–17.

Sørensen A, Mayntz D, Raubenheimer D, Simpson SJ. Protein-leverage in mice: the geometry of macronutrient balancing and consequences for fat deposition. *Obesity* (2008) 16:566–71. doi:10.1038/oby.2007.58

White B, Du F, Higginbotham D. Low dietary protein is associated with an increase in food intake and a decrease in the in vitro release of radiolabeled glutamate and GABA from the lateral hypothalamus. *Nutr Neurosci* (2003) 6:361–7. doi:10.1080/10284150310001640365

Bensaïd A, Tomé D, L'Heureux-Bourdon D, Even P, Gietzen D, Morens CE, et al. A high-protein diet enhances satiety without conditioned taste aversion in the rat. *Physiol Behav* (2003) 78:311–20. doi:10.1016/S0031-9384(02)00977-0

L'Heureux-Bouron D, Tome D, Bensaid A, Morens C, Gaudichon C, Fromentin G. A very high 70%-protein diet does not induce conditioned taste aversion in rats. *J Nutr* (2004) 134:1512–5.

Simpson SJ, Le Couteur DG, Raubenheimer D. Putting the balance back in diet. *Cell* (2015) 161:18–23. doi:10.1016/j.cell.2015.02.033

Simpson SJ, Batley R, Raubenheimer D. Geometric analysis of macronutrient intake in humans: the power of protein? *Appetite* (2003) 41:123–40. doi:10.1016/S0195-6663(03)00049-7

White B, He B, Dean R, Martin R. Low protein diets increase neuropeptide Y gene expression in the basomedial hypothalamus of rats. *J Nutr* (1994) 124:1152–60.

Laeger T, Albarado DC, Burke SJ, Trosclair L, Hedgepeth JW, Berthoud H-R, et al. Metabolic responses to dietary protein restriction require an increase in FGF21 that is delayed by the absence of GCN2. *Cell Rep* (2016) 16:707–16. doi:10.1016/j.celrep.2016.06.044

Cherkasova VA, Hinnebusch AG. Translational control by TOR and TAP42 through dephosphorylation of eIF2alpha kinase GCN2. *Genes Dev* (2003) 17:859–72. doi:10.1101/gad.1069003

Rodland GE, Tvegard T, Boye E, Grallert B. Crosstalk between the Tor and Gcn2 pathways in response to different stresses. *Cell Cycle* (2014) 13:453–61. doi:10.4161/cc.27270

Cornu M, Oppliger W, Albert V, Robitaille AM, Trapani F, Quagliata L, et al. Hepatic mTORC1 controls locomotor activity, body temperature, and lipid metabolism through FGF21. *Proc Natl Acad Sci U S A* (2014) 111:11592–9. doi:10.1073/pnas.1412047111

Harper A, Peters J. Protein intake, brain amino acid and serotonin concentrations and protein self-selection. *J Nutr* (1989) 119:677–89.

Jean C, Rome S, Aattouri N, Fromentin G, Achagiotis CL, Tome D. Nutrient metabolism metabolic evidence for adaptation to a high protein diet in rats. *J Nutr* (2001) 131:91–8.

Morens C, Gaudichon C, Fromentin G, Marsset-Baglieri A, Bensaïd A, Larue-Achagiotis C, et al. Daily delivery of dietary nitrogen to the periphery is stable in rats adapted to increased protein intake. *Am J Physiol Endocrinol Metab* (2001) 281:E826–36.

Morens C, Gaudichon C, Metges CC, Fromentin G, Baglieri A, Even PC, et al. A high-protein meal exceeds anabolic and catabolic capacities in rats adapted to a normal protein diet. *J Nutr* (2000) 130:2312–21.

Davidenko O, Darcel N, Fromentin G, Tomé D. Control of protein and energy intake – brain mechanisms. *Eur J Clin Nutr* (2013) 67:455–61. doi:10.1038/ejcn.2013.73

L'Heureux-Bouron D, Tomé D, Rampin O, Even PC, Larue-Achagiotis C, Fromentin G. Total subdiaphragmatic vagotomy does not suppress high pro- tein diet-induced food intake depression in rats. *J Nutr* (2003) 133:2639–42.

Pillot B, Duraffourd C, Bégeot M, Joly A, Luquet S, Houberdon I, et al. Role of hypothalamic melanocortin system in adaptation of food intake to food protein increase in mice. *PLoS One* (2011) 6:e19107. doi:10.1371/journal.pone.0019107

Solon-Biet SM, Mitchell SJ, de Cabo R, Raubenheimer D, Le Couteur DG, Simpson SJ. Macronutrients and caloric intake in health and longevity. *J Endocrinol* (2015) 226:R17–28. doi:10.1530/JOE-15-0173

8

Hypothalamic Inflammation and Energy Balance Disruptions: Spotlight on Chemokines

Ophélia Le Thuc[1,2,3]*, Katharina Stobbe*[1]*, Céline Cansell*[1]*, Jean-Louis Nahon*[1]*,*
Nicolas Blondeau[1] *and Carole Rovère*[1]*

[1] CNRS, Institut de Pharmacologie Moléculaire et Cellulaire, Université Côte d'Azur, Valbonne, France, [2] Helmholtz Diabetes Center (HDC), German Center for Diabetes Research (DZD), Helmholtz Zentrum München, Neuherberg, Germany, [3] Division of Metabolic Diseases, Technische Universität München, Munich, Germany

***Correspondence:**
Carole Rovère
rovere@ipmc.cnrs.fr

The hypothalamus is a key brain region in the regulation of energy balance as it controls food intake and both energy storage and expenditure through integration of humoral, neural, and nutrient-related signals and cues. Many years of research have focused on the regulation of energy balance by hypothalamic neurons, but the most recent findings suggest that neurons and glial cells, such as microglia and astrocytes, in the hypothalamus actually orchestrate together several metabolic functions. Because glial cells have been described as mediators of inflammatory processes in the brain, the existence of a causal link between hypothalamic inflammation and the deregulations of feeding behavior, leading to involuntary weight loss or obesity for example, has been suggested. Several inflammatory pathways that could impair the hypothalamic control of energy balance have been studied over the years such as, among others, toll-like receptors and canonical cytokines. Yet, less studied so far, chemokines also represent interesting candidates that could link the aforementioned pathways and the activity of hypothalamic neurons. Indeed, chemokines, in addition to their role in attracting immune cells to the inflamed site, have been suggested to be capable of neuromodulation. Thus, they could disrupt cellular activity together with synthesis and/or secretion of multiple neurotransmitters/mediators involved in the maintenance of energy balance. This review discusses the different inflammatory pathways that have been identified so far in the hypothalamus in the context of feeding behavior and body weight control impairments, with a particular focus on chemokines signaling that opens a new avenue in the understanding of the major role played by inflammation in obesity.

Keywords: neuroinflammation, hypothalamus, chemokines, energy balance, metabolic diseases, high-fat diet, obesity, anorexia

INTRODUCTION

Energy balance is finely regulated *via* a bidirectional communication between the brain and the peripheral organs. One brain area is particularly important in this regulation: the hypothalamus. The hypothalamus shelters, in its different nuclei, several neuronal populations producing peptides that are either orexigenic or anorexigenic. The activity of these neuropeptidergic circuits is, among others, modulated by peripheral signals, of neural or hormonal nature, or by nutrients themselves (**Figure 1**). Thus, it would make sense that the function of these neuropeptidergic circuits would be impaired in case of feeding behavior deregulation, whether it is a loss of appetite or a food overconsumption. Numerous studies, based either on lesion, pharmacological, or genetic approaches, indeed confirmed this [for review see Ref. (1)]. Interestingly, hypothalamic inflammation has already been linked to energy balance disruptions: high-grade hypothalamic inflammation has been associated to involuntary weight loss and, on the contrary, low-grade hypothalamic inflammation has been associated to obesity (2, 3). Importantly, these feeding behavior deregulations represent major public health issues, especially obesity. Indeed, obesity, which keeps developing since the end of the 20th century, is often associated to potentially deadly comorbidities such as diabetes, cardiovascular diseases, liver diseases, and cancers. Yet, a loss of appetite, consecutive to some inflammatory pathologies such as cancer, can also have severe consequences, as it can impair recovery by inducing a deficit in energy.

Hence, understanding the molecular mechanisms linking hypothalamic inflammation and feeding behavior deregulations could, in the long-term, allow identifying potential therapeutic targets. As previously mentioned, we will focus in this review on hypothalamic inflammation, even though peripheral inflammation is also often associated with energy balance deregulations: in involuntary weight loss, inflammation is rather firstly systemic and a consequence of a primary pathology. In obesity, both systemic and hypothalamic inflammations have been described, and even if this is still debated, recent studies suggest that hypothalamic inflammation precedes systemic inflammation associated to the obese state (4–6).

In this context, in particular when there is systemic inflammation, it is important to understand how the periphery and the brain can communicate, especially regarding inflammatory signals. The most described brain–periphery communication pathways are the neural and the humoral pathways. The neural pathway involves primarily the vagus nerve—which expresses cytokine receptors—and the dorso-vagal complex, whereas the humoral pathway involves circulating cytokines that are overexpressed with inflammation and that can (1) bind to their receptors on the membrane of endothelial cells, (2) get to the brain at the level of the circumventricular organs and of the choroid plexus when the blood–brain barrier (BBB) is incomplete, or

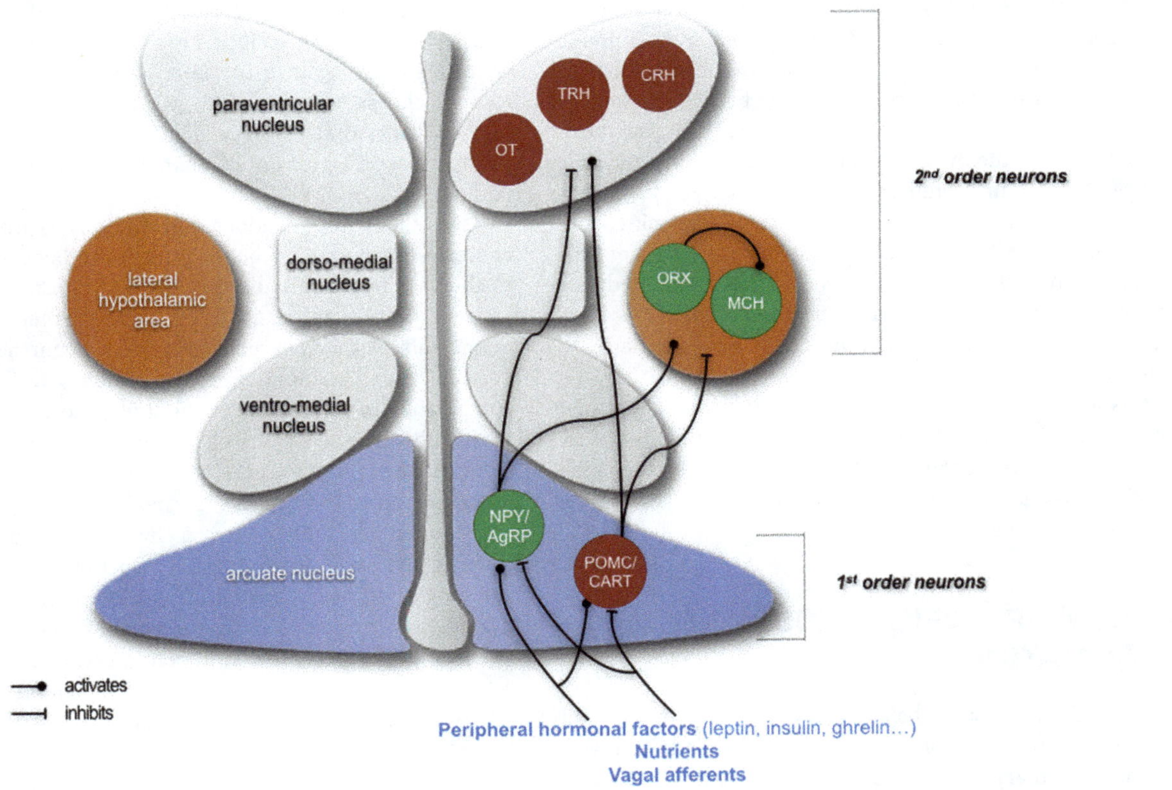

FIGURE 1 | Simplified schematics summarizing the neuropeptidergic hypothalamic networks that are involved in homeostatic regulation of feeding behavior. Signals giving indications about the energy status of an organism are emitted from the periphery and are first integrated by first-order neurons located in the arcuate nucleus, producing either orexigenic neuropeptides (NPY and AgRP) or anorexigenic peptides (POMC and CART). These neurons project to second-order neurons, such as neurons producing the anorexigenic factors oxytocin (OT), thyrotropin-releasing hormone (TRH), and corticotropin-releasing hormone (CRH) in the paraventricular nucleus and neurons producing orexigenic peptides orexin (ORX) and melanin-concentrating hormone (MCH) in the lateral hypothalamus. The integration of peripheral signals by these neuropeptidergic systems participates in the homeostatic regulation of feeding behavior and the maintenance of a suitable weight by ensuring an appropriate food intake as well as appropriate energy intake and expenditure. In green: neurons producing orexigenic peptides; in red: neurons producing anorexigenic peptides. Adapted from Le Thuc and Rovère (7).

(3) reach directly the brain thanks to the increased BBB permeability induced by inflammation (8). However, one must also consider the cellular pathway, which involves the infiltration of immune cells and activation of microglia in the brain parenchyma, and also the microbiota pathway, for example.

Studies that aimed to identify inflammatory mediators allowing bidirectional communication between the periphery and the brain during inflammation mainly focused on the role of peripheral cytokines. Yet, it has been suggested that in the context of disruptions of proper control of food intake and body weight, the central production of inflammatory mediators is more important than the peripheral one, or at least "necessary," in particular in the models of inflammation induced by the bacterial lipopolysaccharide (LPS), where it has been suggested that its effects do not require the signaling from peripheral cytokines (9–11).

Hence, in the context of disruptions of proper energy balance control by hypothalamic circuits, a group of pro-inflammatory mediators might be as relevant as the canonical cytokines, if not more, downstream of the latter: the chemokines. Chemokines are a subgroup of cytokines, small (8–14 kDa) heparin-binding proteins, mainly described for their chemoattractant properties for immune cells to the affected site.

Chemokines and their receptors are suspected to be mediators of the effects of neuroinflammation, from attraction of immune cells to behavioral changes. Beyond participating in the immune response, chemokines and their receptors (the "chemokinergic system") are constitutively expressed in the brain, in a specific manner, both area wise and cell type wise. Interestingly, it is comparable to the neurotransmitters or neuropeptidergic systems (12, 13). Furthermore, the chemokinergic system has been demonstrated to interact with the neurotransmitter and neuropeptidergic systems (14, 15) and some recent studies suggest that the chemokinergic system is able to directly modulate neuronal activity (16–18). Thus, the chemokinergic system could be responsible for the behavioral changes associated to inflammation.

In this review, we discuss how inflammation, with a focus on chemokines, can participate in the deregulation of the hypothalamic control of energy balance and body weight: first, in appetite and weight loss and, second, in the establishment and/or the development of obesity.

INVOLUNTARY WEIGHT LOSS AND INFLAMMATION

Weight loss illustrates an unbalance between energy intake and energy expenditure in favor of expenditure. While both involuntary and voluntary weight losses can be caused by a decrease in food intake or an increase in energy expenditure (increase in basal metabolism, e.g., thermogenesis), only an involuntary weight loss can be explained by an uncontrolled decrease in food intake or by an increase in energy expenditure.

There are multiple possible causes for an involuntary weight loss. This weight loss can be a symptom of a severe primary disease such as cancer, where it is particularly preoccupying when it reaches or exceeds 10% in 1 year. In most cases, one can link an involuntary weight loss to psychic troubles, such as depression, that can induce a sustainable loss of appetite, thus weight loss. Excessive consumption of certain substances (e.g., drugs of abuse and alcohol) can also induce an involuntary weight loss. Yet, a weight loss is only considered "involuntary" when it is not a consequence that can be expected from a specific medical treatment of a known medical condition (19). Moreover, aging is often associated to a loss of appetite which induces, in the long-term, severe malnutrition and, obviously, weight loss. This can also be associated to sarcopenia, a geriatric syndrome characterized by loss of muscle mass and function (19). However, as previously mentioned, an involuntary weight loss can have organic causes such as gastrointestinal diseases [e.g., Crohn's disease, celiac disease (weight loss related to food malabsorption), and digestive ulcer], cardiovascular, endocrine, autoimmune, infectious diseases (e.g., HIV infection, hepatitis, and tuberculosis), neurological diseases (e.g., dementia and Parkinson's disease), or cancer (19, 20). In the case of cancer, weight loss is one of the first symptoms with 50% of patients with cancer reporting weight loss (21). It should be noted that the majority of the abovementioned organic causes are commonly associated with "high-grade"—in other words high-intensity—inflammation. Interestingly, even if benign and time-restricted, numerous pathological states are strongly inflammatory and associated to a reduced appetite or "anorexia." This anorexia is part of a classical defense mechanism of an organism against infection, lesions, etc., that is referred to as "sickness behavior" (22, 23). Sickness behavior involves various behavioral changes that primarily affect mood and energy balance, which develop parallel to infection or to another pathology (22).

Like other strategies adopted by the body to promote healing, anorexia is supposed to be temporary and beneficial. However, in the case of chronic diseases such as cancers, both appetite and weight loss can persist, leading to a further degraded state of the subject (hypoglycemic malaise, amenorrhea in women, decalcification leading to more fragile bones, teeth falling, etc.), comparable, in some aspects only linked to undernutrition, to what is observed with anorexia nervosa (24). Prolonged anorexia, irrespective of its type and its causes, is often a contributory factor to the onset of cachexia. Cachexia is a complex syndrome that cannot be fully reversed by conventional nutritional support and leads to progressive functional impairment, i.e., pathological thinness, associated with deep asthenia and organs dysfunction [decreased muscle strength, fatigue, adipose tissue (AT) dystrophy, etc.] (25, 26). Hence, cachexia can be defined as a complex syndrome in which inflammation leads to early satiety and anorexia, decreased fat mass, and weakness (25, 26). Prolonged loss of appetite may even be fatal. One can then assume that inflammation, here high-grade, could disrupt the proper functioning of the hypothalamic systems that are involved, and thus the regulation of feeding behavior. Hence, considering the serious consequences of unresolved anorexia, it is important to better understand the mechanisms linking inflammation and the cerebral centers that control energy homeostasis, because if the link between high-grade inflammation and loss of appetite and weight is established and extensively recognized, the underlying molecular mechanisms have not yet been fully resolved.

Inflammatory Pathways in the Hypothalamus and Involuntary Weight Loss

In the hypothalamus, some studies have been able to identify some inflammatory pathways, involving different cell types, to be relevant for weight loss.

At the molecular level, as previously mentioned, the literature related to the deregulation of the control of energy balance in the anorexia–cachexia syndrome has focused on the role of pro-inflammatory cytokines, such as interleukin (IL)-1β, IL-6, and TNF-α. It has been shown that pro-inflammatory cytokines, whose production can be induced by infectious agents affecting peripheral organs, notably by LPS—the most commonly used model for modeling disease behavior and anorexia associated with inflammation (27)—participate in the induction of sickness behavior.

Some studies deciphering the kinetic aspects of the effect of central or peripheral cytokine injection suggest that pro-inflammatory mediators exert their effect primarily at the central level versus periphery (28, 29). Numerous studies have focused on IL-1β and have shown that its intracerebroventricular (ICV) injection induces profound behavioral changes in rodents (30). Furthermore, the central role of cytokine signaling at the central level has been confirmed, for example, by the fact that the central injection of the IL-1β receptor antagonist prevents the effects induced by the peripheral injection of this cytokine (31, 32). In addition, some studies suggest that inflammatory inducers such as LPS are not capable of directly inducing sickness behavior and require downstream actors such as cytokines. Indeed, for example, unlike the central injection of LPS, central injection of IL-1 is able to induce sickness behavior in mice whose LPS toll-like receptor (TLR) 4 is non-functional (33).

As mentioned earlier, cytokines, involved in the induction and regulation of sickness behavior at the central level, can be released into the circulation by the immune cells (8) or directly produced by neurons and glial cells in the central nervous system (CNS) (34–39). In the context of systemic diseases, the central effects of these cytokines appear to be independent of the place of their secretion. As previously mentioned, when produced in the periphery, cytokines have the following two main pathways to act on the brain: a neural pathway and a humoral pathway. Most cytokines act in a paracrine manner at the site of infection, suggesting that neural afferents may be the target of pro-inflammatory cytokines. Interestingly, the perineural sheath of the vagus nerve contains immune cells that are capable of producing IL-1, in particular in response to LPS (40). Furthermore, the sensory neurons of the vagus nerve express IL-1 receptors and it has been shown that this cytokine stimulates the sensory activity of the vagus nerve (40). Vagotomy experiments have demonstrated the importance of the vagus nerve in the transmission of information from the periphery to the brain: for example, after injection of LPS or IL-1 at the periphery, vagal afferents are involved in the induction of the sickness behavior and in the neural activation of the brainstem, the hypothalamus, and the limbic structures (40).

Chronic administration of cytokines can reproduce the characteristics of anorexia–cachexia syndrome (38, 41–44), while blocking the signaling of one of them, such as TNF, by the use of neutralizing antibodies, inhibits its development (42, 45, 46). Similarly, administration of an IL-1 receptor antagonist prevents anorexia in cancer animal models (47). Some studies have suggested that endogenous brain IL-1 is a mediator of LPS-induced anorexia by acting on the expression of cytokines in the hypothalamus (9). In addition, it appears that IL-1β can act on ARC POMC neurons (48) and that TNF-α indirectly increases energy expenditure *via* β3 adrenergic signaling in the brown AT (thermogenesis) (49). By different approaches, it has been shown that interfering with mediators of inflammation coincides with a reduction in hypothalamic inflammation and prevents weight loss in animal models of anorexia: for example, the inhibition of the "adenosine monophosphate protein kinase" in the hypothalamus reduces hypothalamic inflammation, which is accompanied by an increase in food intake in the case of cancer-associated anorexia, allowing better overall survival (50). Interestingly, in the context of cancer-associated cachexia, the administration of ghrelin, an appetite-stimulating hormone, increases food intake and is accompanied by a decrease in IL-1β (51).

Focusing on the LPS-induced anorexia model, it is interesting to underline that some studies suggest that this loss of appetite is independent from the vagal afferents and that it only depends on central inflammatory mechanisms, where the central effects of peripheral LPS could be, among others, mediated by some cytokines and/or *via* receptors for LPS expressed by some brain cells (11, 52). Indeed, microglia expresses TLR4, through which LPS has been shown to exert some of its effects (53–56). Furthermore, Hines and colleagues have shown that disrupting TLR4 signaling prevents microglial activation, inhibits the production of cytokines, and prevents the development of the sickness behavior that are induced by peripheral LPS (57). In contrast, a recent study by Reis et al. has shown that if microglia and TLR4 are necessary for LPS to acutely induce inhibitory effects on orexigenic agouti-related peptide (AgRP)/neuropeptide Y (NPY) neurons, conversely, LPS can actually acutely increase the firing activity of anorexigenic pro-opiomelanocortin (POMC) neurons in a microglia/TLR4-independent manner (58). In addition, the same study presents results which further supports that mediators of inflammation such as microglia and TLR4 can, at least acutely, affect basal food intake and hormonal-dependent modulation of feeding behavior. Indeed, the inhibition of microglia alone, *via* ICV injection of minocycline, leads to an increase in food intake, comparable to the one induced by ICV ghrelin (58). Interestingly, the co-injection of ghrelin and minocycline does not synergistically increase food intake. This implies that the inhibition of microglia itself, as it increases food intake, interferes or prevents ghrelin's orexigenic effects (58).

Changes in gene expression of hypothalamic anorexigenic and orexigenic neuropeptides were assessed in mice or rats that received LPS IP injections (59–61). Generally, peripheral LPS appears, initially, to reduce the expression of the orexigenic peptides and, on the contrary, to increase that of the anorexigenic peptides. In later stages, the expression of orexigenic peptides increases again, probably to promote food intake and compensate for weight loss.

Some authors have used other models to study to understand links between inflammation in the brain and the induction of sickness behavior.

For example, Jang and colleagues sought to determine the mechanisms behind anorexia and weight loss associated with illness *via* administration, in mice, of either bacterial or viral products: LPS and human immunodeficiency virus-1 transactivator protein (Tat), respectively (62). They found in both cases that pro-inflammatory cytokines such as IL-β, IL-6, and TNF-α were upregulated in the hypothalamus. Furthermore, AtT-20 and SH-SY5Y cells treated with either Tat or LPS exhibit increased POMC transcriptional activity. In addition, the injection of Tat or LPS in the hypothalamus of mice induces in both cases a decrease in food intake and in body weight. They identified POMC as a potential mediator of illness-induced anorexia and as a possible downstream target of NF-κB. Indeed, they showed through different approaches that the NF-κB pathway in the melanocortin system plays an important role in illness-induced anorexia and body weight loss: both administration of AgRP, an endogenous melanocortin antagonist and the inhibition of the NF-κB pathway specifically in the POMC neurons ($Ikk\beta^{\Delta Pomc}$ mice), significantly blunted the effects of Tat and LPS on food intake and body weight. Interestingly, the authors also present results suggesting that leptin-induced anorexia is also dependent on the NF-κB pathway (62).

Another study has shown that a pathway involving TLR2 participates in the induction of sickness behavior through a microglia-POMC neurons axis (63). In this publication, the authors show, by ICV injection of Pam3CSK4, a specific synthetic TLR2 agonist that TLR2 central signaling is able to trigger sickness behavior through activation of microglial cells, which express TLR2, and *via* the NF-κB and COX pathways. The authors also show that activation of central TLR2 is able to modify the synaptic architecture in the ARC, especially at the level of the POMC neurons: it reduces the rate of GABAergic contacts on POMC neurons, whereas it increases the vesicular glutamate transporter 2 (vGLUT2) contacts on POMC soma, translating an increased excitatory state, in correlation with an increased microglial occupancy.

In addition, Murray et al. used the peripheral administration of the viral mimetic poly I:C to induce type-I interferons (IFN-I) overexpression in the brain. Using IFN-I receptor 1 (IFNAR1)-deficient mice, the results of the authors present suggest that IFN-I are involved in the induction of sickness behavior, including anorexia, whereas IL-6 participates in sickness behavior but not in anorexia (64).

Furthermore, a local increase in serotonin levels in the hypothalamus has already been linked to anorexia and cachexia (65–67) and a recent study showed that inflammation induced by peripheral treatment by either IL-6 and/or TNF-α is associated with an impairment in local serotonin turnover in the hypothalamus, a decrease in NPY and AgRP gene expressions, and a decrease in food intake in comparison to control conditions (68). Authors were able to identify upstream inflammatory regulators including interferon gamma (IFN-γ), transforming growth factor beta (TGF-β), IL-6, and IKBKG, an enzyme crucial for the activation of the NF-κB pathway. This study thus suggests that peripheral inflammation reaches the hypothalamus where it impairs serotonin turnover, which is associated to a decrease in food intake.

Taken together, numerous studies support the hypothesis that inflammation at the hypothalamic level is able to disrupt the proper function of neuropeptidergic circuits of the hypothalamus and thus to induce an involuntary weight loss.

However, mediators linking inflammation and its consequences at the level of central systems regulating energy homeostasis, and ultimately on weight, have not been determined with certainty, and one may note that the nature of the mediators responsible for the central effects of IL-1β has been especially poorly described. Thus, chemokines can represent interesting candidates to study further understanding of the underlying mechanisms.

Chemokines in the Modulation of Hypothalamic Neuropeptidergic Circuits in Inflammation-Associated Involuntary Weight Loss

So far, very few studies have sought to determine if chemokines have a role in the induction of involuntary weight loss associated with inflammation by impairing the homeostatic regulation of energy balance by hypothalamic neuropeptidergic circuits.

A study published in 1994 by Plata-Salamán and Borkoski aimed to investigate how chemokines could act on the regulation of feeding. Indeed, as previously mentioned, chemokines are produced in multiple types of cells as a response to pathological conditions such as infection, inflammation, injury, and trauma. Among the stimuli that can induce the release of these chemokines, we can list LPS, and also the IL-1β, TNF-α, and IFN, which have been associated to food intake suppression by direct action on the CNS. Thus, the authors aimed to determine if chemokines could be involved, as downstream mediators, in the decrease in food intake induced by inflammatory signals such as LPS. In order to do so, they used, in rats, ICV microinfusion of different chemokines from two different subfamilies: CXC and CC, also known as the α and β subfamilies. This way, they tested the effect of CXC-motif chemokine ligand (CXCL)-1, 4, 7, 8, 10 and CC-motif chemokine ligand (CCL)-2–4, 5. Even though it is at a lesser extent than the cytokine IL-1β, their results indeed identify certain chemokines as capable of acutely decreasing food intake: CXCL4, CXCL8, CXCL10, CCL2, and CCL5. Interestingly, in their model, these chemokines would affect feeding behavior at different time scales: if they all reduced food intake in the 2 h following injection, only CXCL8, CXCL4, and CCL2 were able to reduce food intake over the whole dark phase and only CXCL8 and CXCL4 were able to decrease the total daily food intake (69). This study is particularly important as it sets chemokines as contributors, in the brain, to the effects of infection/inflammation on feeding behavior. Nevertheless, no mechanistic insights were then provided.

As previously acknowledged, very few studies aimed at better characterizing how chemokines could modulate feeding behavior after this study by Plata-Salamán and Borkoski.

Yet, in a recent study from our laboratory (70), we sought to identify and characterize chemokines that could possibly deregulate the hypothalamic circuits to alter food intake and energy balance in anorexia and weight loss. We thus assessed the gene expression of several pro-inflammatory mediators in the hypothalamus of mice that had received an acute ICV injection of LPS. After confirmation of LPS-induced inflammation in our mice by observing the overexpression of several pro-inflammatory mediators, we then identified ligands of the chemokine receptors CCR (CC-motif chemokine receptor)-2 and 5 as the most overexpressed. Among them, CCL2 (also known as monocyte chemoattractant protein 1) caught our attention as it has been described as particularly important in the context of LPS-induced neuroinflammation and suggested to be able to reduce food intake (69, 71–73). Thus, we focused on the central signaling of CCL2 and its receptor CCR2 and could demonstrate that it is mandatory for both metabolic and behavioral changes induced by LPS (70). Indeed, inhibiting CCR2 signaling by combined ICV injection of a specific antagonist of CCR2, INCB3344, together with LPS, prevents the weight loss that is induced by ICV injection of LPS alone. Similarly, the weight loss induced by ICV injection of LPS is reduced in mice deficient for CCR2 in comparison to control animals. Experiments in metabolic cages demonstrate that central injection of LPS decreases both food intake and locomotor activity, whereas it increases fat oxidation and induces a shift in used energy substrate in favor of lipids versus carbohydrates. These two last points probably illustrate an increased use of the energy stocked in the AT as lipids. Interestingly, these LPS effects highlighted by the metabolic cages experiments were also reduced when interfering with central CCR2 signaling by co-ICV injection of LPS and INCB3344.

We then identified the neurons, which produce melanin-concentrating hormone (MCH), a peptide known to elicit food intake and to decrease energy consumption, as targets for CCL2 (74). After ICV injection of LPS, we observed a sustained decrease in gene expression and protein levels of MCH, which is blunted/prevented by pharmacological (using INCB3344) or genetic inhibition of CCL2 signaling. Interestingly, we found that, similar to LPS, ICV injection of CCL2 promotes neuroinflammation, together with a decrease in both MCH expression and body weight. Immunostaining experiments showed that 70% of the MCH neurons of the lateral hypothalamus (LHA) express CCL2 receptor. These neurons responded to CCL2 by decreasing both electrical activity and MCH release. Thus, it seems that the inhibition of the MCH system by LPS depends primarily of the central signaling of CCR2. Moreover, in experiments of perifusion of hypothalamic explants treated with KCl and CCL2, MCH secretion is totally inhibited, while co-application of KCl and INCB3344 only, leads to enhanced secretion of MCH. This suggests that endogenous CCL2 could participate, in normal conditions, in modulating MCH system and thus energy balance regulation.

Thus, it appears that the central CCL2/CCR2 axis is able to directly act on neurons producing the orexigenic peptide MCH by reducing their activity and both the expression and secretion of the peptide, leading to a reduced food intake and to an increased use of energy stores. Hence, the central CCL2/CCR2 axis, by acting through MCH neurons, appears as a major actor in appetite and weight loss associated with LPS-induced inflammation (**Figures 2** and **3**). This study was the first to demonstrate that a chemokine can play a role, at the central level, in energy balance deregulation, by acting directly on neuropeptidergic systems in the hypothalamus.

OBESITY AND INFLAMMATION

As previously mentioned, interestingly, inflammation is also a characteristic for an opposite disorder of the energy balance disorder of the regulation of food intake and body weight: obesity. Yet, different from the inflammation associated to involuntary weight loss, this inflammation is of low intensity, also referred to as a "low-grade" inflammation (79). Obesity is characterized by an excessive fat mass distributed throughout the body that can be harmful to health [source: World Health Organization

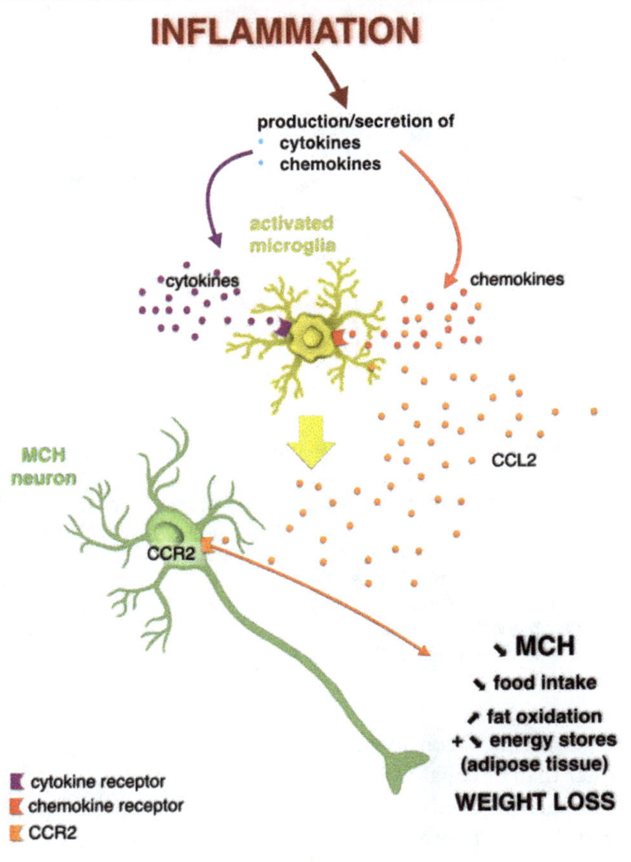

FIGURE 2 | Potential action of the CC-motif chemokine ligand (CCL) 2/CCR2 signaling pathway on melanin-concentrating hormone (MCH) neurons in a weight loss model induced by a central injection of lipopolysaccharide. Hypothalamic inflammation is characterized by overexpression of inflammatory mediators such as cytokines and chemokines. It is possible that these bind to their receptors expressed by glial cells such as microglia, which then activated, can produce even more cytokines and chemokines, including CCL2. However, it is not excluded that CCL2 could act directly on MCH neurons that expressed its receptor in the lateral hypothalamus. This would result in a decreased MCH neuronal activity and in a decreased secretion of this neuropeptide, which is associated to a loss of appetite, an increased fat oxidation, likely reflecting a decrease in energy stores in adipose tissue, and thus a loss of weight. Adapted from Le Thuc and Rovère (7).

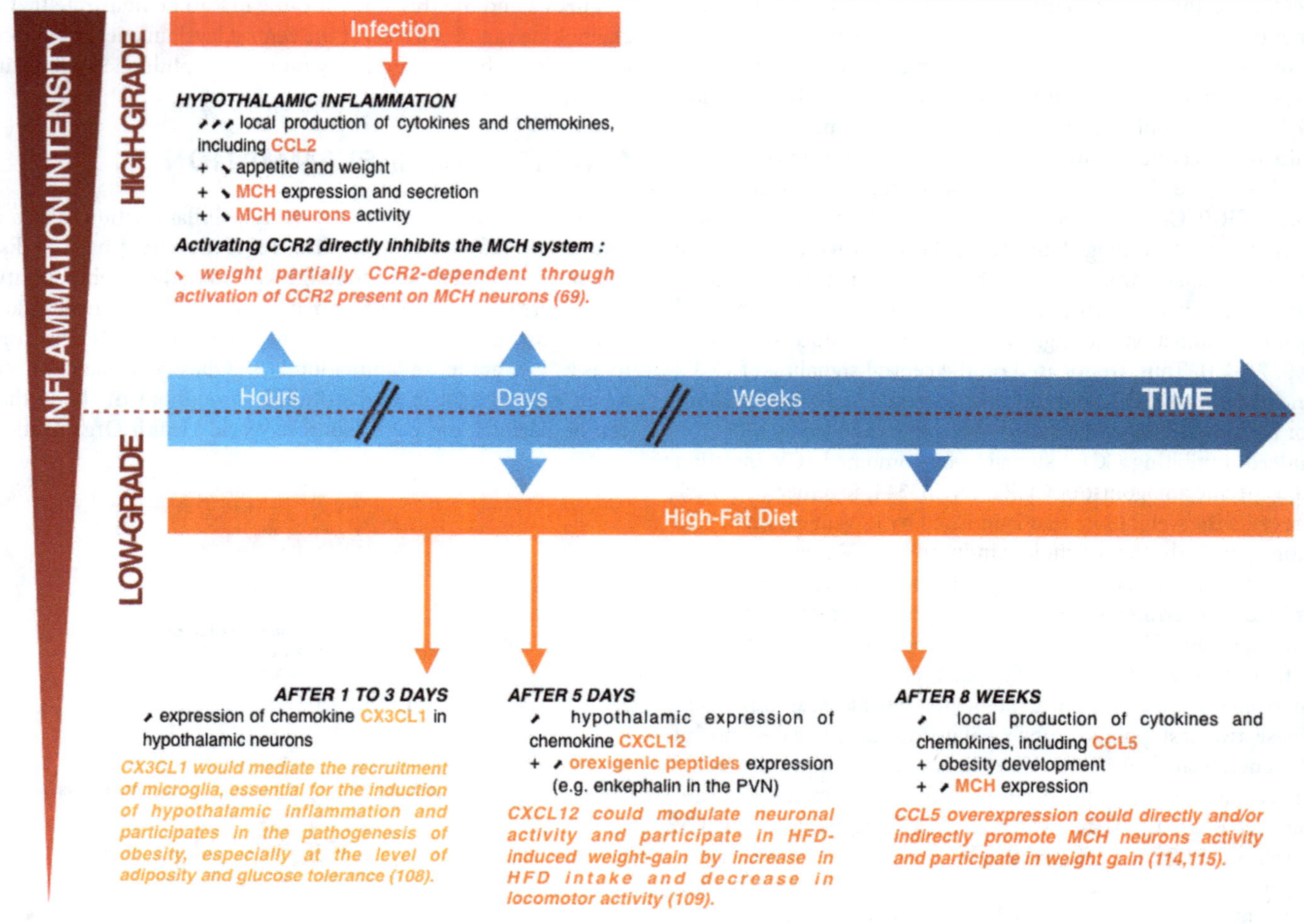

FIGURE 3 | Summary diagram showing the links between hypothalamic inflammation and deregulation of weight. *Upper part*: when lipopolysaccharide induces high-grade hypothalamic inflammation, there is an acute and increase in local production of cytokines and chemokines, including CC-motif chemokine ligand (CCL) 2 (a few hours to a few days) associated with weight loss (a manifestation of the sickness behavior associated with a high-intensity infection). This weight loss is partially dependent on the CCL2/CCR2 signaling pathway, by direct inhibition of the lateral hypothalamus (LHA) neurons producing the orexigenic peptide melanin-concentrating hormone (MCH) (70). *Lower part*: short (1–5 days) or prolonged (several weeks) high-fat diet (HFD) consumption is associated with chronic low-grade hypothalamic inflammation that appears to be linked to the development of obesity, together with an overexpression of orexigenic neuropeptides such as enkephalin in the paraventricular nucleus or MCH in the LHA. The chemokine CX3CL1 appears essential to the induction of hypothalamic inflammation, with an important role in the recruitment of microglia, whereas the chemokines CXC-motif chemokine ligand 12 and CCL5 could modulate neuronal activity and participate in HFD-induced weight loss (75–78). Adapted from Le Thuc and Rovère (7).

(WHO)]. One is considered obese if one's body mass index is greater than or equal to 30 (80, 81). Worldwide, close to 13% of the population were obese in 2014 and the prevalence of obesity nearly doubled between 1980 and 2014 (source: WHO). Obesity is a concern as it represents a risk factor for chronic diseases such as cardiovascular diseases (hypertension, heart disease, and stroke), diabetes, hepatic steatosis, respiratory diseases, musculoskeletal disorders (osteoarthritis, etc.), certain cancers (endometrium, breast, colorectal, etc.), and neurodegenerative disorders (79–81). Furthermore, childhood obesity, which is progressing in an alarming manner, can promote respiratory difficulties, high blood pressure, the emergence of markers of cardiovascular disease, fractures, insulin resistance, and psychological problems. All these aspects in turn increase the risk of adult obesity, premature death, and disability in adulthood (source: WHO).

While the development of obesity may be explained by some genetic aspects or be consecutive to a primary disease and/or its treatment (hormonal and/or psychological factors, drugs, etc.), its most common cause is a change in the population's life-style. This encompasses an increase in sedentariness and hypercaloric diets overconsumption, where the excess in calories intake most often comes from lipids and also carbohydrates (80, 81). As obesity represents a major and growing public health issue, it becomes important to identify and understand its causes and mechanisms. Therefore, understanding the role played by inflammation, both peripheral and central, in the establishment and/or development of obesity and its comorbidities might allow to identify new potential targets in the fight against obesity.

The inflammation associated to obesity exhibits several specificities: first, as mentioned previously, it is low grade and chronic. So far, it has been mostly described in peripheral tissues

(AT, liver, pancreas, etc.). Nevertheless, more recently, it has been shown to also occur in the CNS: a hypercaloric challenge, especially a high-fat diet (HFD), even on the short term, can induce an inflammation in the hypothalamus that is sustained in models of nutritional obesity (82).

Obesity and Peripheral Inflammation

Studies have associated inflammation and obesity for a long time (79). Yet this inflammation is not "typical," as it cannot be associated to the cardinal signs of redness, swelling, heat, and pain. Thus, the inflammation associated to obesity is of different nature. First, it is aseptic: it is caused by the overconsumption of specific nutrients (lipids and carbohydrates); thus, the trigger of this inflammation can be considered to be of metabolic nature. Interestingly, not only the trigger of this inflammation is metabolic, but this inflammation first targets the cells that specialized in metabolism: e.g., adipocytes, hepatocytes, pancreatic β-cells, and myocytes (but also the neurons of the peptidergic systems involved in the regulation of feeding behavior, as detailed further). Hence, this inflammation is often referred to as "metabolic inflammation" or "metainflammation" (79).

The characteristics of the inflammation associated with obesity, in periphery at least, are: (i) being of metabolic nature—it is induced by nutrients and is orchestrated by "metabolic" cells; (ii) being low grade, with moderate and localized overexpression of pro-inflammatory mediators; (iii) creating an impaired milieu where the tissue "composition" in terms of immune cells favors an inflammatory environment in the tissues; and (iv) being sustained in time, without any apparent resolution (79). Furthermore, peripheral metabolic inflammation associated with obesity is deleterious at many levels and, as a consequence of poor eating habits favoring the obese phenotype, inflammation itself promotes tissue dysfunctions, which also contribute to development of obesity, including resistance to insulin and leptin.

Obesity and Hypothalamic Inflammation

In the context of nutritional obesity, inflammatory pathways are not only activated in peripheral tissues but also activated in central areas involved in the control of energy metabolism, especially in the hypothalamus. Several questions then deserve to be asked and answered such as "What are the signals that induce this inflammation?" and "Is inflammation a cause or a consequence of obesity?"

The relationship between nutritional obesity and hypothalamic inflammation was first described by De Souza and his collaborators (83). The authors demonstrated in rats that a 4-month period of HFD feeding activates inflammatory pathways in the mediobasal hypothalamus (MBH), such as JNK and NF-κB, leading to the production of canonical pro-inflammatory cytokines such as IL-1β, TNF-α, and IL-6 and to deficiencies in insulin and leptin signaling. These observations on hypothalamic inflammation associated to nutritional obesity were confirmed in rats, obese mice, and non-human primates (82, 84–92). Interestingly, some studies have shown that the inflammation induced by the consumption of HFD, likely a response to overnutrition, develops much faster in the hypothalamus than in the peripheral tissues. Indeed, inflammation in the AT, for example, is only observable after several weeks or even months, whereas in the hypothalamus, the consumption of a HFD during a much more restricted period of 24–72 h is enough to induce overexpression of pro-inflammatory cytokines and gliosis—which corresponds to an activation and proliferation of glial cells such as microglia and astrocytes, an inflammation hallmark in the brain (82).

Thus, it appears that the inflammation induced by the excess of nutrients in the hypothalamus precedes the establishment of obesity, as well as peripheral inflammation and metabolic disturbances. It is worth mentioning that the gliosis induced by the consumption of a HFD for a short-period of time (2–3 weeks) is actually reversible, whereas it reappears after longer periods of HFD consumption (8 months) (82). This suggests that the initial short-term gliosis is rather a protective mechanism induced to protect against the "injury" induced by the overload of fat, which is in line with the known roles of these cells, and that with time, the consumption of HFD triggers a durable gliosis and inflammation that would then play a major role in the development of the pathophysiology induced by overnutrition. For example, a study by Dalvi et al. further supports that acute gliosis associated with a moderate period of HFD feeding would actually be protective: as long as the inflammation is restricted to glial cells, the organism seems to attempt to limit brain injury by overexpressing in parallel some protective factors such as the heat shock protein 70 and the ciliary neurotrophic factor. After a longer period of HFD feeding, overexpression of inflammatory mediators within the neurons suggests an exhaustion of neuroprotective mechanism in the hypothalamus, leading to a deregulation of the expression of certain neuropeptides that will favor a positive energy balance (93).

What is the signal that triggers hypothalamic inflammation? It has been suggested that it is the excess of nutrients, which are major physiological regulators of hypothalamic neural networks, that induces the establishment of inflammation at the level of the hypothalamus. Some studies attribute the triggering of hypothalamic inflammation to, more especially, saturated fatty acids (SFA), especially long-chain SFA, due to their accumulation in the hypothalamus when consuming HFD, which could, among others, induce inflammatory signaling by activating the TLR4 pathway. It is interesting to note that other fatty acids, such as long-chain polyunsaturated fatty acids, appear, conversely to long-chain SFA, to be beneficial, especially in the diet-induced obesity (DIO) context, as they have anti-inflammatory properties (94–97). In contrast, not only nutrients but also hormones seem to play a role in the regulation of glial cells function. Indeed, as illustrated by a study by Gao et al., showing that monogenic obese mice with deficient leptin signaling [*ob/ob* (leptin deficient) and *db/db* (leptin receptor mutation)] exhibit less microglial activation than wild-type controls both on chow and on HFD (98). The authors further demonstrated that the lack of leptin signaling affects also the microglial function in the hypothalamus as the expression of several inflammatory mediators is reduced (98). This indicates that the signaling of leptin, already described as a pro-inflammatory adipokine (99), could affect microglial activation. Other mechanisms have been proposed as mediators of the hypothalamic inflammation associated with overnutrition such as the endoplasmic reticulum stress (86, 100, 101). Similarly, oxidative stress could be an initiating factor and participate in the maintenance of the hypothalamic inflammation induced by nutrition. Indeed, at the periphery, oxidative stress, along with the production of reactive oxygen species (ROS), has been shown to precede severe metabolic disturbances and insulin resistance (102). Yet, the brain alone uses a large amount of the oxygen and calories consumed by the body, making it particularly vulnerable to excessive ROS production and oxidative stress. Indeed, mitochondria naturally produce ROS in physiological conditions, especially during the oxidation of nutrients such as glucose or fatty acids (103), and it has been shown that an excessive production of ROS in the hypothalamus occurs in the obese rat. This impairs not only the local detection of glucose but also the associated physiological response, such as peripheral insulin secretion (104). Autophagy is another possible pathway. It is a cellular process allowing the elimination of damaged cytoplasmic elements and organelles in order to maintain internal homeostasis and structural integrity and also plays a key role in cellular responses to metabolic stress. Under conditions of overnutrition, endoplasmic reticulum stress and oxidative stress can induce autophagy (105, 106). Impairing the pathways of autophagy can increase food intake and weight, in association with overactivation of the IKKβ/NF-κB pathway in the hypothalamus, illustrating the connection between autophagic and inflammatory pathways in the hypothalamus.

Over the recent years, the importance of the role played in hypothalamic inflammation in the onset of metabolic disorders in obesity was indeed underlined and the potential of counteracting inflammation in the hypothalamus as a strategy in the fight against obesity was highlighted.

For example, a recent study by Douglass and colleagues demonstrates that astrocytes in the MBH of HFD-fed mice mediate hypothalamic inflammation together with DIO *via* their own inflammatory signaling (107). Indeed, the authors showed that the inducible and specific deletion of IKKβ in astrocytes, which should blunt astrocytic inflammatory capacity, reduces the mice susceptibility to DIO (reduced weight gain and fat mass associated with a decrease in food intake and an increase in energy expenditure), improves glucose tolerance and insulin sensitivity (according to glucose and insulin tolerance tests), and finally, reduces HFD-induced astrocytosis in the MBH.

Furthermore, it has been shown that subcutaneous application of liraglutide or canagliflozin (an inhibitor of the sodium-glucose cotransporter 2) in obese and insulin-resistant rodents is able to disrupt the activation of microglial cells in the hypothalamus, which is associated with an improvement of insulin and glucose homeostasis. In addition, when the ICV injection of IL-4 in HFD-fed rats increases further HFD-induced inflammation in the hypothalamus and causes excessive weight gain, the ICV injection of an IKKβ/NF-κB blocker allows, on the contrary, to prevent hypothalamic inflammation, which is associated with both a decrease in body weight and fat mass and improvements in glucose metabolism and general energy homeostasis in DIO animals (86, 108–111).

Another study by André et al. shows that overnutrition will induce, in addition to an increase in body weight and in adiposity, an increase in the number of microglial cells in the ARC. The authors show the inhibition of microglia expansion in the ARC, achieved by the central delivery of an antimitotic drug, allows to limit food intake and the increase in body weight and in adiposity and also to restore leptin sensitivity. This is associated with a "predictable" inhibition of the upregulation of inflammatory pathways in the ARC that is normally associated with overnutrition, but also in periphery (112).

Taken together, studies studying the hypothalamic inflammation associated with obesity support that this inflammation plays a key role in the metabolic dysfunctions associated with obesity and represents a very interesting target.

Research aiming to understand how the central regulation of energy balance is altered in the context of overnutrition has mainly focused on neurons so far. Yet, as previously mentioned, since hypothalamic inflammation, especially its gliosis feature, has been associated to overnutrition, a strong interest in the role of glial cells (mainly microglia and astrocytes) emerged more recently. Interestingly, these glial cells, once activated, are capable of overproducing, locally, pro-inflammatory mediators such as cytokines and chemokines that can, in turn, affect the neuropeptidergic systems of the hypothalamus, potentially participating in the onset of obesity.

Interestingly, chemokines and their receptors have been demonstrated to be expressed by glial cells, and also by neurons. Especially, chemokine receptors appear to be more expressed by neurons than cytokine receptors in some nuclei of the hypothalamus, allowing to ask the following question: "Could not chemokines act as one of the latest inflammatory mediator that would link inflammation to the disruption of the proper functioning of the neuropeptidergic systems involved in the regulation of the energy balance to promote weight gain and thus the development of obesity?"

Chemokines in the Modulation of Hypothalamic Neuropeptidergic Circuits in DIO

As it was the case in the context of hypothalamic inflammation and involuntary weight loss, only few studies have aimed to determine and understand if and how chemokines are able to alter the function of hypothalamic neuropeptidergic circuits and thus participate in the development and/or the maintenance of obesity.

A study by Morari and colleagues has identified fractalkine (or CX3CL1) as involved in the early activation of hypothalamic inflammation in a murine model of DIO, likely through recruitment of microglial cells which express CX3CR1, the receptor for CX3CL1 (75). In this study, the authors show that, early after HFD introduction to the mice (1–3 days), CX3CL1 is induced in hypothalamic neurons of obesity-prone mice, unlike what was observed in obesity-resistant mice. Interestingly, the inhibition of CX3CL1 in the MBH by an approach of small interfering RNA allows a reduction in inflammation, glucose intolerance, and diet-induced adiposity (no significant difference in body weight was observed though). It suggests that CX3CL1, mediating early recruitment of microglia induced by HFD and thus participating in the induction of hypothalamic inflammatory response, participates in the pathogenesis of obesity as it impairs glucose tolerance and adiposity (**Figure 3**).

In addition, one recent study highlights the role of the axis CXCL12/CXC-motif chemokine receptor 4 (CXCR4) in the paraventricular nucleus (PVN) of the hypothalamus in mediating both neuronal and behavioral effects of the consumption of a HFD in rats (76). In more details, the authors show that a 5-day consumption of a HFD induces an overexpression of CXCL12 and its receptors CXCR4 and CXCR7 both in the PVN and in the perifornical lateral hypothalamus (PFLH). The authors also show that HFD is able to induce an overexpression of orexigenic neuropeptides enkephalin and galanin in the PVN and orexin (ORX) and MCH in the PFLH. Moreover, HFD is associated with an increase in the number of CXCR4$^+$ cells in the PVN. Conversely, in the arcuate nucleus, the levels of CXCL12 and CXCR4 were too low to be detected. The ICV injection of CXCL12, next to the hypothalamus, is able to recapitulate the effects of HFD consumption: (1) it reduces novelty-induced locomotor activity, as a 5-day HFD feeding period does; (2) it is associated to an increase in gene expression of enkephalin in the PVN; and (3) it induces an acute increase in calorie intake (by overconsumption of the HFD only and no consumption of chow diet, as rats had access to both diets). This last point interestingly suggests that CXCL12 could participate in the control ingestive behavior, especially since some different studies also previously demonstrated that CXCL12 could affect other systems such as the MCH and vasopressin in the hypothalamus or dopamine in the substantia nigra (18, 113, 114). Taken together, these results suggest that CXCL12 could modulate the activity of orexigenic peptide-producing neurons, especially the encephalin neurons in the PVN. This would favor HFD intake and decrease locomotor activity and, thus, participate in HFD-induced weight gain (**Figure 3**).

The chemokine CCL5, also known as RANTES for Regulated on Activation, Normal T Cell Expressed and Secreted, has already been linked to obesity-associated inflammation in periphery. Indeed, obesity is associated with an increase in CCL5 secretion and gene expression in AT in obese human and mice. There, CCL5 is suspected to mediate the increase in the local accumulation of T cells and macrophages, which is involved in the complex genesis of chronic inflammation (115, 116). In addition, our joint study with Dr. Karine Clément's team proposed CCL5 as biomarker of weight evolution in patients undergoing bariatric bypass surgery Roux-en-Y as its levels were nearly eightfold higher in the serum of obese patients than in the one of control patients. CCL5 seems to be the only chemokine of which serum levels appear to be correlated with caloric intake in patients undergoing bariatric bypass surgery Roux-en-Y: they rapidly decrease after surgery, as caloric intake decreases and, later on, when patient's caloric intake and body weight start increasing again, they also increase again (77). This justified further interest in the potential role of CCL5 as a modulator of the activity of hypothalamic neurons regulating food intake and which could possibly promote the establishment and/or development of obesity. Thus, our group characterized its expression profile, both at the peripheral and hypothalamic levels in a model of nutritional obesity in mice. In this model, we found both peripheral and central inflammations, as evidenced by the overexpression of canonical pro-inflammatory mediators in the serum and hypothalamus. CCL5 was also found to be overexpressed in the periphery and in the hypothalamus of obese animals (78). An ICV injection of CCL5 on the expression of orexigenic peptides MCH and ORX seems able to increase the expression of both ORX and MCH, transiently for ORX and in a more stable and persistent manner for MCH. Furthermore, it would appear that CCL5 is capable of depolarizing MCH neurons, thus facilitating their activation (78). These results indeed suggest that CCL5 is acutely able to modify the activity of the hypothalamic orexigenic MCH system. Taken together, these results suggest that the overexpression of CCL5 would promote the overactivation of hypothalamic MCH neurons and thus participate in weight gain (**Figure 3**). Whether CCL5 is a cause or a consequence of obesity, or if it could effectively disrupt the proper function of the neuropeptidergic circuits of the hypothalamus, which regulate energy balance and promote the establishment of obesity, is nevertheless still matter of investigation.

CONCLUSION

As of today, a substantial amount of publications supports that hypothalamic inflammation mediates disruptions in the hypothalamic control of energy homeostasis, especially regarding body weight regulation. If some pathways and cellular actors have been identified, mechanisms are still ill-described and poorly understood.

Chemokines have long been considered as essential mediators of the inflammatory response, but more particularly because of their ability to activate and attract immune cells to the affected site. However, at the central level, the literature has also attributed to chemokines and their receptors, beyond their role in the attraction of leukocytes in the cerebral parenchyma, important roles in neuronal survival as in neurotoxicity, cerebral development, communication between immune and glial cells, and also communication between neurons and glial cells (since all these cell types have been shown to be able to express the actors of the chemokinergic system) and also in neuromodulation (15, 18).

Several studies now support the hypothesis that chemokines are actually able to modulate the activity of certain neurons. We and others were able to demonstrate that their overexpression is able to deregulate the neuropeptidergic systems of the hypothalamus, which participate in the regulation of the energy balance and participate in the development of deregulations of the latter, whether it is an excessive weight loss or gain (**Figure 3**). Moreover, this does not, in any way, exclude that, under physiological conditions, the chemokines are actors of this regulation. These studies on chemokine central signaling now identify chemokines as novel potential therapeutic targets against deregulations of the energy balance.

AUTHOR CONTRIBUTIONS

OLT conceived and wrote the manuscript. OLT also made the figures. OLT and KS realized the bibliography researches. CC, JLN, NB, and CR critically appraised and revised the manuscript and figures. All authors listed made substantial, direct, and intellectual contribution to the work and gave permission for this manuscript to be published.

FUNDING

Studies from the authors' laboratory were funded by the CNRS, the Fondation pour la Recherche Médicale (DEQ20150331738 and DRM20101220421), and the French Government (National Research Agency, ANR) through the "Investments for the Future" LABEX SIGNALIFE: program reference # ANR-11-LABX-0028-01.

REFERENCES

Waterson MJ, Horvath TL. Neuronal regulation of energy homeostasis: beyond the hypothalamus and feeding. *Cell Metab* (2015) 22:962–70. doi:10.1016/j.cmet.2015.09.026

Velloso LA, Araújo EP, de Souza CT. Diet-induced inflammation of the hypothalamus in obesity. *Neuroimmunomodulation* (2008) 15:189–93. doi:10.1159/000153423

Braun TP, Marks DL. Pathophysiology and treatment of inflammatory anorexia in chronic disease. *J Cachexia Sarcopenia Muscle* (2010) 1:135–45. doi:10.1007/s13539-010-0015-1

Dorfman MD, Thaler JP. Hypothalamic inflammation and gliosis in obesity. *Curr Opin Endocrinol Diabetes Obes* (2015) 22:325–30. doi:10.1097/MED.0000000000000182

Cesar HC, Pisani LP. Fatty-acid-mediated hypothalamic inflammation and epigenetic programming. *J Nutr Biochem* (2017) 42:1–6. doi:10.1016/j.jnutbio.2016.08.008

Wisse BE, Schwartz MW. Does hypothalamic inflammation cause obesity? *Cell Metab* (2009) 10:241–2. doi:10.1016/j.cmet.2009.09.003

Le Thuc O, Rovère C. [Hypothalamic inflammation and energy balance deregulations: focus on chemokines]. *Biol Aujourdhui* (2016) 210(4):211–25. doi:10.1051/jbio/2016026

Wispelwey B, Lesse AJ, Hansen EJ, Scheld WM. *Haemophilus influenzae* lipopolysaccharide-induced blood brain barrier permeability during experimental meningitis in the rat. *J Clin Invest* (1988) 82:1339–46. doi:10.1172/JCI113736

Layé S, Gheusi G, Cremona S, Combe C, Kelley K, Dantzer R, etal. Endogenous brain IL-1 mediates LPS-induced anorexia and hypothalamic cytokine expression. *Am J Physiol Regul Integr Comp Physiol* (2000) 279:R93–8.

Grossberg AJ, Scarlett JM, Marks DL. Hypothalamic mechanisms in cachexia. *Physiol Behav* (2010) 100:478–89. doi:10.1016/j.physbeh.2010.03.011

Wisse BE, Ogimoto K, Tang J, Harris MK, Raines EW, Schwartz MW. Evidence that lipopolysaccharide-induced anorexia depends upon central, rather than peripheral, inflammatory signals. *Endocrinology* (2007) 148:5230–7. doi:10.1210/en.2007-0394

Banisadr G, Quéraud-Lesaux F, Boutterin MC, Pélaprat D, Zalc B, Rostène W, et al. Distribution, cellular localization and functional role of CCR2 chemok- ine receptors in adult rat brain. *J Neurochem* (2002) 81:257–69. doi:10.1046/ j.1471-4159.2002.00809.x

vanderMeerP,UlrichAM,González-ScaranoF,LaviE.Immunohistochemical analysis of CCR2, CCR3, CCR5, and CXCR4 in the human brain: potential mechanisms for HIV dementia. *Exp Mol Pathol* (2000) 69:192–201. doi:10.1006/exmp.2000.2336

Adler MW, Rogers TJ. Are chemokines the third major system in the brain? *J Leukoc Biol* (2005) 78:1204–9. doi:10.1189/jlb.0405222

Rostène W, Dansereau M-A, Godefroy D, Van Steenwinckel J, Réaux- Le Goazigo A, Mélik-Parsadaniantz S, et al. Neurochemokines: a menage a trois providing new insights on the functions of chemok- ines in the central nervous system. *J Neurochem* (2011) 118:680–94. doi:10.1111/j.1471-4159.2011.07371.x

Guyon A, Banisadr G, Rovère C, Cervantes A, Kitabgi P, Melik Parsadaniantz S, et al. Complex effects of stromal cell-derived factor-1α on melanin-concentrating hormone neuron excitability. *Eur J Neurosci* (2005) 21:701–10. doi:10.1111/j.1460-9568.2005.03890.x

Guyon A, Rovère C, Cervantes A, Allaeys I, Nahon JL. Stromal cell-derived factor-1alpha directly modulates voltage-dependent currents of the action potential in mammalian neuronal cells. *J Neurochem* (2005) 93:963–73. doi:10.1111/j.1471-4159.2005.03083.x

Callewaere C, Banisadr G, Desarménien MG, Mechighel P, Kitabgi P, Rostène WH, et al. The chemokine SDF-1/CXCL12 modulates the firing pattern of vasopressin neurons and counteracts induced vasopressin release through CXCR4. *Proc Natl Acad Sci U S A* (2006) 103:8221–6. doi:10.1073/pnas.0602620103

Wong CJ. Involuntary weight loss. *Med Clin* (2014) 98:625–43. doi:10.1016/j.mcna.2014.01.012

Vanderschueren S, Geens E, Knockaert D, Bobbaers H. The diagnostic spectrum of unintentional weight loss. *Eur J Intern Med* (2005) 16:160–4. doi:10.1016/j.ejim.2005.01.004

Tan BH, Fearon KC. Cachexia: prevalence and impact in medicine. *Curr Opin Clin Nutr Metab Care* (2008) 11:400–7. doi:10.1097/MCO.0b013e328300ecc1

Dantzer R. Cytokine, sickness behavior, and depression. *Neurol Clin* (2006) 24:441–60. doi:10.1016/j.ncl.2006.03.003

van Niekerk G, Isaacs AW, Nell T, Engelbrecht AM. Sickness-associated anorexia: Mother Nature's idea of immunonutrition? *Mediators Inflamm* (2016) 2016:8071539. doi:10.1155/2016/8071539

Mehler PS, Brown C. Anorexia nervosa – medical complications. *J Eat Disord* (2015) 3:11. doi:10.1186/s40337-015-0040-8

Muscaritoli M, Anker SD, Argiles J, Aversa Z, Bauer JM, Biolo G, et al. Consensus definition of sarcopenia, cachexia and pre-cachexia: joint document elaborated by special interest groups (SIG) "cachexia-anorexia in chronic wasting diseases" and "nutrition in geriatrics". *Clin Nutr* (2010) 29:154–9. doi:10.1016/j.clnu.2009.12.004

Müller TD, Perez-Tilve D, Tong J, Pfluger PT, Tschöp MH. Ghrelin and its potential in the treatment of eating/wasting disorders and cachexia. *J Cachexia Sarcopenia Muscle* (2010) 1:159–67. doi:10.1007/s13539-010-0012-4

Alexander C, Rietschel ET. Bacterial lipopolysaccharides and innate immunity. *J Endotoxin Res* (2001) 7:167–202. doi:10.1177/096805190100 70030101

Banks WA, Farr SA, La Scola ME, Morley JE. Intravenous human interleukin-1alpha impairs memory processing in mice: dependence on blood-brain barrier transport into posterior division of the septum. *J Pharmacol Exp Ther* (2001) 299:536–41.

Kent S, Bluthé R-M, Kelley KW, Dantzer R. Sickness behavior as a new target for drug development. *Trends Pharmacol Sci* (1992) 13:24–8. doi:10.1016/0165-6147(92)90012-U

Spadaro F, Dunn AJ. Intracerebroventricular administration of interleukin-1 to mice alters investigation of stimuli in a novel environment. *Brain Behav Immun* (1990) 4:308–22. doi:10.1016/0889-1591(90)90034-N

Kent S, Kelley KW, Dantzer R. Effects of lipopolysaccharide on food-motivated behavior in the rat are not blocked by an inter- leukin-1 receptor antagonist. *Neurosci Lett* (1992) 145:83–6. doi:10.1016/0304-3940(92)90209-P

Kent S, Bluthé RM, Dantzer R, Hardwick AJ, Kelley KW, Rothwell NJ, et al. Different receptor mechanisms mediate the pyrogenic and behavioral effects of interleukin 1. *Proc Natl Acad Sci U S A* (1992) 89:9117–20. doi:10.1073/pnas.89.19.9117

Johnson RW, Gheusi G, Segreti S, Dantzer R, Kelley KW. C3H/HeJ mice are refractory to lipopolysaccharide in the brain. *Brain Res* (1997) 752:219–26. doi:10.1016/S0006-8993(96)01454-0

Hopkins SJ, Rothwell NJ. Cytokines and the nervous system. I: expression and recognition. *Trends Neurosci* (1995) 18:83–8. doi:10.1016/0166-2236(95)80029-2

Rothwell NJ, Hopkins SJ. Cytokines and the nervous system II: actions and mechanisms of action. *Trends Neurosci* (1995) 18:130–6. doi:10.1016/ 0166-2236(95)93890-A

Licinio J, Wong ML. Pathways and mechanisms for cytokine signaling of the central nervous system. *J Clin Invest* (1997) 100:2941–7. doi:10.1172/ JCI119846

Sternberg EM. Neural-immune interactions in health and disease. *J Clin Invest* (1997) 100:2641–7. doi:10.1172/JCI119807

Mantovani G, Macciò A, Lai P, Massa E, Ghiani M, Santona MC. Cytokine involvement in cancer anorexia/cachexia: role of megestrol acetate and medroxyprogesterone acetate on cytokine downregulation and improvement of clinical symptoms. *Crit Rev Oncog* (1998) 9:99–106. doi:10.1615/ CritRevOncog.v9.i2.10

Haslett PA. Anticytokine approaches to the treatment of anorexia and cachexia. *Semin Oncol* (1998) 25:53–7.

Konsman JP, Parnet P, Dantzer R. Cytokine-induced sickness behaviour: mechanisms and implications. *Trends Neurosci* (2002) 25:154–9. doi:10.1016/ S0166-2236(00)02088-9.

Gelin J, Moldawer LL, Lönnroth C, Sherry B, Chizzonite R, Lundholm K. Role of endogenous tumor necrosis factor alpha and interleukin 1 for experimental tumor growth and the development of cancer cachexia. *Cancer Res* (1991) 51:415–21.

Matthys P, Billiau A. Cytokines and cachexia. *Nutrition* (1997) 13:763–70. doi:10.1016/S0899-9007(97)00185-8

Moldawer LL, Rogy MA, Lowry SF. The role of cytokines in cancer cachexia. *JPEN J Parenter Enteral Nutr* (1992) 16:43S–9S. doi:10.1177/014860719201 600602

Tisdale MJ. Biology of cachexia. *J Natl Cancer Inst* (1997) 89:1763–73. doi:10.1093/jnci/89.23.1763

Noguchi Y, Yoshikawa T, Matsumoto A, Svaninger G, Gelin J. Are cytokines possible mediators of cancer cachexia? *Surg Today* (1996) 26:467–75. doi:10.1007/BF00311551

Sherry BA, Gelin J, Fong Y, Marano M, Wei H, Cerami A, et al. Anticachectin/ tumor necrosis factor-alpha antibodies attenuate development of cachexia in tumor models. *FASEB J* (1989) 3:1956–62.

Laviano A, Gleason JR, Meguid MM, Yang ZJ, Cangiano C, Rossi Fanelli F. Effects of intra-VMN mianserin and IL-1ra on meal number in anorectic tumor-bearing rats. *J Investig Med* (2000) 48:40–8.

Scarlett JM, Jobst EE, Enriori PJ, Bowe DD, Batra AK, Grant WF, et al. Regulation of central melanocortin signaling by interleukin-1 beta. *Endocrinology* (2007) 148:4217–25. doi:10.1210/en.2007-0017

Arruda AP, Milanski M, Coope A, Torsoni AS, Ropelle E, Carvalho DP, et al. Low-grade hypothalamic inflammation leads to defective thermogenesis, insulin resistance, and impaired insulin secretion. *Endocrinology* (2011) 152:1314–26. doi:10.1210/en.2010-0659

Ropelle ER, Pauli JR, Zecchin KG, Ueno M, de Souza CT, Morari J, et al. A central role for neuronal adenosine 5'-monophosphate-activated protein kinase in cancer-induced anorexia. *Endocrinology* (2007) 148:5220–9. doi:10.1210/en.2007-0381

DeBoer MD, Zhu XX, Levasseur P, Meguid MM, Suzuki S, Inui A, et al. Ghrelin treatment causes increased food intake and retention of lean body mass in a rat model of cancer cachexia. *Endocrinology* (2007) 148:3004–12. doi:10.1210/en.2007-0016

Ueta Y, Hashimoto H, Onuma E, Takuwa Y, Ogata E. Hypothalamic neuropeptides and appetite response in anorexia-cachexia animal. *Endocr J* (2007) 54:831–8. doi:10.1507/endocrj.KR-111

Gay NJ, Gangloff M, Weber AN. Toll-like receptors as molecular switches. *Nat Rev Immunol* (2006) 6:693–8. doi:10.1038/nri1916

Lien E, Means TK, Heine H, Yoshimura A, Kusumoto S, Fukase K, et al. Toll-like receptor 4 imparts ligand-specific recognition of bacterial lipopolysaccharide. *J Clin Invest* (2000) 105:497–504. doi:10.1172/JCI8541

Chakravarty S, Herkenham M. Toll-like receptor 4 on nonhematopoietic cells sustains CNS inflammation during endotoxemia, independent of systemic cytokines. *J Neurosci* (2005) 25:1788–96. doi:10.1523/JNEUROSCI.4268-04.2005

Lehnardt S, Lachance C, Patrizi S, Lefebvre S, Follett PL, Jensen FE, et al. The toll-like receptor TLR4 is necessary for lipopolysaccharide-induced oligodendrocyte injury in the CNS. *J Neurosci* (2002) 22:2478–86.

Hines DJ, Choi HB, Hines RM, Phillips AG, MacVicar BA. Prevention of LPS-induced microglia activation, cytokine production and sickness behavior with TLR4 receptor interfering peptides. *PLoS One* (2013) 8:e60388. doi:10.1371/journal.pone.0060388

Reis WL, Yi C-X, Gao Y, Tschöp MH, Stern JE. Brain innate immunity regulates hypothalamic arcuate neuronal activity and feeding behavior. *Endocrinology* (2015) 156:1303–15. doi:10.1210/en.2014-1849

Gayle D, Ilyin SE, Plata-Salamán CR. Feeding status and bacterial LPS- induced cytokine and neuropeptide gene expression in hypothalamus. *Am J Physiol* (1999) 277:R1188–95.

Ogimoto K, Harris MK, Wisse BE. MyD88 is a key mediator of anorexia, but not weight loss, induced by lipopolysaccharide and interleukin-1 beta. *Endocrinology* (2006) 147:4445–53. doi:10.1210/en.2006-0465

Sergeyev V, Broberger C, Hökfelt T. Effect of LPS administration on the expression of POMC, NPY, galanin, CART and MCH mRNAs in the rat hypothalamus. *Brain Res Mol Brain Res* (2001) 90:93–100. doi:10.1016/ S0169-328X(01)00088-2

Jang P-G, Namkoong C, Kang GM, Hur M-W, Kim S-W, Kim GH, et al. NF-kappaB activation in hypothalamic pro-opiomelanocortin neurons is essential in illness- and leptin-induced anorexia. *J Biol Chem* (2010) 285:9706–15. doi:10.1074/jbc.M109.070706

Jin S, Kim JG, Park JW, Koch M, Horvath TL, Lee BJ. Hypothalamic TLR2 triggers sickness behavior via a microglia-neuronal axis. *Sci Rep* (2016) 6:29424. doi:10.1038/srep29424

Murray C, Griffin ÉW, O'Loughlin E, Lyons A, Sherwin E, Ahmed S, et al. Interdependent and independent roles of type I interferons and IL-6 in innate immune, neuroinflammatory and sickness behaviour responses to systemic poly I:C. *Brain Behav Immun* (2015) 48:274–86. doi:10.1016/j. bbi.2015.04.009

Dwarkasing JT, Boekschoten MV, Argilès JM, van Dijk M, Busquets S, Penna F, et al. Differences in food intake of tumour-bearing cachectic mice are associated with hypothalamic serotonin signalling. *J Cachexia Sarcopenia Muscle* (2015) 6:84–94. doi:10.1002/jcsm.12008

Laviano A, Inui A, Meguid MM, Molfino A, Conte C, Rossi Fanelli F. NPY and brain monoamines in the pathogenesis of cancer anorexia. *Nutrition* (2008) 24:802–5. doi:10.1016/j.nut.2008.06.005

Meguid MM, Ramos EJB, Laviano A, Varma M, Sato T, Chen C, et al. Tumor anorexia: effects on neuropeptide Y and monoamines in paraventricular nucleus. *Peptides* (2004) 25:261–6. doi:10.1016/j.peptides.2004.01.012

Dwarkasing JT, Witkamp RF, Boekschoten MV, Laak MC, Heins MS, Norren K. Increased hypothalamic serotonin turnover in inflammation-induced anorexia. *BMC Neurosci* (2016) 17:26. doi:10.1186/s12868-016-0260-0

Plata-Salamán CR, Borkoski JP. Chemokines/intercrines and central regulation of feeding. *Am J Physiol* (1994) 266:R1711–5.

Le Thuc O, Cansell C, Bourourou M, Denis RG, Stobbe K, Devaux N, et al. Central CCL2 signaling onto MCH neurons mediates metabolic and behavioral adaptation to inflammation. *EMBO Rep* (2016) 17:1738–52. doi:10.15252/embr.201541499

Cazareth J, Guyon A, Heurteaux C, Chabry J, Petit-Paitel A. Molecular and cellular neuroinflammatory status of mouse brain after systemic lipopolysaccharide challenge: importance of CCR2/CCL2 signaling. *J Neuroinflammation* (2014) 11:132. doi:10.1186/1742-2094-11-132

Conductier G, Blondeau N, Guyon A, Nahon J-L, Rovère C. The role of monocyte chemoattractant protein MCP1/CCL2 in neuroinflammatory diseases. *J Neuroimmunol* (2010) 224:93–100. doi:10.1016/j.jneuroim.2010.05.010

Thompson WL, Karpus WJ, Van Eldik LJ. MCP-1-deficient mice show reduced neuroinflammatory responses and increased peripheral inflamma- tory responses to peripheral endotoxin insult. *J Neuroinflammation* (2008) 5:35. doi:10.1186/1742-2094-5-35

Nahon JL. The melanocortins and melanin-concentrating hormone in the central regulation of feeding behavior and energy homeostasis. *C R Biol* (2006) 329:623–38; discussion 653–5. doi:10.1016/j.crvi.2006.03.021

Morari J, Anhe GF, Nascimento LF, de Moura RF, Razolli D, Solon C, et al. Fractalkine (CX3CL1) is involved in the early activation of hypothalamic inflammation in experimental obesity. *Diabetes* (2014) 63:3770–84. doi:10.2337/db13-1495

Poon K, Barson JR, Ho HT, Leibowitz SF. Relationship of the chemok- ine, CXCL12, to effects of dietary fat on feeding-related behaviors and hypothalamic neuropeptide systems. *Front Behav Neurosci* (2016) 10:51. doi:10.3389/fnbeh.2016.00051

Dalmas E, Rouault C, Abdennour M, Rovere C, Rizkalla S, Bar-Hen A, et al. Variations in circulating inflammatory factors are related to changes in calorie and carbohydrate intakes early in the course of surgery-induced weight reduction. *Am J Clin Nutr* (2011) 94:450–8. doi:10.3945/ajcn.111.013771

Le Thuc O, Blondeau N, Rouaud F, Poitou C, Clement K, Guyon A, et al. Role of the chemokine RANTES/CCL5 in the establishment of high-fat diet-induced obesity in mice. *9th FENS Forum of Neuroscience*. Milan (2014).

Gregor MF, Hotamisligil GS. Inflammatory mechanisms in obesity. *Annu Rev Immunol* (2011) 29:415–45. doi:10.1146/annurev-immunol-031210-101322

Williams EP, Mesidor M, Winters K, Dubbert PM, Wyatt SB. Overweight and obesity: prevalence, consequences, and causes of a growing public health problem. *Curr Obes Rep* (2015) 4:363–70. doi:10.1007/s13679-015-0169-4

Smith KB, Smith MS. Obesity statistics. *Prim Care* (2016) 43:121–35,ix. doi:10.1016/j.pop.2015.10.001

Thaler JP, Yi C-X, Schur EA, Guyenet SJ, Hwang BH, Dietrich MO, et al. Obesity is associated with hypothalamic injury in rodents and humans. *J Clin Invest* (2012) 122:153–62. doi:10.1172/JCI59660

De Souza CT, Araujo EP, Bordin S, Ashimine R, Zollner RL, Boschero AC, et al. Consumption of a fat-rich diet activates a proinflammatory response and induces insulin resistance in the hypothalamus. *Endocrinology* (2005) 146:4192–9. doi:10.1210/en.2004-1520

Kleinridders A, Schenten D, Konner AC, Belgardt BF, Mauer J, Okamura T, et al. MyD88 signaling in the CNS is required for development of fatty acid-induced leptin resistance and diet-induced obesity. *Cell Metab* (2009) 10:249–59. doi:10.1016/j.cmet.2009.08.013

Valdearcos M, Robblee MM, Benjamin DI, Nomura DK, Xu AW, Koliwad SK. Microglia dictate the impact of saturated fat consumption on hypothalamic inflammation and neuronal function. *Cell Rep* (2014) 9:2124–38. doi:10.1016/j.celrep.2014.11.018

Zhang X, Zhang G, Zhang H, Karin M, Bai H, Cai D. Hypothalamic IKKbeta/NF-kappaB and ER stress link overnutrition to energy imbalance and obesity. *Cell* (2008) 135:61–73. doi:10.1016/j.cell.2008.07.043

Posey KA, Clegg DJ, Printz RL, Byun J, Morton GJ, Vivekanandan-Giri A, et al. Hypothalamic proinflammatory lipid accumulation, inflammation, and insulin resistance in rats fed a high-fat diet. *Am J Physiol Endocrinol Metab* (2009) 296:E1003–12. doi:10.1152/ajpendo.90377.2008

Grayson BE, Levasseur PR, Williams SM, Smith MS, Marks DL, Grove KL. Changes in melanocortin expression and inflammatory pathways in fetal offspring of nonhuman primates fed a high-fat diet. *Endocrinology* (2010) 151:1622–32. doi:10.1210/en.2009-1019

Holland WL, Bikman BT, Wang L-P, Yuguang G, Sargent KM, Bulchand S, et al. Lipid-induced insulin resistance mediated by the proinflammatory receptor TLR4 requires saturated fatty acid-induced ceramide biosynthesis in mice. *J Clin Invest* (2011) 121:1858–70. doi:10.1172/JCI43378

Maric T, Woodside B, Luheshi GN. The effects of dietary saturated fat on basal hypothalamic neuroinflammation in rats. *Brain Behav Immun* (2014) 36:35–45. doi:10.1016/j.bbi.2013.09.011

Morselli E, Fuente-Martin E, Finan B, Kim M, Frank A, Garcia-Caceres C, et al. Hypothalamic PGC-1α protects against high-fat diet exposure by regulating ERα. *Cell Rep* (2014) 9:633–45. doi:10.1016/j.celrep.2014.09.025

Weissmann L, Quaresma PGF, Santos AC, de Matos AHB, Pascoal VDÁB, Zanotto TM, et al. IKKε is key to induction of insulin resistance in the hypothalamus, and its inhibition reverses obesity. *Diabetes* (2014) 63:3334–45. doi:10.2337/db13-1817

Dalvi PS, Chalmers JA, Luo V, Han DY, Wellhauser L, Liu Y, et al. High fat induces acute and chronic inflammation in the hypothalamus: effect of high- fat diet, palmitate and TNF-alpha on appetite-regulating NPY neurons. *Int J Obes (Lond)* (2017) 41:149–58. doi:10.1038/ijo.2016.183

Zhang W, Hu X, Yang W, Gao Y, Chen J. Omega-3 polyunsaturated fatty acid supplementation confers long-term neuroprotection against neonatal hypoxic-ischemic brain injury through anti-inflammatory actions. *Stroke* (2010) 41:2341–7. doi:10.1161/STROKEAHA.110.586081

Buckley JD, Howe PRC. Long-chain omega-3 polyunsaturated fatty acids may be beneficial for reducing obesity – a review. *Nutrients* (2010) 2:1212–30. doi:10.3390/nu2121212

Cintra DE, Ropelle ER, Moraes JC, Pauli JR, Morari J, de Souza CT, et al. Unsaturated fatty acids revert diet-induced hypothalamic inflammation in obesity. *PLoS One* (2012) 7:e30571. doi:10.1371/journal.pone.0030571

Oliveira V, Marinho R, Vitorino D, Santos GA, Moraes JC, Dragano N, et al. Diets containing alpha-linolenic (omega 3) or oleic (omega 9) fatty acids res- cues obese mice from insulin resistance. *Endocrinology* (2015) 156:4033–46. doi:10.1210/en.2014-1880

Gao Y, Ottaway N, Schriever SC, Legutko B, García-Cáceres C, de la Fuente E, et al. Hormones and diet, but not body weight, control hypothalamic microglial activity. *Glia* (2014) 62:17–25. doi:10.1002/ glia.22580

Fantuzzi G, Faggioni R. Leptin in the regulation of immunity, inflammation, and hematopoiesis. *J Leukoc Biol* (2000) 68:437–46.

Hotamisligil GS. Endoplasmic reticulum stress and the inflammatory basis of metabolic disease. *Cell* (2010) 140:900–17. doi:10.1016/j.cell.2010. 02.034

Purkayastha S, Zhang H, Zhang G, Ahmed Z, Wang Y, Cai D. Neural dysregulation of peripheral insulin action and blood pressure by brain endoplasmic reticulum stress. *Proc Natl Acad Sci U S A* (2011) 108:2939–44. doi:10.1073/pnas.1006875108

Matsuzawa-Nagata N, Takamura T, Ando H, Nakamura S, Kurita S, Misu H, et al. Increased oxidative stress precedes the onset of high-fat diet-induced insulin resistance and obesity. *Metabolism* (2008) 57:1071–7. doi:10.1016/j.metabol.2008.03.010

Leloup C, Casteilla L, Carrière A, Galinier A, Benani A, Carneiro L, et al. Balancing mitochondrial redox signaling: a key point in metabolic regulation. *Antioxid Redox Signal* (2011) 14:519–30. doi:10.1089/ars.2010.3424

Colombani A-L, Carneiro L, Benani A, Galinier A, Jaillard T, Duparc T, et al. Enhanced hypothalamic glucose sensing in obesity: alteration of redox signaling. *Diabetes* (2009) 58:2189–97. doi:10.2337/db09-0110

Butler D, Bahr BA. Oxidative stress and lysosomes: CNS-related con- sequences and implications for lysosomal enhancement strategies and induction of autophagy. *Antioxid Redox Signal* (2006) 8:185–96. doi:10.1089/ars.2006.8.185

Yorimitsu T, Nair U, Yang Z, Klionsky DJ. Endoplasmic reticulum stress triggers autophagy. *J Biol Chem* (2006) 281:30299–304. doi:10.1074/jbc.M607007200

Douglass JD, Dorfman MD, Fasnacht R, Shaffer LD, Thaler JP. Astrocyte IKKbeta/NF-kappaB signaling is required for diet-induced obesity and hypothalamic inflammation. *Mol Metab* (2017) 6:366–73. doi:10.1016/j.molmet.2017.01.010

Benzler J, Ganjam GK, Pretz D, Oelkrug R, Koch CE, Legler K, et al. Central inhibition of IKKbeta/NF-kappaB signaling attenuates high-fat diet-induced obesity and glucose intolerance. *Diabetes* (2015) 64:2015–27. doi:10.2337/ db14-0093

Barreto-Vianna AR, Aguila MB, Mandarim-de-Lacerda CA. Effects of liraglutide in hypothalamic arcuate nucleus of obese mice. *Obesity (Silver Spring)* (2016) 24:626–33. doi:10.1002/oby.21387

Naznin F, Sakoda H, Okada T, Tsubouchi H, Waise TM, Arakawa K, et al. Canagliflozin, a sodium glucose cotransporter 2 inhibitor, attenuates obesity-induced inflammation in the nodose ganglion, hypothalamus, and skeletal muscle of mice. *Eur J Pharmacol* (2017) 794:37–44. doi:10.1016/j.ejphar.2016.11.028

Oh-I S, Thaler JP, Ogimoto K, Wisse BE, Morton GJ, Schwartz MW. Central administration of interleukin-4 exacerbates hypothalamic inflammation and weight gain during high-fat feeding. *Am J Physiol Endocrinol Metab* (2010) 299:E47–53. doi:10.1152/ajpendo.00026.2010

André C, Guzman-Quevedo O, Rey C, émus-Borel JR, Clark S, Castellanos-Jankiewicz A, et al. Inhibiting microglia expansion prevents diet-induced hypothalamic and peripheral inflammation. *Diabetes* (2017) 66:908–19. doi:10.2337/db16-0586

Guyon A, Rovere C, Cervantes A, Allaeys I, Nahon JL. Stromal cell-derived factor-1alpha directly modulates voltage-dependent currents of the action potential in mammalian neuronal cells. *J Neurochem* (2005) 93:963–73. doi:10.1111/j.1471-4159.2005.03083.x

Skrzydelski D, Guyon A, Dauge V, Rovere C, Apartis E, Kitabgi P, et al. The chemokine stromal cell-derived factor-1/CXCL12 activates the nigrostriatal dopamine system. *J Neurochem* (2007) 102:1175–83. doi:10.1111/j.1471-4159.2007.04639.x

Keophiphath M, Rouault C, Divoux A, Clement K, Lacasa D. CCL5 promotes macrophage recruitment and survival in human adipose tissue. *Arterioscler Thromb Vasc Biol* (2009) 30:39–45. doi:10.1161/atvbaha.109. 197442

Wu H, Ghosh S, Perrard XD, Feng L, Garcia GE, Perrard JL, et al. T-cell accumulation and regulated on activation, normal T cell expressed and secreted upregulation in adipose tissue in obesity. *Circulation* (2007) 115:1029–38. doi:10.1161/circulationaha.106.638379

9

The Neuroendocrine Regulation of Food Intake in Fish

Helene Volkoff *

Departments of Biology and Biochemistry, Memorial University of Newfoundland, St. John's, NL, Canada

***Correspondence:**
Helene Volkoff
hvolkoff@mun.ca

Fish are the most diversified group of vertebrates and, although progress has been made in the past years, only relatively few fish species have been examined to date, with regards to the endocrine regulation of feeding in fish. In fish, as in mammals, feeding behavior is ultimately regulated by central effectors within feeding centers of the brain, which receive and process information from endocrine signals from both brain and peripheral tissues. Although basic endocrine mechanisms regulating feeding appear to be conserved among vertebrates, major physiological differences between fish and mammals and the diversity of fish, in particular in regard to feeding habits, digestive tract anatomy and physiology, suggest the existence of fish- and species-specific regulating mechanisms. This review provides an overview of hormones known to regulate food intake in fish, emphasizing on major hormones and the main fish groups studied to date.

Keywords: fish, hormones, feeding, appetite, diversity, brain, intestine

INTRODUCTION

Feeding is a complex behavior consisting of food ingestion itself as well as foraging or appetitive behaviors (which reflect motivation to consume food; Keen-Rhinehart et al., 2013; Woods and Begg, 2016). Feeding is ultimately regulated by central feeding centers of the brain, which receive and process information from endocrine signals from both brain and periphery. These signals consist of hormones that increase (e.g., orexin; neuropeptide Y-NPY) or inhibit, (e.g., cocaine and amphetamine regulated transcript-CART; proopiomelanocortin-POMC) feeding. Feeding centers are also influenced by metabolic and neural peripheral signals providing information on meal ingestion and nutritional status (Volkoff, 2006; Volkoff et al., 2009a,b; Rui, 2013; Sobrino Crespo et al., 2014).

Fish are the most diversified group of vertebrates, with 33,200 species identified to date (FishBase, 2016), the bony fish (teleosts) containing more than half of all vertebrate species (Nelson, 2006). However, only relatively few fish species have been examined to date, with regards to their physiology, in particular feeding. The large numbers of fish species, habitats, feeding habits and digestive tract anatomy and physiology, as well as the number of extrinsic and intrinsic factors affecting feeding behavior and physiology (Volkoff et al., 2009a; Hoskins and Volkoff, 2012) most probably result in complex species-specific feeding regulating mechanisms in fish, with a number of hormones and tissues involved.

Research on the endocrine regulation of feeding in fish has progressed in recent years. New fish appetite-regulating hormones and species other than traditional models (such as goldfish, salmon and zebrafish) are gradually being examined. In addition, traditional techniques such as brain lesions and injections and biochemical purification of peptides, although still useful and being used, have been complemented by new approaches such as gene expression studies, quantitative PCR, genomics (microarrays, RNA-seq), proteomics and metabolomics, transgenesis, gene knockout and silencing, and *in vitro* (cell and tissue culture, perifusion) studies.

The field of fish feeding endocrine physiology is evolving very rapidly and up-to-date reviews are often lacking. One of the first reviews on the endocrine regulation of feeding by R.E. Peter in 1979 (Peter, 1979) mostly focused on growth and growth hormone (GH) but predicted regions of the brain that might be responsible for feeding regulation in fish. In 1986, Matty's review described early data on the effects of GH, thyroid hormones, insulin, and gonadal steroids on feeding (Matty, 1986). Ten years later, Le Bail and Boeuf's review formulated hypotheses on mammalian hormones (e.g., leptin) that might putatively regulate feeding in fish (Le Bail and Boeuf, 1997). In the early twenty-first century, a number of reviews report recent advances on the field and include an increasing number of hormones (e.g., NPY, orexins, CART), some more comparative (Lin et al., 2000; de Pedro and Björnsson, 2001; Volkoff et al., 2005; Gorissen et al., 2006; Volkoff, 2011; Hoskins and Volkoff, 2012), some more focused on a single species (e.g., goldfish Matsuda, 2009; Matsuda et al., 2011a) or a particular group of fish (e.g., elasmobranchs Demski, 2012), some focused on growth (Won and Borski, 2013), and some on aquaculture and behavior (Papoutsoglou, 2012).

The purpose of this review is to provide an up-to-date, brief overview of the hormones regulating food intake in fish, emphasizing on recent studies, major brain hormones and the main fish groups studied thus far.

OVERVIEW OF REGULATION OF FOOD INTAKE

In fish, as in mammals (Sobrino Crespo et al., 2014), feeding behavior is regulated by specific regions in the brain, the so-called feeding centers. Early pioneer studies using stimulation and lesion experiments in teleosts (reviewed in Peter, 1979) and elasmobranchs (reviewed in Demski, 2012) seemed to indicate that the hypothalamic area was involved in feeding and that the brain control of feeding in fish might use mechanisms similar to those in mammals. However, whereas in mammals, the feeding centers appear to be restricted to the hypothalamus, evidence indicates that they might be more widespread in fish brains (Cerda-Reverter and Canosa, 2009).

Feeding centers are under the influence of hormones produced by the brain and the periphery. Neurohormones secreted by the brain, in particular the hypothalamic area, regulate energy balance by inhibiting (anorexigenic factors) or stimulating (orexigenic factors) feeding. Peripheral chemical (e.g., glucose) or endocrine (e.g., gastrointestinal hormones) factors released in the blood cross the blood brain barrier and have a direct action on feeding centers. Peripheral sensory information (mechanical or endocrine) carried by the vagus nerve can also affect feeding centers, via innervation from the brainstem (Volkoff, 2011).

HORMONES INVOLVED IN FOOD INTAKE

The list of hormones regulating feeding in vertebrates is long and increasingly so. Here, focus will be placed on major hormones and newly examined appetite-regulating factors (but not on their receptors), and the phylogeny of the fish species examined to date. **Table 1**, **Figure 1** summarize the hormones that have been examined in fish and their possible effects on feeding.

Major Appetite Regulating Factors

Central Orexigenic Factors

Agouti-related protein (or peptide, AgRP)

AgRP is a peptide released by hypothalamic NPY/AgRP neurons and is an endogenous antagonist of the melanocortin receptors MC3R and MC4R. AgRP plays a crucial role in the regulation of energy balance, as it increases food intake, by antagonizing the effects of the anorexigenic POMC product, α-melanocyte-stimulating hormone (α-MSH) (Sohn, 2015; Takeuchi, 2016).

In fish, AgRP has been identified in several species, including teleosts (e.g., goldfish *Carassius auratus* Cerdá-Reverter and Peter, 2003 and zebrafish *Danio rerio* Song et al., 2003, Atlantic salmon *Salmo salar* Murashita et al., 2009a, and seabass *Dicentrarchus labrax* Agulleiro et al., 2014, pufferfish *Takifugu rubripes* Klovins et al., 2004; Kurokawa et al., 2006), who have two genes products (AgRP1 and AgRP2; Cérda-Reverter et al., 2011) and Holocephali (Chimaeriforme, elephant fish *Callorhinchus milii* Västermark and Schioth, 2011).

AgRP appears to act as an orexigenic factor in Cypriniformes, as fasting increases hypothalamic *AgRP* expression in goldfish (Cerdá-Reverter and Peter, 2003), zebrafish (Song et al., 2003), and Ya fish *Schizothorax prenanti* (Wei et al., 2013). In addition, transgenic zebrafish overexpressing AgRP exhibit obesity, increased growth and adipocyte hypertrophy (Song and Cone, 2007). GH-transgenic common carp *Cyprinus carpio*, which display increased food intake, have higher hypothalamic AgRP1 mRNA expression levels than non-transgenic fish, further suggesting an orexigenic action (Zhong et al., 2013). However, this is contradicted by another study in carp showing that brain AgRP mRNA expression decreases after fasting and increases after re-feeding (Wan et al., 2012). In seabass (Perciforme), long-term fasting increases hypothalamic expression of AgRP1 but decreases that of AgRP2 (Agulleiro et al., 2014), suggesting an isoform-specific orexigenic action.

Within Salmoniformes, there is conflicting data with regards to the actions of AgRP. In Arctic charr *Salvelinus alpinus*, non-feeding fish have higher brain AgRP expression levels than feeding fish (Striberny et al., 2015) and transgenic coho salmon *Oncorhynchus kisutch*, which display increased feeding, have higher brain AgRP1 levels of mRNA than wild-type fish (Kim et al., 2015), suggesting an orexigenic role for AgRP. However, in Atlantic salmon, AgRP-1 brain mRNA levels decrease after fasting (Murashita et al., 2009a) and increase after feeding (Valen et al., 2011), rather pointing to an anorexigenic role.

Galanin

Galanin is a peptide expressed in both central nervous system and GIT, that regulates diverse physiological functions in

TABLE 1 | List of major hormones (in alphabetical order) potentially involved in the regulation of feeding in fish (by order, family and species studied).

Hormone	Order	Family	Species	Major references	Effect on feeding
AgRP	Cypriniforme	Cyprinidae	Common carp (*Cyprinus carpio*)	Zhong et al., 2013	+
			Common carp (*Cyprinus carpio*)	Wan et al., 2012	– ?
			Goldfish (*Carassius auratus*)	Cerdá-Reverter and Peter, 2003	+
			Ya fish (*Schizothorax prenanti*)	Wei et al., 2013	+
			Zebrafish (*Danio rerio*)	Song et al., 2003; Song and Cone, 2007	+
	Salmoniforme	Salmonidae	Atlantic salmon (*Salmo salar*)	Murashita et al., 2009a; Valen et al., 2011	–
			Arctic charr (*Salvelinus alpinus*)	Striberny et al., 2015	+
			Coho salmon (*Oncorhynchus kisutch*)	Kim et al., 2015	+
	Perciforme	Moronidae	Sea bass (*Dicentrarchus labrax*)	Agulleiro et al., 2014	+
Amylin	Cypriniforme	Cyprinidae	Goldfish (*Carassius auratus*)	Thavanathan and Volkoff, 2006	–
Apelin	Characiforme	Characidae	Blind cavefish (*Astyanax mexicanus*)	Penney and Volkoff, 2014	+
		Serrasalmidae	Red-bellied piranha (*Pygocentrus nattereri*)	Volkoff, 2014a	+
	Cyprinoforme	Cyprinidae	*Cyprinus carpio* and *Capoetta trutta*	Köprücü and Algül, 2015	?
			Goldfish (*Carassius auratus*)	Volkoff and Wyatt, 2009; Wong et al., 2013; Volkoff, 2014a; Zhang et al., 2016b	+
			Ya fish (*Schizothorax prenanti*)	Lin et al., 2014a	+
	Perciforme	Labridae	Cunner (*Tautogolabrus adspersus*)	Hayes and Volkoff, 2014	– ?
AVT (arginine vasotocin)	Salmoniforme	Salmonidae	Rainbow trout (*Oncorhynchus mykiss*)	Gesto et al., 2014	–
CART	Beloniformes	Adrianichthyidae	Medaka (*Oryzias latipes*)	Murashita and Kurokawa, 2011	–
	Characiforme	Characidae	Blind cavefish (*Astyanax mexicanus*)	Penney and Volkoff, 2014	–
			Dourado (*Salminus brasiliensis*)	Volkoff et al., 2016	0
		Serrasalmidae	Pacu (*Piaractus mesopotamicus*)	Volkoff et al., 2017	–
			Pirapitinga (*Piaractus brachypomus*)	Volkoff, 2015a	?
			Red-bellied piranha (*Pygocentrus nattereri*)	Volkoff, 2014a	–
	Cypriniforme	Cyprinidae	Common carp (*Cyprinus carpio*)	Wan et al., 2012	–
			Goldfish (*Carassius auratus*)	Abbott and Volkoff, 2011; Volkoff, 2012, 2014b; Zhang et al., 2016b	–
			Grass carp (*Ctenopharyngodon idellus*)	Zhou et al., 2013; Liu et al., 2014	–
			Zebrafish (*Danio rerio*)	Mukherjee et al., 2012; Nishio et al., 2012; Akash et al., 2014; Manuel et al., 2014, 2015; Libran-Perez et al., 2014; Woods et al., 2014; Guillot et al., 2016	–
	Gadiforme	Gadidae	Atlantic cod (*Gadus morhua*)	Kehoe and Volkoff, 2007	– ?
	Perciforme	Labridae	Cunner (Tautogolabrus adspersus)	Babichuk and Volkoff, 2013	–
	Pleuronectiformes	Pleuronectidae	Atlantic halibut (*Hippoglossus hippoglossus*)	Gomes et al., 2014	0
			Winter flounder (*Pseudopleuronectes americanus*)	MacDonald and Volkoff, 2009a	0
		Soleidae	Senegalese sole (*Solea senegalensis*)	Bonacic et al., 2015	–
	Rajiforme (elasmobranch)	Rajidae	Winter skate (*Raja ocellata*)	MacDonald and Volkoff, 2009b	0
	Salmoniforme	Salmonidae	Atlantic salmon (*Salmo salar*)	Murashita et al., 2009a; Burt et al., 2013; Kousoulaki et al., 2013	–
			Arctic Charr (*Salvelinus alpinus*)	Striberny et al., 2015	0
			Rainbow trout (*Oncorhynchus mykiss*)	Figueiredo-Silva et al., 2012; MacDonald et al., 2014	–

(Continued)

TABLE 1 | Continued

Hormone	Order	Family	Species	Major references	Effect on feeding
	Siluriforme	Clariidae	African sharptoothcatfish (*Clarias gariepinus*)	Subhedar et al., 2011	–
			Walking catfish (*Clarias batrachus*)	Barsagade et al., 2010	–
		Ictaluridae	Channel catfish (Ictalurus punctatus)	Kobayashi et al., 2008; Peterson et al., 2012	–
CCK	Characiforme	Characidae	Blind cavefish (Astyanax fasciatus mexicanus)	Wall and Volkoff, 2013	–
			Dourado (*Salminus brasiliensis)*	Pereira et al., 2015; Volkoff et al., 2016	–
			Thin dogfish (*Oligosarcus hepsetus)*	Vieira-Lopes et al., 2013	–
		Serrasalmidae	Pacu (*Piaractus mesopotamicus*)	Volkoff et al., 2017	–
			Pirapitinga (*Piaractus brachypomus)*	Volkoff, 2015a	–
			Red-bellied piranha (*Pygocentrus nattereri*)	Volkoff, 2014a	–
	Cypriniforme	Cyprinidae	Blunt snout bream (*Megalobrama amblycephala*)	Ping et al., 2013; Ji et al., 2015	–
			Common carp (*Cyprinus carpio*)	Zhong et al., 2013	–
			Goldfish (*Carassius auratus*)	Kang et al., 2010, 2011; Tinoco et al., 2015	–
			Grass carp (*Ctenopharyngodon idella*) juveniles	Liu et al., 2013	–
			Zebrafish (*Danio rerio*)	Koven and Schulte, 2012; Tian et al., 2015	–
	Gadiforme	Gadidae	Atlantic cod larvae (*Gadus morhua*)	Tillner et al., 2013	–
	Perciforme	Carangidae	Yellowtail (*Seriola quinqueradiata*)	Furutani et al., 2013; Hosomi et al., 2014	–
		Cichlidae	*Astatotilapia burtoni*	Grone et al., 2012	–
		Labridae	Cunner (*Tautogolabrus adspersus*)	Babichuk and Volkoff, 2013; Hayes and Volkoff, 2014	–
		Moronidae	Sea bass (*Dicentrarchus labrax*) larvae	Tillner et al., 2014	–
		Sciaenidae	Yellow croaker *(Larimichthys crocea*) larvae	Cai et al., 2015	–
		Sparidae	White sea bream (*Diplodus sargus)*	Micale et al., 2012	–
	Pleuronectiforme	Pleuronectidae	Atlantic halibut (*Hippoglossus hippoglossus*)	Kamisaka et al., 2001	–
			Olive flounder (*Paralichthys olivaceus*)	Kurokawa et al., 2000	–
			Winter flounder (*Pseudopleuronectes americanus*)	MacDonald and Volkoff, 2009a	–
	Salmoniforme	Salmonidae	Atlantic salmon (*Salmo salar*)	Valen et al., 2011	–
	Siluriforme	Ictaluridae	Channel catfish (*Ictalurus punctatus*)	Peterson et al., 2012	–
CRF/UCN system	Acipenseriformes	Acipenseridae	Siberian sturgeon (*Acipenser baerii*)	Zhang et al., 2016c	–
	Cypriniforme	Cyprinidae	Goldfish (*Carassius auratus*)	De Pedro et al., 1993	–
			Ya fish (*Schizothorax prenanti*)	Wang et al., 2014	–
	Salmoniforme	Salmonidae	Rainbow trout (*Oncorhynchus mykiss*)	Bernier and Craig, 2005; Ortega et al., 2013	–
Endocannabinoid system	Cypriniforme	Cyprinidae	Goldfish (*Carassius auratus*)	Cottone et al., 2013	+ ?
			Goldfish (*Carassius auratus)*	Cottone et al., 2009	+
	Perciforme	Sparidae	Sea bream (*Sparus aurata)*	Piccinetti et al., 2010	+
	Pleuronectiforme	Soleidae	Sole (*Solea solea*)	Palermo et al., 2013	?
Galanin	Cypriniforme	Cyprinidae	Goldfish (*Carassius auratus*)	de Pedro et al., 1995; Volkoff and Peter, 2001b; Unniappan et al., 2004	+
			Tench (*Tinca tinca*)	Guijarro et al., 1999	+
			Zebrafish (*Danio rerio*)	Li et al., 2013	+

(Continued)

TABLE 1 | Continued

Hormone	Order	Family	Species	Major references	Effect on feeding
Ghrelin	Anguilliformes	Anguillidae	Japanese eel (*Anguilla japonica*)	Lee et al., 2015	?
	Characiforme	Serrasalmidae	Pirapitinga (*Piaractus brachypomus*)	Volkoff, 2015a	?
			Red-bellied piranha (*Pygocentrus nattereri*)	Volkoff, 2015b	+
	Cypriniforme	Cyprinidae	Bunnei (*Barbus sharpeyi*)	Mabudi et al., 2011	?
			Gibel carp (*Carassius auratus gibelio*)	Zhou et al., 2016	+
			Goldfish (*Carassius auratus*)	Unniappan et al., 2002; Kang et al., 2011; Nisembaum et al., 2014; Blanco et al., 2016a,b	+
			Grass carp (*Ctenopharyngodon idella*)	Liu et al., 2014	+
			Zebrafish (*Danio rerio*)	Koven and Schulte, 2012	+
	Lepidosireniforme (dipnoid)	Protopteridae	West African lungfish (*Protopterus annectens*)	Kaiya et al., 2014	?
	Perciforme	Cichlidae	Tilapia (*Oreochromis mossambicus*)	Schwandt et al., 2010; Upton and Riley, 2013	+
		Scombridae	Pacific bluefin tuna (*Thunnus orientalis*)	Suda et al., 2012	?
	Pleuronectiforme	Pleuronectidae	Atlantic halibut (*Hippoglossus hippoglossus*)	Einarsdottir et al., 2011; Gomes et al., 2014	+
		Scophthalmidae	Juvenile turbot (*Scophthalmus maximus*)	Song et al., 2015	+
	Salmoniforme	Salmonidae	Atlantic salmon (*Salmo salar*)	Hevrøy et al., 2011; Vikesa et al., 2015	?
			Brown trout (*Salmo trutta*)	Tinoco et al., 2014a	+ ?
			Coho salmon (*Oncorhynchus kisutch*)	Kim et al., 2015	+
			Rainbow trout (*Oncorhynchus mykiss*)	Velasco et al., 2016	?
			Rainbow trout (*Oncorhynchus mykiss*)	Jönsson et al., 2010	–
	Siluriforme	Bagridae	Yellow catfish (*Pelteobagrus fulvidraco*)	Zhang et al., 2016a	+
		Ictaluridae	Channel catfish (*Ictalurus punctatus*)	Peterson et al., 2012	0
GnRH	Cypriniforme	Cyprinidae	Goldfish (*Carassius auratus*)	Hoskins et al., 2008; Matsuda et al., 2008	–
			Ya fish (*Schizothorax prenanti*)	Wang et al., 2014	–
			Zebrafish (*Danio rerio*)	Nishiguchi et al., 2012	–
	Gadiforme	Gadidae	Atlantic cod (*Gadus morhua*)	Tuziak and Volkoff, 2013a	0
	Pleuronectiforme	Pleuronectidae	Winter flounder (*Pseudopleuronectes americanus*)	Tuziak and Volkoff, 2013b	–
Kisspeptin	Cypriniforme	Cyprinidae	Goldfish (*Carassius auratus*)	Mawhinney, 2007	0
	Perciforme	Moronidae	Sea bass (*Dicentrarchus labrax*)	Escobar et al., 2016	+ ?
Leptin	Beloniforme	Adrianichthyidae	Medaka (*Oryzias latipes*)	Chisada et al., 2014	–
	Characiforme	Serrasalmidae	Pacu (*Piaractus mesopotamicus*)	Volkoff et al., 2017	0 ?
			Pirapitinga (*Piaractus brachypomus*)	Volkoff, 2015a	?
			Red-bellied piranha (*Pygocentrus nattereri*)	Volkoff, 2015b	0 ?
	Cypriniforme	Cyprinidae	Blunt snout bream *Megalobrama amblycephala*	Xu et al., 2016	–
			Common carp (Cyprinus carpio)	Bernier et al., 2012	–
			Goldfish (*Carassius auratus*)	Volkoff et al., 2003; Vivas et al., 2011; Tinoco et al., 2012, 2014b; Yan et al., 2016	–
			Grass carp (*Ctenopharyngodon idellus*)	Lu et al., 2015; Li et al., 2010	–
			Grass carp (*Ctenopharyngodon idellus*)	Li A. et al., 2016	?
			Topmouth culter (*Culter alburnus*)	Wang et al., 2013	?
			White-clouds minnow (Tanichthys albonubes)	Chen et al., 2016b	–
			Zebrafish (*Danio rerio*)	Tian et al., 2015; Cui et al., 2016; Michel et al., 2016	–

(Continued)

TABLE 1 | Continued

Hormone	Order	Family	Species	Major references	Effect on feeding
	Gadiforme	Lotidae	Burbot (*Lota lota*)	Nieminen et al., 2003	+ ?
	Gymnotiforme	Sternopygidae	Electric fish (*Eigenmannia virescens*)	Sinnett and Markham, 2015	?
	Perciforme	Carangidae	Golden pompano (*Trachinotus blochii*)	Wu et al., 2016	?
		Centrarchidae	Green sunfish (*Lepomis cyanellus*)	Johnson et al., 2000	+ ?
		Cichlidae	Tilapia (*Oreochromis mossambicus*)	Baltzegar et al., 2014; Douros et al., 2014	?
			Nile tilapia (*Oreochromis niloticus*)	Shpilman et al., 2014	?
		Labridae	Orange-spotted grouper (*Epinephelus coioides*)	Huang et al., 2014	?
		Labridae	Orange-spotted grouper (*Epinephelus coioides*)	Zhang et al., 2013	?
		Moronidae	European sea bass (*Dicentrarchus labrax*)	Gambardella et al., 2012	?
			Striped bass (*Morone saxatilis*)	Won et al., 2012	−
		Percichthyidae	Mandarin fish (*Siniperca chuatsi*)	Yuan et al., 2016	?
			Murray cod (*Maccullochella peelii peelii*)	Ettore et al., 2012 Varricchio et al., 2012	?
		Scombridae	Mackerel (*Scomber japonicus*)	Ohga et al., 2015	?
	Pleuronectiformes	Paralichthyidae	Fine flounder (*Paralichthys adspersus*)	Fuentes et al., 2012	+
	Salmoniforme	Salmonidae	Atlantic salmon (*Salmo salar*)	Rønnestad et al., 2010; Murashita et al., 2011; Trombley et al., 2012, 2014; Kullgren et al., 2013; Moen and Finn, 2013	?
			Arctic charr (*Salvelinus alpinus*)	Froiland et al., 2012; Jørgensen et al., 2013	?
			Rainbow trout (*Oncorhynchus mykiss*)	Gong et al., 2016	−
			Rainbow trout (*Oncorhynchus mykiss*)	Varricchio et al., 2012; Francis et al., 2014; MacDonald et al., 2014; Johansson and Björnsson, 2015; Salmeron et al., 2015; Johansson et al., 2016; Pfundt et al., 2016	?
	Siluriforme	Bagridae	Yellow catfish (*Pelteobagrus fulvidraco*)	Gong et al., 2013; Song et al., 2015; Zheng et al., 2015	?
MCH	Beloniforme	Adrianichthyidae	Medaka (*Oryzias latipes*)	Qu et al., 1996	0
	Carcharhiniforme	Sphyrnidae	Scalloped hammerhead shark (*Sphyrna lewini*)	Mizusawa et al., 2012	0
	Characiforme	Serrasalmidae	Red-bellied piranha (*Pygocentrus nattereri*)	Pérez Sirkin et al., 2013	?
	Cypriniforme	Cyprinidae	Goldfish (*Carassius auratus*)	Shimakura et al., 2006; Matsuda et al., 2007a	−
			Ya fish (*Schizothorax prenanti*)	Wang et al., 2016	+
	Gadiforme	Gadidae	Atlantic cod (*Gadus morhua*)	Tuziak and Volkoff, 2013a; Tuziak et al., 2014	+
	Pleuronectiforme	Pleuronectidae	Barfin flounder (*Verasper moseri*)	Takahashi et al., 2004; Amiya et al., 2008	+
			Olive flounder (*Paralichthys olivaceus*)	Kang and Kim, 2013b	+
			Starry flounder (*Platichthys stellatus*)	Kang and Kim, 2013a	+
			Winter flounder (*Pseudopleuronectes americanus*)	Tuziak and Volkoff, 2012	+
Nesfatin-1	Cypriniforme	Cyprinidae	Goldfish (*Carassius auratus*)	Gonzalez et al., 2010; Kerbel and Unniappan, 2012; Blanco et al., 2016a; Sundarrajan et al., 2016	−
			Zebrafish (*Danio rerio*)	Hatef et al., 2015	−
			Ya fish (*Schizothorax prenanti*)	Lin et al., 2014b	−
	Salmoniforme	Salmonidae	Rainbow trout (*Oncorhynchus mykiss*)	Caldwell et al., 2014	0
Neuromedin S	Cypriniforme	Cyprinidae	Zebrafish (*Danio rerio*)	Chen et al., 2016a	+ ?
Neuropepide B	Perciforme	Cichlidae	Nile tilapia (*Oreochromis niloticus*)	Yang et al., 2014	+ ?

(Continued)

TABLE 1 | Continued

Hormone	Order	Family	Species	Major references	Effect on feeding
NMU	Cypriniforme	Cyprinidae	Common carp (*Cyprinus carpio*)	Kono et al., 2012	?
	Cypriniforme	Cyprinidae	Goldfish (*Carassius auratus*)	Maruyama et al., 2008, 2009	–
	Perciforme	Labridae	Orange-spotted grouper (*Epinephelus coioides*)	Li et al., 2015	–
NPY	Characiforme	Characidae	Dourado (*Salminus brasiliensis*)	Pereira et al., 2015	+ ?
	Chimaeriformes	Callorhinchidae	Elephant fish (*Callorhinchus milii*)	Larsson et al., 2009	+ ?
	Cypriniforme	Cyprinidae	Blunt snout bream (*Megalobrama amblycephala*)	Xu et al., 2016	+
			Goldfish (*Carassius auratus*)	Lopez-Patino et al., 1999; de Pedro et al., 2000; Narnaware et al., 2000; Hoskins and Volkoff, 2012	+
			Grass carp (*Ctenopharyngodon idellus*)	He et al., 2013; Zhou et al., 2013; Jin et al., 2015	+
			Jian carp (*Cyprinus carpio* var. Jian)	Tang et al., 2014	+
			Ya fish (*Schizothorax prenanti*)	Wei et al., 2014	+
			Zebrafish (*Danio rerio*)	Yokobori et al., 2012; Dalmolin et al., 2015	+
	Gadiforme	Gadidae	Atlantic cod (*Gadus morhua*)	Kehoe and Volkoff, 2007; Tuziak et al., 2014	+
			Atlantic cod (*Gadus morhua*)	Kortner et al., 2011	?
	Gonorynchiforme actinopterygii	Chanidae	Milkfish (*Chanos chanos*)	Lin et al., 2016	?
	Perciforme	Carangidae	Yellowtail (*Seriola quinqueradiata*)	Hosomi et al., 2014	+
		Cichlidae	*Astatotilapia burtoni*	Grone et al., 2012	+
		Labridae	Cunner (*Tautogolabrus adspersus*)	Babichuk and Volkoff, 2013	+
			Orange-spotted grouper (*Epinephelus coioides*)	Tang et al., 2013	+
		Moronidae	Sea bass (*Dicentrarchus labrax*)	Leal et al., 2013	+
		Percichthyidae	Mandarin fish (*Siniperca chuatsi*)	Sun et al., 2014	?
		Rachycentridae	Cobia (*Rachycentron canadum*)	Van Nguyen et al., 2013	+
		Osphronemidae	Snakeskin gourami (*Trichogaster pectoralis*)	Boonanuntanasarn et al., 2012	+
	Pleuronectiforme	Pleuronectidae	Olive flounder (*Paralichthys olivaceus*)	Wang et al., 2015	+
		Paralichthyidae	Brazilian flounder (*Paralichthys orbignyanus*)	Campos et al., 2012	+
	Salmoniforme	Salmonidae	Atlantic salmon (*Salmo salar*)	Silverstein et al., 1998; Valen et al., 2011; Figueiredo-Silva et al., 2012	+
	Salmoniforme	Salmonidae	Chinook salmon (*Oncorhynchus tshawytscha*)	Silverstein et al., 1998	+
		Salmonidae	Rainbow trout (*Oncorhynchus mykiss*)	Aldegunde and Mancebo, 2006	+
	Siluriformes	Ictaluridae	Channel catfish (*Ictalurus punctatus*)	Silverstein and Plysetskaya, 2000; Peterson et al., 2012; Schroeter et al., 2015	+
	Tetraodontiformes	Tetraodontidae	Tiger Puffer (*Takifugu rubripes*)	Kamijo et al., 2011	+
Obestatin	Cypriniforme	Cyprinidae	Grass carp (*Ctenopharyngodon idellus*)	Yuan et al., 2015	– ?
Octadecaneuropeptide (ODN)	Cypriniforme	Cyprinidae	Goldfish (*Carassius auratus*)	Matsuda et al., 2007b, 2010, 2011b	–
Orexin	Characiforme	Characidae	Blind cavefish (*Astyanax fasciatus mexicanus*)	Wall and Volkoff, 2013; Penney and Volkoff, 2014	+
			Dourado (*Salminus brasiliensis*)	Volkoff et al., 2016	+
		Serrasalmidae	Pacu (*Piaractus mesopotamicus*)	Volkoff et al., 2017	+
			Pirapitinga (*Piaractus brachypomus*)	Volkoff, 2015a	?

(Continued)

TABLE 1 | Continued

Hormone	Order	Family	Species	Major references	Effect on feeding
			Red-bellied piranha (*Pygocentrus nattereri*)	Pérez Sirkin et al., 2013; Suzuki and Yamamoto, 2013; Volkoff, 2014a	+
	Cypriniforme	Cyprinidae	Goldfish (*Carassius auratus*)	Abbott and Volkoff, 2011; Facciolo et al., 2011; Hoskins and Volkoff, 2012; Crudo et al., 2013; Volkoff, 2013, 2014b; Nisembaum et al., 2014; D'angelo et al., 2016	+
			Zebrafish (*Danio rerio*)	Panula, 2010; Yokobori et al., 2011; Elbaz et al., 2012; Pavlidis et al., 2015; Sterling et al., 2015	+
	Gadiforme	Gadidae	Cod (*Gadus morhua*)	Tuziak et al., 2014; Le et al., 2016	+
	Perciforme	Cichlidae	*Astatotilapia burtoni*	Grone et al., 2012	+
			Cichlasoma dimerus	Pérez Sirkin et al., 2013	?
			Nile tilapia (*Oreochromis niloticus*)	Chen et al., 2011	+
		Labridae	Cunner (*Tautogolabrus adspersus*)	Babichuk and Volkoff, 2013; Hayes and Volkoff, 2014	+
			Orange-spotted grouper (*Epinephelus coioides*)	Yan et al., 2011	+
			Ornate wrasse (*Thalassoma pavo*)	Facciolo et al., 2009	+
	Pleuronectiforme	Pleuronectidae	Winter flounder (*Pseudopleuronectes americanus*)	Buckley et al., 2010	+
			Barfin Flounder (*Verasper moseri*)	Amiya et al., 2012	+
	Polypteriformes actinopterygian	Polypteridae	*Polypterus senegalus* and *Erpetoichthys calabaricus*	López et al., 2014	?
	Rajiformes	Rajidae	Winter skate (*Leucoraja ocellata*)	MacDonald and Volkoff, 2010	+
	Salmoniforme	Salmonidae	Rainbow trout (*Oncorhynchus mykiss*)	Varricchio et al., 2015	?
PACAP	Cypriniforme	Cyprinidae	Goldfish (*Carasisus auratus*)	Matsuda et al., 2005; Matsuda and Maruyama, 2007	–
			Grass carp (*Ctenopharyngodon idellus*)	Zhou et al., 2013	– ?
	Gadiforme	Gadidae	Cod (*Gadus morhua*)	Xu and Volkoff, 2009	– ?
POMC/α-MSH	Cypriniforme	Cyprinidae	Goldfish (*Carasisus auratus*)	Cerdá-Reverter et al., 2003; Kang et al., 2010; Kojima et al., 2010; Yan et al., 2016	–
			Zebrafish (*Danio rerio*)	Shanshan et al., 2016	–
			Zebrafish (*Danio rerio*)	Dalmolin et al., 2015	+
	Pleuronectiforme	Pleuronectidae	Barfin flounder (*Verasper moseri*)	Takahashi et al., 2005	0
			Halibut (*Hippoglossus hippoglossus*)	Gomes et al., 2015	?
			Olive flounder (*Paralichthys olivaceus*)	Kang and Kim, 2015	0
	Salmoniforme	Salmonidae	Atlantic salmon (*Salmo salar*)	Valen et al., 2011	–
			Coho salmon (*Oncorhynchus kisutch*)	Kim et al., 2015	0
			Coho salmon (*Oncorhynchus kisutch*)	Leder and Silverstein, 2006; White et al., 2016	–
PrRP	Cypriniforme	Cyprinidae	Goldfish (*Carassius auratus*)	Kelly and Peter, 2006	–
	Perciforme	Gobidae	Mudskipper (*Periophtalmus modestus*)	Sakamoto et al., 2002; Tachibana and Sakamoto, 2014	+ ?
PYY	Acipenseriformes	Acipenseridae	Siberian sturgeon (*Acipenser baerii*)	Chen et al., 2015	–
	Characiforme	Characidae	Blind cavefish (*Astyanax fasciatus mexicanus*)	Wall and Volkoff, 2013	–
		Serrasalmidae	Red-bellied piranha (*Pygocentrus nattereri*)	Volkoff, 2014a	–
	Clupeiformes	Engraulidae	Tapertail anchovy (*Coilia nasus*)	Yang et al., 2016	+ ?

(Continued)

TABLE 1 | Continued

Hormone	Order	Family	Species	Major references	Effect on feeding
	Cypriniforme	Cyprinidae	Goldfish (*Carassius auratus*)	Gonzalez and Unniappan, 2010	−
			Grass carp (*Ctenopharyngodon idellus*)	Chen et al., 2013, 2014	−
	Perciforme	Carangidae	Yellowtail (*Seriola quinqueradiata*)	Murashita et al., 2006, 2007	+ ?
	Salmoniforme	Salmonidae	Atlantic salmon (*Salmo salar*)	Murashita et al., 2009a; Valen et al., 2011; Kousoulaki et al., 2013	0
	Siluriforme	Ictaluridae	Channel catfish (*Ictalurus punctatus*)	Schroeter et al., 2015	0 ?
Secretoneurin	Cypriniforme	Cyprinidae	Goldfish (*Carassius auratus*)	Trudeau et al., 2012; Mikwar et al., 2016	+
Spexin	Cypriniforme	Cyprinidae	Goldfish (*Carassius auratus*)	Wong et al., 2013	−
	Perciforme	Labridae	Orange-spotted grouper (*Epinephelus coioides*)	Li S. et al., 2016	−
Thyroid axis	Acipenseriformes	Acipenseridae	Amur sturgeon (*Acipenser schrenckii*)	Li et al., 2012	?
	Cypriniforme	Cyprinidae	Goldfish (*Carassius auratus*)	Sinha et al., 2012	+
			Goldfish (*Carassius auratus*)	Abbott and Volkoff, 2011; Goodyear, 2012	+ ?
	Siluriforme	Ictaluridae	Channel catfish (*Ictalurus punctatus*)	Pohlenz et al., 2013	+

The effects on feeding are described as stimulatory (+), inhibitory (−), not detected (0) or unknown/uncertain (?).

mammals, including arousal/sleep, feeding, energy metabolism, and reproduction (Merchenthaler, 2010). Galanin and its receptors have been identified in a number of fish species (see review in Mensah et al., 2010). Central injections of galanin stimulate feeding in Cypriniformes (both goldfish de Pedro et al., 1995; Volkoff and Peter, 2001b, and tench, *Tinca tinca* Guijarro et al., 1999). In goldfish, brain galanin mRNA expression is not affected by fasting but increases post-prandially in unfed fish (Unniappan et al., 2004) and in zebrafish, fasting up-regulates brain mRNA expression of galanin receptors (Li et al., 2013). These data suggest that the galanin system is involved in the regulation of feeding in Cypriniformes, and perhaps other fish.

Melanin concentrating hormone (MCH)

Melanin concentrating hormone is a peptide originally isolated from the pituitary of chum salmon (*Oncorhynchus keta*) as a hormone involved in body color change (Kawauchi et al., 1983). MCH was later isolated in mammals and shown to stimulate feeding (Qu et al., 1996). In fish, the role of MCH as an appetite regulator is still unclear.

In Cypriniformes, early immunoreativity (ir) studies in goldfish showed the presence of MCH in neuron populations related to the regulation of feeding and of sleep and arousal (Huesa et al., 2005). In goldfish, central injections of MCH decrease feeding but have no effect on locomotor activity (Shimakura et al., 2006), anti-MCH serum treatments increase feeding (Matsuda et al., 2007a), and the number of certain hypothalamic neuronal cell bodies containing MCH-ir decreases in fasted fish (Matsuda et al., 2007a), altogether suggesting an anorexigenic role for MCH in this species. However, in Ya fish, MCH hypothalamic mRNA expression is higher in fasted compared to fed fish, suggesting an orexigenic role (Wang et al., 2016). Data on Gadiformes and Pleuronectiformes also seem to suggest an appetite-stimulating role for MCH: MCH brain mRNA levels increase during fasting in both Atlantic cod *Gadus morhua* (Tuziak and Volkoff, 2013a) and winter flounder *Pseudopleuronectes americanus* (Tuziak and Volkoff, 2012), and in cod fed diets with relatively high amounts of plant (camelina) material (Tuziak et al., 2014). In starry (*Platichthys stellatus*; Kang and Kim, 2013b), olive (*Paralichthys olivaceus*; Kang and Kim, 2013a) and Barfin (*Verasper moseri;* Takahashi et al., 2004) flounders, fish placed in light backgrounds have enhanced appetite and growth, which is concomitant with increased expression levels of MCH mRNA and/or numbers of MCH neurons in the brain. However, in medaka *Oryzias latipes*, transgenic fish overexpressing MCH have normal growth and feeding behavior (Qu et al., 1996) and in the scalloped hammerhead shark *Sphyrna lewini*, hypothalamic MCH mRNA levels are not affected by fasting (Mizusawa et al., 2012), suggesting little or no role of MCH in feeding regulation of Beloniformes and sharks.

Neuronal relationship between MCH- and NPY-containing neurons have been shown in goldfish (Matsuda et al., 2009) and MCH treatment increases orexin mRNA expression and decreases NPY mRNA expression in cultured goldfish forebrain slices (Matsuda et al., 2009), suggesting an interaction of MCH with appetite regulators in goldfish. Similarly, in red-bellied piranha *Pygocentrus nattereri*, orexin and MCH co-localize in pituitary and brain (Suzuki et al., 2007), and in Barfin flounder, close contacts are seen between orexin- and MCH-ir cell bodies and fibers in the hypothalamus, suggesting an interaction between the two systems and a possible role for MCH in the modulation of locomotion and feeding (Amiya et al., 2008).

Neuropeptide Y (NPY)

Neuropeptide Y (NPY) belongs to the NPY family of peptides, which also includes, peptide YY and pancreatic polypeptide (PP)

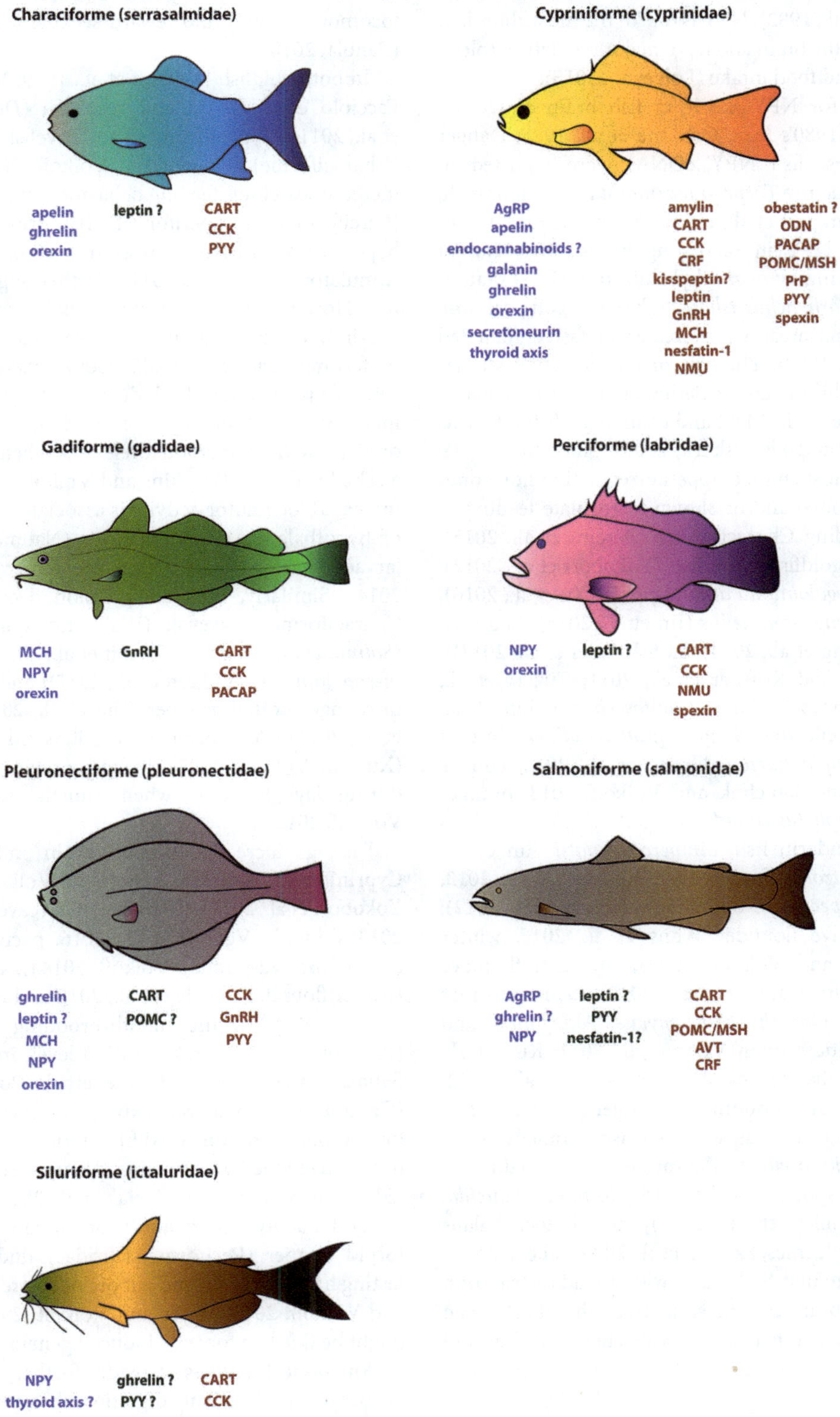

FIGURE 1 | Major appetite regulators known for seven of the most studied representative fish families (serrasalmidae, cyprinidae, gadidae, labridae, pleuronectidae, salmonidae, and ictaluridae). Factors in blue (far left) and in red (far right) under the fish diagrams represent putative orexigenic and anorexigenic factors, respectively. Factors in green (middle) represent factors with no established effect on feeding. A "?" indicates uncertainty with regards to the role of a given factor in regulating feeding.

(Holzer et al., 2012). Originally isolated from mammalian brain extracts (Tatemoto et al., 1982), NPY is one of the most abundant neuropeptides within the brain and has a major regulatory role in energy homeostasis and food intake (Loh et al., 2015).

Although reports for NPY-like ir in fish brain and other tissues appear in the 1980's (e.g., Osborne et al., 1985; Danger et al., 1990), the first fish NPY cDNAs were reported in goldfish and the electric ray *Torpedo marmorata* (elasmobranch, Torpediniformes; Blomqvist et al., 1992). One of the first studies showing the role of NPY in regulating in fish was that of Silverstein et al., showing by *in situ* hybridization (ISH) that, in chinook salmon (*Oncorhynchus tshawytscha*) and coho salmon, NPY-like mRNA signal areas were greater in fasted than fed fish (Silverstein et al., 1998). The first *in vivo* injection studies were performed in goldfish (Lopez-Patino et al., 1999; de Pedro et al., 2000; Narnaware et al., 2000) and channel catfish *Ictalurus punctatus* (Silverstein and Plysetskaya, 2000). Since then, NPY has been one of the most studied appetite-regulating hormones in fish. It has been cloned and/or shown to regulate feeding in several groups, including Characiformes (Pereira et al., 2015), Cypriniformes [(e.g., goldfish, zebrafish (Yokobori et al., 2012), blunt snout bream *Megalobrama amblycephala* (Xu et al., 2016), grass carp *Ctenopharyngodon idellus* (Jin et al., 2015), Jian carp (*Cyprinus carpio*) (Tang et al., 2014), Ya fish (Wei et al., 2014)], Gadiformes (Atlantic cod Kortner et al., 2011; Tuziak et al., 2014); Gonorynchiformes (milkfish *Chanos chanos*, Lin et al., 2016); Perciformes (yellowtail *Seriola quinqueradiata* Hosomi et al., 2014, *Astatotilapia burtoni* Grone et al., 2012, cunner *Tautogolabrus adspersus* Babichuk and Volkoff, 2013, orange-spotted grouper *Epinephelus coioides* Tang et al., 2013, sea bass Leal et al., 2013, mandarin fish, *Siniperca chuatsi* Sun et al., 2014, cobia *Rachycentron canadum* Van Nguyen et al., 2013, gourami *Trichogaster pectoralis* Boonanuntanasarn et al., 2012); Pleuronectiformes (olive flounder Wang et al., 2015, winter flounder MacDonald and Volkoff, 2009a, Brazilian flounder *Paralichthys orbignyanus* Campos et al., 2012), Salmoniformes (e.g., rainbow trout *Oncorhynchus mykiss* Aldegunde and Mancebo, 2006, Atlantic salmon Valen et al., 2011; Kim et al., 2015), Siluriformes (channel catfish, Peterson et al., 2012; Schroeter et al., 2015); Tetraodontiformes (tiger puffer *Takifugu rubripes* Kamijo et al., 2011) as well as elasmobranchs [(e.g., winter skate *Leucoraja ocellata*, Rajiforme (MacDonald and Volkoff, 2009b) and spotted catshark (*Scyliorhinus canicula*, Carcharhiniforme) Mulley et al., 2014)] and holocephalans (elephant fish Chimaeriformes; Larsson et al., 2009). The majority of these studies indicate that NPY has a widespread distribution and is present in both brain and intestinal tract, that it acts as an orexigenic factor and that its expression is affected by feeding and fasting.

Orexin

Orexins (also called hypocretins) are neuropeptides originally isolated in rats (Sakurai, 2014), that have since been identified in several fish species. The first direct evidence of an orexigenic action of orexins was shown via intracerebroventricular (ICV) injections in goldfish (Volkoff et al., 1999). As in mammals (Tsujino and Sakurai, 2009; Sakurai, 2014), orexins increase not only appetite and feeding behavior but also locomotor activity and reward-seeking/foraging behavior in fish (Panula, 2010).

In both goldfish (Volkoff et al., 1999; Nakamachi et al., 2006; Facciolo et al., 2011) and zebrafish (*Danio rerio*) (Yokobori et al., 2011) (Cypriniformes), and cavefish (*Astyanax mexicanus*) (Characiforme) (Penney and Volkoff, 2014), orexin injections increase searching/feeding behaviors. In orange-spotted grouper (Perciforme), intraperitoneal (IP) orexin injections increase hypothalamic mRNA expression levels of NPY, a major appetite stimulator (Yan et al., 2011), further suggesting an orexigenic role. However, in ornate wrasse (*Thalassoma pavo)* (Perciforme), orexin IP injections induce increases in locomotion but decreases in feeding (Facciolo et al., 2009), suggesting that the major role of orexin might be induction of hyperactivity rather than increasing food ingestion. Indeed, in goldfish, hypothalamic orexin mRNA expression levels peak when fish are active prior to a scheduled meal (Hoskins and Volkoff, 2012) and in zebrafish, increased locomotor activity is associated with increased activity of hypothalamic orexin neurons (Naumann et al., 2010) and larvae overexpressing orexin are hyperactive (Woods et al., 2014). Similarly, orexin expression decreases post-feeding in Characiformes [cavefish (Wall and Volkoff, 2013), dourado (*Salminus brasiliensis*) (Volkoff et al., 2016) and pacu (*Piaractus mesopotamicus*) (Volkoff et al., 2017)] and is higher at mealtime in orange-spotted grouper (Yan et al., 2011) and tilapia (Chen et al., 2011) (Perciformes), as well as Atlantic cod (Gadiforme) (Xu and Volkoff, 2007). In cod, orexin levels are also higher during daylight hours, when animals are active (Hoskins and Volkoff, 2012).

Fasting increases orexin brain mRNA expression in Cypriniformes (goldfish Abbott and Volkoff, 2011 and zebrafish Yokobori et al., 2011), Characiformes (cavefish Wall and Volkoff, 2013, dourado Volkoff et al., 2016, pacu Volkoff et al., 2017, and red-bellied piranha Volkoff, 2014a), and Pleuronectiformes (winter flounder Buckley et al., 2010 and Barfin flounder Amiya et al., 2012). In the mouth-brooding *Astatotilapia burtoni* (Perciforme), brain orexin mRNA levels increase in non-feeding females carrying eggs (Grone et al., 2012). In Atlantic cod (Gadiforme), orexin brain expression levels are higher in fish fed low rations than in fish fed high rations (Xu and Volkoff, 2007) or in fish fed the 30% camelina (plant) meal diet compared to fish fed a control (fish) diet (Tuziak et al., 2014), suggesting an effect of food quality and quantity on orexin expression. However, torpid cunner (Peciforme, labridae) undergoing a long-term fasting have low brain and gut orexin expression levels (Babichuk and Volkoff, 2013; Hayes and Volkoff, 2014), but this decrease might be due to a toprpor-induced general metabolic shutdown.

Anatomical studies provide further evidence for a role of orexin in nutrient digestion/abrorption and growth. In several fish species, e.g., pirapitinga (*Piaractus brachypomus*) (Characiforme) (Volkoff, 2015a), cunner (Perciforme) (Hayes and Volkoff, 2014) and rainbow trout (Salmoniforme) (Varricchio et al., 2015), orexin mRNA/protein expression is high in the gastrointestinal tract, suggesting a role of the orexin system in regulating feeding and digestive processes. Among Perciformes, in Japanese sea perch (*Lateolabrax japonicus*), orexin-like ir is present in pituitary GH-containing cells, suggesting a control of growth by the orexin system (Suzuki et al., 2007) and in *Cichlasoma dimerus*, orexin-ir fibers are present in both hypothalamus and in pituitary, suggesting a neuroendocrine control of pituitary secretions (Pérez Sirkin et al., 2013).

In addition to teleosts, orexin has been examined in the primitive bony fish birchir *Polypterus senegalus* and rope fish *Erpetoichthys calabaricus* (Chondrosteans, Polypteriformes) for which the brain orexin ir patterns are similar to that of other fish examined (López et al., 2014) and in the Chondrichthyan winter skate (Rajiforme), in which fasting increases hypothalamic orexin expression (MacDonald and Volkoff, 2010).

Overall, it appears that in all fish species studied to date, orexin is related to both food intake and appetitive/searching behavior and perhaps to growth.

Anorexigenic Factors

CART

CART is a peptide which transcript expression is regulated by administration of cocaine or amphetamine in rodents (Vicentic and Jones, 2007; Subhedar et al., 2014) and amphetamine in goldfish (Volkoff, 2013). CART acts as an anorexigenic factor in mammals (Larsen and Hunter, 2006), and was first identified and shown to be anorexigenic in goldfish (Volkoff and Peter, 2000, 2001a).

Two CART isoforms have been identified in goldfish (Volkoff and Peter, 2001a) and common carp (Wan et al., 2012), and 4 in zebrafish (Akash et al., 2014) whereas, to date, only one form has been isolated for grass carp (Zhou et al., 2013; Liu et al., 2014), Characiformes [pirapitinga (serrasalmidae) (Volkoff, 2015a), pacu (serrasasalmidae) (Volkoff et al., 2017) and dourado (characidae) (Volkoff et al., 2016), red bellied piranha (serrasalmidae) (Volkoff, 2014a)], Salmoniformes [Atlantic salmon (Murashita et al., 2009a), rainbow trout (Figueiredo-Silva et al., 2012), Arctic charr (Striberny et al., 2015) and lake trout (*Salvelinus namaycush*) (Volkoff et al., 2007)], Siluriformes (channel catfish Kobayashi et al., 2008), Gadiformes (Atlantic cod Kehoe and Volkoff, 2007), Perciformes (cunner Babichuk and Volkoff, 2013), winter flounder (MacDonald and Volkoff, 2009a) and Atlantic halibut (*Hippoglossus hippoglossus*) (Gomes et al., 2015) (Pleuronectiformes), venomous toadfish *Thalassophryne nattereri* (Batrachoidiforme) (Magalhaes et al., 2006), rainbow smelt (*Osmerus mordax*) (Osmeriforme), pufferfishes (*Takifugu rubripes* and *Tetraodon nigroviridis*, Tetraodontiforme) and stickleback *Gasterosteus aculeatus* (Gasterosteiforme) (cited in Murashita et al., 2009a). However, six forms of CART have been identified in the medaka (Beloniforme) (Murashita and Kurokawa, 2011) and seven forms in Senegalese sole *Solea senegalensis* (Pleuronectiforme), the highest number of CART genes reported to date in a vertebrate species (Bonacic et al., 2015). The only elasmobranch CART identified to date is that of winter skate (Rajiforme) (MacDonald and Volkoff, 2009b).

CART injections induce a decrease in food intake and an increase in locomotion in goldfish (Volkoff and Peter, 2000) and enhance responsiveness to sensory stimuli in zebrafish larvae (Woods et al., 2014), suggesting that CART is involved in feeding/searching behaviors in cyprinids.

Fasting/food restriction decreases CART brain expression in Cypriniformes (goldfish Volkoff and Peter, 2001a, zebrafish Nishio et al., 2012; Guillot et al., 2016 and common carp, Wan et al., 2012), most Characiformes (red-bellied piranha Volkoff, 2014a, and pacu Volkoff et al., 2017), most Salmoniformes (Atlantic salmon, Murashita et al., 2009a; Kousoulaki et al., 2013, rainbow trout Figueiredo-Silva et al., 2012), Atlantic cod (Kehoe and Volkoff, 2007), cunner (Perciforme) (Babichuk and Volkoff, 2013), medaka (CART3) (Murashita and Kurokawa, 2011), and Siluriformes (channel catfish Kobayashi et al., 2008, African sharptooth catfish *Clarias gariepinus* Subhedar et al., 2011), suggesting an anorexigenic role for CART in teleost fish. Postprandial increases in CART brain expression have been shown in Senegalese sole (CART1a, CART 2a and CART4) (Bonacic et al., 2015), pacu (Volkoff et al., 2017), dourado (Volkoff et al., 2016), channel catfish (Peterson et al., 2012) but not in cod (Kehoe and Volkoff, 2007).

However, in Arctic charr, CART hypothalamic expression is similar throughout the seasonal feeding cycles (Striberny et al., 2015) and fasting does not affect CART expression in either dourado (Volkoff et al., 2016), winter flounder (MacDonald and Volkoff, 2009a) or Atlantic halibut larvae (Gomes et al., 2015), and in lake trout, fish exposed to the pesticide tebufenozide and control fish have similar food intakes, despite higher CART mRNA brain expression levels in exposed fish (Volkoff et al., 2007). In winter skate, 2 weeks of fasting have no effects on brain CART expression (MacDonald and Volkoff, 2009b), suggesting that CART might not have a major feeding-regulating role in elasmobranchs.

CART expression does not appear to be affected by diet, as in both cod fed a camelina (plant) diet (Tuziak et al., 2014) or rotifers or zooplankton (Katan et al., 2016) and pacu fed soybean concentrate (Volkoff et al., 2017), similar CART brain expression are seen between experimental and control fish.

Overall, there is a large interspecific variation in the number of forms and responses to fasting in the CART system in fish, although most studies tend to show that CART is mostly a central factor that might act as an appetite inhibitor.

Pro-opiomelanocortin (POMC) family of peptides

Proopiomelanocortin (POMC) is a common precursor that is processed post-translationally to generate melanocortin peptides [α-, β-, and γ-melanocyte-stimulating hormone (α-, β-, γ-MSH)], adrenocorticotropic hormone (ACTH) and other hormones that include β-endorphin (β-END) and β-lipotropic hormone (β-LPH) (Adan et al., 2006; Takahashi, 2016). POMC is mainly produced in the vertebrate pituitary, but is also found in brain, in particular the arcuate nucleus (ARC) of the hypothalamus. Receptors for melanocortin peptides include five subtypes (MC1R- MC5R) (Takahashi, 2016). In mammals, POMC and α-MSH have been shown to be involved in the regulation of appetite and energy homeostasis: POMC neurons suppress appetite by releasing α-MSH, which is an agonist at the anorectic melanocortin-4 receptor (MC4R) (Adan et al., 2006; Cone, 2006; Sohn, 2015).

Teleost fish lack γ-MSH and the POMC gene encodes an extra MSH (δ-MSH) in elasmobranchs (Cérda-Reverter et al., 2011). Fish POMC was first identified in Salmoniformes (Kawauchi, 1983; Kitahara et al., 1988) and Cypriniformes (Arends et al., 1998), followed by the identification of several forms in other fish species. As in other vertebrates, fish POMC is mainly expressed in the pituitary gland, but also within the lateral tuberal nucleus, which is equivalent to the mammalian ARC (Cérda-Reverter et al., 2011). POMC, α-MSH and the MC4R have been shown to regulate feeding in a few fish species.

In goldfish, fasting does not seem to affect hypothalamic POMC mRNA expression levels (Cerdá-Reverter et al., 2003), but ICV administration of [Nle4, d-Phe7]- α-MSH, a melanocortin agonist, inhibits food intake (Cerdá-Reverter et al., 2003), suggesting the melanocortin system participates in central regulation of food intake in Cypriniformes (Cerdá-Reverter et al., 2003). In addition, ICV injections of a MSH (MC4R) receptor agonist (melanotan II) suppress hypothalamic NPY expression (Kojima et al., 2010), and hypothalamic α-MSH-containing neurons are in close contact to NPY-containing nerve fibers, suggesting that the anorexigenic actions of the melanocortin system are mediated in part by an inhibition of the NPY system. In zebrafish larvae, although early ISH studies could not detect fasting-induced changes in hypothalamic POMC transcript levels (Song et al., 2003), more recent qPCR studies indicate that POMCa expression decreases in starved fish (Shanshan et al., 2016). In addition, GH-transgenic zebrafish, who have increased feeding, display down-regulation of POMC (Dalmolin et al., 2015), consistent with an anorexigenic role for POMC-derived peptides in Cypriniformes.

Similarly, in salmonids, POMC/α-MSH appears to have an anorexigenic role. In coho salmon, IP injections of α-MSH decrease food intake (White et al., 2016), in rainbow trout, fasting induces a decrease in hypothalamic expression of POMC-A1 (but not POMC-A2 or POMC-B) (Leder and Silverstein, 2006), and in Atlantic salmon, expression of both POMC-A1 and POMC-B increase after feeding (Valen et al., 2011). Interestingly, α-MSH treatment does not affect feeding of GH-transgenic coho salmon (White et al., 2016), despite similar hypothalamic POMC and MC4R mRNA expression levels compared to non-transgenic fish (Kim et al., 2015), suggesting that the actions of α-MSH might be inhibited by high expression levels of GH and/or AgRP.

In both olive (Kang and Kim, 2015) and Barfin flounder (Takahashi et al., 2005) (Pleuronectiformes), pituitary POMC-C (isoforms 1, 2, and 3) mRNAs are not affected by fasting, suggesting pituitary POMC might not directly related to appetite regulation. However, in fasted halibut larvae, whole brain POMC-C mRNA expression is higher in unfed fish 30 min after re-feeding compared to continuously fed fish (Gomes et al., 2015), suggesting a short-term regulation of appetite. Given the small number of studies available, and the variation in experimental protocols (adults vs. larvae, pituitary vs. brain, long-term vs. short-term feeding), conclusions are difficult to drawn regarding the role of POMC in flatfish.

Major Peripheral Factors

Ghrelin

Originally discovered in rat stomach as an endogenous ligand to the GH secretagogue-receptor (Kojima et al., 1999) ghrelin is the only known orexigenic factor in the GIT of mammals (Higgins et al., 2007). In the 2000's, a ghrelin-like peptide which stimulated GH release was first described in Nile tilapia (*Oreochromis mossambicus*; Shepherd et al., 2000) and a ghrelin-ir peptide was first detected in burbot (*Lota lota*) plasma (Mustonen et al., 2002). Using goldfish as a model, Unniappan et al. provided the first fish ghrelin cDNA sequence and the first evidence of an orexigenic role for ghrelin in fish, as central injections of ghrelin stimulated food intake (Unniappan et al., 2002). Subsequent studies on several fish species reported sequences for ghrelin and confirmed its role as an appetite stimulator in fish (see Jönsson, 2013 for a review), including other Cypriniformes [e.g., goldfish (Kang et al., 2011; Nisembaum et al., 2014; Blanco et al., 2016a); gibel carp (*Carassius auratus gibelio*) (Zhou et al., 2016); *Schizothorax davidi* (Zhou et al., 2014)], Characiformes (red-bellied piranha Volkoff, 2015b), Perciformes (Nile tilapia Schwandt et al., 2010), for which fasting-induced and periprandial changes in expression/protein levels occur. In Salmoniformes, there is contradictory evidence. In rainbow trout, central ghrelin injections and long-term peripheral treatment both decrease food intake compared to controls (Jönsson et al., 2010) and in Atlantic salmon, ghrelin plasma levels are lower in fasted fish compared with fed fish (Hevrøy et al., 2011) and show no clear periprandial changes (Vikesa et al., 2015), suggesting that ghrelin might have little effect or an inhibitory effect on feeding of in salmonids. In contrast, in brown trout (*Salmo truta*), ghrelin treatment increases foraging activity (Tinoco et al., 2014a). In rainbow trout, ICV ghrelin injections induce changes in parameters related to hepatic lipid metabolism (Velasco et al., 2016), suggesting a role of ghrelin in metabolism and nutrient storage. In yellow catfish (*Pelteobagrus fulvidraco*) (Siluriforme), although fasting increases ghrelin expression (Zhang et al., 2016a), no periprandial differences in plasma or stomach ghrelin expression are observed (Peterson et al., 2012).

It thus seems that the role of ghrelin in the regulation of feeding and metabolism of fish is still unclear, and might be species- and form-specific, so that further studies on more species are required.

Anorexigenic Factors

Cholecystokinin (CCK)

In mammals, CCK inhibits food intake and induces the release of digestive enzymes from intestine/pancreas and gallbladder (Boguszewski et al., 2010; Dockray, 2012).

In fish, CCK was first shown to have a role in digestion, as, for example, it stimulated contraction of the gallbadder in coho (Vigna and Gorbman, 1977) and Atlantic (Aldman and Holmgren, 1987) salmon, as well as bluegill (*Lepomis macrochirus*), killifish (*Fundulus heteroclitus*), and the holostean bowfin (*Amia calva*) (Rajjo et al., 1988), stimulated lipase secretion in the stomachless killifish (Honkanen et al., 1988) and inhibited gastric secretion in Atlantic cod (Holstein, 1982). The first direct evidence of the actions of CCK on feeding was provided by injections in goldfish (Himick and Peter, 1994), followed by cloning of goldfish CCK cDNA (Peyon et al., 1998) and the demonstration of periprandial variations in CCK mRNA expression levels (Peyon et al., 1999). Subsequently, a number of studies have characterized CCK in several fish, including other Cypriniformes (e.g., common carp Zhong et al., 2013; zebrafish Koven and Schulte, 2012; Tian et al., 2015; grass carp; blunt snout bream Ping et al., 2013; Ji et al., 2015), Characiformes (e.g., cavefish Wall and Volkoff, 2013, dourado Pereira et al., 2015; Volkoff et al., 2016, thin dogfish *Oligosarcus hepsetus* Vieira-Lopes et al., 2013, pirapitinga Volkoff, 2015a, red-bellied piranha Volkoff, 2014a, pacu Volkoff et al., 2017), Salmoniformes (e.g., Atlantic salmon Valen et al., 2011), Gadiformes (Atlantic cod Tillner et al., 2013), Perciformes [e.g., yellowtail (Furutani et al., 2013; Hosomi et al., 2014); *Astatotilapia burtoni* (Grone et al., 2012); cunner (Babichuk and Volkoff, 2013; Hayes and Volkoff, 2014); sea bass (Tillner et al., 2014); yellow croaker (*Larimichthys crocea*) (Cai et al., 2015); white sea bream, *Diplodus sargus* (Micale et al., 2012, 2014)], Pleuronectiformes (e.g., winter flounder (MacDonald and Volkoff, 2009a), Atlantic halibut Kamisaka et al., 2001, olive flounder Kurokawa et al., 2000) and Siluriformes (channel catfish Peterson et al., 2012).

Overall, in all fish species studied to date, CCK appears to have similar roles in feeding and digestive processes to its role in mammals, i.e., it acts as a satiety/appetite-inhibiting factor and induces the release of digestive enzymes from the GIT.

Leptin

Leptin, a peptide originally cloned in obese *ob/ob* mice (Zhang et al., 1994), is secreted in mammals mainly by white adipose tissue, and its blood levels are proportional to body fat content (Park and Ahima, 2015). Leptin is a multifunctional hormone in both mammals (Park and Ahima, 2015) and fish (see review by Gorissen and Flik, 2014) and is involved in the regulation of not only food intake and body weight, but also reproduction, development and stress responses.

First hints of a role of leptin in fish were provided by reports of a decrease in feeding in goldfish ICV-injected with human leptin (Volkoff et al., 2003). The first fish leptin was identified in the pufferfish genome in 2005 by synteny studies (Kurokawa et al., 2005), followed by isolation of zebrafish, medaka, and carp leptins (Huising et al., 2006b). Since then, leptins have been identified in several fish species and shown to have multiple physiological functions (reviewed in Copeland et al., 2011; Angotzi et al., 2013; Londraville et al., 2014). As opposed to mammals who have a single leptin gene, several fish species have several leptin gene paralogs (e.g., lepA and lepB). Also in contrast to mammals, where subcutaneous fat is the main source of leptin, fish leptin is expressed in several tissues including liver and intestine, which is consistent with the fact that fish generally store lipids in intra-abdominal regions and liver (Birsoy et al., 2013).

Most studies on fish leptin have been conducted in Cypriniformes, in particular goldfish and zebrafish, and Salmoniformes. In goldfish, leptin injections decrease feeding and locomotor behavior (Volkoff et al., 2003; de Pedro et al., 2006; Vivas et al., 2011; Tinoco et al., 2012) in part by stimulating anorexigenic sytems (e.g., CART, CCK, and POMC) and inhibiting orexigenic ones (e.g., orexin, NPY, AgRP) (Volkoff et al., 2003; Yan et al., 2016). Similarly, in rainbow trout (Salmoniforme), central leptin administration suppresses food intake and increases the hypothalamic expressions of CART and POMC (Gong et al., 2016). Leptin treatment also inhibits feeding in grass carp (Li et al., 2010) (Cypriniforme) and increases energy expenditure in zebrafish larvae (Renquist et al., 2013). In Atlantic salmon (Salmoniforme), chronic IP treatment with leptin induces a decrease in growth rates (Murashita et al., 2011), and in hybrid striped bass (*Morone saxatilis* × *Morone chrysops*) (Perciforme), leptin treatment increases hepatic IGF-1 mRNA expression (Won et al., 2016), suggesting that leptin affects metabolism and growth.

Hepatic/gut/brain leptin increases in expressions are seen post-prandially in goldfish (Tinoco et al., 2012, 2014b), common carp (Huising et al., 2006a) and zebrafish (Tian et al., 2015) (Cypriniformes) as well as pacu (Volkoff et al., 2017) (Characiforme). However, in rainbow trout plasma leptin levels decrease post-feeding (Johansson and Björnsson, 2015).

There is a great variability in results with regards to fasting-induced changes in the leptin system. In goldfish, no significant differences in either brain or liver leptin expressions are seen between control, overfed and fasting fish, suggesting nutritional status does not affect the leptin system in goldfish (Tinoco et al., 2012). Similarly, leptin expression is not affected by fasting in the liver of common carp (Huising et al., 2006a) (Cyrpiniforme) and Nile tilapia (Shpilman et al., 2014) (Perciforme) or in the brains of red-bellied piranha (Volkoff, 2015b) and pacu (Volkoff et al., 2017) (Characiformes). However, fasting/food restriction increases hepatic leptin expression in white-clouds mountain minnow (*Tanichthys albonubes*, Cypriniforme; Chen et al., 2016b), in most Perciformes examined (orange-spotted grouper Zhang et al., 2013, mandarin fish Yuan et al., 2016, and mackerel *Scomber japonicus* Ohga et al., 2015, European sea bass Gambardella et al., 2012), in Arctic charr (Jørgensen et al., 2013) and Atlantic salmon (Rønnestad et al., 2010; Trombley et al., 2012; Moen and Finn, 2013) (Salmoniformes). In contrast, decreases in leptin expression are seen in liver of zebrafish (lepA) (Gorissen et al., 2009) and striped bass (*Morone saxatilis*) (lepB, perciforme) (Won et al., 2012) and intestine of red-bellied piranha (Volkoff, 2015b), and in blunt snout bream (Cypriniforme), higher feeding rates are associated with increased leptin pituitary expression (Xu et al., 2016). Whereas plasma leptin levels increase following fasting in rainbow trout (Salmeron et al., 2015; Johansson et al., 2016; Pfundt et al., 2016), Atlantic salmon (Trombley et al., 2012) and fine flounder *Paralichthys adspersus* (Pleuronectiforme) (Fuentes et al., 2012, 2013), they have been shown to decrease in earlier studies in fasted burbot (*Lota lota*) (Gadiforme) (Nieminen et al., 2003) and green sunfish (*Lepomis cyanellus*) (Perciforme) (Johnson et al., 2000).

In fish, leptin has been linked to metabolism. For example, in zebrafish, knocking down lepA decreases metabolic rate (Dalman et al., 2013) and in golden pompano, *Trachinotus blochii* (Perciforme), lepA gene polymorphisms are associated with different body weights, heights and lengths (Wu et al., 2016). Whereas in mammals, leptin acts as an adipostat and its plasma levels are proportional to the amount of body fat, there is little evidence for such a role in fish. In topmouth culter *Culter alburnus* (Cyprinoforme), leptin mRNA expression is lower in wild populations, who have more muscle fat content than cultured fish (Wang et al., 2013), in grass carp, fish fed high fat diets have higher leptin expression (Li A. et al., 2016) than control fish, and in medaka, leptin receptor null-mutants have higher food intake and larger deposits of visceral fat than that of wild-type fish (Chisada et al., 2014), suggesting a correlation between leptin levels and fat. However, results from other studies seem to contradict this hypothesis: leptin receptor null adult zebrafish do not exhibit increased feeding or adiposity (Michel et al., 2016); In rainbow trout, leptin levels are higher in lean fish than fat fish (Salmeron et al., 2015; Johansson et al., 2016; Pfundt et al., 2016), and in Arctic charr, neither hepatic leptin expression nor plasma leptin levels correlate with fish adiposity (Froiland et al., 2012; Jørgensen et al., 2013); In murray cod *Maccullochella peelii peelii* (Perciforme), fish fed different experimental diets containing fish oil with or without vegetable oil have similar leptin levels (Ettore et al., 2012; Varricchio et al., 2012); In yellow catfish (Siluriforme), IP injections of human leptin reduce hepatic lipid content and the activities of lipogenic enzymes (Song et al., 2015) but Zn deficiency, which tends to increase hepatic and muscle lipid contents, does not affect leptin mRNA levels (Zheng et al., 2015).

Zebrafish lacking a functional leptin receptor have alterations in insulin and glucose levels, suggesting a role of leptin in the control of glucose homeostasis (Michel et al., 2016), which is consistent with data showing that leptin gene expression is induced by glucose in grass carp (Lu et al., 2015) and that leptin injections increase plasma glucose levels in Nile tilapia (Baltzegar et al., 2014).

Interestingly, in the Gymnotiforme *Eigenmannia virescens,* intramuscular injections of leptin increase electric organ discharges (EOD) amplitude in food-deprived but not well-fed fish, suggesting that leptin mediates EOD responses to metabolic stress in electric fish (Sinnett and Markham, 2015).

Overall, there seems to be a great species-specific variability in the functions of leptin with regards to the regulation of feeding and metabolism in fish, perhaps due to different lipid metabolism and storage areas among fish species.

Peptide YY

Peptide YY consists of two forms, PYYa and PYYb (previously called PY) (Wahlestedt and Reis, 1993; Cerdá-Reverter and Larhammar, 2000; Sundström et al., 2013) and is a brain-gut peptide that acts as an anorexigenic signal in mammals (Blevins et al., 2008; Karra et al., 2009; Zhang et al., 2012). Interestingly, one of the first studies showing an effect of PYY on feeding in mammals used fish PYY (Balasubramaniam et al., 1992). PYY was first shown to be present in the gastrointestinal tract of fish by immunochemical methods in the 1980's (daddy sculpin *Cottus scorpius* and Baltic sea cod *Gadus morhua callarias* El-Salhy, 1984) and first cloned and detected in the brain by ISH in an Agnatha, the river lamprey (*Lampetra fluviatilis*; Söderberg et al., 1994). The first indirect evidence of a role for PYY in feeding in fish was provided in sea bass, in which PYY transcripts were detected in brain areas regulating feeding (Cerdá-Reverter et al., 2000) and the first direct evidence of an anorexigenic role for PYY in fish was provided by IP injections of goldfish PYY in goldfish (Gonzalez and Unniappan, 2010). Peripheral injections of species-specific PYY also decrease food intake in another cyprinid, the grass carp (Chen et al., 2013) and in Siberian sturgeon *Acipenser baerii* (Acipenseriformes) (Chen et al., 2015). However, in channel catfish (Siluriformes), human PYY injections do not affect food intake or plasma glucose levels or hypothalamic POMC expression (Schroeter et al., 2015), suggesting perhaps that species-specific PYYs are needed to elicit an effect on feeding.

Fasting induces decreases in brain PYY expression in both goldfish (Gonzalez and Unniappan, 2010) and Ya fish (Yuan et al., 2014) (Cypriniformes) and in PPY intestinal expression in red-bellied piranha (Characiforme,) (Volkoff, 2014a), suggesting a role in satiety. However, fasting does not affect brain PYY expression in either cavefish (Characiforme) (Wall and Volkoff, 2013) or red-bellied piranha (Volkoff, 2014a), either brain or gut PYY mRNA expression in Atlantic salmon (Salmoniforme) (Murashita et al., 2009b), and induces increases in PYY gut expression in both yellowtail (Perciformes) (Murashita et al., 2006, 2007) and Japanese grenadier anchovy *Coilia nasus* (Clupeiformes) (Yang et al., 2016).

PYY mRNA expression increases post-feeding in the brain of goldfish (Gonzalez and Unniappan, 2010) and Ya fish (Yuan et al., 2014), cave fish (Wall and Volkoff, 2013) and Siberian sturgeon (Chen et al., 2015), in the intestine of grass carp (Chen et al., 2014) and in whole larval Atlantic halibut (Pleuronectiformes) (Gomes et al., 2015). However, in Atlantic salmon, brain PYY expression shows no periprandial changes (Valen et al., 2011; Kousoulaki et al., 2013), perhaps suggesting that PYY does not play a major role as a short-term satiety factor in salmonids.

Overall, it appears that in most fish examined to date, PYY might acts as an anorectic/satiety peptide, although this does not seem to hold true for all fish species (e.g., salmon, yellowtail, or catfish).

Other Hormones and Systems

Hypothalamus-Pituitary-Thyroid Axis (HPT Axis)

The hypothalamic-pituitary-thyroid (HPT) axis regulates levels of thyroid hormones, which are essential for a number of biological functions, including food intake and energy expenditure. Hormones produced by the axis consist of thyrotropin releasing hormone (TRH), thyroid stimulating hormone (TSH) and thyroid hormones (triiodothyronine T_3 and thyroxine T_4) secreted by the hypothalamus, the pituitary and the thyroid gland, respectively (Fekete and Lechan, 2014).

In goldfish (Cypriniforme), ICV injections of TRH increase feeding and locomotor behaviors and the hypothalamic mRNA expressions of both orexin and CART (Abbott and Volkoff, 2011), and IP injections of T_4 increase food intake and locomotion (Goodyear, 2012), suggesting an orexigenic role. Fasting increases TRH hypothalamic mRNA levels (Abbott and Volkoff, 2011), further suggesting that the HPT axis regulates feeding in goldfish. In Amur sturgeon, *Acipenser schrenckii* (Acipenseriforme), lower serum levels of thyroid hormones are seen in fish placed in high-density groups who display low feeding rates (Li et al., 2012). However, decreases in plasma levels of thyroid hormones are seen in fasted goldfish [T_3] (Sinha et al., 2012) and in fasted channel catfish [T_4 and T_3] (Gaylord et al., 2001), suggesting that food deprivation might decrease the activity of the HPT at the level of thyroid hormone synthesis and secretion, similar to what is observed in mammals (Boelen et al., 2008). A decrease in circulating thyroid hormones might inhibit the thyroid hormone negative feedback action on hypothalamic cells and contribute to the increase in hypothalamic TRH expression levels seen in goldfish. Overall, these data suggest that, in fish, TRH and thyroid hormones might affect feeding and metabolism and that nutritional status might affect the HPT axis.

Reproductive Hypothalamus-Pituitary-Gonad (HPG) Axis

Gonadotropin releasing hormone (GnRH)

GnRH is a hypothalamic hormone that stimulates the release of pituitary gonadotropins, which in turn stimulate the release of gonadal steroids. Three major forms of GnRH are present in fish, GnRH 1, 2, and 3 (Roch et al., 2014). GnRH appears to act as an anorexigenic hormone, as in goldfish, ICV injections with GnRH2 not only stimulate spawning (Hoskins et al., 2008) but also decrease food intake (Hoskins et al., 2008; Matsuda et al., 2008) and hypothalamic orexin mRNA expression (Hoskins et al., 2008). Similarly, in zebrafish, ICV injections of GnRH2 decrease food intake (Nishiguchi et al., 2012). In addition, in goldfish, treatment with orexin stimulate feeding, inhibit spawning behavior, and decrease brain GnRH2 expression, suggesting a coordinated control of feeding and reproduction by the orexin and GnRH systems (Hoskins et al., 2008).

In winter flounder, fasting reduces both brain GnRH2 and GnRH3, but not GnRH1, mRNA expression levels (Tuziak and Volkoff, 2013b) and in zebrafish, GnRH2 brain mRNA levels increase in overfed fish (Nishiguchi et al., 2012). However, in Atlantic cod, neither GnRH2 nor GnRH3 brain transcripts are influenced by food deprivation (Tuziak and Volkoff, 2013a), suggesting that the role of GnRHs in the regulation of feeding might be species- and form-specific.

RFamides

RFamide peptides, first isolated in invertebrate species in the late 1970's and later found in vertebrates, act as neurotransmitters and neuromodulators. In vertebrates, the RFamide peptide family consists of PRL-releasing peptides (PrRP), PQRFamide peptides (neuropeptide FF, NPFF), pyroglutamylated RFamide peptide (QRFP)/26RFamides, LPXRFamide peptides (gonadotropin-inhibitory hormone, GnIH, in lower vertebrates, RFamide-related peptide-3, RFRP-3, in mammals) and kisspeptins (Tsutsui and Ubuka, 2013; Osugi et al., 2016). RFamides have been shown to regulate several physiological functions in vertebrates, including feeding (Bechtold and Luckman, 2007; Quillet et al., 2016). A number of RFamides have been identified in fish, although most have been examined for their role in reproduction and are not yet well characterized with regards to their potential role as feeding regulators.

In goldfish, IP or ICV administration of PrRP decrease food intake, and hypothalamic PrRP mRNA expression increases post-prandially and after food deprivation, suggesting an anorexigenic role for PrRP in goldfish (Kelly and Peter, 2006). In line with this hypothesis, in the euryhaline fish mudskipper (*Periophthalmus modestus*, Perciforme, gobidae), freshwater fish have lower food intake/growth rates than saltwater fish and higher brain and intestine PrRP mRNA expressions, suggesting that PrRP is involved in the regulation of feeding and energy homeostasis in this species (Sakamoto et al., 2002; Tachibana and Sakamoto, 2014).

Two neuropeptide FF receptor 1 (NPFFR1) genes have been identified in carp and shown to display variations in expression associated with growth-related traits (Peng et al., 2016). As NPFF1 is receptor for neuropeptide FF (NPFF) and the LPXRFamide peptide RFamide-related peptide (RFRP), which are involved in control of feeding behavior in both invertebrates and vertebrates, these data suggest that NPFFR1s might be related to the regulation of growth and body weight in common carp (Peng et al., 2016). Similarly, in seabass, LPXRFamide-ir cells and/or fibers are present in feeding, gustatory, sensory, and behavioral centers of the brain, suggesting that it could be involved in the regulation of foraging/feeding behavior (Paullada-Salmerón et al., 2016).

In goldfish, hypothalamic expression of 26RFa increases in fasted animals (Liu et al., 2009) and IP injections of human RFRP-3 decrease food intake (Mawhinney, 2007), indicating that these neuropeptides might regulate food intake and energy balance in cyprinid fish.

In sea bass, food-restricted male fish display an increase in both kisspeptin and kisspeptin receptor expressions in both pituitary and hypothalamus (Escobar et al., 2016), suggesting the kisspeptin system is affected by nutritional status. However, in goldfish, IP injections of mammalian kisspeptin appear to have no effect on feeding (Mawhinney, 2007).

CRF and the Hypothalamus-Pituitary-Interrenal (HPI) Axis

The major endocrine components of the hypothalamic–pituitary–adrenal (HPA) axis (or interrenal, HPI in lower vertebrates) are hypothalamic corticotropin-releasing factor (CRF, or corticotropin-releasing hormone, CRH), pituitary adrenocorticotropin (ACTH) and glucocorticoids (e.g., cortisol, corticosterone) from the adrenal/interrenal gland. CRF mediates the release of ACTH, which in turn stimulates the release of steroids by the adrenal/interrenal gland (Smith and Vale, 2006). The HPI axis regulates numerous physiological functions, including metabolic functions (e.g., blood glucose levels during fasting), food intake, reproduction, growth, and immunity. Urocortins (UCN) 1 (also termed urotensin 1 in fishes), 2, and 3 belong to a recently discovered family of CRF-related peptides, which functions are still not well characterized (Majzoub, 2006).

The role of the HPI axis in the regulation of feeding of fish has been examined in several fish species. In goldfish, ICV injections of CRF decrease feeding (De Pedro et al., 1993) and increase locomotor activity (Matsuda et al., 2013). In Ya fish, fasting decreases CRF brain expression levels (Wang et al., 2014) and goldfish exposed to the toxin fluoxetine have low food intake and increased brain expression of CRF (Mennigen et al., 2010), further suggesting an anorexigenic role for CRF in cyprinids. In goldfish, feeding fish with a diet containing low cortisol levels or implanting fish with cortisol-containing pellets result in higher food intake and CRF mRNA levels, compared to controls (Bernier et al., 2004). These results and others suggest that stress, cortisol and CRF can modulate food intake in Cypriniformes (Bernier et al., 2004).

In rainbow trout, CRF and urotensin 1 are anorexigenic, as ICV injections of either peptides inhibit feeding (Ortega et al., 2013). In addition, hypoxia stress suppresses appetite and increases forebrain CRF and urotensin mRNA levels, suggesting that, in Salmoniformes, CRF-related peptides might mediate the hypoxia-induced reduction in food intake (Bernier and Craig, 2005).

In Siberian sturgeon, IP injections of urocortin 3 inhibit feeding, and UCN3 brain mRNA expression levels increase post-feeding and decrease during fasting, suggesting that UCN3 acts as a satiety/anorexigenic factor in fish (Zhang et al., 2016c).

For more extensive reviews on the regulation of feeding by the HPI, please refer to previously published works, including (Bernier and Peter, 2001; Bernier, 2006; Flik et al., 2006; Lowry and Moore, 2006; Backström and Winberg, 2013).

"Novel" Appetite-Regulating Peptides

Amylin

Amylin (or islet amyloid polypeptide, IAPP), a hormone co-secreted with insulin from pancreatic β-cells, inhibits feeding in mammals (Riediger et al., 2003). In fish, the role of amylin in feeding has only been examined in goldfish. In this species, IP or ICV amylin treatments decrease food intake whereas ICV injections of an amylin receptor antagonist (AC 187) stimulate feeding (Thavanathan and Volkoff, 2006), suggesting an anorexigenic role for amylin in fish.

Apelin

Apelin is a peptide first identified in bovine stomach as a ligand for the orphan receptor APJ, with close identity to the angiotensin II (Ang II) receptor (Tatemoto et al., 1998; Habata et al., 1999) and subsequently shown to be involved in multiple physiological processes (see O'Carroll et al., 2013, for review) including feeding and metabolism in mammals: for example, apelin injections decrease food intake (O'Shea et al., 2003), and in adipocytes, apelin expression is inhibited by fasting (Boucher et al., 2005) and its secretion is regulated by insulin (Boucher et al., 2005).

In fish, apelin appear to be orexigenic: apelin injections increase food intake in goldfish (Volkoff and Wyatt, 2009) and cavefish (Penney and Volkoff, 2014). Fasting induces increases in brain apelin mRNA expression in Ya-fish (Lin et al., 2014a) and red-bellied piranha (Volkoff, 2014a). Moreover, in goldfish, the obesogen factor tributyltin (TBT) stimulates food intake and also increases brain apelin expression (Zhang et al., 2016b). In cavefish, IP injections of apelin increase orexin brain expression, and CCK injections induce a decrease in brain apelin expression (Penney and Volkoff, 2014), an indication that apelin interacts with other appetite regulators. Similarly, brain injections of the anorexigenic factor spexin reduce apelin brain expression (Wong et al., 2013) and *in vitro* treatment of brain fragments with apelin increase expressions of orexigenic peptides—i.e., orexin—and decrease CART expression (Volkoff, 2014b). Overall, the data suggest an orexigenic role for apelin in Cypriniformes. In cunner (Perciforme), summer fasting decreases intestinal apelin mRNA levels (Hayes and Volkoff, 2014), suggesting that GIT apelin might not be involved in the regulation of feeding. In common carp- but not in trout barb *Capoeta trutta*-, there is a negative correlation between apelin levels and body weight (Köprücü and Algül, 2015), suggesting that apelin might not be involved in metabolic processes leading to weight gain in some species.

Arginine Vasotocin

Arginine vasotocin (AVT) is the mammalian homolog of arginine vasopressin (AVP), and has been shown to have diverse and complex roles in fish physiology, including regulation of metabolic processes, stress responses and several behaviors (Balment et al., 2006). In rainbow trout, AVT treatments decrease feeding, and increase plasma levels of cortisol and glucose, brain serotonergic activity, and hypothalamic levels of POMC and CART, suggesting it acts as an anorexigenic factor in fish (Gesto et al., 2014).

Endocanabinoid System

In mammals, the endocannabinoid system (ECS), which consists of cannabinoid receptors (CB1 and CB2) and endogenous cannabinoids, is involved in the regulation of several physiological functions, including feeding and energy balance (Pagotto et al., 2006).

In goldfish, CB1 and CB2 are both expressed in brain, where CB1 co-localizes with NPY (Cottone et al., 2013). Treatment with low doses of the endocannabinoid receptor agonist anandamide (AEA) increases food intake (Valenti et al., 2005), and food deprivation increases CB1 and AEA brain mRNA levels (Cottone et al., 2009), suggesting the involvement of the ECS in the control of energy intake in Cypriniforme. Similarly, in sea bream *Sparus aurata* (Perciforme), AEA administered via water increases food intake and NPY brain mRNA levels (Piccinetti et al., 2010). In common sole, *Solea solea* (Pleuronectiforme), feeding fish with dietary nucleotides reduce CB1 brain transcript levels, suggesting that feeding and diets modulate the ECS (Palermo et al., 2013).

Nesfatin-1

Nesfatin-1, discovered in 2006 in mammals, is a peptide secreted from hypothalamic nuclei related to appetite regulation, from the precursor non-esterified fatty acid/nucleobinding 2 (NUCB2), and has been shown to reduce feeding and water intake in mammals (Ayada et al., 2015). In fish, the role of nesfatin-1 as an appetite regulator has been examined in Cypriniformes and Salmoniformes.

In goldfish, nesfatin-1 has been shown to be involved in the regulation of feeding and metabolism: nesfatin-1-like and ghrelin-like ir co-localize in both enteroendocrine and hypothalamic cells; IP or ICV injections of nesfatin-1 inhibit both food intake and brain expressions of ghrelin and NUCB2; and fasting increases both hepatic and hypothalamic NUCB2 mRNA levels (Gonzalez et al., 2010; Kerbel and Unniappan, 2012). In addition, NUCB2 mRNA levels increase in liver and hypothalamus in fish fed fat-enriched diets and decrease in gut after long-term feeding with a high-protein diet, suggesting that macronutrients regulate the expression of NUCB2/nesfatin-1 (Blanco et al., 2016a). In zebrafish, two isoforms of NUCB2 (NUCB2A and NUCB2B) exist, and both mRNAs decrease in the brain post-prandially and after food deprivation, suggesting an anorexigenic role for nesfatin-1 (Hatef et al., 2015). In Ya-fish, NUCB2A mRNA levels increase post-prandially in both hypothalamus and intestine, and fasting induces a decrease in NUCB2A mRNA levels in the hypothalamus, but an increase in the hepatopancreas, suggesting anorexigenic and metabolic roles (Lin et al., 2014b). However, in rainbow trout (*Oncorhynchus mykiss*), plasma nesfatin-1 levels are similar between fed and fasted females (Caldwell et al., 2014).

Neuropeptide B, Neuromedin S, and Neuromedin U

Neuropepide B (NPB), and neuromedins S (NMS) and U (NMU) are newly discovered mammalian short peptides that have been shown to affect feeding in fish.

NPB has been characterized in Nile tilapia (Perciforme), where it is expressed in brain and spinal cord. In this species, fasting increases NPB brain mRNA expression, and IP injections of NPB increase brain mRNA expression of NPY and CCK and inhibit pituitary GH expression, suggesting NPB is involved in feeding and growth in fish (Yang et al., 2014).

In both zebrafish (Chen et al., 2016a) and orange-spotted grouper (Li et al., 2015), an NMS-related protein (NMS-RP) has been identified that appears to act as an orexigenic factor. In both species, IP administration of species-specific NMS-RP increases both NPY and orexin expressions, and hypothalamic levels of NMS mRNA increase after food deprivation.

NMU has been characterized in Cypriniformes (carp, goldfish) and Perciformes (orange-spotted grouper). In both common carp (Kono et al., 2012) and goldfish (Maruyama et al., 2008), several forms of NMU (3–5) have been isolated and their mRNA expressions shown to decrease upon fasting, suggesting a role in feeding and metabolism (Kono et al., 2012). Similarly, in orange-spotted grouper, hypothalamic NMU mRNA levels decrease in fasted fish and increase post-feeding (Li et al., 2015), suggesting an anorexigenic role. In goldfish, central injections of NMU inhibit feeding and locomotor behaviors (Maruyama et al., 2008) and increase brain CRF mRNA expression levels (Maruyama et al., 2009) and in grouper, IP injections of NMU down-regulate hypothalamic NPY expression (Li et al., 2015), suggesting that the anorexigenic actions of NMU are mediated by the CRF system and an inhibition of the NPY system.

Obestatin

Obestatin, a gastrointestinal peptide discovered in 2005, is derived from the same precursor as ghrelin and inhibits food intake in mammals (Cowan et al., 2016). In grass carp, although IP injections of an obestatin-like peptide alone do not affect food intake or the expression levels of NPY, CART, or POMC, when co-injected with ghrelin, it blocks ghrelin-induced stimulation of appetite and up-regulation of expressions of NPY and NPY receptors (Yuan et al., 2015), suggesting that obestatin might inhibit the ghrelin system in Cypriniformes.

Octadecaneuropeptide

The octadecaneuropeptide (ODN) is a peptide belonging to the family of endozepines and is generated through the cleavage of diazepam-binding inhibitor (DBI) in the mammalian central nervous system (CNS) (Tonon et al., 2006). ODN acts as an inverse agonist of central-type benzodiazepine receptors (CBR) and inhibits food intake in rodents (do Rego et al., 2006).

Immunocytochemical methods first showed the presence in brain and pituitary of rainbow trout (Malagon et al., 1992) and more recently in the agnathan Atlantic hagfish, *Myxine glutinosa* (Myxiniforme, myxinidae; Candiani et al., 2000). Central injections of goldfish ODN inhibit food intake (Matsuda et al., 2007b) and stimulate locomotor activity (Matsuda et al., 2011b), and increase POMC brain mRNA levels (Matsuda et al., 2010), suggesting that the anorexigenic actions of ODN are in part mediated by the melanocortin system.

Pituitary Adenylate Cyclase Activating Polypeptide (PACAP)

Originally identified in the ovine hypothalamus (Miyata et al., 1989), pituitary adenylate cyclase-activating polypeptide (PACAP) belongs to the secretin/glucagon family of peptides that also includes secretin, glucagon, glucagon-like peptides and vasoactive intestinal peptide (Sherwood et al., 2000). In rodents, central injections of PACAP decrease food intake (Morley et al., 1992).

PACAP has been cloned in several fish, including Anguilliformes European eel (*Anguilla anguilla*) (Montero et al., 1998), Cypriniformes (e.g., zebrafish Sherwood et al., 2007, goldfish Matsuda et al., 1997), Gadiformes (cod Xu and Volkoff, 2009), Pleuronectiformes (e.g., olive flounder Nam et al., 2013), Salmoniformes (e.g., Atlantic salmon Parker et al., 1993), and Siluriformes (Thai catfish *Clarias macrocephalus* McRory et al., 1995, darkbarbel catfish *Pelteobagrus vachelli* Xu et al., 2012) as well as elasmobranchs (e.g., marbled electric ray *Torpedo marmorata* Agnese et al., 2016, stingray *Dasyatis akajei* Matsuda et al., 1998). In several fish, PACAP stimulates GH secretion by pituitary cells (see review in Gahete et al., 2009), but its role in regulating feeding is still unclear. In goldfish, central or peripheral PACAP injections inhibit food intake (Matsuda et al., 2005) and locomotor activity (Matsuda et al., 2006) and these actions might be mediated in part by the stimulation of POMC and CRH pathways (Matsuda and Maruyama, 2007). Similarly, in grass carp, central NPY injections decrease brain PACAP expression (Zhou et al., 2013), suggesting an anorexigenic role for PACAP in Cypriniformes. In Atlantic cod, PACAP inhibits intestinal smooth muscle contractions (Olsson and Holmgren, 2000), and although brain expression levels are not affected by 30 days of food deprivation, they increase after during the re-feeding period (Xu and Volkoff, 2009), suggesting that PACAP is involved in the regulation of feeding and digestive processes (Xu and Volkoff, 2009).

Secretoneurin

Secretoneurin (SN) is a short peptide derived from a secretogranin-II (SgII, also called chromogranin C) precursor protein (Zhao et al., 2009). In goldfish, ICV injections of the SN increase food intake and locomotor behavior (Trudeau et al., 2012), increase mRNA levels of hypothalamic NPY and decrease hypothalamic CART. In addition, fasting increases telencephalon SgII mRNA levels (Mikwar et al., 2016), suggesting that, in fish, SN might act as an orexigenic factor.

Spexin

Spexin (SPX) is a peptide identified in 2007 in mammalian adipose tissue. SPX expression is down-regulated in obese humans and rats, and subcutaneous injections of SPX reduce food intake and increase locomotion (Walewski et al., 2014).

In goldfish, SPX appear to act as an anorexigenic factor: brain injections of SPX inhibit both basal and NPY- or orexin-induced food consumption, decrease brain expressions of orexigenic factors (NPY, AgRP, and apelin) and increase that of anorexigenic factors (CCK, CART, POMC, MCH, and CRH), and brain SPX mRNA levels increase post-prandially (Wong et al., 2013). Similarly, in the orange-spotted grouper, IP administration of SPX increases hypothalamic mRNA levels of POMC and inhibits orexin expression, suggesting an anorexigenic role (Li S. et al., 2016). However, grouper SPX hypothalamic expression increases following long-term food deprivation (Li S. et al., 2016), suggesting that spexin might be a short-term satiety factor rather than a long-term hunger signal.

CONCLUDING REMARKS

Although the basic mechanisms regulating feeding seem to be relatively conserved between mammals and fish, it must be kept in mind that major physiological differences exist between these two groups. Fish are ectotherms and thus have lower metabolic rates than mammals and more sensitive to environmental changes, their physiology changing with their fluctuating surroundings. They also have different means of energy/nutrient storage (e.g., fat storage in liver rather than subcutaneous adipose tissue), and different growth patterns (as opposed to mammals, fish continue to grow after sexual maturity), suggesting that the endocrine regulation of energy balance, feeding and growth in fish differs from that of mammals.

Comparative studies at the genome level have revealed conserved sequences for appetite regulators across mammalian and fish species, indicating potentially conserved biological functions. Whereas the genome of all vertebrates is the result of two rounds (2R) of whole genome duplication (WGD) occurring in early vertebrate evolution, additional WGDs occurred in the teleost fish ancestor (3R) and most recently in certain teleost lineages (4R, e.g., salmonidae and cyprinidae), leading to the presence of increased gene copy numbers and multiple protein isoforms with potentially different physiological functions (Glasauer and Neuhauss, 2014), making the fish model potentially more complex. One must thus keep in mind that fish feeding-regulating hormones might not always have the same function as their mammalian homologs.

Fish are an extremely diversified group, with a great variability in feeding habits and requirements as well gut morphology and digestion processes. Fish can be carnivores, herbivores, omnivores or detritivores, with different feeding habits often seen within the same family (e.g., herbivore Mbuna cichlids and carnivore Nile tilapia in cichlidae; herbivore/omnivore pacu and carnivore piranha in serrasalmidae). Different fish species not only require different compositions of food, but also different amounts of food and feeding frequencies (Moore, 1941). Diet and feeding habits is reflected in the anatomy and physiology of the gastrointestinal tract. For example, carnivores or omnivores (such as most Characiformes and Siluriformes) have stomachs, pyloric caeca, and relatively short and straight intestines, whereas herbivores or detrivores (e.g., Cypriniformes and Cyprinodontiformes) may lack both stomach and caeca and have long and convoluted intestines (Leknes, 2015). Different diets and guts translate into different digestive enzyme profiles and different methods of nutrient storage (Day et al., 2011), as seen for lipids (e.g., in muscle in "oily" fish such as salmon and herring vs. liver in "lean" fish such as cod and flatfish), which usage might also be affected by reproductive stages and modes (guarding vs. non guarding; mature vs. immature; oviparous vs. viviparous).

Given the high diversity within fish, one should thus be careful when generalizing results from one species to all fish. Comparative studies establishing similarities and differences among species should be valuable to understand mechanisms regulating feeding. However, the large number of species poses the problem of the model species to choose. To date, most studies examining the neuroendocrine regulation of fish still use "classical" model species, i.e., cyprinids and salmonids. These somewhat differ from most fishes, as they display polyploidy, and might not represent a "perfect" model, but they are easily available and maintained, as their different holding conditions, habitats and diets, are well known. However, new species, in particular commercially important aquaculture species such as Perciformes (the largest teleost order) and Pleuronectiformes have recently been examined.

The increasing number of studies and species examined often generates conflicting and sometimes contradictory results. This variability might express true differences between species, but contradictory data also occur within same species. This variability might have several reasons. First, there is a great variability in the nature and nomenclature of isoforms examined (e.g., within CART forms). Second, when comparing studies, it is sometimes difficult to compare results obtained using different protocols (e.g., different lengths of fasting) and techniques (e.g., mRNA vs. protein vs. plasma levels), in particular because changes in gene expression do not necessarily translate into different protein levels or circulating levels. Finally, fish used between studies are often of different ages (e.g., larval vs. adult), sexual maturity (immature vs. mature spawning or non-spawning) or even environmental conditions (e.g., temperatures, photoperiods), all of these factors influencing feeding.

Even in mammals, the regulation of appetite is not yet fully understood. Using a comparative approach involving multiple fish species, perhaps choosing representative families/species from each fish group, and complementary methods might help us start drawing accurate models for the endocrine regulation of feeding in fish.

AUTHOR CONTRIBUTIONS

HV designed this review, including table and figure, researched, acquired and analyzed all the information, drafted and revised the manuscript, and approved the version to be published. To HV's knowledge, information contained in this review and studies cited within it have been appropriately checked for accuracy or integrity.

ACKNOWLEDGMENTS

Many investigators have made contributions to the understanding of endocrinology of feeding in fish and some of their works are not cited in this review, due to space constraints. Research in the HV's laboratory is supported by a Natural Sciences and Engineering Research Council (NSERC) Discovery Grant (# 261414-03).

REFERENCES

Abbott, M., and Volkoff, H. (2011). Thyrotropin Releasing Hormone (TRH) in goldfish (*Carassius auratus*): role in the regulation of feeding and locomotor behaviors and interactions with the orexin system and cocaine- and amphetamine regulated transcript (CART). *Horm. Behav.* 59, 236–245. doi: 10.1016/j.yhbeh.2010.12.008

Adan, R. A., Tiesjema, B., Hillebrand, J. J., la Fleur, S. E., Kas, M. J., and de Krom, M. (2006). The MC4 receptor and control of appetite. *Br. J. Pharmacol.* 149, 815–827. doi: 10.1038/sj.bjp.0706929

Agnese, M., Valiante, S., Rosati, L., Andreuccetti, P., and Prisco, M. (2016). Pituitary adenylate cyclase-activating peptide (PACAP) and PAC1 receptor in the testis of cartilaginous fish *Torpedo marmorata*: a molecular and phylogenetic study. *Comp. Biochem. Physiol. Part B Biochem. Mol. Biol.* 191, 26–35. doi: 10.1016/j.cbpb.2015.09.002

Agulleiro, M. J., Cortes, R., Leal, E., Rios, D., Sanchez, E., and Cerda-Reverter, J. M. (2014). Characterization, tissue distribution and regulation by fasting of the agouti family of peptides in the sea bass (*Dicentrarchus labrax*). *Gen. Comp. Endocrinol.* 205, 251–259. doi: 10.1016/j.ygcen.2014.02.009

Akash, G., Kaniganti, T., Tiwari, N. K., Subhedar, N. K., and Ghose, A. (2014). Differential distribution and energy status-dependent regulation of the four CART neuropeptide genes in the zebrafish brain. *J. Comp. Neurol.* 522, 2266–2285. doi: 10.1002/cne.23532

Aldegunde, M., and Mancebo, M. (2006). Effects of neuropeptide Y on food intake and brain biogenic amines in the rainbow trout (*Oncorhynchus mykiss*). *Peptides* 27, 719–727. doi: 10.1016/j.peptides.2005.09.014

Aldman, G., and Holmgren, S. (1987). Control of gallbladder motility in the rainbow trout, *Salmo gairdneri*. *Fish Physiol. Biochem.* 4, 143–155. doi: 10.1007/BF02110881

Amiya, N., Amano, M., Iigo, M., Yamanome, T., Takahashi, A., and Yamamori, K. (2008). Interaction of orexin/hypocretin-like immunoreactive neurons with melanin-concentrating hormone and alpha-melanocyte-stimulating hormone neurons in brain of a pleuronectiform fish, barfin flounder. *Fish. Sci.* 74, 1040–1046. doi: 10.1111/j.1444-2906.2008.01622.x

Amiya, N., Mizusawa, K., Kobayashi, Y., Yamanome, T., Amano, M., and Takahashi, A. (2012). Food deprivation increases the expression of the prepro-orexin gene in the hypothalamus of the Barfin flounder, *Verasper moseri*. *Zool. Sci.* 29, 43–48. doi: 10.2108/zsj.29.43

Angotzi, A. R., Stefansson, S. O., Nilsen, T. O., Rathore, R. M., and Rønnestad, I. (2013). Molecular cloning and genomic characterization of novel Leptin-like genes in salmonids provide new insight into the evolution of the Leptin gene family. *Gen. Comp. Endocrinol.* 187, 48–59. doi: 10.1016/j.ygcen.2013.03.022

Arends, R. J., Vermeer, H., Martens, G. J., Leunissen, J. A. M., Wendelaar Bonga, S. E., and Flik, G. (1998). Cloning and expression of two proopiomelanocortin mRNAs in the common carp (*Cyprinus carpio* L.). *Mol. Cell. Endocrinol.* 143, 23–31. doi: 10.1016/S0303-7207(98)00139-7

Ayada, C., Toru, U., and Korkut, Y. (2015). Nesfatin-1 and its effects on different systems. *Hippokratia* 19, 4–10.

Babichuk, N. A., and Volkoff, H. (2013). Changes in expression of appetite-regulating hormones in the cunner (*Tautogolabrus adspersus*) during short-term fasting and winter torpor. *Physiol. Behav.* 120C, 54–63. doi: 10.1016/j.physbeh.2013.06.022

Backstrom, T., and Winberg, S. (2013). Central corticotropin releasing factor and social stress. *Front. Neurosci.* 7:117. doi: 10.3389/fnins.2013.00117

Balasubramaniam, A., Rigel, D. F., Chance, W. T., and Fischer, J. E. (1992). Central and peripheral effects of sculpin pancreatic polypeptide and anglerfish peptide Y in rats. *Pept. Res.* 5, 106–109.

Balment, R. J., Lu, W., Weybourne, E., and Warne, J. M. (2006). Arginine vasotocin a key hormone in fish physiology and behaviour: a review with insights from mammalian models. *Gen. Comp. Endocrinol.* 147, 9–16. doi: 10.1016/j.ygcen.2005.12.022

Baltzegar, D. A., Reading, B. J., Douros, J. D., and Borski, R. J. (2014). Role for leptin in promoting glucose mobilization during acute hyperosmotic stress in teleost fishes. *J. Endocrinol.* 220, 61–72. doi: 10.1530/JOE-13-0292

Barsagade, V. G., Mazumdar, M., Singru, P. S., Thim, L., Clausen, J. T., and Subhedar, N. (2010). Reproductive phase-related variations in cocaine- and amphetamine-regulated transcript (CART) in the olfactory system, forebrain, and pituitary of the female catfish, *Clarias batrachus* (Linn.). *J. Comp. Neurol.* 518, 2503–2524. doi: 10.1002/cne.22349

Bechtold, D. A., and Luckman, S. M. (2007). The role of RFamide peptides in feeding. *J. Endocrinol.* 192, 3–15. doi: 10.1677/JOE-06-0069

Bernier, N. J. (2006). The corticotropin-releasing factor system as a mediator of the appetite-suppressing effects of stress in fish. *Gen. Comp. Endocrinol.* 146, 45–55. doi: 10.1016/j.ygcen.2005.11.016

Bernier, N. J., and Craig, P. M. (2005). CRF-related peptides contribute to stress response and regulation of appetite in hypoxic rainbow trout. *Am. J. Physiol.* 289, R982–R990. doi: 10.1152/ajpregu.00668.2004

Bernier, N. J., Gorissen, M., and Flik, G. (2012). Differential effects of chronic hypoxia and feed restriction on the expression of leptin and its receptor, food intake regulation and the endocrine stress response in common carp. *J. Exp. Biol.* 215, 2273–2282. doi: 10.1242/Jeb.066183

Bernier, N. J., and Peter, R. E. (2001). The hypothalamic-pituitary-interrenal axis and the control of food intake in teleost fish. *Comp. Biochem. Physiol. Part B* 129, 639–644. doi: 10.1016/S1096-4959(01)00360-8

Bernier, N. J., Bedard, N., and Peter, R. E. (2004). Effects of cortisol on food intake, growth, and forebrain neuropeptide Y and corticotropin-releasing factor gene expression in goldfish. *Gen. Comp. Endocrinol.* 135, 230–240. doi: 10.1016/j.ygcen.2003.09.016

Birsoy, K., Festuccia, W. T., and Laplante, M. (2013). A comparative perspective on lipid storage in animals. *J. Cell Sci.* 126(Pt 7), 1541–1552. doi: 10.1242/jcs.104992

Blanco, A. M., Bertucci, J. I., Delgado, M. A.J., Valenciano, A. I., and Unniappan, S. (2016a). Tissue-specific expression of ghrelinergic and NUCB2/nesfatin-1 systems in goldfish (*Carassius auratus*) is modulated by macronutrient composition of diets. *Comp. Biochem. Physiol. Part A Mol. Integr. Physiol.* 195, 1–9. doi: 10.1016/j.cbpa.2016.01.016

Blanco, A. M., Gomez-Boronat, M., Redondo, I., Valenciano, A. I., and Delgado, M. J. (2016b). Periprandial changes and effects of short- and long-term fasting on ghrelin, GOAT, and ghrelin receptors in goldfish (*Carassius auratus*). *J. Comp. Physiol.* 186, 727–738. doi: 10.1007/s00360-016-0986-0

Blevins, J. E., Chelikani, P. K., Haver, A. C., and Reidelberger, R. D. (2008). PYY(3-36) induces Fos in the arcuate nucleus and in both catecholaminergic and non-catecholaminergic neurons in the nucleus tractus solitarius of rats. *Peptides* 29, 112–119. doi: 10.1016/j.peptides.2007.11.003

Blomqvist, A. G., Söderberg, C., Lundell, I., Milner, R. J., and Larhammar, D. (1992). Strong evolutionary conservation of neuropeptide Y: sequences of chicken, goldfish, and *Torpedo marmorata* DNA clones. *Proc. Natl. Acad. Sci. U.S.A.* 89, 2350–2354. doi: 10.1073/pnas.89.6.2350

Boelen, A., Wiersinga, W. M., and Fliers, E. (2008). Fasting-induced changes in the hypothalamus-pituitary-thyroid axis. *Thyroid* 18, 123–129. doi: 10.1089/thy.2007.0253

Boguszewski, C. L., Paz-Filho, G., and Velloso, L. A. (2010). Neuroendocrine body weight regulation: integration between fat tissue, gastrointestinal tract, and the brain. *Endokrynol. Polska* 61, 194–206.

Bonacic, K., Martínez, A., Martín-Robles, Á. J., Muñoz-Cueto, J. A., and Morais, S. (2015). Characterization of seven cocaine- and amphetamine-regulated transcripts (CARTs) differentially expressed in the brain and peripheral tissues of *Solea senegalensis* (Kaup). *Gen. Comp. Endocrinol.* 224, 260–272. doi: 10.1016/j.ygcen.2015.08.017

Boonanuntanasarn, S., Jangprai, A., and Yoshizaki, G. (2012). Characterization of neuropeptide Y in snakeskin gourami and the change in its expression due to feeding status and melanocortin 4 receptor expression. *Gen. Comp. Endocrinol.* 179, 184–195. doi: 10.1016/j.ygcen.2012.07.024

Boucher, J., Masri, B., Daviaud, D., Gesta, S., Guigne, C., Mazzucotelli, A., et al. (2005). Apelin, a newly identified adipokine up-regulated by insulin and obesity. *Endocrinology* 146, 1764–1771. doi: 10.1210/en.2004-1427

Buckley, C., MacDonald, E. E., Tuziak, S. M., and Volkoff, H. (2010). Molecular cloning and characterization of two putative appetite regulators in winter flounder (*Pleuronectes americanus*): preprothyrotropin-releasing hormone (TRH) and preproorexin (OX). *Peptides* 31, 1737–1747. doi: 10.1016/j.peptides.2010.05.017

Burt, K., Hamoutene, D., Perez-Casanova, J., Gamperl, A. K., and Volkoff, H. (2013). The effect of intermittent hypoxia on growth, appetite and some aspects of the immune response of Atlantic salmon (*Salmo salar*). *Aquac. Res.* 45, 124–137. doi: 10.1111/J.1365-2109.2012.03211.X

Cai, Z. N., Li, W. J., Mai, K. S., Xu, W., Zhang, Y. J., and Ai, Q. H. (2015). Effects of dietary size-fractionated fish hydrolysates on growth, activities of digestive enzymes and aminotransferases and expression of some protein metabolism related genes in large yellow croaker (*Larimichthys crocea*) larvae. *Aquaculture* 440, 40–47. doi: 10.1016/j.aquaculture.2015.01.026

Caldwell, L. K., Pierce, A. L., Riley, L. G., Duncan, C. A., and Nagler, J. J. (2014). Plasma nesfatin-1 is not affected by long-term food restriction and does not predict rematuration among iteroparous female rainbow trout (*Oncorhynchus mykiss*). *PLoS ONE* 9:e85700. doi: 10.1371/journal.pone.0085700

Campos, V. F., Robaldo, R. B., Deschamps, J. C., Seixas, F. K., McBride, A. J. A., Marins, L. F., et al. (2012). Neuropeptide Y gene expression around meal time in the Brazilian flounder *Paralichthys orbignyanus*. *J. Biosci.* 37, 227–232. doi: 10.1007/s12038-012-9205-7

Candiani, S., Augello, A., Oliveri, D., and Pestarino, M. (2000). Immunoreactive endozepine-like peptides in the brain and pituitary of the Atlantic hagfish, *Myxine glutinosa*. *Histochem. J.* 32, 415–421. doi: 10.1023/A:1004091204806

Cérda-Reverter, J. M., Agulleiro, M. J. R. R. G., Sánchez, E., Ceinos, R., and Rotllant, J. (2011). Fish melanocortin system. *Eur. J. Pharmacol.* 660, 53–60. doi: 10.1016/j.ejphar.2010.10.108

Cerda-Reverter, J. M., and Canosa, L. F. (2009). "Neuroendocrine systems of the fish brain," in *Fish Physiology*, eds N. J. Bernier, G. Van Der Kraak, A. P. Farrell, and C. J. Brauner (Academic Press), 3–74.

Cerdá-Reverter, J. M., and Larhammar, D. (2000). Neuropeptide Y family of peptides: structure, anatomical expression, function, and molecular evolution. *Biochem. Cell Biol.* 78, 371–392. doi: 10.1139/o00-004

Cerdá-Reverter, J. M., and Peter, R. E. (2003). Endogenous melanocortin antagonist in fish: structure, brain mapping, and regulation by fasting of the goldfish agouti-related protein gene. *Endocrinology* 144, 4552–4561. doi: 10.1210/en.2003-0453

Cerdá-Reverter, J. M., Martinez-Rodriguez, G., Anglade, I., Kah, O., and Zanuy, S. (2000). Peptide YY (PYY) and fish pancreatic peptide Y (PY) expression in the brain of the sea bass (*Dicentrarchus labrax*) as revealed by in situ hybridization. *J. Comp. Neurol.* 426, 197–208. doi: 10.1002/1096-9861(20001016)426:2<197::AID-CNE3>3.0.CO;2-3

Cerdá-Reverter, J. M., Schioth, H. B., and Peter, R. E. (2003). The central melanocortin system regulates food intake in goldfish. *Regul. Pept.* 115, 101–113. doi: 10.1016/S0167-0115(03)00144-7

Chen, H., Huang, H., Chen, X., Deng, S. P., Zhu, C., Huang, H., et al. (2016a). Structural and functional characterization of neuromedin S in the teleost fish, zebrafish (*Danio rerio*). *Comp. Biochem. Physiol. B Biochem. Mol. Biol.* 191, 76–83. doi: 10.1016/j.cbpb.2015.09.007

Chen, H., Zhang, X., Hao, J., Chen, D., Liu, J., Gao, Y., et al. (2015). Molecular cloning, expression analysis, and appetite regulatory effect of peptide YY in Siberian sturgeon (*Acipenser baerii*). *Gene* 563, 172–179. doi: 10.1016/j.gene.2015.03.028

Chen, T., Chen, S., Ren, C., Hu, C., Tang, D., and Yan, A. (2016b). Two isoforms of leptin in the White-clouds Mountain minnow (*Tanichthys albonubes*): differential regulation by estrogen despite similar response to fasting. *Gen. Comp. Endocrinol.* 225, 174–184. doi: 10.1016/j.ygcen.2015.08.002

Chen, W.-B., Wang, X., Zhou, Y.-L., Dong, H.-Y., Lin, H.-R., and Li, W.-S. (2011). Molecular cloning, tissue distribution and the expression in the regulation of food intake of prepro-orexin in Nile tilapia (*Oreochromis niloticus*). *Zool. Res.* 32, 285–292. doi: 10.3724/SP.J.1141.2011.03285

Chen, Y., Pandit, N. P., Fu, J., Li, D., and Li, J. (2014). Identification, characterization and feeding response of peptide YYb (PYYb) gene in grass carp (*Ctenopharyngodon idellus*). *Fish Physiol. Biochem.* 40, 45–55. doi: 10.1007/s10695-013-9822-6

Chen, Y., Shen, Y., Pandit, N. P., Fu, J., Li, D., and Li, J. (2013). Molecular cloning, expression analysis, and potential food intake attenuation effect of peptide YY in grass carp (*Ctenopharyngodon idellus*). *Gen. Comp. Endocrinol.* 187, 66–73. doi: 10.1016/j.ygcen.2013.03.029

Chisada, S.-I., Kurokawa, T., Murashita, K., Rønnestad, I., Taniguchi, Y., Toyoda, A., et al. (2014). Leptin receptor-deficient (knockout) medaka, *Oryzias latipes*, show chronical up-regulated levels of orexigenic neuropeptides, elevated food intake and stage specific effects on growth and fat allocation. *Gen. Comp. Endocrinol.* 195, 9–20. doi: 10.1016/j.ygcen.2013.10.008

Cone, R. D. (2006). Studies on the Physiological functions of the melanocortin system. *Endocr. Rev.* 27, 736–749. doi: 10.1210/er.2006-0034

Copeland, D. L., Duff, R. J., Liu, Q., Prokop, J., and Londraville, R. L. (2011). Leptin in teleost fishes: an argument for comparative study. *Front. Physiol.* 2:26. doi: 10.3389/fphys.2011.00026

Cottone, E., Guastalla, A., Pomatto, V., Campantico, E., Palermo, F., Magni, A. M., et al. (2009). Interplay of the endocannabinoid system with neuropeptide Y and corticotropin-releasing factor in the goldfish forebrain. *Ann. N. Y. Acad. Sci.* 1163, 372–375. doi: 10.1111/j.1749-6632.2009.04432.x

Cottone, E., Pomatto, V., Cerri, F., Campantico, E., Mackie, K., Delpero, M., et al. (2013). Cannabinoid receptors are widely expressed in goldfish: molecular cloning of a CB2-like receptor and evaluation of CB1 and CB2 mRNA expression profiles in different organs. *Fish Physiol. Biochem.* 39, 1287–1296. doi: 10.1007/s10695-013-9783-9

Cowan, E., Burch, K. J., Green, B. D., and Grieve, D. J. (2016). Obestatin as a key regulator of metabolism and cardiovascular function with emerging therapeutic potential for diabetes. *Br. J. Pharmacol.* 173, 2165–2181. doi: 10.1111/bph.13502

Crudo, M., Zizza, M., Panula, P., Canonaco, M., and Facciolo, R. M. (2013). Orexin-A influences mRNA expression of some glutamatergic receptor subtypes in *Carassius auratus* (Actinopterygii: Cyprinidae). *Ital. J. Zool.* 80, 329–336. doi: 10.1080/11250003.2013.823246

Cui, Y., Lv, S., Liu, J., Nie, S., Chen, J., Dong, Q., et al. (2016). Chronic perfluorooctanesulfonic acid exposure disrupts lipid metabolism in zebrafish. *Hum. Exp. Toxicol.* pii:0960327116646615. doi: 10.1177/0960327116646615

Dalman, M. R., Liu, Q., King, M. D., Bagatto, B., and Londraville, R. L. (2013). Leptin expression affects metabolic rate in zebrafish embryos (*D-rerio*). *Front. Physiol.* 4:160. doi: 10.3389/fphys.2013.00160

Dalmolin, C., Almeida, D. V., Figueiredo, M. A., and Marins, L. F. (2015). Food intake and appetite control in a GH-transgenic zebrafish. *Fish Physiol. Biochem.* 41, 1131–1141. doi: 10.1007/s10695-015-0074-5

D'angelo, L., Castaldo, L., De Girolamo, P., Lucini, C., Paolucci, M., Pelagalli, A., et al. (2016). Orexins and receptor OX2R in the gastroenteric apparatus of two teleostean species: *Dicentrarchus labrax* and *Carassius auratus*. *Anat. Rec.* 299, 1121–1129. doi: 10.1002/ar.23374

Danger, J. M., Tonon, M. C., Jenks, B. G., Saint-Pierre, S., Martel, J. C., Fasolo, A., et al. (1990). Neuropeptide Y: localization in the central nervous system and neuroendocrine functions. *Fundam. Clin. Pharmacol.* 4, 307–340. doi: 10.1111/j.1472-8206.1990.tb00497.x

Day, R. D., German, D. P., Manjakasy, J. M., Farr, I., Hansen, M. J., and Tibbetts, I. R. (2011). Enzymatic digestion in stomachless fishes: how a simple gut accommodates both herbivory and carnivory. *J. Comp. Physiol. B* 181, 603–613. doi: 10.1007/s00360-010-0546-y

De Pedro, N., Alonso-Gómez, A. L., Gancedo, B., Delgado, M. J., and Alonso-Bedate, M. (1993). Role of corticotropin-releasing factor (CRF) as a food intake regulator in goldfish. *Physiol. Behav.* 53, 517–520. doi: 10.1016/0031-9384(93)90146-7

de Pedro, N., and Björnsson, B. T. (2001). "Regulation of Food Intake by Neuropeptides and Hormones," in *Food Intake in Fish*, eds. D. Houlihan, T. Boujard, and M. Jobling (Hoboken, NJ; New Jersey, NJ: Blackwell Science Ltd), 269–296.

de Pedro, N., Cespedes, M. V., Delgado, M. J., and Alonso-Bedate, M. (1995). The galanin-induced feeding stimulation is mediated via alpha 2-adrenergic receptors in goldfish. *Regul. Pept.* 57, 77–84. doi: 10.1016/0167-0115(95)91255-4

de Pedro, N., López-Patiño, M. A., Guijarro, A. I., Pinillos, M. L., Delgado, M. J., and Alonso-Bedate, M. (2000). NPY receptors and opioidergic system are involved in NPY-induced feeding in goldfish. *Peptides* 21, 1495–1502. doi: 10.1016/S0196-9781(00)00303-X

de Pedro, N., Martinez-Alvarez, R., and Delgado, M. J. (2006). Acute and chronic leptin reduces food intake and body weight in goldfish (*Carassius auratus*). *J. Endocrinol.* 188, 513–520. doi: 10.1677/joe.1.06349

Demski, L. S. (2012). The neural control of feeding in elasmobranchs: a review and working model. *Environ. Biol. Fish.* 95, 169–183. doi: 10.1007/s10641-011-9827-x

do Rego, J.-C., Orta, M.-H., Leprince, J., Tonon, M.-C., Vaudry, H., and Costentin, J. (2006). Pharmacological characterization of the receptor mediating the anorexigenic action of the octadecaneuropeptide: evidence for an endozepinergic tone regulating food intake. *Neuropsychopharmacology* 32, 1641–1648. doi: 10.1038/sj.npp.1301280

Dockray, G. J. (2012). Cholecystokinin. *Curr. Opin. Endocrinol. Diabetes Obes.* 19, 8–12. doi: 10.1097/MED.0b013e32834eb77d

Douros, J. D., Baltzegar, D. A., Breves, J. P., Lerner, D. T., Seale, A. P., Grau, E. G., et al. (2014). Prolactin is a major inhibitor of hepatic Leptin A synthesis and secretion: studies utilizing a homologous Leptin A ELISA in the tilapia. *Gen. Comp. Endocrinol.* 207, 86–93. doi: 10.1016/J.Ygcen.2014.03.007

Einarsdottir, I. E., Power, D. M., Jonsson, E., and Bjornsson, B. T. (2011). Occurrence of ghrelin-producing cells, the ghrelin receptor and Na^{+}, K^{+}-ATPase in tissues of Atlantic halibut (*Hippoglossus hippoglossus*) during early development. *Cell Tissue Res.* 344, 481–498. doi: 10.1007/S00441-011-1158-X

Elbaz, I., Yelin-Bekerman, L., Nicenboim, J., Vatine, G., and Appelbaum, L. (2012). Genetic ablation of hypocretin neurons alters behavioral state transitions in zebrafish. *J. Neurosci.* 32, 12961–12972. doi: 10.1523/JNEUROSCI.1284-12.2012

El-Salhy, M. (1984). Occurrence of polypeptide YY (PYY) and pancreatic polypeptide (PP) in the gastrointestinal tract of the bony fish. *Biomed. Res.* 5, 441–444.

Escobar, S., Felip, A., Zanuy, S., and Carrillo, M. (2016). Is the kisspeptin system involved in responses to food restriction in order to preserve reproduction in pubertal male sea bass (*Dicentrarchus labrax*)? *Comp. Biochem. Physiol. Part A* 199, 38–46. doi: 10.1016/j.cbpa.2016.05.005

Ettore, V., Finizia, R., Elena, C., Giovanni, T., David, F., Paolo, D. G., et al. (2012). Immunohistochemical and immunological detection of ghrelin and leptin in rainbow trout *Oncorhynchus mykiss* and murray cod *Maccullochella peelii peelii* as affected by different dietary fatty acids. *Microsc. Res. Tech.* 75, 771–780. doi: 10.1002/jemt.21124

Facciolo, R. M., Crudo, M., Giusi, G., Alo, R., and Canonaco, M. (2009). Light- and dark-dependent orexinergic neuronal signals promote neurodegenerative phenomena accounting for distinct behavioral responses in the teleost *Thalassoma pavo*. *J. Neurosci. Res.* 87, 748–757. doi: 10.1002/jnr.21886

Facciolo, R. M., Crudo, M., Zizza, M., Giusi, G., and Canonaco, M. (2011). Feeding behaviors and ORXR-beta-GABA(A)R subunit interactions in *Carassius auratus*. *Neurotoxicol. Teratol.* 33, 641–650. doi: 10.1016/j.ntt.2011.09.008

Fekete, C., and Lechan, R. M. (2014). Central regulation of hypothalamic-pituitary-thyroid axis under physiological and pathophysiological conditions. *Endocr. Rev.* 35, 159–194. doi: 10.1210/er.2013-1087

Figueiredo-Silva, A. C., Saravanan, S., Schrama, J. W., Kaushik, S., and Geurden, I. (2012). Macronutrient-induced differences in food intake relate with hepatic oxidative metabolism and hypothalamic regulatory neuropeptides in rainbow trout (*Oncorhynchus mykiss*). *Physiol. Behav.* 106, 499–505. doi: 10.1016/j.physbeh.2012.03.027

FishBase (2016). *World Wide Web Electronic Publication*, eds R. Froese and D. Pauly. Available online at: http://www.fishbase.org, version (01/2016).

Flik, G., Klaren, P. H., Van den Burg, E. H., Metz, J. R., and Huising, M. O. (2006). CRF and stress in fish. *Gen. Comp. Endocrinol.* 146, 36–44. doi: 10.1016/j.ygcen.2005.11.005

Francis, D. S., Thanuthong, T., Senadheera, S. P. S. D., Paolucci, M., Coccia, E., De Silva, S. S., et al. (2014). n-3 LC-PUFA deposition efficiency and appetite-regulating hormones are modulated by the dietary lipid source during rainbow trout grow-out and finishing periods. *Fish Physiol. Biochem.* 40, 577–593. doi: 10.1007/S10695-013-9868-5

Froiland, E., Jobling, M., Bjornsson, B. T., Kling, P., Ravuri, C. S., and Jorgensen, E. H. (2012). Seasonal appetite regulation in the anadromous Arctic charr: evidence for a role of adiposity in the regulation of appetite but not for leptin in signalling adiposity. *Gen. Comp. Endocrinol.* 178, 330–337. doi: 10.1016/j.ygcen.2012.06.017

Fuentes, E. N., Kling, P., Einarsdottir, I. E., Alvarez, M., Valdes, J. A., Molina, A., et al. (2012). Plasma leptin and growth hormone levels in the fine flounder (*Paralichthys adspersus*) increase gradually during fasting and decline rapidly after refeeding. *Gen. Comp. Endocrinol.* 177, 120–127. doi: 10.1016/j.ygcen.2012.02.019

Fuentes, E. N., Safian, D., Einarsdottir, I. E., Valdes, J. A., Elorza, A. A., Molina, A., et al. (2013). Nutritional status modulates plasma leptin, AMPK and TOR activation, and mitochondrial biogenesis: implications for cell metabolism and growth in skeletal muscle of the fine flounder. *Gen. Comp. Endocrinol.* 186, 172–180. doi: 10.1016/j.ygcen.2013.02.009

Furutani, T., Masumoto, T., and Fukada, H. (2013). Molecular cloning and tissue distribution of cholecystokinin-1 receptor (CCK-1R) in yellowtail *Seriola quinqueradiata* and its response to feeding and *in vitro* CCK treatment. *Gen. Comp. Endocrinol.* doi: 10.1016/j.ygcen.2013.02.003

Gahete, M. D., Durán-Prado, M., Luque, R. M., Martínez-Fuentes, A. J., Quintero, A., Gutiérrez-Pascual, E., et al. (2009). Understanding the multifactorial control of growth hormone release by somatotropes. *Ann. N. Y. Acad. Sci.* 1163, 137–153. doi: 10.1111/j.1749-6632.2008.03660.x

Gambardella, C., Gallus, L., Amaroli, A., Terova, G., Masini, M. A., and Ferrando, S. (2012). Fasting and re-feeding impact on leptin and aquaglyceroporin 9 in the liver of European sea bass (*Dicentrarchus labrax*). *Aquaculture* 354–355, 1–6. doi: 10.1016/j.aquaculture.2012.04.043

Gaylord, T. G., MacKenzie, D. S., and Gatlin, D. M. (2001). Growth performance, body composition and plasma thyroid hormone status of channel catfish (*Ictalurus punctatus*) in response to short-term feed deprivation and refeeding. *Fish Physiol. Biochem.* 24, 73–79. doi: 10.1023/A:1011199518135

Gesto, M., Soengas, J. L., Rodriguez-Illamola, A., and Miguez, J. M. (2014). Arginine vasotocin treatment induces a stress response and exerts a potent anorexigenic effect in rainbow trout, *Oncorhynchus mykiss*. *J. Neuroendocrinol.* 26, 89–99. doi: 10.1111/jne.12126

Glasauer, S. M., and Neuhauss, S. C. (2014). Whole-genome duplication in teleost fishes and its evolutionary consequences. *Mol. Genet. Genomics* 289, 1045–1060. doi: 10.1007/s00438-014-0889-2

Gomes, A. S., Jordal, A. E., Olsen, K., Harboe, T., Power, D. M., and Ronnestad, I. (2015). Neuroendocrine control of appetite in Atlantic halibut (*Hippoglossus hippoglossus*): changes during metamorphosis and effects of feeding. *Comp. Biochem. Physiol. Part A Mol. Integr. Physiol.* 183, 116–125. doi: 10.1016/j.cbpa.2015.01.009

Gomes, A. S., Kamisaka, Y., Harboe, T., Power, D. M., and Ronnestad, I. (2014). Functional modifications associated with gastrointestinal tract organogenesis during metamorphosis in Atlantic halibut (*Hippoglossus hippoglossus*). *BMC Dev. Biol.* 14:11. doi: 10.1186/1471-213X-14-11

Gong, N., Jonsson, E., and Björnsson, B. T. (2016). Acute anorexigenic action of leptin in rainbow trout is mediated by the hypothalamic Pi3k pathway. *J. Mol. Endocrinol.* 56, 227–238. doi: 10.1530/JME-15-0279

Gong, Y., Luo, Z., Zhu, Q.-L., Zheng, J.-L., Tan, X.-Y., Chen, Q.-L., et al. (2013). Characterization and tissue distribution of leptin, leptin receptor and leptin receptor overlapping transcript genes in yellow catfish *Pelteobagrus fulvidraco*. *Gen. Comp. Endocrinol.* 182, 1–6. doi: 10.1016/j.ygcen.2012.11.006

Gonzalez, R., and Unniappan, S. (2010). Molecular characterization, appetite regulatory effects and feeding related changes of peptide YY in goldfish. *Gen. Comp. Endocrinol.* 166, 273–279. doi: 10.1016/j.ygcen.2009.09.008

Gonzalez, R., Kerbel, B., Chun, A., and Unniappan, S. (2010). Molecular, cellular and physiological evidences for the anorexigenic actions of Nesfatin-1 in goldfish. *PLoS ONE* 5:e15201. doi: 10.1371/journal.pone.0015201

Goodyear, K. (2012). *Effects of Thyroid Hormone Injections on Feeding and Appetite-Regulating Hormones in Goldfish (Carassius auratus).* Honours thesis, Memorial University of Newfoundland.

Gorissen, M. H. A. G., Flik, G., and Huising, M. O. (2006). Peptides and proteins regulating food intake: a comparative view. *Anim. Biol.* 56, 447–473. doi: 10.1163/157075606778967829

Gorissen, M., and Flik, G. (2014). Leptin in teleostean fish, towards the origins of leptin physiology. *J. Chem. Neuroanat.* 61–62, 200–206. doi: 10.1016/J.Jchemneu.2014.06.005

Gorissen, M., Bernier, N. J., Nabuurs, S. B., Flik, G., and Huising, M. O. (2009). Two divergent leptin paralogues in zebrafish (*Danio rerio*) that originate early in teleostean evolution. *J. Endocrinol.* 201, 329–339. doi: 10.1677/JOE-09-0034

Grone, B. P., Carpenter, R. E., Lee, M., Maruska, K. P., and Fernald, R. D. (2012). Food deprivation explains effects of mouthbrooding on ovaries and steroid hormones, but not brain neuropeptide and receptor mRNAs, in an African cichlid fish. *Horm. Behav.* 62, 18–26. doi: 10.1016/j.yhbeh.2012.04.012

Guijarro, A. I., Delgado, M. J., Pinillos, M. L., López-Pati-o, M. A., Alonso-Bedate, M., and De Pedro, N. (1999). Galanin and β-endorphin as feeding regulators in cyprinids: effect of temperature. *Aquat. Res.* 30, 483–489. doi: 10.1046/j.1365-2109.1999.00360.x

Guillot, R., Cortés, R., Navarro, S., Mischitelli, M., Garcia-Herranz, V., Sanchez, E., et al. (2016). Behind melanocortin antagonist overexpression in the zebrafish brain: a behavioral and transcriptomic approach. *Horm. Behav.* 82, 87–100. doi: 10.1016/j.yhbeh.2016.04.011

Habata, Y., Fujii, R., Hosoya, M., Fukusumi, S., Kawamata, Y., Hinuma, S., et al. (1999). Apelin, the natural ligand of the orphan receptor APJ, is abundantly secreted in the colostrum. *Biochim. Biophys. Acta* 1452, 25–35. doi: 10.1016/S0167-4889(99)00114-7

Hatef, A., Shajan, S., and Unniappan, S. (2015). Nutrient status modulates the expression of nesfatin-1 encoding nucleobindin 2A and 2B mRNAs in zebrafish gut, liver and brain. *Gen. Comp. Endocrinol.* 215, 51–60. doi: 10.1016/j.ygcen.2014.09.009

Hayes, J., and Volkoff, H. (2014). Characterization of the endocrine, digestive and morphological adjustments of the intestine in response to food deprivation and torpor in cunner, *Tautogolabrus adspersus*. *Comp. Biochem. Physiol. Part A* 170C, 46–59. doi: 10.1016/j.cbpa.2014.01.014

He, S., Liang, X.-F., Li, L., Sun, J., and Shen, D. (2013). Differential gut growth, gene expression and digestive enzyme activities in young grass carp (*Ctenopharyngodon idella*) fed with plant and animal diets. *Aquaculture* 410, 18–24. doi: 10.1016/j.aquaculture.2013.06.015

Hevrøy, E. M., Azpeleta, C., Shimizu, M., Lanzen, A., Kaiya, H., Espe, M., et al. (2011). Effects of short-term starvation on ghrelin, GH-IGF system, and IGF-binding proteins in Atlantic salmon. *Fish Physiol. Biochem.* 37, 217–232. doi: 10.1007/s10695-010-9434-3

Higgins, S. C., Gueorguiev, M., and Korbonits, M. R. (2007). Ghrelin, the peripheral hunger hormone. *Ann. Med.* 39, 116–136. doi: 10.1080/07853890601149179

Himick, B. A., and Peter, R. E. (1994). CCK/gastrin-like immunoreactivity in brain and gut, and CCK suppression of feeding in goldfish. *Am. J. Physiol. Regul. Integr. Comp. Physiol. 267*, R841–R851.

Holstein, B. (1982). Inhibition of gastric acid secretion inthe Atlantic cod, *Gadus morhua*, by sulphated and desulphated gastrin, caerulein, and CCK-octapeptide. *Acta Physiol. Scand.* 114, 453–459. doi: 10.1111/j.1748-1716.1982.tb07009.x

Holzer, P., Reichmann, F., and Farzi, A. (2012). Neuropeptide Y, peptide YY and pancreatic polypeptide in the gut-brain axis. *Neuropeptides* 46, 261–274. doi: 10.1016/j.npep.2012.08.005

Honkanen, R. E., Crim, J. W., and Patton, J. S. (1988). Effects of cholecystokinin peptides on digestive enzymes in killifish *in vivo*. *Comp. Biochem. Physiol. A* 89, 655–660. doi: 10.1016/0300-9629(88)90849-3

Hoskins, L. J., and Volkoff, H. (2012). The comparative endocrinology of feeding in fish: insights and challenges. *Gen. Comp. Endocrinol.* 176, 327–335. doi: 10.1016/j.ygcen.2011.12.025

Hoskins, L. J., Xu, M., and Volkoff, H. (2008). Interactions between gonadotropin-releasing hormone (GnRH) and orexin in the regulation of feeding and reproduction in goldfish (*Carassius auratus*). *Horm. Behav.* 54, 379–385. doi: 10.1016/j.yhbeh.2008.04.011

Hosomi, N., Furutani, T., Takahashi, N., Masumoto, T., and Fukada, H. (2014). Yellowtail neuropeptide Y: molecular cloning, tissue distribution, and response to fasting. *Fish. Sci.* 80, 483–492. doi: 10.1007/s12562-014-0711-4

Huang, H., Wei, Y., Meng, Z. N., Zhang, Y., Liu, X. C., Guo, L., et al. (2014). Polymorphisms of leptin-b gene associated with growth traits in orange-spotted grouper (*Epinephelus coioides*). *Int. J. Mol. Sci.* 15, 11996–12006. doi: 10.3390/Ijms150711996

Huesa, G., van den Pol, A. N., and Finger, T. E. (2005). Differential distribution of hypocretin (orexin) and melanin-concentrating hormone in the goldfish brain. *J. Comp. Neurol.* 488, 476–491. doi: 10.1002/cne.20610

Huising, M. O., Geven, E. J. W., Kruiswijk, C. P., Nabuurs, S. B., Stolte, E. H., Spanings, F. A. T., et al. (2006a). Increased leptin expression in common carp (*Cyprinus carpio*) after food intake but not after fasting or feeding to satiation. *Endocrinology* 147, 5786–5797. doi: 10.1210/en.2006-0824

Huising, M. O., Kruiswijk, C. P., and Flik, G. (2006b). Phylogeny and evolution of class-I helical cytokines. *J. Endocrinol.* 189, 1–25. doi: 10.1677/joe.1.06591

Ji, W., Ping, H.-C., Wei, K.-J., Zhang, G.-R., Shi, Z.-C., Yang, R.-B., et al. (2015). Ghrelin, neuropeptide Y (NPY) and cholecystokinin (CCK) in blunt snout bream (*Megalobrama amblycephala*): cDNA cloning, tissue distribution and mRNA expression changes responding to fasting and refeeding. *Gen. Comp. Endocrinol.* 223, 108–119. doi: 10.1016/j.ygcen.2015.08.009

Jin, Y., Tian, L. X., Xie, S. W., Guo, D. Q., Yang, H. J., Liang, G. Y., et al. (2015). Interactions between dietary protein levels, growth performance, feed utilization, gene expression and metabolic products in juvenile grass carp (*Ctenopharyngodon idella*). *Aquaculture* 437, 75–83. doi: 10.1016/j.aquaculture.2014.11.031

Johansson, M., and Björnsson, B. T. (2015). Elevated plasma leptin levels of fasted rainbow trout decrease rapidly in response to feed intake. *Gen. Comp. Endocrinol.* 214, 24–29. doi: 10.1016/j.ygcen.2015.02.020

Johansson, M., Morgenroth, D., Einarsdottir, I. E., Gong, N., and Bjornsson, B. T. (2016). Energy stores, lipid mobilization and leptin endocrinology of rainbow trout. *J. Comp. Physiol. B Biochem. Syst. Environ. Physiol.* 186, 759–773. doi: 10.1007/s00360-016-0988-y

Johnson, R. M., Johnson, T. M., and Londraville, R. L. (2000). Evidence for leptin expression in fishes. *J. Exp. Zool.* 286, 718–724. doi: 10.1002/(SICI)1097-010X(20000601)286:7<718::AID-JEZ6>3.0.CO;2-I

Jönsson, E. (2013). The role of ghrelin in energy balance regulation in fish. *Gen. Comp. Endocrinol.* 187, 79–85. doi: 10.1016/j.ygcen.2013.03.013

Jönsson, E., Kaiya, H., and Björnsson, B. T. (2010). Ghrelin decreases food intake in juvenile rainbow trout (*Oncorhynchus mykiss*) through the central anorexigenic corticotropin-releasing factor system. *Gen. Comp. Endocrinol.* 166, 39–46. doi: 10.1016/j.ygcen.2009.11.001

Jørgensen, E. H., Martinsen, M., Strøm, V., Hansen, K. E., Ravuri, C. S., Gong, N., et al. (2013). Long-term fasting in the anadromous Arctic charr is associated with downregulation of metabolic enzyme activity and upregulation of leptin A1 and SOCS expression in the liver. *J. Exp. Biol.* 216(Pt 17), 3222–3230. doi: 10.1242/jeb.088344

Kaiya, H., Konno, N., Kangawa, K., Uchiyama, M., and Miyazato, M. (2014). Identification, tissue distribution and functional characterization of the ghrelin receptor in West African lungfish, *Protopterus annectens*. *Gen. Comp. Endocrinol.* 209, 106–117. doi: 10.1016/J.Ygcen.2014.07.021

Kamijo, M., Kojima, K., Maruyama, K., Konno, N., Motohashi, E., Ikegami, T., et al. (2011). Neuropeptide Y in Tiger Puffer (*Takifugu rubripes*): distribution, cloning, characterization, and mRNA expression responses to prandial condition. *Zool. Sci.* 28, 882–890. doi: 10.2108/zsj.28.882

Kamisaka, Y., Totland, G. K., Tagawa, M., Kurokawa, T., Suzuki, T., Tanaka, M., et al. (2001). Ontogeny of cholecystokinin-immunoreactive cells in the digestive tract of *Atlantic halibut, Hippoglossus hippoglossus*, larvae. *Gen. Comp. Endocrinol.* 123, 31–37. doi: 10.1006/gcen.2001.7653

Kang, D. Y., and Kim, H. C. (2013a). Functional characterization of two melanin-concentrating hormone genes in the color camouflage, hypermelanosis, and appetite of starry flounder. *Gen. Comp. Endocrinol.* 189, 74–83. doi: 10.1016/j.ygcen.2013.04.025

Kang, D. Y., and Kim, H. C. (2013b). Influence of density and background color to stress response, appetite, growth, and blind-side hypermelanosis of flounder, *Paralichthys olivaceus. Fish Physiol. Biochem.* 39, 221–232. doi: 10.1007/s10695-012-9693-2

Kang, D. Y., and Kim, H. C. (2015). Functional relevance of three proopiomelanocortin (POMC) genes in darkening camouflage, blind-side hypermelanosis, and appetite of *Paralichthys olivaceus. Comp. Biochem. Physiol. Part B* 179, 44–56. doi: 10.1016/j.cbpb.2014.09.002

Kang, K. S., Yahashi, S., Azuma, M., and Matsuda, K. (2010). The anorexigenic effect of cholecystokinin octapeptide in a goldfish model is mediated by the vagal afferent and subsequently through the melanocortin- and corticotropin-releasing hormone-signaling pathways. *Peptides* 31, 2130–2134. doi: 10.1016/j.peptides.2010.07.019

Kang, K. S., Yahashi, S., and Matsuda, K. (2011). The effects of ghrelin on energy balance and psychomotor activity in a goldfish model: an overview. *Int. J. Pept.* 2011:171034. doi: 10.1155/2011/171034

Karra, E., Chandarana, K., and Batterham, R. L. (2009). The role of peptide YY in appetite regulation and obesity. *J. Physiol.* 587, 19–25. doi: 10.1113/jphysiol.2008.164269

Katan, T., Nash, G. W., Rise, M. L., Hall, J. R., Fernandes, J. M. O., Boyce, D., et al. (2016). A little goes long way: improved growth in Atlantic cod (*Gadus morhua*) fed small amounts of wild zooplankton. *Aquaculture* 451, 271–282. doi: 10.1016/j.aquaculture.2015.09.014

Kawauchi, H. (1983). Chemistry of proopiocortin-related peptides in the salmon pituitary. *Arch. Biochem. Biophys.* 227, 343–350. doi: 10.1016/0003-9861(83)90462-9

Kawauchi, H., Kawazoe, I., Tsubokawa, M., Kishida, M., and Baker, B. I. (1983). Characterization of melanin-concentrating hormone in chum salmon pituitaries. *Nature* 305, 321–323. doi: 10.1038/305321a0

Keen-Rhinehart, E., Ondek, K., and Schneider, J. E. (2013). Neuroendocrine regulation of appetitive ingestive behavior. *Front. Neurosci.* 7:213. doi: 10.3389/fnins.2013.00213

Kehoe, A. S., and Volkoff, H. (2007). Cloning and characterization of neuropeptide Y (NPY) and cocaine and amphetamine regulated transcript (CART) in Atlantic cod (*Gadus morhua*). *Comp. Biochem. Physiol. A Mol. Integr. Physiol.* 146, 451–461. doi: 10.1016/j.cbpa.2006.12.026

Kelly, S. P., and Peter, R. E. (2006). Prolactin-releasing peptide, food intake, and hydromineral balance in goldfish. *Am. J. Physiol. Regul. Integr. Comp. Physiol.* 291, R1474–R1481. doi: 10.1152/ajpregu.00129.2006

Kerbel, B., and Unniappan, S. (2012). Nesfatin-1 suppresses energy intake, co-localises ghrelin in the brain and gut, and alters ghrelin, cholecystokinin and orexin mRNA expression in goldfish. *J. Neuroendocrinol.* 24, 366–377. doi: 10.1111/j.1365-2826.2011.02246.x

Kim, J.-H., Leggatt, R. A., Chan, M., Volkoff, H., and Devlin, R. H. (2015). Effects of chronic growth hormone overexpression on appetite-regulating brain gene expression in coho salmon. *Mol. Cell. Endocrinol.* 413, 178–188. doi: 10.1016/j.mce.2015.06.024

Kitahara, N., Nishizawa, T., Iida, K., Okazaki, H., Andoh, T., and Soma, G.-I. (1988). Absence of a a-melanocyte-stimulating hormone sequence in proopiomelanocortin mRNA of chum salmon *Oncorhynchus keta. Comp. Biochem. Physiol. Part B Comp. Biochem.* 91, 365–370. doi: 10.1016/0305-0491(88)90155-1

Klovins, J., Haitina, T., Fridmanis, D., Kilianova, Z., Kapa, I., Fredriksson, R., et al. (2004). The melanocortin system in Fugu: determination of POMC/AGRP/MCR gene repertoire and synteny, as well as pharmacology and anatomical distribution of the MCRs. *Mol. Biol. Evol.* 21, 563–579. doi: 10.1093/molbev/msh050

Kobayashi, Y., Peterson, B. C., and Waldbieser, G. C. (2008). Association of cocaine- and amphetamine-regulated transcript (CART) messenger RNA level, food intake, and growth in channel catfish. *Comp. Biochem. Physiol. Part A* 151, 219–225. doi: 10.1016/j.cbpa.2008.06.029

Kojima, K., Amiya, N., Kamijo, M., Kageyama, H., Uchiyama, M., Shioda, S., et al. (2010). Relationship between alpha-melanocyte-stimulating hormone-and neuropeptide Y-containing neurons in the goldfish hypothalamus. *Gen. Comp. Endocrinol.* 167, 366–372. doi: 10.1016/j.ygcen.2009.12.004

Kojima, M., Hosoda, H., Date, Y., Nakazato, M., Matsuo, H., and Kangawa, K. (1999). Ghrelin is a growth-hormone-releasing acylated peptide from stomach. *Nature* 402, 656–660. doi: 10.1038/45230

Kono, T., Hamasuna, S., Korenaga, H., Iizasa, T., Nagamine, R., Ida, T., et al. (2012). The role of neuromedin U during inflammatory response in the common carp. *Fish Shellfish Immunol.* 32, 151–160. doi: 10.1016/j.fsi.2011.11.004

Köprücü, S., and Algül, S. (2015). Comparatively examining of the apelin-13 levels in the *Capoeta trutta* (Heckel, 1843) and *Cyprinus carpio* (Linnaeus, 1758). *J. Anim. Physiol. Anim. Nutr.* 99, 210–214. doi: 10.1111/jpn.12240

Kortner, T. M., Overrein, I., Oie, G., Kjorsvik, E., and Arukwe, A. (2011). The influence of dietary constituents on the molecular ontogeny of digestive capability and effects on growth and appetite in Atlantic cod larvae (*Gadus morhua*). *Aquaculture* 315, 114–120. doi: 10.1016/j.aquaculture.2010.04.008

Kousoulaki, K., Ronnestad, I., Olsen, H. J., Rathore, R., Campbell, P., Nordrum, S., et al. (2013). Krill hydrolysate free amino acids responsible for feed intake stimulation in Atlantic salmon (*Salmo salar*). *Aquac. Nutr.* 19(Suppl. 1, Sp. Iss. SI), 47–61. doi: 10.1111/anu.12094

Koven, W., and Schulte, P. (2012). The effect of fasting and refeeding on mRNA expression of PepT1 and gastrointestinal hormones regulating digestion and food intake in zebrafish (*Danio rerio*). *Fish Physiol. Biochem.* 38, 1565–1575. doi: 10.1007/s10695-012-9649-6

Kullgren, A., Jutfelt, F., Fontanillas, R., Sundell, K., Samuelsson, L., Wiklander, K., et al. (2013). The impact of temperature on the metabolome and endocrine metabolic signals in Atlantic salmon (*Salmo salar*). *Comp. Biochem. Physiol. A Mol. Integr. Physiol.* 164, 44–53. doi: 10.1016/J.Cbpa.2012.10.005

Kurokawa, T., Murashita, K., and Uji, S. (2006). Characterization and tissue distribution of multiple agouti-family genes in pufferfish, *Takifugu rubripes. Peptides* 27, 3165–3175. doi: 10.1016/j.peptides.2006.09.013

Kurokawa, T., Suzuki, T., and Andoh, T. (2000). Development of cholecystokinin and pancreatic polypeptide endocrine systems during the larval stage of Japanese flounder, *Paralichthys olivaceus. Gen. Comp. Endocrinol.* 120, 8–16. doi: 10.1006/gcen.2000.7512

Kurokawa, T., Uji, S., and Suzuki, T. (2005). Identification of cDNA coding for a homologue to mammalian leptin from pufferfish, *Takifugu rubripes. Peptides* 26, 745–750. doi: 10.1016/j.peptides.2004.12.017

Larsen, P. J., and Hunter, R. G. (2006). The role of CART in body weight homeostasis. *Peptides* 27, 1981–1986. doi: 10.1016/j.peptides.2005.11.027

Larsson, T. A., Tay, B.-H., Sundstrom, G., Fredriksson, R., Brenner, S., Larhammar, D., et al. (2009). Neuropeptide Y-family peptides and receptors in the elephant shark, *Callorhinchus milii* confirm gene duplications before the gnathostome radiation. *Genomics* 93, 254–260. doi: 10.1016/j.ygeno.2008.10.001

Le, H. T., Angotzi, A. R., Ebbesson, L. O., Karlsen, O., and Ronnestad, I. (2016). The ontogeny and brain distribution dynamics of the appetite regulators NPY, CART and OX in larval Atlantic cod (*Gadus morhua* L.). *PLoS ONE* 11:e0153743. doi: 10.1371/journal.pone.0153743

Le Bail, P.-Y., and Boeuf, G. (1997). What hormones may regulate appetite in fish? *Aquat. Living Resour.* 10, 371–379.

Leal, E., Fernández-Durán, B., Agulleiro, M. J., Conde-Siera, M., Miguez, J. M., and Cerda-Reverter, J. M. (2013). Effects of dopaminergic system activation on feeding behavior and growth performance of the sea bass (*Dicentrarchus labrax*): a self-feeding approach. *Horm. Behav.* 64, 113–121. doi: 10.1016/j.yhbeh.2013.05.008

Leder, E. H., and Silverstein, J. T. (2006). The pro-opiomelanocortin genes in rainbow trout (*Oncorhynchus mykiss*): duplications, splice variants, and differential expression. *J. Endocrinol.* 188, 355–363. doi: 10.1677/joe.1.06283

Lee, N., Kim, D., Lee, B., Kim, S., and Kim, K. (2015). Distribution of ghrelin immunoreactivity in artificially reared Japanese eel, *Anguilla japonica*, leptocephalus and metamorphosed glass eel. *J. Environ. Biol.* 36, 521–529.

Leknes, I. L. (2015). Mucin in epithelial cells in oesophagus and stomach of black tetra, *Gymnocorymbus ternetzi* (Characidae, Teleostei). *Zoomorphology* 134, 269–277. doi: 10.1007/s00435-015-0256-9

Li, A., Yuan, X., Liang, X.-F., Liu, L., Li, J., Li, B., et al. (2016). Adaptations of lipid metabolism and food intake in response to low and high fat diets in juvenile grass carp (*Ctenopharyngodon idellus*). *Aquaculture* 457, 43–49. doi: 10.1016/j.aquaculture.2016.01.014

Li, D., Liu, Z. D., and Xie, C. X. (2012). Effect of stocking density on growth and serum concentrations of thyroid hormones and cortisol in Amur sturgeon,

Acipenser schrenckii. *Fish Physiol. Biochem.* 38, 511–520. doi: 10.1007/s10695-011-9531-y

Li, G. G., Liang, X. F., Xie, Q. L., Li, G. Z., Yu, Y., and Lai, K. S. (2010). Gene structure, recombinant expression and functional characterization of grass carp leptin. *Gen. Comp. Endocrinol.* 166, 117–127. doi: 10.1016/j.ygcen.2009.10.009

Li, L., Wei, S., Huang, Q., Feng, D., Zhang, S., and Liu, Z. (2013). A novel galanin receptor 1a gene in zebrafish: tissue distribution, developmental expression roles in nutrition regulation. *Comp. Biochem. Physiol. Part B* 164, 159–167. doi: 10.1016/j.cbpb.2012.12.004

Li, S., Liu, Q., Xiao, L., Chen, H., Li, G., Zhang, Y., et al. (2016). Molecular cloning and functional characterization of spexin in orange-spotted grouper (*Epinephelus coioides*). *Comp. Biochem. Physiolo. Part B* 196–197, 85–91. doi: 10.1016/j.cbpb.2016.02.009

Li, S., Xiao, L., Liu, Q., Zheng, B., Chen, H., Liu, X., et al. (2015). Distinct functions of neuromedin U and neuromedin S in orange-spotted grouper. *J. Mol. Endocrinol.* 55, 95–106. doi: 10.1530/JME-15-0018

Libran-Perez, M., Velasco, C., Lopez-Patino, M. A., Miguez, J. M., and Soengas, J. L. (2014). Counter-regulatory response to a fall in circulating fatty acid levels in rainbow trout. Possible involvement of the hypothalamus-pituitary-interrenal axis. *PLoS ONE* 9:e113291. doi: 10.1371/journal.pone.0113291

Lin, F., Wu, H., Chen, H., Xin, Z., Yuan, D., Wang, T., et al. (2014a). Molecular and physiological evidences for the role in appetite regulation of apelin and its receptor APJ in Ya-fish (*Schizothorax prenanti*). *Mol. Cell. Endocrinol.* 396, 46–57. doi: 10.1016/j.mce.2014.08.009

Lin, F., Zhou, C., Chen, H., Wu, H., Xin, Z., Liu, J., et al. (2014b). Molecular characterization, tissue distribution and feeding related changes of NUCB2A/nesfatin-1 in Ya-fish (*Schizothorax prenanti*). *Gene* 536, 238–246. doi: 10.1016/j.gene.2013.12.031

Lin, X., Volkoff, H., Narnaware, Y., Bernier, N. J., Peyon, P., and Peter, R. E. (2000). Brain regulation of feeding behavior and food intake in fish. *Comp. Biochem. Physiol. Part A* 126, 415–434. doi: 10.1016/S1095-6433(00)00230-0

Lin, X., Wang, P., Ou, Y., Li, J., and Wen, J. (2016). An immunohistochemical study on endocrine cells in the neuroendocrine system of the digestive tract of milkfish *Chanos chanos* (Forsskal, 1775). *Aquac. Res.* doi: 10.1111/are.12979. [Epub ahead of print].

Liu, L., Liang, X.-F., Li, J., Yuan, X., Zhou, Y., and He, Y. (2014). Feed intake, feed utilization and feeding-related gene expression response to dietary phytic acid for juvenile grass carp (*Ctenopharyngodon idellus*). *Aquaculture* 424, 201–206. doi: 10.1016/j.aquaculture.2013.12.044

Liu, Y., Li, S. S., Huang, X. G., Lu, D. Q., Liu, X. C., Ko, W. H., et al. (2013). Identification and characterization of a motilin-like peptide and its receptor in teleost. *Gen. Comp. Endocrinol.* 186, 85–93. doi: 10.1016/J.Ygcen.2013.02.018

Liu, Y., Zhang, Y., Li, S., Huang, W., Liu, X., Lu, D., et al. (2009). Molecular cloning and functional characterization of the first non-mammalian 26RFa/QRFP orthologue in Goldfish, *Carassius auratus*. *Mol. Cell. Endocrinol.* 303, 82–90. doi: 10.1016/j.mce.2009.01.009

Loh, K., Herzog, H., and Shi, Y.-C. (2015). Regulation of energy homeostasis by the NPY system. *Trends Endocrinol. Metabol.* 26, 125–135. doi: 10.1016/j.tem.2015.01.003

Londraville, R. L., Macotela, Y., Duff, R. J., Easterling, M. R., Liu, Q., and Crespi, E. J. (2014). Comparative endocrinology of leptin: assessing function in a phylogenetic context. *Gen. Comp. Endocrinol.* 203, 146–157. doi: 10.1016/j.ygcen.2014.02.002

López, J. M., Sanz-Morello, B., and González, A. (2014). Organization of the orexin/hypocretin system in the brain of two basal actinopterygian fishes, the cladistians *Polypterus senegalus* and *Erpetoichthys calabaricus*. *Peptides* 61, 23–37. doi: 10.1016/j.peptides.2014.08.011

López-Patiño, M. A., Guijarro, A. I., Isorna, E., Delgado, M. J., Alonso-Bedate, M., and de Pedro, N. (1999). Neuropeptide Y has a stimulatory action on feeding behavior in goldfish (*Carassius auratus*). *Eur. J. Pharmacol.* 377, 147–153. doi: 10.1016/S0014-2999(99)00408-2

Lowry, C. A., and Moore, F. L. (2006). Regulation of behavioral responses by corticotropin-releasing factor. *Gen. Comp. Endocrinol.* 146, 19–27. doi: 10.1016/j.ygcen.2005.12.006

Lu, R.-H., Zhou, Y., Yuan, X.-C., Liang, X.-F., Fang, L., Bai, X.-L., et al. (2015). Effects of glucose, insulin and triiodothyroxine on leptin and leptin receptor expression and the effects of leptin on activities of enzymes related to glucose metabolism in grass carp (*Ctenopharyngodon idella*) hepatocytes. *Fish Physiol. Biochem.* 41, 981–989. doi: 10.1007/s10695-015-0063-8

Mabudi, H., Jamili, S., Majd, N. E., Vosoughi, G., Fatemi, M. R., and Rashed, S. (2011). The effects of ghrelin on ovary histology in *Barbus sharpeyi*. *J. Anim. Physiol. Anim. Nutr. (Berl.)* 95, 599–602. doi: 10.1111/j.1439-0396.2010.01089.x

MacDonald, E. E., and Volkoff, H. (2010). Molecular cloning and characterization of preproorexin in winter skate (*Leucoraja ocellata*). *Gen. Comp. Endocrinol.* 169, 192–196. doi: 10.1016/j.ygcen.2010.09.014

MacDonald, E., and Volkoff, H. (2009a). Cloning, distribution and effects of season and nutritional status on the expression of neuropeptide Y (NPY), cocaine and amphetamine regulated transcript (CART) and cholecystokinin (CCK) in winter flounder (*Pseudopleuronectes americanus*). *Horm. Behav.* 56, 58–65. doi: 10.1016/j.yhbeh.2009.03.002

MacDonald, E., and Volkoff, H. (2009b). Neuropeptide Y (NPY), cocaine- and amphetamine-regulated transcript (CART) and cholecystokinin (CCK) in winter skate (*Raja ocellata*): cDNA cloning, tissue distribution and mRNA expression responses to fasting. *Gen. Comp. Endocrinol.* 161, 252–261. doi: 10.1016/j.ygcen.2009.01.021

MacDonald, L. E., Alderman, S. L., Kramer, S., Woo, P. T. K., and Bernier, N. J. (2014). Hypoxemia-induced leptin secretion: a mechanism for the control of food intake in diseased fish. *J. Endocrinol.* 221, 441–455. doi: 10.1530/Joe-13-0615

Magalhaes, G. S., Junqueira-de-Azevedo, I. L. M., Lopes-Ferreira, M., Lorenzini, D. M., Ho, P. L., and Moura-da-Silva, A. M. (2006). Transcriptome analysis of expressed sequence tags from the venom glands of the fish *Thalassophryne nattereri*. *Biochimie* 88, 693–699. doi: 10.1016/j.biochi.2005.12.008

Majzoub, J. A. (2006). Corticotropin-releasing hormone physiology. *Eur. J. Endocrinol.* 155(suppl. 1), S71–S76. doi: 10.1530/eje.1.02247

Malagon, M., Vallarino, M., Tonon, M. C., and Vaudry, H. (1992). Localization and characterization of diazepam-binding inhibitor (DBI)-like peptides in the brain and pituitary of the trout (*Salmo gairdneri*). *Brain Res.* 576, 208–214. doi: 10.1016/0006-8993(92)90682-Y

Manuel, R., Gorissen, M., Roca, C. P., Zethof, J., van de Vis, H., Flik, G., et al. (2014). Inhibitory avoidance learning in zebrafish (*Danio rerio*): effects of shock intensity and unraveling differences in task performance. *Zebrafish* 11, 341–352. doi: 10.1089/zeb.2013.0970

Manuel, R., Gorissen, M., Stokkermans, M., Zethof, J., Ebbesson, L. O., Vis, H. V., et al. (2015). The effects of environmental enrichment and age-related differences on inhibitory avoidance in zebrafish (*Danio rerio* Hamilton). *Zebrafish* 12, 152–165. doi: 10.1089/zeb.2014.1045

Maruyama, K., Konno, N., Ishiguro, K., Wakasugi, T., Uchiyama, M., Shioda, S., et al. (2008). Isolation and characterisation of four cDNAs encoding neuromedin U (NMU) from the brain and gut of goldfish, and the inhibitory effect of a deduced NMU on food intake and locomotor activity. *J. Neuroendocrinol.* 20, 71–78. doi: 10.1111/j.1365-2826.2007.01615.x

Maruyama, K., Wada, K., Ishiguro, K., Shimakura, S.-I., Wakasugi, T., Uchiyama, M., et al. (2009). Neuromedin U-induced anorexigenic action is mediated by the corticotropin-releasing hormone receptor-signaling pathway in goldfish. *Peptides* 30, 2483–2486. doi: 10.1016/j.peptides.2009.08.013

Matsuda, K. (2009). Recent advances in the regulation of feeding behavior by neuropeptides in fish. *Ann. N. Y. Acad. Sci.* 1163, 241–250. doi: 10.1111/j.1749-6632.2008.03619.x

Matsuda, K., and Maruyama, K. (2007). Regulation of feeding behavior by pituitary adenylate cyclase-activating polypeptide (PACAP) and vasoactive intestinal polypeptide (VIP) in vertebrates. *Peptides* 28, 1761–1766. doi: 10.1016/j.peptides.2007.03.007

Matsuda, K., Arimura, A., Shioda, S., Takei, Y., Shimomura, H., and Uchiyama, M. (1997). "Pituitary adenylate-cyclase activating polypeptide (PACAP) in fishes: purification, distribution and physiological function," in *Advances in Comparative Endocrinology*, eds S. Kawashima and S. Kikuyama (Tome: Monduzzi Editore), 687–691.

Matsuda, K., Hagiwara, Y., Shibata, H., Sakashita, A., and Wada, K. (2013). Ovine corticotropin-releasing hormone (oCRH) exerts an anxiogenic-like action in the goldfish, *Carassius auratus*. *Gen. Comp. Endocrinol.* 188, 118–122. doi: 10.1016/j.ygcen.2013.01.001

Matsuda, K., Kang, K. S., Sakashita, A., Yahashi, S., and Vaudry, H. (2011a). Behavioral effect of neuropeptides related to feeding regulation in fish. *Ann. N. Y. Acad. Sci.* 1220, 117–126. doi: 10.1111/j.1749-6632.2010.05884.x

Matsuda, K., Kojima, K., Shimakura, S., Miura, T., Uchiyama, M., Shioda, S., et al. (2009). Relationship between melanin-concentrating hormone- and neuropeptide Y-containing neurons in the goldfish hypothalamus. *Comp. Biochem. Physiol. Part A* 153, 3–7. doi: 10.1016/j.cbpa.2008.10.002

Matsuda, K., Kojima, K., Wada, K., Maruyama, K., Leprince, J., Tonon, M. C., et al. (2010). The anorexigenic action of the octadecaneuropeptide (ODN) in goldfish is mediated through the MC4R- and subsequently the CRH receptor-signaling pathways. *J. Mol. Neurosci.* 42, 74–79. doi: 10.1007/s12031-010-9346-9

Matsuda, K., Maruyama, K., Nakamachi, T., Miura, T., and Shioda, S. (2006). Effects of pituitary adenylate cyclase-activating polypeptide and vasoactive intestinal polypeptide on food intake and locomotor activity in the goldfish, *Carassius auratus*. *Ann. N. Y. Acad. Sci.* 1070, 417–421. doi: 10.1196/annals.1317.054

Matsuda, K., Maruyama, K., Nakamachi, T., Miura, T., Uchiyama, M., and Shioda, S. (2005). Inhibitory effects of pituitary adenylate cyclase-activating polypeptide (PACAP) and vasoactive intestinal peptide (VIP) on food intake in the goldfish, *Carassius auratus*. *Peptides* 26, 1611–1616. doi: 10.1016/j.peptides.2005.02.022

Matsuda, K., Nakamura, K., Shimakura, S.-I., Miura, T., Kageyama, H., Uchiyama, M., et al. (2008). Inhibitory effect of chicken gonadotropin-releasing hormone II on food intake in the goldfish, *Carassius auratus*. *Horm. Behav.* 54, 83–89. doi: 10.1016/j.yhbeh.2008.01.011

Matsuda, K., Shimakura, S. I., Miura, T., Maruyama, K., Uchiyama, M., Kawauchi, H., et al. (2007a). Feeding-induced changes of melanin-concentrating hormone (MCH)-like immunoreactivity in goldfish brain. *Cell Tissue Res.* 328, 375–382. doi: 10.1007/s00441-006-0347-5

Matsuda, K., Wada, K., Azuma, M., Leprince, J., Tonon, M. C., Sakashita, A., et al. (2011b). The Octadecaneuropeptide exerts an anxiogenic-like action in goldfish. *Neuroscience* 181, 100–108. doi: 10.1016/j.neuroscience.2011.02.058

Matsuda, K., Wada, K., Miura, T., Maruyama, K., Shimakura, S. I., Uchiyama, M., et al. (2007b). Effect of the diazepam-binding inhibitor-derived peptide, octadecaneuropeptide, on food intake in goldfish. *Neuroscience* 150, 425–432. doi: 10.1016/j.neuroscience.2007.09.012

Matsuda, K., Yoshida, T., Nagano, Y., Kashimoto, K., Yatohgo, T., Shimomura, H., et al. (1998). Purification and primary structure of pituitary adenylate cyclase activating polypeptide (PACAP) from the brain of an elasmobranch, stingray, *Dasyatis akajei*. *Peptides* 19, 1489–1495. doi: 10.1016/S0196-9781(98)00091-6

Matty, A. J. (1986). Nutrition, hormones and growth. *Fish Physiol. Biochem.* 2, 141–150. doi: 10.1007/BF02264082

Mawhinney, R. M. S. (2007). *The Effect of Intracerebroventricular Injections of Kisspeptin and Human RFRP-3 on the Feeding Behaviour of Goldfish, Carassius auratus. Honours* thesis, Memorial University of Newfoundland.

McRory, J. E., Parker, D. B., Ngamvongchon, S., and Sherwood, N. M. (1995). Sequence and expression of cDNA for pituitary adenylate cyclase activating polypeptide (PACAP) and growth hormone-releasing hormone (GHRH)-like peptide in catfish. *Mol. Cell. Endocrinol.* 108, 169–177. doi: 10.1016/0303-7207(94)03467-8

Mennigen, J. A., Sassine, J., Trudeau, V. L., and Moon, T. W. (2010). Waterborne fluoxetine disrupts feeding and energy metabolism in the goldfish *Carassius auratus*. *Aquat. Toxicol.* 100, 128–137. doi: 10.1016/j.aquatox.2010.07.022

Mensah, E. T., Volkoff, H., and Unniappan, S. (2010). Galanin systems in non-mammalian vertebrates with special focus on fishes. *EXS* 102, 243–262. doi: 10.1007/978-3-0346-0228-0_17

Merchenthaler, I. (2010). Galanin and the neuroendocrine axes. *EXS* 102, 71–85. doi: 10.1007/978-3-0346-0228-0_7

Micale, V., Campo, S., D'Ascola, A., Guerrera, M. C., Levanti, M. B., Germana, A., et al. (2012). Cholecystokinin in white sea bream: molecular cloning, regional expression, and immunohistochemical localization in the gut after feeding and fasting. *PLoS ONE* 7:e52428. doi: 10.1371/journal.pone.0052428

Micale, V., Campo, S., D'Ascola, A., Guerrera, M. C., Levanti, M. B., Germana, A., et al. (2014). Cholecystokinin: how many functions? Observations in seabreams. *Gen. Comp. Endocrinol.* 205, 166–167. doi: 10.1016/j.ygcen.2014.02.019

Michel, M., Page-McCaw, P. S., Chen, W., and Cone, R. D. (2016). Leptin signaling regulates glucose homeostasis, but not adipostasis, in the zebrafish. *Proc. Natl Acad. Sci. U.S.A* 113, 3084–3089. doi: 10.1073/pnas.1513212113

Mikwar, M., Navarro-Martin, L., Xing, L., Volkoff, H., Hu, W., and Trudeau, V. L. (2016). Stimulatory effect of the secretogranin-11 derived peptide secretoneurin on food intake and locomotion in female goldfish (*Carassius auratus*). *Peptides* 78, 42–50. doi: 10.1016/j.peptides.2016.01.007

Miyata, A., Arimura, A., Dahl, R. R., Minamino, N., Uehara, A., Jiang, L., et al. (1989). Isolation of a novel 38 residue-hypothalamic polypeptide which stimulates adenylate cyclase in pituitary cells. *Biochem. Biophys. Res. Commun.* 164, 567–574. doi: 10.1016/0006-291X(89)91757-9

Mizusawa, K., Amiya, N., Yamaguchi, Y., Takabe, S., Amano, M., Breves, J. P., et al. (2012). Identification of mRNAs coding for mammalian-type melanin-concentrating hormone and its receptors in the scalloped hammerhead shark *Sphyrna lewini*. *Gen. Comp. Endocrinol.* 179, 78–87. doi: 10.1016/j.ygcen.2012.07.023

Moen, A.-G. G., and Finn, R. N. (2013). Short-term, but not long-term feed restriction causes differential expression of leptins in Atlantic salmon. *Gen. Comp. Endocrinol.* 183, 83–88. doi: 10.1016/j.ygcen.2012.09.027

Montero, M., Yon, L., Rousseau, K., Arimura, A., Fournier, A., Dufour, S., et al. (1998). Distribution, characterization, and growth hormone-releasing activity of pituitary adenylate cyclase-activating polypeptide in the European eel, *Anguilla anguilla*. *Endocrinology* 139, 4300–4310. doi: 10.1210/en.139.10.4300

Moore, W. G. (1941). Studies on the feeding habits of fishes. *Ecology* 22, 91–96. doi: 10.2307/1930015

Morley, J. E., Horowitz, M., Morley, P. M. K., and Flood, J. F. (1992). Pituitary adenylate cyclase activating polypeptide (PACAP) reduces food intake in mice. *Peptides* 13, 1133–1135. doi: 10.1016/0196-9781(92)90019-Y

Mukherjee, A., Subhedar, N. K., and Ghose, A. (2012). Ontogeny of the cocaine- and amphetamine-regulated transcript (CART) neuropeptide system in the brain of zebrafish, *Danio rerio*. *J. Comp. Neurol.* 520, 770–797. doi: 10.1002/cne.22779

Mulley, J. F., Hargreaves, A. D., Hegarty, M. J., Heller, R. S., and Swain, M. T. (2014). Transcriptomic analysis of the lesser spotted catshark (*Scyliorhinus canicula*) pancreas, liver and brain reveals molecular level conservation of vertebrate pancreas function. *BMC Genomics* 15:1074. doi: 10.1186/1471-2164-15-1074

Murashita, K., and Kurokawa, T. (2011). Multiple cocaine- and amphetamine-regulated transcript (CART) genes in medaka, *Oryzias latipes*: cloning, tissue distribution and effect of starvation. *Gen. Comp. Endocrinol.* 170, 494–500. doi: 10.1016/j.ygcen.2010.11.005

Murashita, K., Fukada, H., Hosokawa, H., and Masumoto, T. (2006). Cholecystokinin and peptide Y in yellowtail (*Seriola quinqueradiata*): molecular cloning, real-time quantitative RT-PCR, and response to feeding and fasting. *Gen. Comp. Endocrinol.* 145, 287–297. doi: 10.1016/j.ygcen.2005.09.008

Murashita, K., Fukada, H., Hosokawa, H., and Masumoto, T. (2007). Changes in cholecystokinin and peptide Y gene expression with feeding in yellowtail (*Seriola quinqueradiata*): relation to pancreatic exocrine regulation. *Comp. Biochem. Physiol. Part B Biochem. Mol. Biol.* 146, 318–325. doi: 10.1016/j.cbpb.2006.11.009

Murashita, K., Jordal, A. E. O., Nilsen, T. O., Stefansson, S. O., Kurokawa, T., Bjornsson, B. T., et al. (2011). Leptin reduces Atlantic salmon growth through the central pro-opiomelanocortin pathway. *Comp. Biochem. Physiol. A Mol. Integr. Physiol.* 158, 79–86. doi: 10.1016/j.cbpa.2010.09.001

Murashita, K., Kurokawa, T., Ebbesson, L. O. E., Stefansson, S. O., and Ronnestad, I. (2009a). Characterization, tissue distribution, and regulation of agouti-related protein (AgRP), cocaine- and amphetamine-regulated transcript (CART) and neuropeptide Y (NPY) in Atlantic salmon (*Salmo salar*). *Gen. Comp. Endocrinol.* 162, 160–171. doi: 10.1016/j.ygcen.2009.03.015

Murashita, K., Kurokawa, T., Nilsen, T. O., and Rønnestad, I. (2009b). Ghrelin, cholecystokinin, and peptide YY in Atlantic salmon (*Salmo salar*): molecular cloning and tissue expression. *Gen. Comp. Endocrinol.* 160, 223–235. doi: 10.1016/j.ygcen.2008.11.024

Mustonen, A. M., Nieminen, P., and Hyvarinen, H. (2002). Leptin, ghrelin, and energy metabolism of the spawning burbot (*Lota lota*, L.). *J. Exp. Zool.* 293, 119–126. doi: 10.1002/jez.10142

Nakamachi, T., Matsuda, K., Maruyama, K., Miura, T., Uchiyama, M., Funahashi, H., et al. (2006). Regulation by orexin of feeding behaviour and locomotor activity in the goldfish. *J. Neuroendocrinol.* 18, 290–297. doi: 10.1111/j.1365-2826.2006.01415.x

Nam, B. H., Moon, J. Y., Kim, Y. O., Kong, H. J., Kim, W. J., Kim, D. G., et al. (2013). Structural and functional characterization of pituitary adenylyl cyclase-activating polypeptide (PACAP)/PACAP-related peptide (PRP) and its receptor in olive flounder (Paralichthys olivaceus). *Comp. Biochem. Physiol. B Biochem. Mol. Biol.* 164, 18–28. doi: 10.1016/j.cbpb.2012.09.003

Narnaware, Y. K., Peyon, P. P., Lin, X., and Peter, R. E. (2000). Regulation of food intake by neuropeptide Y in goldfish. *Am. J. Physiol. Regul. Integr. Comp. Physiol.* 279, R1025–R1034.

Naumann, E. A., Kampff, A. R., Prober, D. A., Schier, A. F., and Engert, F. (2010). Monitoring neural activity with bioluminescence during natural behavior. *Nat. Neurosci.* 13, 513–520. doi: 10.1038/nn.2518

Nelson, J. S. (2006). *Fishes of the World.* New Jersey, NJ: John Wiley & Sons.

Nieminen, P., Mustonen, A.-M., and Hyvarinen, H. (2003). Fasting reduces plasma leptin- and ghrelin-immunoreactive peptide concentrations of the burbot (*Lota lota*) at 2C but not at 10C. *Zool. Sci.* 20, 1109–1115. doi: 10.2108/zsj.20.1109

Nisembaum, L. G., de Pedro, N., Delgado, M. J., and Isorna, E. (2014). Crosstalking between the "gut-brain" hormone ghrelin and the circadian system in the goldfish. Effects on clock gene expression and food anticipatory activity. *Gen. Comp. Endocrinol.* 205, 287–295. doi: 10.1016/j.ygcen.2014.03.016

Nishiguchi, R., Azuma, M., Yokobori, E., Uchiyama, M., and Matsuda, K. (2012). Gonadotropin-releasing hormone 2 suppresses food intake in the zebrafish, *Danio rerio. Front. Endocrinol.* 3:122. doi: 10.3389/fendo.2012.00122

Nishio, S., Gibert, Y., Berekelya, L., Bernard, L., Brunet, F., Guillot, E., et al. (2012). Fasting induces CART down-regulation in the zebrafish nervous system in a cannabinoid receptor 1-dependent manner. *Mol. Endocrinol.* 26, 1316–1326. doi: 10.1210/me.2011-1180

O'Carroll, A.-M., Lolait, S. J., Harris, L. E., and Pope, G. R. (2013). The apelin receptor APJ: journey from an orphan to a multifaceted regulator of homeostasis. *J. Endocrinol.* 219, R13–R35. doi: 10.1530/JOE-13-0227

Ohga, H., Matsumori, K., Kodama, R., Kitano, H., Nagano, N., Yamaguchi, A., et al. (2015). Two leptin genes and a leptin receptor gene of female chub mackerel (*Scomber japonicus*): molecular cloning, tissue distribution and expression in different obesity indices and pubertal stages. *Gen. Comp. Endocrinol.* 222, 88–98. doi: 10.1016/j.ygcen.2015.06.002

Olsson, C., and Holmgren, S. (2000). PACAP and nitric oxide inhibit contractions in the proximal intestine of the Atlantic cod, *Gadus morhua. J. Exp. Biol.* 203, 575–583.

Ortega, V. A., Lovejoy, D. A., and Bernier, N. J. (2013). Appetite-suppressing effects and interactions of centrally administered corticotropin-releasing factor, urotensin I and serotonin in rainbow trout (*Oncorhynchus mykiss*). *Front. Neurosci.* 7:196. doi: 10.3389/fnins.2013.00196

Osborne, N. N., Patel, S., Terenghi, G., Allen, J. M., Polak, J. M., and Bloom, S. R. (1985). Neuropeptide Y (NPY)-like immunoreactive amacrine cells in retinas of frog and goldfish. *Cell Tissue Res.* 241, 651–656. doi: 10.1007/BF00214587

O'Shea, M., Hansen, M. J., Tatemoto, K., and Morris, M. J. (2003). Inhibitory effect of apelin-12 on nocturnal food intake in the rat. *Nutr. Neurosci.* 6, 163–167. doi: 10.1080/1028415031000111273

Osugi, T., Son, Y. L., Ubuka, T., Satake, H., and Tsutsui, K. (2016). RFamide peptides in agnathans and basal chordates. *Gen. Comp. Endocrinol.* 227, 94–100. doi: 10.1016/j.ygcen.2015.06.012

Pagotto, U., Marsicano, G., Cota, D., Lutz, B., and Pasquali, R. (2006). The emerging role of the endocannabinoid system in endocrine regulation and energy balance. *Endocr. Rev.* 27, 73–100. doi: 10.1210/er.2005-0009

Palermo, F. A., Cardinaletti, G., Cocci, P., Tibaldi, E., Polzonetti-Magni, A., and Mosconi, G. (2013). Effects of dietary nucleotides on acute stress response and cannabinoid receptor 1 mRNAs in sole, *Solea solea. Comp. Biochem. Physiol. Part A* 164, 477–482. doi: 10.1016/j.cbpa.2012.12.005

Panula, P. (2010). Hypocretin/orexin in fish physiology with emphasis on zebrafish. *Acta Physiol.* 198, 381–386. doi: 10.1111/j.1748-1716.2009.02038.x

Papoutsoglou, S. E. (2012). The role of the brain in farmed fish. *Rev. Aquac.* 4, 1–10. doi: 10.1111/j.1753-5131.2012.01056.x

Park, H.-K., and Ahima, R. S. (2015). Physiology of leptin: energy homeostasis, neuroendocrine function and metabolism. *Metabolism* 64, 24–34. doi: 10.1016/j.metabol.2014.08.004

Parker, D. B., Coe, I. R., Dixon, G. H., and Sherwood, N. M. (1993). Two salmon neuropeptides encoded by one brain cDNA are structurally related to members of the glucagon superfamily. *Eur. J. Biochem.* 215, 439–448. doi: 10.1111/j.1432-1033.1993.tb18051.x

Paullada-Salmerón, J. A., Cowan, M., Aliaga-Guerrero, M., Gomez, A., Zanuy, S., Mananos, E., et al. (2016). LPXRFa peptide system in the European sea bass: a molecular and immunohistochemical approach. *J. Comp. Neurol.* 524, 176–198. doi: 10.1002/cne.23833

Pavlidis, M., Theodoridi, A., and Tsalafouta, A. (2015). Neuroendocrine regulation of the stress response in adult zebrafish, *Danio rerio. Prog. Neuropsychopharmacol. Biol. Psychiatry* 60, 121–131. doi: 10.1016/j.pnpbp.2015.02.014

Peng, W., Xu, J., Zhang, Y., Feng, J., Dong, C., Jiang, L., et al. (2016). An ultra-high density linkage map and QTL mapping for sex and growth-related traits of common carp (*Cyprinus carpio*). *Sci. Rep.* 6:26693. doi: 10.1038/srep26693

Penney, C. C., and Volkoff, H. (2014). Peripheral injections of cholecystokinin, apelin, ghrelin and orexin in cavefish (*Astyanax fasciatus* mexicanus): effects on feeding and on the brain expression levels of tyrosine hydroxylase, mechanistic target of rapamycin and appetite-related hormones. *Gen. Comp. Endocrinol.* 196, 34–40. doi: 10.1016/j.ygcen.2013.11.015

Pereira, R. T., Costa, L. S., Oliveira, I. R., Araujo, J. C., Aerts, M., Vigliano, F. A., et al. (2015). Relative distribution of gastrin-, CCK-8-, NPY- and CGRP-immunoreactive cells in the digestive tract of dorado (*Salminus brasiliensis*). *Tissue Cell* 47, 123–131. doi: 10.1016/j.tice.2015.01.009

Pérez Sirkin, D. I., Suzuki, H., Cánepa, M. M., and Vissio, P. G. (2013). Orexin and neuropeptide Y: tissue specific expression and immunoreactivity in the hypothalamus and preoptic area of the cichlid fish *Cichlasoma dimerus. Tissue Cell* 45, 452–459. doi: 10.1016/j.tice.2013.09.001

Peter, R. E. (1979). "The brain and feeding behavior," in *Fish Physiology,* Vol. VIII, eds. H. Ws, R. Dj, and B. Jr. (New York, NY: Academic Press), 121–159.

Peterson, B. C., Waldbieser, G. C., Riley, L. G., Upton, K. R., Kobayashi, Y., and Small, B. C. (2012). Pre- and postprandial changes in orexigenic and anorexigenic factors in channel catfish (*Ictalurus punctatus*). *Gen. Comp. Endocrinol.* 176, 231–239. doi: 10.1016/j.ygcen.2012.01.022

Peyon, P., Lin, X. W., Himick, B. A., and Peter, R. E. (1998). Molecular cloning and expression of cDNA encoding brain preprocholecystokinin in goldfish. *Peptides* 19, 199–210. doi: 10.1016/S0196-9781(97)00296-9

Peyon, P., Saied, H., Lin, X., and Peter, R. E. (1999). Postprandial, seasonal and sexual variations in cholecystokinin gene expression in goldfish brain. *Brain Res. Mol. Brain Res.* 74, 190–196. doi: 10.1016/S0169-328X(99)00282-X

Pfundt, B., Mielenz, B., Sanver, F., Pfeffer, E., Sauerwein, H., and Mielenz, M. (2016). Effects of largely different feeding intensities on serum insulin-like growth factor-1 concentrations, quantified by enzyme immunoassay, leptin and growth hormone receptor 1 mRNA in rainbow trout (*Oncorhynchus mykiss*). *Aquac. Nutr.* 22, 586–596. doi: 10.1111/anu.12282

Piccinetti, C. C., Migliarini, B., Petrosino, S., Di Marzo, V., and Carnevali, O. (2010). Anandamide and AM251, via water, modulate food intake at central and peripheral level in fish. *Gen. Comp. Endocrinol.* 166, 259–267. doi: 10.1016/j.ygcen.2009.09.017

Ping, H. C., Feng, K., Zhang, G. R., Wei, K. J., Zou, G. W., and Wang, W. M. (2013). Ontogeny expression of ghrelin, neuropeptide Y and cholecystokinin in blunt snout bream, *Megalobrama amblycephala. J. Anim. Physiol. Anim. Nutr.* doi: 10.1111/jpn.12084

Pohlenz, C., Buentello, A., Miller, T., Small, B. C., MacKenzie, D. S., and Gatlin, D. M. (2013). Effects of dietary arginine on endocrine growth factors of channel catfish, *Ictalurus punctatus. Comp. Biochem. Physiol. A Mol. Integr. Physiol.* 166, 215–221. doi: 10.1016/J.Cbpa.2013.06.016

Qu, D., Ludwig, D. S., Gammeltoft, S., Piper, M., Pelleymounter, M. A., Cullen, M. J., et al. (1996). A role for melanin-concentrating hormone in the central regulation of feeding behaviour. *Nature* 380, 243–247. doi: 10.1038/380243a0

Quillet, R., Ayachi, S., Bihel, F., Elhabazi, K., Ilien, B., and Simonin, F. (2016). RF-amide neuropeptides and their receptors in Mammals: pharmacological properties, drug development and main physiological functions. *Pharmacol. Ther.* 160, 84–132. doi: 10.1016/j.pharmthera.2016.02.005

Rajjo, I. M., Vigna, S. R., and Crim, J. W. (1988). Actions of cholecystokinin-related peptides on the gallbladder of bony fishes *in vitro. Comp. Biochem. Physiol. C* 90, 267–273. doi: 10.1016/0742-8413(88)90132-6

Renquist, B. J., Zhang, C., Williams, S. Y., and Cone, R. D. (2013). Development of an assay for high-throughput energy expenditure monitoring in the zebrafish. *Zebrafish* 10, 343–352. doi: 10.1089/zeb.2012.0841

Riediger, T., Zuend, D., Becskei, C., and Lutz, T. A. (2003). The anorectic hormone amylin contributes to feeding-related changes of neuronal activity in key structures of the gut-brain axis. *Am. J. Physiol. Regul. Integr. Comp. Physiol.* 286, R114–R122. doi: 10.1152/ajpregu.00333.2003

Roch, G. J., Busby, E. R., and Sherwood, N. M. (2014). GnRH receptors and peptides: skating backward. *Gen. Comp. Endocrinol.* 209, 118–134. doi: 10.1016/j.ygcen.2014.07.025

Rønnestad, I., Nilsen, T. O., Murashita, K., Angotzi, A. R., Moen, A. G. G., Stefansson, S. O., et al. (2010). Leptin and leptin receptor genes in Atlantic salmon: cloning, phylogeny, tissue distribution and expression correlated to long-term feeding status. *Gen. Comp. Endocrinol.* 168, 55–70. doi: 10.1016/j.ygcen.2010.04.010

Rui, L. (2013). Brain regulation of energy balance and body weight. *Rev. Endocr. Metabol. Disord.* 14, 387–407. doi: 10.1007/s11154-013-9261-9

Sakamoto, T., Iwata, K., and Ando, M. (2002). Growth hormone and prolactin expression during environmental adaptation of gobies. *Fish. Sci.* 68, 757–760. doi: 10.2331/fishsci.68.sup1_757

Sakurai, T. (2014). Roles of orexins in the regulation of body weight homeostasis. *Obes. Res. Clin. Pract.* 8, e414–e420. doi: 10.1016/j.orcp.2013.12.001

Salmerón, C., Johansson, M., Angotzi, A. R., Rønnestad, I., Jonsson, E., Bjornsson, B. T., et al. (2015). Effects of nutritional status on plasma leptin levels and *in vitro* regulation of adipocyte leptin expression and secretion in rainbow trout. *Gen. Comp. Endocrinol.* 210, 114–123. doi: 10.1016/j.ygcen.2014.10.016

Schroeter, J. C., Fenn, C. M., and Small, B. C. (2015). Elucidating the roles of gut neuropeptides on channel catfish feed intake, glycemia, and hypothalamic NPY and POMC expression. *Comp. Biochem. Physiol. Part A Mol. Integr. Physiol.* 188, 168–174. doi: 10.1016/j.cbpa.2015.06.031

Schwandt, S. E., Peddu, S. C., and Riley, L. G. (2010). Differential roles for octanoylated and decanoylated ghrelins in regulating appetite and metabolism. *Int. J. Pept.* 2010:275804. doi: 10.1155/2010/275804

Shanshan, L., Cuizhen, Z., and Gang, P. (2016). Effects of starvation on the expression of feeding related neuropeptides in the larval zebrafish hypothalamus. *Yi Chuan* 38, 821–830. doi: 10.16288/j.yczz.16-087

Shepherd, B. S., Eckert, S. M., Parhar, I. S., Vijayan, M. M., Wakabayashi, I., Hirano, T., et al. (2000). The hexapeptide KP-102 (D-ala-D-beta-Nal-ala-trp-D-phe-lys-NH(2)) stimulates growth hormone release in a cichlid fish (*Ooreochromis mossambicus*). *J. Endocrinol.* 167, R7–R10. doi: 10.1677/joe.0.167R007

Sherwood, N. M., Adams, B. A., Isaac, E. R., Wu, S., and Fradinger, E. A. (2007). Knocked down and out: PACAP in development, reproduction and feeding. *Peptides* 28, 1680–1687. doi: 10.1016/j.peptides.2007.03.008

Sherwood, N. M., Krueckl, S. L., and McRory, J. E. (2000). The origin and function of the pituitary adenylate cyclase-activating polypeptide (PACAP)/Glucagon superfamily. *Endocr. Rev.* 21, 619–670. doi: 10.1210/er.21.6.619

Shimakura, S., Marayama, K., Miura, T., Uchiyama, M., Kawauchi, H., Takahashi, A., et al. (2006). Effect of melanin-concentrating hormone on feeding behavior and locomotor activity in the goldfish, *Carassius auratus*. *Regul. Pept.* 135, 156–156.

Shpilman, M., Hollander-Cohen, L., Ventura, T., Gertler, A., and Levavi-Sivan, B. (2014). Production, gene structure and characterization of two orthologs of leptin and a leptin receptor in tilapia. *Gen. Comp. Endocrinol.* 207, 74–85. doi: 10.1016/j.ygcen.2014.05.006

Silverstein, J. T., and Plysetskaya, E. M. (2000). The effects of NPY and insulin on food intake regulation in fish. *Am. Zool.* 40, 296–308. doi: 10.1093/icb/40.2.296

Silverstein, J. T., Breininger, J., Baskin, D. G., and Plisetskaya, E. M. (1998). Neuropeptide Y-like gene expression in the salmon brain increases with fasting. *Gen. Comp. Endocrinol.* 110, 157–165. doi: 10.1006/gcen.1998.7058

Sinha, A. K., Liew, H. J., Diricx, M., Kumar, V., Darras, V. M., Blust, R., et al. (2012). Combined effects of high environmental ammonia, starvation and exercise on hormonal and ion-regulatory response in goldfish (*Carassius auratus* L.). *Aquat. Toxicol.* 114, 153–164. doi: 10.1016/j.aquatox.2012.02.027

Sinnett, P. M., and Markham, M. R. (2015). Food deprivation reduces and leptin increases the amplitude of an active sensory and communication signal in a weakly electric fish. *Horm. Behav.* 71, 31–40. doi: 10.1016/j.yhbeh.2015.03.010

Smith, S. M., and Vale, W. W. (2006). The role of the hypothalamic-pituitary-adrenal axis in neuroendocrine responses to stress. *Dialogues Clin. Neurosci.* 8, 383–395.

Sobrino Crespo, C., Perianes Cachero, A., Puebla Jimenez, L., Barrios, V., and Arilla Ferreiro, E. (2014). Peptides and food intake. *Front. Endocrinol.* 5:58. doi: 10.3389/fendo.2014.00058

Söderberg, C., Pieribone, V. A., Dahlstrand, J., Brodin, L., and Larhammar, D. (1994). Neuropeptide role of both peptide YY and neuropeptide Y in vertebrates suggested by abundant expression of their mRNAS in a cyclostome brain. *J. Neurosci. Res.* 37, 633–640. doi: 10.1002/jnr.490370510

Sohn, J. W. (2015). Network of hypothalamic neurons that control appetite. *BMB Rep.* 48, 229–233. doi: 10.5483/BMBRep.2015.48.4.272

Song, Y., and Cone, R. D. (2007). Creation of a genetic model of obesity in a teleost. *FASEB J.* 21, 2042–2049. doi: 10.1096/fj.06-7503com

Song, Y., Golling, G., Thacker, T. L., and Cone, R. D. (2003). Agouti-related protein (AGRP) is conserved and regulated by metabolic state in the zebrafish, *Danio rerio*. *Endocrine* 22, 257–265. doi: 10.1385/ENDO:22:3:257

Song, Y.-F., Wu, K., Tan, X.-Y., Zhang, L.-H., Zhuo, M.-Q., Pan, Y.-X., et al. (2015). Effects of recombinant human leptin administration on hepatic lipid metabolism in yellow catfish *Pelteobagrus fulvidraco*: *in vivo* and *in vitro* studies. *Gen. Comp. Endocrinol.* 212, 92–99. doi: 10.1016/j.ygcen.2015.01.022

Sterling, M. E., Karatayev, O., Chang, G. Q., Algava, D. B., and Leibowitz, S. F. (2015). Model of voluntary ethanol intake in zebrafish: effect on behavior and hypothalamic orexigenic peptides. *Behav. Brain Res.* 278, 29–39. doi: 10.1016/J.Bbr.2014.09.024

Striberny, A., Ravuri, C. S., Jobling, M., and Jorgensen, E. H. (2015). Seasonal differences in relative gene expression of putative central appetite regulators in Arctic charr (*Salvelinus alpinus*) do not reflect its annual feeding cycle. *PLoS ONE* 10:e0138857. doi: 10.1371/journal.pone.0138857

Subhedar, N. K., Nakhate, K. T., Upadhya, M. A., and Kokare, D. M. (2014). CART in the brain of vertebrates: circuits, functions and evolution. *Peptides* 54, 108–130. doi: 10.1016/j.peptides.2014.01.004

Subhedar, N., Barsagade, V. G., Singru, P. S., Thim, L., and Clausen, J. T. (2011). Cocaine- and amphetamine-regulated transcript peptide (CART) in the telencephalon of the catfish, *Clarias gariepinus*: distribution and response to fasting, 2-deoxy-D-glucose, glucose, insulin, and leptin treatments. *J. Comp. Neurol.* 519, 1281–1300. doi: 10.1002/cne.22569

Suda, A., Kaiya, H., Nikaido, H., Shiozawa, S., Mishiro, K., and Ando, H. (2012). Identification and gene expression analyses of ghrelin in the stomach of Pacific bluefin tuna (*Thunnus orientalis*). *Gen. Comp. Endocrinol.* 178, 89–97. doi: 10.1016/J.Ygcen.2012.04.026

Sun, J., He, S., Liang, X. F., Li, L., Wen, Z., Zhu, T., et al. (2014). Identification of SNPs in NPY and LEP and the association with food habit domestication traits in mandarin fish. *J. Genet.* 93, e118–e122. doi: 10.1007/s12041-014-0442-4

Sundarrajan, L., Blanco, A. M., Bertucci, J. I., Ramesh, N., Canosa, L. F., and Unniappan, S. (2016). Nesfatin-1-Like peptide encoded in nucleobindin-1 in goldfish is a novel anorexigen modulated by sex steroids, Macronutrients and daily rhythm. *Sci. Rep.* 6:28377. doi: 10.1038/srep28377

Sundström, G., Larsson, T. A., Xu, B., Heldin, J., and Larhammar, D. (2013). Interactions of zebrafish peptide YYb with the neuropeptide Y-family receptors Y4, Y7, Y8a, and Y8b. *Front. Neurosci.* 7:29. doi: 10.3389/fnins.2013.00029

Suzuki, H., Miyoshi, Y., and Yamamoto, T. (2007). Orexin-A (hypocretin 1)-like immunoreactivity in growth hormone-containing cells of the Japanese seaperch (*Lateolabrax japonicus*) pituitary. *Gen. Comp. Endocrinol.* 150, 205–211. doi: 10.1016/j.ygcen.2006.08.008

Suzuki, H., and Yamamoto, T. (2013). Orexin-B-like immunoreactivity localizes in both luteinizing-hormone-containing cells and melanin-concentrating hormone-containing fibers in the red-bellied piranha (*Pygocentrus nattereri*) pituitary. *Cell Tissue Res.* 351, 175–182. doi: 10.1007/S00441-012-1516-3

Tachibana, T., and Sakamoto, T. (2014). Functions of two distinct prolactin-releasing peptides evolved from a common ancestral gene. *Front. Endocrinol.* 5:170. doi: 10.3389/fendo.2014.00170

Takahashi, A. (2016). "Chapter 16 - proopiomelanocortin family A2 - Takei, Yoshio," in *Handbook of Hormones*, eds H. Ando and K. Tsutsui (San Diego, CA: Academic Press), e116–e113.

Takahashi, A., Amano, M., Itoh, T., Yasuda, A., Yamanome, T., Amemiya, Y., et al. (2005). Nucleotide sequence and expression of three subtypes of proopiomelanocortin mRNA in barfin flounder. *Gen. Comp. Endocrinol.* 141, 291–303. doi: 10.1016/j.ygcen.2005.01.010

Takahashi, A., Tsuchiya, K., Yamanome, T., Amano, M., Yasuda, A., Yamamori, K., et al. (2004). Possible involvement of melanin-concentrating hormone in food intake in a teleost fish, barfin flounder. *Peptides* 25, 1613–1622. doi: 10.1016/j.peptides.2004.02.022

Takeuchi, S. (2016). "Subchapter 8B - Agouti-Related Protein A2 - Takei, Yoshio," in *Handbook of Hormones*, eds. H. Ando and K. Tsutsui (San Diego, CA: Academic Press), 70–71.

Tang, Y., Li, H., Li, J., Yu, F., and Yu, J. (2014). Characterization and expression analysis of two distinct neuropeptide Ya paralogues in Jian carp (*Cyprinus carpio* var. *Jian). Fish Physiol. Biochem.* 40, 1709–1719. doi: 10.1007/s10695-014-9961-4

Tang, Z., Sun, C., Yan, A., Wu, S., Qin, C., Zhang, Y., et al. (2013). Genes involved in fatty acid metabolism: molecular characterization and hypothalamic mRNA response to energy status and neuropeptide Y treatment in the orange-spotted grouper *Epinephelus coioides*. *Mol. Cell. Endocrinol.* 376, 114–124. doi: 10.1016/j.mce.2013.06.020

Tatemoto, K., Carlquist, M., and Mutt, V. (1982). Neuropeptide Y: a novel brain peptide with structural similarities to peptide YY and pancreatic polypeptide. *Nature* 296, 659–660. doi: 10.1038/296659a0

Tatemoto, K., Hosoya, M., Habata, Y., Fujii, R., Kakegawa, T., Zou, M.-X., et al. (1998). Isolation and characterization of a novel endogenous peptide ligand for the human APJ receptor. *Biochem. Biophys. Res. Commun.* 251, 471–476. doi: 10.1006/bbrc.1998.9489

Thavanathan, R., and Volkoff, H. (2006). Effects of amylin on feeding of goldfish: interactions with CCK. *Regul. Pept.* 133, 90–96. doi: 10.1016/j.regpep.2005.09.025

Tian, J., He, G., Mai, K. S., and Liu, C. D. (2015). Effects of postprandial starvation on mRNA expression of endocrine-, amino acid and peptide transporter-, and metabolic enzyme-related genes in zebrafish (*Danio rerio*). *Fish Physiol. Biochem.* 41, 773–787. doi: 10.1007/s10695-015-0045-x

Tillner, R., Ronnestad, I., Dhert, P., and Ueberschar, B. (2014). The regulatory loop between gut cholecystokinin and tryptic enzyme activitcxuy in sea bass (*Dicentrarchus labrax*) larvae is influenced by different feeding regimes and trigger substances. *Aquaculture* 420, 139–146. doi: 10.1016/j.aquaculture.2013.10.046

Tillner, R., Ronnestad, I., Harboe, T., and Ueberschar, B. (2013). Hormonal control of tryptic enzyme activity in Atlantic cod larvae (*Gadus morhua*): involvement of cholecystokinin during ontogeny and diurnal rhythm. *Aquaculture* 402, 133–140. doi: 10.1016/j.aquaculture.2013.04.003

Tinoco, A. B., Näslund, J., Delgado, M. J., de Pedro, N., Johnsson, J. I., and Jonsson, E. (2014a). Ghrelin increases food intake, swimming activity and growth in juvenile brown trout (*Salmo trutta*). *Physiol. Behav.* 124, 15–22. doi: 10.1016/j.physbeh.2013.10.034

Tinoco, A. B., Nisembaum, L. G., de Pedro, N., Delgado, M. J., and Isorna, E. (2014b). Leptin expression is rhythmic in brain and liver of goldfish (*Carassius auratus*). Role of feeding time. *Gen. Comp. Endocrinol.* 204, 239–247. doi: 10.1016/j.ygcen.2014.06.006

Tinoco, A. B., Nisembaum, L. G., Isorna, E., Delgado, M. J., and de Pedro, N. (2012). Leptins and leptin receptor expression in the goldfish (*Carassius auratus*). Regulation by food intake and fasting/overfeeding conditions. *Peptides* 34, 329–335. doi: 10.1016/j.peptides.2012.02.001

Tinoco, A. B., Valenciano, A. I., Gomez-Boronat, M., Blanco, A. M., Nisembaum, L. G., De Pedro, N., et al. (2015). Two cholecystokinin receptor subtypes are identified in goldfish, being the CCKAR involved in the regulation of intestinal motility. *Comp. Biochem. Physiol. A Mol. Integr. Physiol.* 187, 193–201. doi: 10.1016/j.cbpa.2015.05.027

Tonon, M.-C., Leprince, J., Gandolfo, P., Compae, V., Pelletier, G., Malagon, M. M., et al. (2006). "Chapter 111 - Endozepines," in *Handbook of Biologically Active Peptides*, ed A. J. Kastin (Burlington, ON: Academic Press), 813–819.

Trombley, S., Maugars, G., Kling, P., Bjornsson, B. T., and Schmitz, M. (2012). Effects of long-term restricted feeding on plasma leptin, hepatic leptin expression and leptin receptor expression in juvenile Atlantic salmon (*Salmo salar* L.). *Gen. Comp. Endocrinol.* 175, 92–99. doi: 10.1016/j.ygcen.2011.10.001

Trombley, S., Mustafa, A., and Schmitz, M. (2014). Regulation of the seasonal leptin and leptin receptor expression profile during early sexual maturation and feed restriction in male Atlantic salmon, *Salmo salar* L., parr. *Gen. Comp. Endocrinol.* 204, 60–70. doi: 10.1016/J.Ygcen.2014.04.033

Trudeau, V. L., Martyniuk, C. J., Zhao, E., Hu, H., Volkoff, H., Decatur, W. A., et al. (2012). Is secretoneurin a new hormone? *Gen. Comp. Endocrinol.* 175, 10–18. doi: 10.1016/j.ygcen.2011.10.008

Tsujino, N., and Sakurai, T. (2009). Orexin/hypocretin: a neuropeptide at the interface of sleep, energy homeostasis, and reward system. *Pharmacol. Rev.* 61, 162–176. doi: 10.1124/pr.109.001321

Tsutsui, K., and Ubuka, T. (2013). "Chapter 107 - gonadotropin-inhibitory hormone," in *Handbook of Biologically Active Peptides, 2nd Edn.* ed A.J. Kastin. (Boston, CA: Academic Press), 802–811.

Tuziak, S. M., and Volkoff, H. (2012). A preliminary investigation of the role of melanin-concentrating hormone (MCH) and its receptors in appetite regulation of winter flounder (*Pseudopleuronectes americanus*). *Mol. Cell. Endocrinol.* 348, 281–296. doi: 10.1016/j.mce.2011.09.015

Tuziak, S. M., and Volkoff, H. (2013a). Melanin-concentrating hormone (MCH) and gonadotropin-releasing hormones (GnRH) in Atlantic cod, *Gadus morhua*: tissue distributions, early ontogeny and effects of fasting. *Peptides* 50, 109–118. doi: 10.1016/j.peptides.2013.10.005

Tuziak, S. M., and Volkoff, H., (2013b). Gonadotrophin-releasing hormone in winter flounder (*Pseudopleuronectes americanus*): molecular characterization, distribution and effects of fasting. *Gen. Comp. Endocrinol.* 184, 9–21. doi: 10.1016/j.ygcen.2012.12.010

Tuziak, S. M., Rise, M. L., and Volkoff, H. (2014). An investigation of appetite-related peptide transcript expression in Atlantic cod (*Gadus morhua*) brain following a *Camelina sativa* meal-supplemented feeding trial. *Gene* 550, 253–263. doi: 10.1016/j.gene.2014.08.039

Unniappan, S., Cerdá-Reverter, J. M., and Peter, R. E. (2004). *In situ* localization of preprogalanin mRNA in the goldfish brain and changes in its expression during feeding and starvation. *Gen. Comp. Endocrinol.* 136, 200–207. doi: 10.1016/j.ygcen.2003.12.010

Unniappan, S., Lin, X., Cervini, L., Rivier, J., Kaiya, H., Kangawa, K., et al. (2002). Goldfish ghrelin: molecular characterization of the complementary deoxyribonucleic acid, partial gene structure and evidence for Its stimulatory role in food intake. *Endocrinology* 143, 4143–4146. doi: 10.1210/en.2002-220644

Upton, K. R., and Riley, L. G. (2013). Acute stress inhibits food intake and alters ghrelin signaling in the brain of tilapia (*Oreochromis mossambicus*). *Domest. Anim. Endocrinol.* 44, 157–164. doi: 10.1016/J.Domaniend.2012.10.001

Valen, R., Jordal, A. E. O., Murashita, K., and Ronnestad, I. (2011). Postprandial effects on appetite-related neuropeptide expression in the brain of Atlantic salmon, *Salmo salar*. *Gen. Comp. Endocrinol.* 171, 359–366. doi: 10.1016/j.ygcen.2011.02.027

Valenti, M., Cottone, E., Martinez, R., De Pedro, N., Rubio, M., Viveros, M. P., et al. (2005). The endocannabinoid system in the brain of *Carassius auratus* and its possible role in the control of food intake. *J. Neurochem.* 95, 662–672. doi: 10.1111/j.1471-4159.2005.03406.x

Van Nguyen, M., Jordal, A. E. O., Espe, M., Buttle, L., Lai, H. V., and Ronnestad, I. (2013). Feed intake and brain neuropeptide Y (NPY) and cholecystokinin (CCK) gene expression in juvenile cobia fed plant-based protein diets with different lysine to arginine ratios. *Comp. Biochem. Physiol. A Mol. Integr. Physiol.* 165, 328–337. doi: 10.1016/j.cbpa.2013.04.004

Varricchio, E., Russo, F., Coccia, E., Mario Turchini, G., Scott Francis, D., and Paolucci, M. (2015). The orexinergic system in rainbow trout *Oncorhynchus mykiss* and its regulation by dietary lipids. *Microsc. Res. Tech.* 78, 707–714. doi: 10.1002/jemt.22528

Varricchio, E., Russo, F., Coccia, E., Turchini, G., Francis, D., De Girolamo, P., et al. (2012). Immunohistochemical and immunological detection of ghrelin and leptin in rainbow trout *Oncorhynchus mykiss* and murray cod *Maccullochella peelii* peelii as affected by different dietary fatty acids. *Microsc. Res. Tech.* 75, 771–780. doi: 10.1002/jemt.21124

Västermark, A., and Schioth, H. B. (2011). The early origin of melanocortin receptors, agouti-related peptide, agouti signalling peptide, and melanocortin receptor-accessory proteins, with emphasis on pufferfishes, elephant shark, lampreys, and amphioxus. *Eur. J. Pharmacol.* 660, 61–69. doi: 10.1016/j.ejphar.2010.10.106

Velasco, C., Librán-Pérez, M., Otero-Rodino, C., Lopez-Patino, M. A., Maguez, J. M., Cerda-Reverter, J. M., et al. (2016). Ghrelin modulates hypothalamic fatty acid-sensing and control of food intake in rainbow trout. *J. Endocrinol.* 228, 25–37. doi: 10.1530/JOE-15-0391

Vicentic, A., and Jones, D. C. (2007). The CART (cocaine- and amphetamine-regulated transcript) system in appetite and drug addiction. *J. Pharmacol. Exp. Ther.* 320, 499–506. doi: 10.1124/jpet.105.091512

Vieira-Lopes, D. A., Pinheiro, N. L., Sales, A., Ventura, A., Araujo, F. G., Gomes, I. D., et al. (2013). Immunohistochemical study of the digestive tract of *Oligosarcus hepsetus*. *World J. Gastroenterol.* 19, 1919–1929. doi: 10.3748/wjg.v19.i12.1919

Vigna, S. R., and Gorbman, A. (1977). Effects of cholecystokinin, gastrin, and related peptides on coho salmon gallbladder contraction *in vitro*. *Am. J. Physiol.* 232, E485–E491.

Vikesa, V., Nankervis, L., Remo, S. C., Waagbo, R., and Hevroy, E. M. (2015). Pre and postprandial regulation of ghrelin, amino acids and IGF1 in Atlantic salmon (*Salmo salar* L.) at optimal and elevated seawater temperatures. *Aquaculture* 438, 159–169. doi: 10.1016/j.aquaculture.2014.12.021

Vivas, Y., Azpeleta, C., Feliciano, A., Velarde, E., Isorna, E., Delgado, M. J., et al. (2011). Time-dependent effects of leptin on food intake and locomotor activity in goldfish. *Peptides* 32, 989–995. doi: 10.1016/j.peptides.2011.01.028

Volkoff, H. (2006). The role of neuropeptide Y, orexins, cocaine and amphetamine-related transcript, cholecystokinin, amylin and leptin in the regulation of feeding in fish. *Comp. Biochem. Physiol. A Mol. Integr. Physiol.* 144, 325–331. doi: 10.1016/j.cbpa.2005.10.026

Volkoff, H. (2011). "Control of appetite in fish," in *Encyclopedia of Fish Physiology*, ed A. P. Farrell (San Diego, CA: Academic Press), 1509–1514.

Volkoff, H. (2012). Sleep and orexins in non mammalian vertebrates. *Vitam. Horm.* 89, 315–339. doi: 10.1016/B978-0-12-394623-2.00017-2

Volkoff, H. (2013). The effects of amphetamine injections on feeding behavior and the brain expression of orexin, CART, tyrosine hydroxylase (TH) and thyrotropin releasing hormone (TRH) in goldfish (*Carassius auratus*). *Fish Physiol. Biochem.* 39, 979–991. doi: 10.1007/s10695-012-9756-4

Volkoff, H. (2014a). Appetite regulating peptides in red-bellied piranha, *Pygocentrus nattereri*: cloning, tissue distribution and effect of fasting on mRNA expression levels. *Peptides* 56C, 116–124. doi: 10.1016/j.peptides.2014.03.022

Volkoff, H. (2014b). *In vitro* assessment of interactions between appetite-regulating peptides in brain of goldfish (*Carassius auratus*). *Peptides* 61, 61–68. doi: 10.1016/j.peptides.2014.09.002

Volkoff, H. (2015a). Cloning and tissue distribution of appetite-regulating peptides in pirapitinga (*Piaractus brachypomus*). *J. Anim. Physiol. Anim. Nutr.* 99, 987–1001. doi: 10.1111/jpn.12318

Volkoff, H. (2015b). Cloning, tissue distribution and effects of fasting on mRNA expression levels of leptin and ghrelin in red-bellied piranha (*Pygocentrus nattereri*). *Gen. Comp. Endocrinol.* 217–218:20–27. doi: 10.1016/j.ygcen.2015.05.004

Volkoff, H., and Peter, R. E. (2000). Effects of CART peptides on food consumption, feeding and associated behaviors in the goldfish, *Carassius auratus*: actions on neuropeptide Y- and orexin A-induced feeding. *Brain Res.* 887, 125–133. doi: 10.1016/S0006-8993(00)03001-8

Volkoff, H., and Peter, R. E. (2001a). Characterization of two forms of cocaine- and amphetamine-regulated transcript (CART) peptide precursors in goldfish: molecular cloning and distribution, modulation of expression by nutritional status, and interactions with leptin. *Endocrinology* 142, 5076–5088. doi: 10.1210/endo.142.12.8519

Volkoff, H., and Peter, R. E. (2001b). Interactions between orexin A, NPY and galanin in the control of food intake of the goldfish, *Carassius auratus*. *Regul. Pept.* 101, 59–72. doi: 10.1016/S0167-0115(01)00261-0

Volkoff, H., and Wyatt, J. L. (2009). Apelin in goldfish (*Carassius auratus*): cloning, distribution and role in appetite regulation. *Peptides* 30, 1434–1440. doi: 10.1016/j.peptides.2009.04.020

Volkoff, H., Bjorklund, J. M., and Peter, R. E. (1999). Stimulation of feeding behavior and food consumption in the goldfish, Carassius auratus, by orexin-A and orexin-B. *Brain Res.* 846, 204–209. doi: 10.1016/S0006-8993(99)02052-1

Volkoff, H., Canosa, L. F., Unniappan, S., Cerda-Reverter, J. M., Bernier, N. J., Kelly, S. P., et al. (2005). Neuropeptides and the control of food intake in fish. *Gen. Comp. Endocrinol.* 142, 3–19. doi: 10.1016/j.ygcen.2004.11.001

Volkoff, H., Eykelbosh, A. J., and Peter, R. E. (2003). Role of leptin in the control of feeding of goldfish *Carassius auratus*: interactions with cholecystokinin, neuropeptide Y and orexin A, and modulation by fasting. *Brain Res.* 972, 90–109. doi: 10.1016/S0006-8993(03)02507-1

Volkoff, H., Hamoutene, D., and Payne, J. F. (2007). *Potential Effects of Tebufenozide on Feeding and Metabolism of Lake Trout (Salvelinus namaycush) Canadian Technical Report of Fisheries and Aquatic* Sciences.

Volkoff, H., Sabioni, R. E., and Cyrino, J. E. P. (2016). Appetite regulating factors in dourado, *Salminus brasiliensis*: cDNA cloning and effects of fasting and feeding on gene expression. *Gen. Comp. Endocrinol.* 237, 34–42. doi: 10.1016/j.ygcen.2016.07.022

Volkoff, H., Sabioni, R. E., Coutinho, L. L., and Cyrino, J. E. (2017). Appetite regulating factors in pacu (*Piaractus mesopotamicus*): tissue distribution and effects of food quantity and quality on gene expression. *Comp. Biochem. Physiol. Part A Mol. Integr. Physiol.* 203, 241–254. doi: 10.1016/j.cbpa.2016.09.022

Volkoff, H., Unniappan, S., and Kelly, S. P. (2009a). "The endocrine regulation of food intake," in *Fish Physiology*, eds N. J. Bernier, G. Van Der Kraak, A. P. Farrell, and C. J. Brauner (Cambridge, MA: Academic Press), 421–465.

Volkoff, H., Xu, M., MacDonald, E., and Hoskins, L. (2009b). Aspects of the hormonal regulation of appetite in fish with emphasis on goldfish, Atlantic cod and winter flounder: notes on actions and responses to nutritional, environmental and reproductive changes. *Comp. Biochem. Physiol. Part A Mol. Integr. Physiol.* 153, 8–12. doi: 10.1016/j.cbpa.2008.12.001

Wahlestedt, C., and Reis, D. J. (1993). Neuropeptide Y-related peptides and their receptors–are the receptors potential therapeutic drug targets? *Annu. Rev. Pharmacol. Toxicol.* 33, 309–352. doi: 10.1146/annurev.pa.33.040193.001521

Walewski, J. L., Ge, F., Lobdell, H., Levin, N., Schwartz, G. J., Vasselli, J., et al. (2014). Spexin is a novel human peptide that reduces adipocyte uptake of long chain fatty acids and causes weight loss in rodents with diet-induced obesity. *Obesity* 22, 1643–1652. doi: 10.1002/oby.20725

Wall, A., and Volkoff, H. (2013). Effects of fasting and feeding on the brain mRNA expressions of orexin, tyrosine hydroxylase (TH), PYY and CCK in the Mexican blind cavefish (*Astyanax fasciatus* mexicanus). *Gen. Comp. Endocrinol.* 183, 44–52. doi: 10.1016/j.ygcen.2012.12.011

Wan, Y., Zhang, Y., Ji, P., Li, Y., Xu, P., and Sun, X. (2012). Molecular characterization of CART, AgRP, and MC4R genes and their expression with fasting and re-feeding in common carp (*Cyprinus carpio*). *Mol. Biol. Rep.* 39, 2215–2223. doi: 10.1007/s11033-011-0970-4

Wang, K., Chen, X. T., Zhao, R. W., Hao, Q. R., Zhang, H., Xu, G. F., et al. (2013). Cloning and analysis of leptin in *Culter alburnus* in Xingkai Lake and down regulating its expression compared to cultured population. *J. Anim. Vet. Adv.* 12, 128–134. doi: 10.3923/javaa.2013.128.134

Wang, Q., Tan, X., Du, S., Sun, W., You, F., and Zhang, P. (2015). Characterization, tissue distribution, and expression of neuropeptide Y in olive flounder Paralichthys olivaceus. *Chinese J. Oceanol. Limnol.* 33, 553–558. doi: 10.1007/s00343-015-4090-1

Wang, T., Yuan, D., Zhou, C., Lin, F., Wei, R., Chen, H., et al. (2016). Molecular characterization of melanin-concentrating hormone (MCH) in *Schizothorax prenanti*: cloning, tissue distribution and role in food intake regulation. *Fish Physiol. Biochem.* 42, 883–893. doi: 10.1007/s10695-015-0182-2

Wang, T., Zhou, C., Yuan, D., Lin, F., Chen, H., Wu, H., et al. (2014). *Schizothorax prenanti* corticotropin-releasing hormone (CRH): molecular cloning, tissue expression, and the function of feeding regulation. *Fish Physiol. Biochem.* 40, 1407–1415. doi: 10.1007/s10695-014-9935-6

Wei, R., Yuan, D., Wang, T., Zhou, C., Lin, F., Chen, H., et al. (2013). Characterization, tissue distribution and regulation of agouti-related protein (AgRP) in a cyprinid fish (*Schizothorax prenanti*). *Gene* 527, 193–200. doi: 10.1016/j.gene.2013.06.003

Wei, R., Zhou, C., Yuan, D., Wang, T., Lin, F., Chen, H., et al. (2014). Characterization, tissue distribution and regulation of neuropeptideY in *Schizothorax prenanti*. *J. Fish Biol.* 85, 278–291. doi: 10.1111/jfb.12413

White, S. L., Volkoff, H., and Devlin, R. H. (2016). Regulation of feeding behavior and food intake by appetite-regulating peptides in wild-type and growth hormone-transgenic coho salmon. *Horm. Behav.* 84, 18–28. doi: 10.1016/j.yhbeh.2016.04.005

Won, E. T., and Borski, R. J. (2013). Endocrine regulation of compensatory growth in fish. *Front. Endocrinol.* 4:74. doi: 10.3389/fendo.2013.00074

Won, E. T., Baltzegar, D. A., Picha, M. E., and Borski, R. J. (2012). Cloning and characterization of leptin in a Perciform fish, the striped bass (*Morone saxatilis*):

control of feeding and regulation by nutritional state. *Gen. Comp. Endocrinol.* 178, 98–107. doi: 10.1016/j.ygcen.2012.04.019

Won, E. T., Douros, J. D., Hurt, D. A., and Borski, R. J. (2016). Leptin stimulates hepatic growth hormone receptor and insulin-like growth factor gene expression in a teleost fish, the hybrid striped bass. *Gen. Comp. Endocrinol.* 229, 84–91. doi: 10.1016/j.ygcen.2016.02.003

Wong, M. K., Sze, K. H., Chen, T., Cho, C. K., Law, H. C., Chu, I. K., et al. (2013). Goldfish spexin: solution structure and novel function as a satiety factor in feeding control. *Am. J. Physiol. Endocrinol. Metabol.* 305, E348–E366. doi: 10.1152/ajpendo.00141.2013

Woods, I. G., Schoppik, D., Shi, V. J., Zimmerman, S., Coleman, H. A., Greenwood, J., et al. (2014). Neuropeptidergic signaling partitions arousal behaviors in zebrafish. *J. Neurosci.* 34, 3142–3160. doi: 10.1523/JNEUROSCI.3529-13.2014

Woods, S. C., and Begg, D. P. (2016). "Regulation of the motivation to eat," in *Behavioral Neuroscience of Motivation*, eds E. H. Simpson and P. D. Balsam (Cham: Springer International Publishing), 15–34.

Wu, C. S., Wu, G. C., Zhang, G. Q., Wang, Q., Luo, J., and Chen, G. H. (2016). Single nucleotide polymorphisms in the leptin-a gene and associations with growth traits in the golden pompano, *Trachinotus blochii*. *J. World Aquac. Soc.* 47, 414–423. doi: 10.1111/jwas.12272

Xu, C., Li, X. F., Tian, H. Y., Jiang, G. Z., and Liu, W. B. (2016). Feeding rates affect growth, intestinal digestive and absorptive capabilities and endocrine functions of juvenile blunt snout bream *Megalobrama amblycephala*. *Fish Physiol. Biochem.* 42, 689–700. doi: 10.1007/s10695-015-0169-z

Xu, M., and Volkoff, H. (2007). Molecular characterization of prepro-orexin in Atlantic cod (*Gadus morhua*): Cloning, localization, developmental profile and role in food intake regulation. *Mol. Cell. Endocrinol.* 271, 28–37. doi: 10.1016/j.mce.2007.03.003

Xu, M., and Volkoff, H. (2009). Cloning, tissue distribution and effects of food deprivation on pituitary adenylate cyclase activating polypeptide (PACAP)/PACAP-related peptide (PRP) and preprosomatostatin 1 (PPSS 1) in Atlantic cod (*Gadus morhua*). *Peptides* 30, 766–776. doi: 10.1016/j.peptides.2008.12.010

Xu, M., Long, L., Chen, L., Qin, J., Zhang, L., Yu, N., et al. (2012). Cloning and differential expression pattern of pituitary adenylyl cyclase-activating polypeptide and the PACAP-specific receptor in darkbarbel catfish *Pelteobagrus vachelli*. *Comp. Biochem. Physiol. Part B Biochem. Mol. Biol.* 161, 41–53. doi: 10.1016/j.cbpb.2011.09.005

Yan, A., Zhang, L., Tang, Z., Zhang, Y., Qin, C., Li, B., et al. (2011). Orange-spotted grouper (*Epinephelus coioides*) orexin: molecular cloning, tissue expression, ontogeny, daily rhythm and regulation of NPY gene expression. *Peptides* 32, 1363–1370. doi: 10.1016/j.peptides.2011.05.004

Yan, A.-F., Chen, T., Chen, S., Ren, C.-H., Hu, C.-Q., Cai, Y.-M., et al. (2016). Goldfish leptin-AI and leptin-AII: function and central mechanism in feeding control. *Int. J. Mol. Sci.* 17:783. doi: 10.3390/ijms17060783

Yang, L., Sun, C., and Li, W. (2014). Neuropeptide B in *Nile tilapia Oreochromis niloticus*: molecular cloning and its effects on the regulation of food intake and mRNA expression of growth hormone and prolactin. *Gen. Comp. Endocrinol.* 200, 27–34. doi: 10.1016/j.ygcen.2014.01.016

Yang, S., Xu, G., Du, F., and Xu, P. (2016). Molecular cloning, tissue and embryonic development expression, and appetite regulatory effect of pancreatic peptide Y in *Coilia nasus*. *Fish. Sci.* 82, 347–355. doi: 10.1007/s12562-015-0960-x

Yokobori, E., Azuma, M., Nishiguchi, R., Kang, K. S., Kamijo, M., Uchiyama, M., et al. (2012). Neuropeptide Y stimulates food intake in the zebrafish, *Danio rerio*. *J. Neuroendocrinol.* 24, 766–773. doi: 10.1111/j.1365-2826.2012.02281.x

Yokobori, E., Kojima, K., Azuma, M., Kang, K. S., Maejima, S., Uchiyama, M., et al. (2011). Stimulatory effect of intracerebroventricular administration of orexin A on food intake in the zebrafish, *Danio rerio*. *Peptides* 32, 1357–1362. doi: 10.1016/j.peptides.2011.05.010

Yuan, D., Zhou, C., Wang, T., Lin, F., Chen, H., Wu, H., et al. (2014). Molecular characterization and tissue expression of peptide YY in *Schizothorax prenanti*: effects of periprandial changes and fasting on expression in the hypothalamus. *Regul. Pept.* 190–191, 32–38. doi: 10.1016/j.regpep.2014.03.004

Yuan, X., Cai, W., Liang, X. F., Su, H., Yuan, Y., Li, A., et al. (2015). Obestatin partially suppresses ghrelin stimulation of appetite in "high-responders" grass carp, *Ctenopharyngodon idellus*. *Comp. Biochem. Physiol. Part A* 184, 144–149. doi: 10.1016/j.cbpa.2015.02.019

Yuan, X., Li, A., Liang, X.-F., Huang, W., Song, Y., He, S., et al. (2016). Leptin expression in mandarin fish *Siniperca chuatsi* (Basilewsky): regulation by postprandial and short-term fasting treatment. *Comp. Biochem. Physiol. Part A Mol. Integr. Physiol.* 194, 8–18. doi: 10.1016/j.cbpa.2016.01.014

Zhang, H., Chen, H., Zhang, Y., Li, S., Lu, D., Zhang, H., et al. (2013). Molecular cloning, characterization and expression profiles of multiple leptin genes and a leptin receptor gene in orange-spotted grouper (*Epinephelus coioides*). *Gen. Comp. Endocrinol.* 181, 295–305. doi: 10.1016/j.ygcen.2012.09.008

Zhang, J., Ma, W., He, Y., Wu, J., Dawar, F. U., Ren, F., et al. (2016a). Sex biased expression of ghrelin and GHSR associated with sexual size dimorphism in yellow catfish. *Gene* 578, 169–176. doi: 10.1016/j.gene.2015.12.017

Zhang, J., Sun, P., Yang, F., Kong, T., and Zhang, R. (2016b). Tributyltin disrupts feeding and energy metabolism in the goldfish (*Carassius auratus*). *Chemosphere* 152, 221–228. doi: 10.1016/j.chemosphere.2016.02.127

Zhang, L., Nguyen, A. D., Lee, I. C. J., Yulyaningsih, E., Riepler, S. J., Stehrer, B., et al. (2012). NPY modulates PYY function in the regulation of energy balance and glucose homeostasis. *Diabetes Obes. Metabol.* 14, 727–736. doi: 10.1111/j.1463-1326.2012.01592.x

Zhang, X., Wu, Y., Hao, J., Zhu, J., Tang, N., Qi, J., et al. (2016c). Intraperitoneal injection urocortin-3 reduces the food intake of *Siberian sturgeon* (*Acipenser baerii*). *Peptides* 85, 80–88. doi: 10.1016/j.peptides.2016.09.007

Zhang, Y., Proenca, R., Maffei, M., Barone, M., Leopold, L., and Friedman, J. M. (1994). Positional cloning of the mouse obese gene and its human homologue. *Nature* 372, 425–432. doi: 10.1038/372425a0

Zhao, E., Zhang, D., Basak, A., and Trudeau, V. L. (2009). New insights into granin-derived peptides: evolution and endocrine roles. *Gen. Comp. Endocrinol.* 164, 161–174. doi: 10.1016/j.ygcen.2009.01.011

Zheng, J. L., Luo, Z., Hu, W., Liu, C. X., Chen, Q. L., Zhu, Q. L., et al. (2015). Different effects of dietary Zn deficiency and excess on lipid metabolism in yellow catfish *Pelteobagrus fulvidraco*. *Aquaculture* 435, 10–17. doi: 10.1016/j.aquaculture.2014.09.011

Zhong, C., Song, Y., Wang, Y., Zhang, T., Duan, M., Li, Y., et al. (2013). Increased food intake in growth hormone-transgenic common carp (*Cyprinus carpio* L.) may be mediated by upregulating Agouti-related protein (AgRP). *Gen. Comp. Endocrinol.* 192, 81–88. doi: 10.1016/j.ygcen.2013.03.024

Zhou, C., Zhang, X., Liu, T., Wei, R., Yuan, D., Wang, T., et al. (2014). *Schizothorax davidi* ghrelin: cDNA cloning, tissue distribution and indication for its stimulatory character in food intake. *Gene* 534, 72–77. doi: 10.1016/j.gene.2013.10.012

Zhou, C., Zheng, J., Lei, L., Yuan, D., Zhu, C., Ye, H., et al. (2016). Evidence that ghrelin may be associated with the food intake of gibel carp (*Carassius auratus* gibelio). *Fish Physiol. Biochem.* doi: 10.1007/s10695-016-0246-y. [Epub ahead of print].

Zhou, Y., Liang, X. F., Yuan, X. C., Li, J., He, Y., Fang, L., et al. (2013). Neuropeptide Y stimulates food intake and regulates metabolism in grass carp, *Ctenopharyngodon idellus*. *Aquaculture* 380, 52–61. doi: 10.1016/j.aquaculture.2012.11.033

10

Ghrelin-Reactive Immunoglobulins in Conditions of Altered Appetite and Energy Balance

Sergueï O. Fetissov[1,2], Nicolas Lucas[1,2] and Romain Legrand[1,2]*

[1] INSERM UMR1073, Nutrition, Gut and Brain Laboratory, Rouen, France, [2] Institute for Research and Innovation in Biomedicine (IRIB), University of Rouen Normandy, Rouen, France

***Correspondence:**
Sergueï O. Fetissov
serguei.fetissov@univ-rouen.fr

Part of circulating ghrelin is bound to immunoglobulins (Ig) protecting it from degradation and preserving its functional activity. This review summarizes the data on ghrelin- and desacyl-ghrelin-reactive IgG in conditions of altered appetite and energy balance. Plasma levels and affinity kinetics of such IgG were compared in patients with obesity and anorexia nervosa (AN) and in animal models of obesity including *ob/ob* mice, high-fat diet-induced obese mice, and obese Zucker rats as well as in mice after chronic food restriction and activity-based anorexia and in rats with methotrexate-induced anorexia. We show that plasmatic IgG in both obese humans and animals are characterized by increased affinity for ghrelin. In contrast, patients with AN and anorectic rodents all show lower affinity of ghrelin- and desacyl-ghrelin-reactive IgG, respectively, the changes which were not observed in non-anorectic, chronically starved mice. We also show that affinity of ghrelin-reactive IgG correlate with plasma levels of ghrelin. These data point to common mechanisms underlying modifications of affinity kinetics properties of ghrelin-reactive IgG during chronic alterations of energy balance in humans and rodents and support a functional role of such autoantibodies in ghrelin-mediated regulation of appetite.

Keywords: ghrelin, desacyl-ghrelin, anorexia, obesity, autoantibodies

INTRODUCTION

Ghrelin is a 28 amino acid acylated enteroendocrine peptide produced mainly in the stomach, which has been isolated and named based on its ability to stimulate growth hormone secretion (1). One of the main properties of ghrelin, independent from growth hormone secretagogue activity, is stimulation of feeding and body weight gain (2–4). Importantly, acylation of the serine 3 residue in the ghrelin's N-terminal by octanoic acid is necessary for binding of the growth hormone secretagogue receptor 1 (GHSR1), designated as ghrelin receptor (5) and biological activity including stimulation of food intake (6–8). However, the active, acylated form of ghrelin is unstable in the circulation and is degraded to desacyl-ghrelin (9, 10). The half-life pharmacokinetics properties of acyl-ghrelin in human plasma are about 10 min (11). The preservation of the acylated ghrelin form in the circulation appears, hence, as a key factor for maintaining its role in regulation of appetite and energy balance. Several mechanisms are involved in the regulation of ghrelin signaling during its production and receptor activation, which can be exploited for development of ghrelin-based therapy of altered appetite (12). Recently, a new regulatory factor of the ghrelin signaling has been identified, which is ghrelin-reactive immunoglobulins (Ig) (13). This review is the first attempt to summarize the data on ghrelin-reactive IgG obtained since their initial identification and the following studies in animal models of altered appetite and energy balance.

METHODS

The review focuses mainly on the data from five papers, all reporting affinity kinetics of ghrelin- and desacyl-ghrelin-reactive IgG. They include a study of patients with hyperphagic obesity and anorexia nervosa (AN) and of *ob/ob* mice by Takagi et al. (13); two studies by François et al. in high-fat diet (HFD)-induced obese mice (14) and in rats with methotrexate (MTX)-induced anorexia (15), a study by Lucas et al. in obese Zucker rats (16) as well as a Legrand et al. study in mice after chronic food-restriction and activity-based anorexia (17). In all mentioned studies, the same protocols of IgG plasma extraction and affinity kinetic assay by the surface plasmon resonance were used as was previously described in details (18). All measurements of ghrelin and desacyl-ghrelin peptides in above mentioned studies were performed using corresponding kits from Mitsubishi Chemical Med Corp. (Tokyo, Japan), selectively detecting acyl- and desacyl-ghrelin with resulting plasma ratios of 1:3 to 1:6 in humans. In the text, we use the terms of ghrelin and acyl-ghrelin as synonyms. For the statistical analysis of ghrelin and ghrelin-reactive IgG properties between different animal models and patients, they are shown as means of folds of changes vs. corresponding controls. In this analysis, we combined two animal models of anorexia including ABA mice and MTX rats and three animal models of obesity including *ob/ob* mice, HFD-induced obese mice, and obese Zucker rats. Group differences shown in **Tables 1–4** and **Figure 1** were analyzed using statistical tests indicated in the legends. We also used the Pearson's test to analyze correlations between plasma levels of ghrelin or desacyl-ghrelin and plasma levels and affinity (KD values) of corresponding IgG.

TABLE 1 | Plasma concentrations of acyl-ghrelin and desacyl-ghrelin in humans and rodents.

	Acyl-ghrelin (pM)		Desacyl-ghrelin (pM)		Acyl/desacyl-ghrelin ratio	
Mean ± SEM						
OB	24.88 ± 5.81	ns	137.7 ± 16.07	ns	1:6	↘$^{\$}$
AN	52.67 ± 7.14	↗$^{\$\$\$}$	249.1 ± 38.32	↗$^{\$\$\$}$	1:4	ns
Ctrl	25.65 ± 3.58		114.7 ± 29.24		1:3	
ob/ob	10.36 ± 0.96	↘$^{\#}$	75.17 ± 10.31	↘*	1:7	ns
Ctrl	13.02 ± 0.90		120.4 ± 17.32		1:8	
HFD	10.21 ± 0.95	ns	117.3 ± 9.75	↘**	1:10	ns
Ctrl	11.92 ± 1.45		196.5 ± 27.95		1:13	
Zucker	17.18 ± 1.59	ns	444.8 ± 33.86	↗*	1:25	ns
Ctrl	16.20 ± 4.38		242.0 ± 55.80		1:16	
ABA	21.58 ± 6.86	ns	1331.0 ± 87.52	↗$^{\$\$}$	1:63	ns
FTR	17.82 ± 5.02	ns	1221.0 ± 120.7	↗$^{\$}$	1:71	↘$^{\$}$
Ctrl	9.14 ± 2.50		195.8 ± 22.50		1:17	
MTX	12.68 ± 2.21	↗**	698.8 ± 95.8	↗*	1:46	ns
Ctrl	7.44 ± 1.08		352.4 ± 27.79		1:46	

Human patients: OB, obese; AN, anorexia nervosa. Rodent models of obesity: ob/ob mice; HFD, high fat diet-induced obese mice and Zucker rats. Rodent models of anorexia and starvation: ABA, activity-based anorexia in mice; FTR, feeding-time restriction in mice; and MTX, methotrexate-induced anorexia in rats. Ctrl, healthy human or rodent controls in corresponding row. Student's t-test or Mann–Whitney test, $^{*}p < 0.05$; $^{**}p < 0.01$; $^{\#}p < 0.10$. *ANOVA with Tukey's posttest or Kruskal–Wallis with Dunn's posttest* $^{\$}p < 0.05$, $^{\$\$}p < 0.01$, $^{\$\$\$}p < 0.001$.

DETECTION OF GHRELIN-REACTIVE IgG

Ghrelin-reactive IgG were first shown to be naturally present in plasma of healthy humans and rodents in 2008 by Fetissov et al. (19). Further studies confirmed and extended this initial finding by including female patients with restrictive AN (20) and with hyperphagic obesity (13). Moreover, a study using plasma samples of a large number of healthy male ($n = 562$) and female ($n = 636$) adolescents also revealed an ubiquitous presence of ghrelin-reactive autoantibodies of both IgG and IgM classes, which mean plasma levels were slightly elevated in girls vs. boys (21). In rodents, ghrelin-reactive IgG were detected in both rats (15, 19) and mice (13, 14, 17). Since the rodents studies were performed only in males, presence of possible sex differences of ghrelin-reactive IgG was not explored. However, it is likely that similarly to humans they may also be increased in female rodents who naturally display elevated plasma levels of total IgG and IgM as well as increased levels of autoantibodies reactive with other neuropeptides, e.g., α-melanocyte-stimulating hormone (α-MSH) (22).

Ghrelin-reactive IgG were also measured in the hypothalamic and liver tissue of C57Bl6 mice, showing their levels at the limit of detection (13). However, if levels of ghrelin-reactive IgG in these tissues of lean mice were stratified according to their exposure to a restraint stress in an EchoMRI instrument, which they had undergone prior to tissue sample for the analysis of their body composition, an increase is observed in both tissues and a decrease in plasma of stressed animals. It suggests that ghrelin-reactive IgG may help transportation of ghrelin mobilized during stress from plasma to its tissue targets.

Desacyl-ghrelin-reactive IgG are also present in humans (13, 20) and rodents (15, 17). Although some part of desacyl-ghrelin-reactive IgG may bind to acyl-ghrelin, they should also have distinct paratopes, because levels of desacyl-ghrelin IgG are often higher than of acyl-ghrelin IgG in human plasma (13, 20) and also because they have different affinity kinetics properties (13). The exact epitopes responsible for plasma IgG binding to ghrelin and desacyl-ghrelin remain to be been studied.

Both "free" and "total" ghrelin- and desacyl-ghrelin-reactive IgG are detected in plasma of humans and rodents. While "free" IgG are measured in physiological buffer, the "total" levels are measured in a high salt buffer, which dissociate immune complexes typically resulting in increased "total" vs. "free" levels of IgG. Accordingly, increased levels of free/total ratios may reflect an increase in IgG available to bind ghrelin or desacyl-ghrelin (**Table 2**).

ORIGIN AND REGULATION OF GHRELIN-REACTIVE IgG

Ghrelin-reactive IgG are natural autoantibodies and, therefore, are produced by germ-like B-cells as a part of native immunity (23). As was postulated by Avrameas, natural autoantibodies may participate in a complex regulatory network, not necessarily

TABLE 2 | Plasma levels of IgG reactive with acyl-ghrelin and desacyl-ghrelin in humans and rodents.

	Acyl-ghrelin-reactive IgG				Desacyl-ghrelin-reactive IgG				Acyl-ghrelin-reactive IgG		Desacyl-ghrelin-reactive IgG	
	Free		Total		Free		Total		Free/total ratio		Free/total ratio	
Mean ± SEM												
OB	0.291 ± 0.050	ns	0.617 ± 0.054	↘$^{\$}$	0.563 ± 0.049	ns	1.250 ± 0.057	ns	1:2.1	↗$^{\$}$	1:2.3	ns
AN	0.288 ± 0.020	ns	0.753 ± 0.049	ns	0.643 ± 0.054	ns	1.364 ± 0.080	ns	1:2.5	ns	1:2.1	ns
Ctrl	0.264 ± 0.020		0.918 ± 0.103		0.584 ± 0.094		1.384 ± 0.101		1:3.2		1:2.4	
ob/ob	0.133 ± 0.025	↘*	0.098 ± 0.013	↘#	n.a.	n.a.	1:0.6	ns	n.a.			
Ctrl	0.207 ± 0.024		0.162 ± 0.028		n.a.	n.a.			1:0.8		n.a.	
HFD	0.504 ± 0.050	ns	0.450 ± 0.033	↘**	n.a.	n.a.	1:0.8	ns	n.a.			
Ctrl	0.589 ± 0.067		0.624 ± 0.059		n.a.	n.a.			1:0.9		n.a.	
Zucker	0.268 ± 0.062	↘*	0.235 ± 0.073	↘*	0.244 ± 0.048	↘#	0.241 ± 0.066	↘*	1:0.6	↗*	1:0.8	↗*
Ctrl	0.715 ± 0.206		1.061 ± 0.259		0.627 ± 0.165		0.975 ± 0.225		1:1.5		1:1.5	
ABA	0.258 ± 0.084	ns	0.340 ± 0.127	ns	0.226 ± 0.091	ns	0.366 ± 0.127	ns	1:1.5	↗£	1:1.4	ns
FTR	0.187 ± 0.045		0.459 ± 0.109		0.242 ± 0.062		0.501 ± 0.127		1:2.4		1:2.0	
Ctrl	0.172 ± 0.052		0.315 ± 0.043		0.238 ± 0.069		0.464 ± 0.080		1:1.9		1:2.0	
MTX	0.063 ± 0.016	↘*	0.041 ± 0.007	↘***	0.070 ± 0.015	↘*	0.031 ± 0.006	↘***	1:0.6	↗***	1:0.4	↗***
Ctrl	0.188 ± 0.043		0.319 ± 0.044		0.223 ± 0.048		0.271 ± 0.036		1:1.7		1:1.2	

*Human patients: OB, obese; AN, anorexia nervosa. Rodent models of obesity: ob/ob mice; HFD, high fat diet-induced obese mice and Zucker rats. Rodent models of anorexia and starvation: ABA, activity-based anorexia in mice; FTR, feeding-time restriction in mice; and MTX, methotrexate-induced anorexia in rats. Ctrl, healthy human or rodent controls in corresponding row. Student's t-test or Mann–Whitney test, *p < 0.05; **p < 0.01; ***p < 0.001; #p < 0.10. ANOVA with Tukey's posttest or Kruskal–Wallis test with Dunns' posttest, $^{\$}p < 0.05$; ABA vs. FTR £p < 0.05.*

TABLE 3 | Affinity kinetics of acyl-ghrelin-reactive IgG in humans and rodents.

	Acyl-ghrelin-reactive IgG					
	Ka (1/Ms)		Kd (1/s)		KD (M)	
Mean ± SEM						
AN	9.36E+04 ± 2.23E+03	ns	3.25E−03 ± 8.04E−04	↗$^{\$}$	4.86E−07 ± 1.20E−07	↗$^{\$\$}$
OB	2.23E+04 ± 1.16E+04	↗$^{\$}$	1.86E−03 ± 3.04E−04	ns	1.91E−07 ± 1.48E−08	ns
Ctrl	6.84E+03 ± 1.19E+03		1.49E−03 ± 1.14E−04		2.54E−07 ± 2.81E±08	
ob/ob	1.01E+05 ± 9.46E+03	ns	1.81E−03 ± 7.81E−05	↘**	2.03E−08 ± 2.88E−09	↘*
Ctrl	8.89E+04 ± 9.08E+03		2.46E−03 ± 1.48E−04		3.02E−08 ± 3.57E−09	
HFD	1.68E+04 ± 4.87E+03	ns	1.58E−03 ± 3.22E−04	ns	1.17E−07 ± 1.18E−08	↘**
Ctrl	1.04E+04 ± 2.06E+03		2.02E−03 ± 2.82E−04		2.55E−07 ± 4.51E−08	
Zucker	1.01E+04 ± 1.54E+03	ns	1.22E−03 ± 1.61E−04	↘*	1.36E−07 ± 2.65E−08	↘*
Ctrl	7.93E+03 ± 6.53E+02		1.70E−03 ± 9.79E−05		2.24E−07 ± 2.50E−08	
ABA	4.72E+04 ± 8.12E+03	↗*,£	5.11E−04 ± 1.07E−04	ns	1.24E−08 ± 2.83E−09	ns
FTR	2.03E+04 ± 6.62E+03	ns	2.51E−04 ± 1.32E−04	ns	1.38E−08 ± 5.61E−09	ns
Ctrl	1.48E+04 ± 5.58E+03		2.45E−03 ± 1.15E−04		1.52E−08 ± 6.15E−09	
MTX	2.00E+03 ± 6.30E+02	ns	1.29E−03 ± 2.28E−04	↗**	1.18E−07 ± 4.92E−07	ns
Ctrl	1.79E+03 ± 5.06E+02		5.97E−04 ± 1.92E−04		5.73E−07 ± 2.49E−08	

*Human patients: OB, obese; AN, anorexia nervosa. Rodent models of obesity: ob/ob mice; HFD, high fat diet-induced obese mice and Zucker rats. Rodent models of anorexia and starvation: ABA, activity-based anorexia in mice; FTR, feeding-time restriction in mice; and MTX, methotrexate-induced anorexia in rats. Ctrl, healthy human or rodent controls in corresponding row. ANOVA with Tukey's posttest or Kruskal–Wallis test with Dunn's posttest, $^{\$}p < 0.05$; AN vs. OB $^{\$\$}p < 0.01$. Student's t-test or Mann–Whitney test vs. Ctrl *p < 0.05; **p < 0.01, vs. RFA £p < 0.05.*

directly related to the immune function but contributing to the homeostatic control (24). The production and affinity maturation of IgG are influenced by a variety of antigens and non-specific immune-stimulatory or inhibitory factors such as cytokines and steroid hormones. Moreover, increased plasma levels of ghrelin-reactive IgG in rats can be induced acutely by gastric electrical stimulation (25), suggesting that they can be stored and released upon a physiological stimulus. It is of interest that gastric electrical stimulation activated c-fos production in numerous lymphoid cells of the gastric mucosa surrounding the enteroendocrine ghrelin-synthetizing cells (26). Strong inhibition of ghrelin-reactive IgG levels in plasma is observed in rats after treatment with MTX, an immunosuppressive agent, which induces intestinal mucositis (15).

TABLE 4 | Affinity kinetics of desacyl-ghrelin-reactive IgG in humans and rodents.

	Desacyl-ghrelin-reactive IgG					
	Ka (1/Ms)		Kd (1/s)		KD (M)	
Mean ± SEM						
AN	1.04E+04 ± 1.02E+03	ns	2.26E−03 ± 3.86E−04	ns	8.61E−07 ± 7.17E−08	ns
OB	2.21E+04 ± 9.80E+03	ns	1.74E−03 ± 4.16E−04	ns	1.47E−07 ± 1.69E−08	ns
Ctrl	1.21E+04 ± 1.28E+03		1.65E−03 ± 1.50E−04		1.51E−07 ± 1.56E−08	
ob/ob	3.73E+03 ± 3.61E+03	↘#	7.23E−03 ± 8.10E−07	ns	9.59E−06 ± 3.76E−06	ns
Ctrl	1.89E+04 ± 9.33E+03		2.68E−05 ± 1.55E−05		4.13E−06 ± 3.38E−06	
HFD	2.72E+03 ± 1.74E+03	ns	1.34E−04 ± 1.30E−04	↘*	3.79E−08 ± 1.47E−08	↘#
Ctrl	1.09E+04 ± 4.71E+03		8.39E−04 ± 3.03E−04		1.38E−07 ± 4.72E−08	
Zucker	2.40E+04 ± 3.55E+03	ns	1.34E−03 ± 3.51E−04	↘*	6.78E−08 ± 2.30E−08	ns
Ctrl	2.85E+04 ± 4.24E+03		2.26E−03 ± 3.05E−04		9.88E−08 ± 2.21E−08	
ABA	1.94E+04 ± 8.06E+03	ns	1.12E−03 ± 2.09E−04	↗$$	9.20E−08 ± 2.34E−08	↗$
FTR	8.32E+03 ± 2.89E+03	ns	3.24E−04 ± 2.03E−04	ns	1.03E−07 ± 5.97E−08	ns
Ctrl	1.74E+04 ± 9.64E+03		2.07E−06 ± 1.20E−06		1.57E−08 ± 1.06E−09	
MTX	2.56E+03 ± 1.55E+03	ns	2.01E−04 ± 1.33E−04	ns	6.97E−08 ± 1.73E−08	↗*
Ctrl	1.71E+02 ± 1.33E+02		1.05E−06 ± 2.16E−07		2.07E−08 ± 5.46E−09	

Human patients: OB, obese; AN, anorexia nervosa. Rodent models of obesity: ob/ob mice; HFD, high fat diet-induced obese mice and Zucker rats. Rodent models of anorexia and starvation: ABA, activity-based anorexia in mice; FTR, feeding-time restriction in mice; and MTX, methotrexate-induced anorexia in rats. Ctrl, healthy human or rodent controls in corresponding row. ANOVA with Tukey's posttest or Kruskal–Wallis test with Dunn's posttest, $^{\$}p < 0.05$; $^{\$\$}p < 0.01$. Student's t-test or Mann–Whitney test, vs. Ctrl $^{*}p < 0.05$; $^{\#}p < 0.10$.

A particular role in production of IgG and other classes of Ig can be played by antigens derived from gut microbiota as a constitutive part of the gastro-intestinal tract in all animals (27). The gut bacterial antigens may also be involved in regulation of production and properties of ghrelin-reactive IgG. In fact, germ-free rats showed elevated plasma levels of ghrelin-reactive IgG (19), supporting a role of some intestinal antigens in tolerization toward ghrelin (28). The molecular basis linking microbial antigens with peptides may relate to the concept of molecular mimicry by cross-reactive autoantibody production (29). Indeed, sequence homology between ghrelin and several proteins from commensal gut microorganisms was shown, e.g., of seven consecutive amino acids present in a protein from *Enterococcus faecalis* (19). A role of molecular mimicry was recently validated as a mechanism underlying production of α-MSH-reactive IgG induced by caseinolytic peptidase B (ClpB) homolog protein from *Escherichia coli* (30). ClpB contains a discontinuous six amino acid homology with α-MSH; immunization of mice with ClpB generates α-MSH-cross reactive IgG (30). Plasma presence of the IgA class of ghrelin-reactive IgG also points to their origin triggered by luminal antigens (19).

Beside the stimulation of antigens from commensal gut microbiota, pathogenic and environmental microorganisms may possibly influence production of ghrelin-reactive IgG. In fact, plasma levels of ghrelin-reactive IgG in healthy adolescents correlate strongly with both IgG and IgM directed against influenza A virus (21). Although the initial *in silico* search for five consecutive amino acids sequence homology did not reveal matches between ghrelin and the Influenza viruses (19), a discontinuous eight amino acid homology for ghrelin is present in the PB1-F2 influenza A protein.

Another example of ghrelin-reactive IgG comes from studies of children with idiopathic short stature by the Lewinski group.

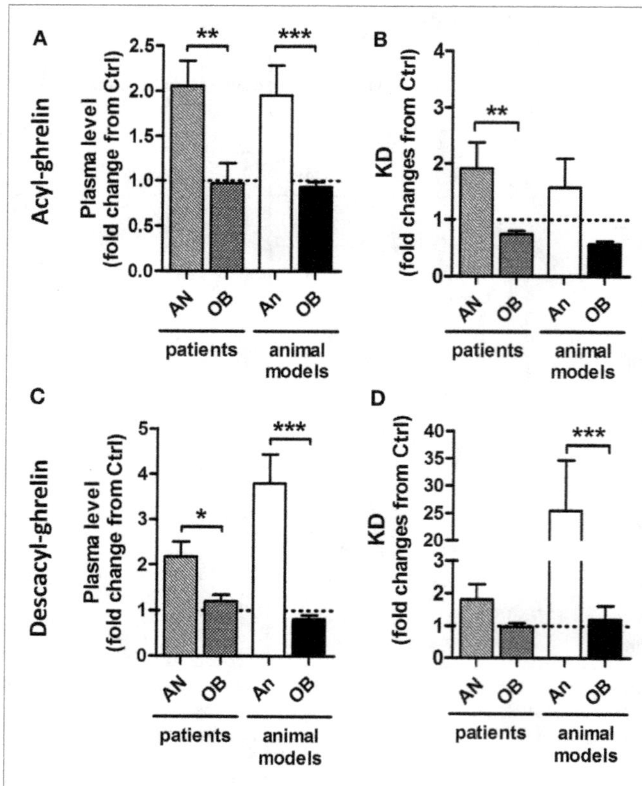

FIGURE 1 | Relative to control (Ctrl) values (1.0) changes in plasma ghrelin and desacyl ghrelin as well as affinity of their reactive IgG in patients and animal models of obesity and anorexia. Changes in plasma levels of acyl-ghrelin **(A)** and desacyl-ghrelin **(C)**. Changes in affinity (dissociation equilibrium constant, KD) of plasmatic IgG for acyl-ghrelin **(B)** and desacyl ghrelin **(D)**. AN, anorexia nervosa patients; An, animal models of anorexia; OB, obese patients or animals. Mann–Whitney tests $^{***}p < 0.001$, $^{**}p < 0.01$, and $^{*}p < 0.05$.

They showed that prevalence of high level IgG reactive with several peptide hormones, including ghrelin, orexin A, leptin, and α-MSH combined, was associated with an increased incidence of *Helicobacter pylori* and/or *Candida albicans* (31). A follow-up study showed that mean plasma levels of ghrelin-reactive IgG were also elevated in children with short stature, but they were not significantly different in patients with growth hormone deficiency (32). Since *H. pylori* is only residing in the stomach, which is the main source of ghrelin, it is of interest to explore possible role of *H. pylori* in production of ghrelin-reactive IgG. In fact, cure of *H. pylori* in humans was accompanied by increased plasma levels of ghrelin (33).

FUNCTIONAL ROLE OF GHRELIN-REACTIVE IgG

An established physiological role of IgG is to protect against infection including their ability to directly neutralize antigens and to trigger cell lysis *via* activation of the complement. While presence of IgG reactive with some peptide hormones have been detected in plasma of healthy humans (34), their possible functional role remained unknown, as previously reviewed (35). Ghrelin-reactive IgG were the first IgG revealing that they have a functional role in the peptide signaling by protecting ghrelin from degradation in plasma (13). In fact, as was shown by an *in vitro* assay, depletion of plasma from IgG resulted in an almost complete loss of acyl-ghrelin, while their reintroduction allowed its full recovery (13). Thus, the main functional role of ghrelin-reactive IgG appears to protect ghrelin from degradation.

Such protection did not reduce the orexigenic activity of ghrelin, because administrations of ghrelin together with plasmatic IgG, stimulated food intake and even enhanced it when IgG were derived from plasma of obese humans or mice (13). Such enhancing effect was explained by a slight, about three times, increase of IgG affinity for ghrelin and the evidence that such IgG are able to transport more active ghrelin in obese patients. Moreover, the KD values of ghrelin-reactive IgG remained in the micromolar range, which would preclude their competition with the nanomolar affinity of ghrelin receptor binding (36).

We show here that KD values of IgG for ghrelin correlate positively with plasma ghrelin concentrations in obese and AN patients as well as in *ob/ob* mice (**Figures 2A,B**). These correlations demonstrate that a decrease in IgG affinity for ghrelin (increase in KD) corresponds to higher ghrelin levels and suggest that properties of ghrelin-reactive IgG may at least partly underlie individual differences in plasma ghrelin levels. An inverse relation is unlikely, because increased antigen concentration should stimulate the affinity maturation of IgG. We also find that plasma levels of ghrelin-reactive free IgG as well as ratios of free/total IgG levels correlate positively with plasma ghrelin (**Figures 2C,D**). In contrast, ghrelin-reactive total IgG correlate negatively with plasma ghrelin (**Figure 2E**). Taken together, these correlations support a carrier role of plasmatic IgG for ghrelin.

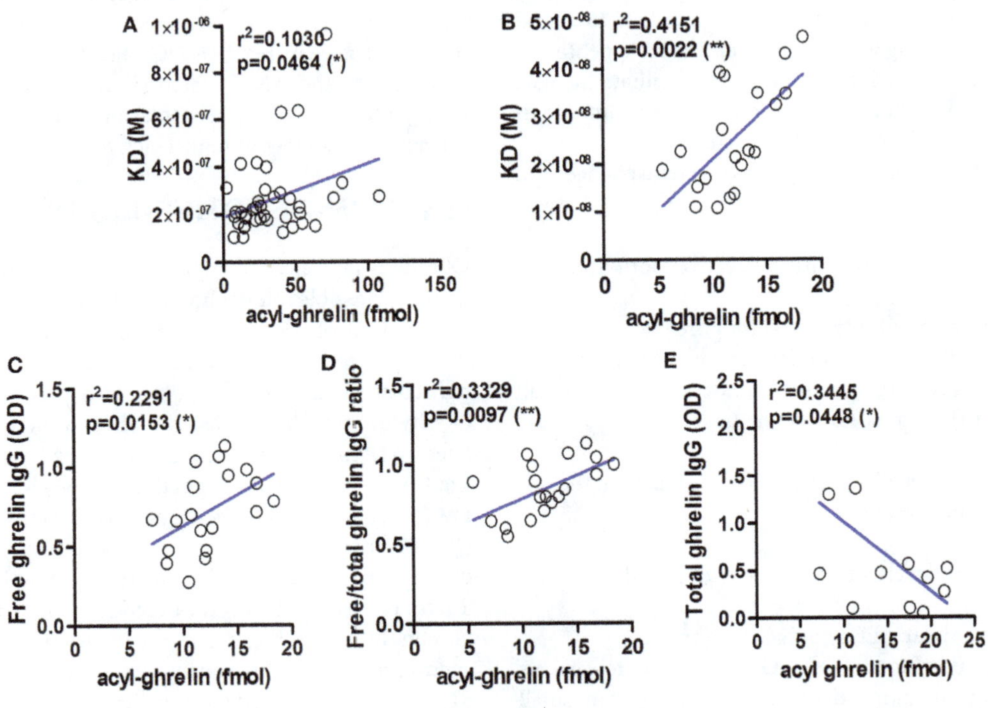

FIGURE 2 | Examples of correlations between affinity and levels of ghrelin-reactive IgG and plasma concentrations of acyl-ghrelin. Correlations between the values of dissociation equilibrium constants (KD) of plasmatic IgG reactive with ghrelin and acyl ghrelin in obese and anorectic patients and controls **(A)** and in *ob/ob* and lean mice **(B)**. Correlations between plasma levels of ghrelin-reactive free IgG **(C)** as well as ratios of their free/total levels **(D)** in ob/ob and lean mice. Correlations between plasma levels of ghrelin-reactive total IgG in Zucker rats **(E)**. *R*-squared and *p*-values for Pearson's correlation tests are shown, $^{**}p < 0.01$ and $^{*}p < 0.05$.

Considering increased functional effects of ghrelin in immune complex with IgG vs. ghrelin alone, the accompanying changes in plasma ghrelin levels during altered energy metabolism can be a "mirror" reflection of the ghrelin's functional activity. Accordingly, increased plasma levels of ghrelin, e.g., in AN patients and in animal models of anorexia (**Figure 1**), may signify ghrelin's inability to form stable immune complexes with IgG and, hence, may result in a functional deficiency of the ghrelin signaling or "ghrelin resistance." Such explanation may appear at first glance as paradoxical, but it gains further support from the corroborating data revealing an enhancing role of IgG in signaling by other peptide hormones such as α-MSH (37, 38).

Thus, the changes in IgG affinity kinetics resulting in a slight increase of affinity can be considered as a gain of function in ghrelin signaling. Taking in account important functional consequences of affinity changes in ghrelin-reactive IgG, it is clear that a simple measurement of their plasma levels is not sufficient and should be combined with the affinity kinetics analysis. Nevertheless, affinity changes should still be taken with caution as a putative biomarker, as long as we do not know if they involve or not any epitope changes that may prevent the availability of the ghrelin N-terminal, necessary for the GHSR1 binding. We do not yet know if presence of IgG in immune complex with ghrelin may play an allosteric role in ghrelin receptor activation, a phenomenon suggested for IgG reactive with α-MSH (37, 38).

To summarize these data, presence of IgG at normal levels and with physiological micromolar affinity for ghrelin in humans appears as a homeostatic factor in regulation of ghrelin signaling. Accordingly, any changes in these factors should lead to alteration of the ghrelin signaling with resulting effects on appetite and body weight regulation. Therefore, in order to facilitate the data interpretation toward an enhanced or diminished ghrelin signaling, the following algorithm can be proposed.

For the enhanced ghrelin signaling one of several changes can be observed:

- Increased plasma levels of ghrelin-reactive both free and total IgG;
- Increased micromolar affinity of IgG for ghrelin;
- Changes in affinity kinetics of IgG for ghrelin toward its increased binding including increased association rate (small Ka) and/or decreased dissociation rate (small Kd).

By the opposite, for the diminished ghrelin signaling, the following changes can be present:

- Decreased plasma levels of ghrelin-reactive both free and total IgG;
- Decreased micromolar affinity of IgG for ghrelin;
- Changes in affinity kinetics of IgG for ghrelin toward its decreased binding including decreased association rate (small Ka) and/or increased dissociation rate (small Kd).

While the functional role of ghrelin-reactive IgG with regard to ghrelin's orexigenic effect can be interpreted as facilitating, the corresponding role of IgG reactive with desacyl-ghrelin is uncertain. As discussed above, IgG may bind to the common central and the C-terminal parts of ghrelin and desacyl-ghrelin and, hence, may transport both types of peptides. In fact, absorption studies of ghrelin- and desacyl-ghrelin-reactive IgG confirmed that they can bind both peptides (20).

Although some studies showed potential anorexigenic effects of desacyl-ghrelin (39, 40), its functional role in the regulation of appetite remains uncertain including direct functional consequences of desacyl-ghrelin transport by IgG toward an unknown putative receptor (41). One alternative possibility is that desacyl-ghrelin may compete with acyl-ghrelin for protective IgG and, thereby, desacyl-ghrelin may have an anorexigenic effect by diminishing the ghrelin signaling *via* reduced formation of ghrelin/IgG immune complexes. Such possibility is of functional importance because starvation preferentially upregulates desacyl-ghrelin, e.g., its ratios to acyl-ghrelin can be increased from 1:20 in *ad libitum* fed mice to more than 1:70 in starved mice (**Table 1**) (17). Functional significance of the affinity kinetics changes in desacyl-ghrelin-reactive IgG is also difficult to interpret owning the same problem of the uncertain role of the desacyl-ghrelin peptide. Whether such changes are different from those obtained for acyl-ghrelin, it suggests that they may concern antibodies primarily targeting the desacylated N-terminal of ghrelin. It is, nevertheless, possible that decreased affinity of IgG for desacyl-ghrelin may be favorable for desacyl-ghrelin competition with ghrelin for ghrelin-protective IgG and, hence, may result in reduced orexigenic activity of ghrelin. Furthermore, we have seen that KD values of desacyl-ghrelin IgG correlate positively with plasma levels of desacyl-ghrelin in animals with anorexia. Significant correlations were also found between plasma levels of desacyl-ghrelin reactive IgG and desacyl-ghrelin in patients with obesity and AN. Such correlations suggest that, similar to acyl-ghrelin, desacyl-ghrelin plasma concentrations can also be regulated by desacyl-ghrelin-reactive IgG.

GHRELIN-REACTIVE-IgG IN OBESITY

Obesity is typically accompanied by increased food intake, suggesting a possible role of ghrelin in the mechanism of hyperphagia (42). Indeed, obese subjects are more sensitive than lean subjects to increase their food intake after ghrelin administration (43). A particular situation may exist in non-hyperphagic HFD-induced obesity in mice that are less sensitive to the ghrelin's orexigenic effect (44). In obese subjects, basal plasma levels of ghrelin measured as total ghrelin (acyl-ghrelin + desacyl-ghrelin) were found low (45, 46) or normal when measured selectively for acyl-ghrelin (13, 47, 48) (**Table 1**). Thus, increased food intake in common obesity cannot be related to increased ghrelin concentrations. There are, nevertheless, some exceptions showing elevated plasma ghrelin in hyperphagic obese patients with the Prader–Willi syndrome (PWS) (49) and hyperphagic obese Zucker rats (50, 51). However, our study showed that obese Zucker rats display elevated desacyl-ghrelin, while acyl-ghrelin remains normal (16) (**Table 1**).

IgG in obese patients showed their ability to better protect ghrelin from degradation by an *in vitro* test and to increase its orexigenic activity after intraperitoneal administrations in rats

(13). Such ghrelin's enhancing properties of IgG in obesity can be explained by its increased affinity, as discussed above. Similarly, increased affinity of IgG for ghrelin was found in genetic animal models of obesity including both *ob/ob* mice (13) and Zucker rats (16) (**Table 3**). Obesity in both rodent's models is due to the deficient leptin signaling and is characterized by hyperphagia. In mice that developed obesity after 2 months of HFD, IgG was also characterized by increased affinity for ghrelin (**Table 3**); however, these mice are not hyperphagic. In contrast to other animal models of obesity and to obese patients, HFD-obese mice also showed an increase in affinity of desacyl-ghrelin IgG (**Table 4**), but the significance of such change is not clear. The affinity kinetic properties of the association and dissociation rates leading to increased affinity were all different between humans and animal models of obesity including increased small *Ka* in obese patients, a decrease of small *Kd* in *ob/ob* mice and Zucker rats, and no significant changes in HFD obese mice (**Table 3**).

Although plasma levels of ghrelin-reactive IgG in obese patients and in all animal models reviewed here were slightly lower than in their non-obese controls (**Table 2**), the free/total ratios of ghrelin-reactive IgG were increased in patients and in Zucker rats (**Table 2**). Interestingly, a recent conference report revealed elevated plasma levels of ghrelin-reactive IgG in children with PWS (52). If confirmed, it will be the only so far known pathological conditions characterized by increased production of ghrelin-reactive IgG.

Taken together, these data suggest that obesity development leads to increased carrying properties of IgG for ghrelin in both obese humans and in animal models of obesity *via* increased affinity (**Figure 1**). Such changes in ghrelin-reactive IgG properties may represent a mechanistic factor underlying enhanced ghrelin signaling leading to hyperphagia and increased adiposity.

GHRELIN-REACTIVE-IgG IN ANOREXIA

Anorexia can be a primary problem in patient with eating disorders such as in restrictive AN, or it can be symptomatic during a chronic disease worsening its outcome. Ghrelin production and its plasma concentration are typically elevated during chronic starvation, accompanied or not by anorexia in both humans and

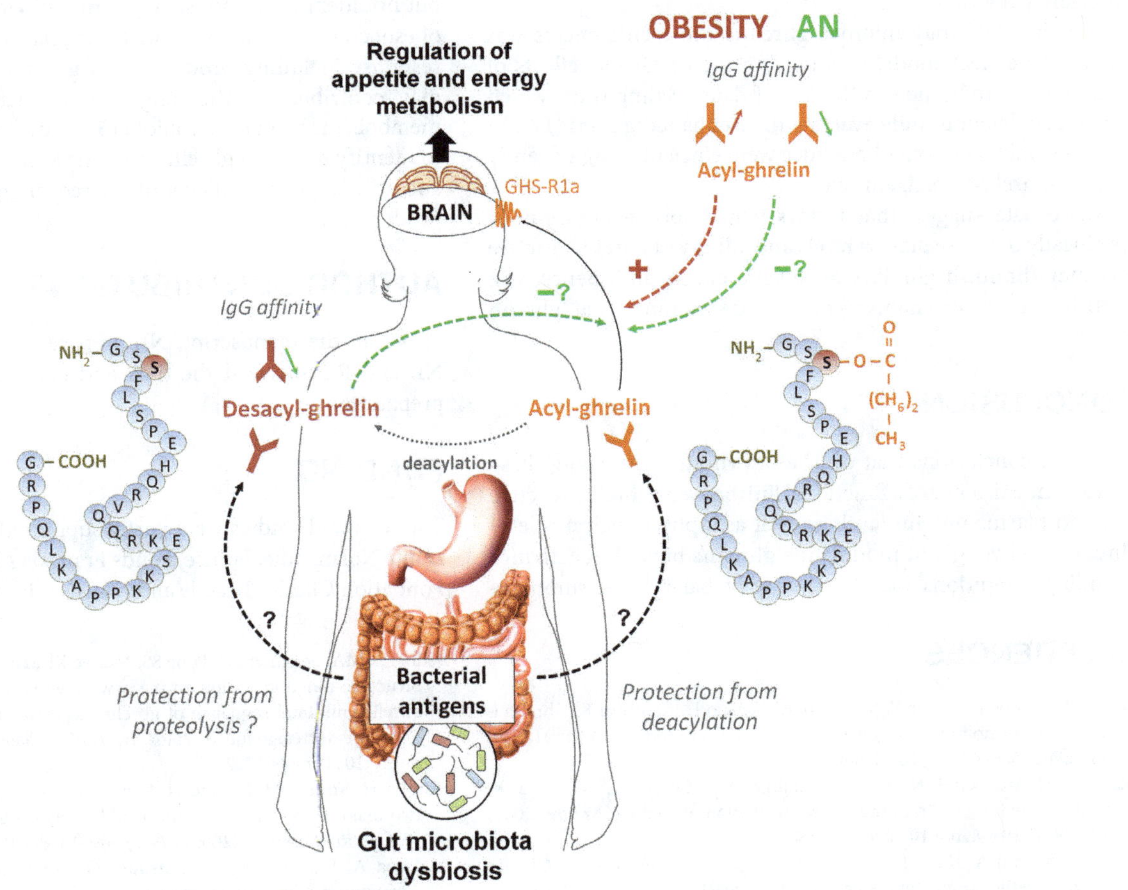

FIGURE 3 | A schematic model summarizing the postulated role of ghrelin-reactive IgG in ghrelin signaling in appetite control during normal and pathological conditions. According this model, acyl-ghrelin is protected by IgG from deacylation, therefore enhancing its orexigenic signaling to the brain. Changes in affinity of IgG for ghrelin in obese patients (increase) and in orexia nervosa patients (decrease) may enhance and diminish, respectively, ghrelin's orexigenic effects. Desacyl-ghrelin may lower orexigenic effect *via* competing with ghrelin for ghrelin-reactive IgG resulting in increased ghrelin degradation. Moreover, decreased affinity of IgG for desacyl ghrelin may favor its dissociation from immune complexes and completion with ghrelin. The origin of changes in affinity of ghrelin- and desacyl ghrelin-reactive IgG is currently unknown but may potentially depend on antigenic stimulation from dysbiotic gut microbiota associated with long-term nutritional modifications in anorexia and obesity.

experimental animals (13, 17, 53–56). Such elevation of plasma ghrelin suggests its homeostatic role in the long-term regulation of energy balance aimed at increased food intake, once food will be available (42). This homeostatic control is obviously not working in anorectic humans and rodents, who display functional "ghrelin resistance." A role of plasmatic IgG in mechanisms of "ghrelin resistance" during anorexia can be suggested based on changes in their properties in an opposite way to obesity. In fact, patients with AN display lower affinity than in controls (**Table 3**), and many AN patients display also low plasma levels of ghrelin-reactive IgG (20). In the ABA and MTX rodent models of anorexia, we did not observe low affinity of IgG for ghrelin but it was present for desacyl-ghrelin (**Tables 3** and **4**). Such decrease of affinity was detected only in ABA mice but not in FTR mice that were starved but did not develop spontaneous anorexia, suggesting a possible contribution of desacyl-ghrelin-reactive IgG in the anorectic phenotype. MTX-treated rats, which develop severe anorexia, were also characterized by strong inhibition of ghrelin-reactive IgG levels (15). As discussed above, lower levels and affinity of IgG for both ghrelin and desacyl-ghrelin may decrease ghrelin's orexigenic effects. Such possibility was not, however, experimentally validated.

Whether IgG may improve ghrelin's orexigenic effects was tested in the ABA model in mice, but the orexigenic effects of treatments were limited to the 3 h of daily feeding time, which was not sufficient to fully evaluate their enhancing roles (17). In any case, only IgG from obese mice were efficient to significantly improve ghrelin's orexigenic effect.

These data suggest that factors which specifically or non-specifically decrease plasma levels and affinity of ghrelin-reactive IgG may diminish ghrelin's orexigenic effects and, hence, will contribute to the mechanisms of anorexia *via* functional "ghrelin resistance."

CONCLUSION

The main conclusions that can be drawn after reviewing these data are the existence of a functional link between ghrelin-reactive IgG and plasma ghrelin levels as well as a physiological role of ghrelin-reactive IgG in modulating ghrelin's biological activities including conditions of altered energy balance. A summary **Figure 3** schematically illustrates the postulated link between ghrelin-reactive IgG and regulation of appetite whereas changes in IgG properties during obesity and anorexia may enhance or diminish ghrelin signaling, while desacyl-ghrelin may compete with ghrelin for IgG which protect ghrelin from deacylation.

Data analysis from patients and several animal models of altered energy balance shows that both obese humans and animals display lower levels of ghrelin-reactive IgG characterized by increased affinity. In contrast, patients with AN and anorectic rodents all show lower affinity of ghrelin- and desacyl-ghrelin-reactive IgG, respectively, the changes which were not observed in non-anorectic chronically starved mice. Such changes in properties of both ghrelin- and desacyl-ghrelin-reactive IgG in patients with obesity and anorexia suggest that they are not a direct consequence of the positive or negative energy balance *per se* but may be a result of some typical changes associated with altered regulation of energy metabolism impacting on the autoantibody production. Although the mechanisms of such common changes are currently unknown, they may potentially involve modifications of gut microbiota leading to altered production of ghrelin-like antigenic molecules. Indeed, typical, but not identical response of gut microbiota to starvation or an obesogenic diet may potentially explain similar autoantibody response including production of ghrelin-reactive IgG, which may contribute to the long-term regulation of host energy metabolisms by gut microbiota (57). Further studies are needed to identify potential ghrelin-mimetic antigens in gut microbiota and to analyze the effects of altered energy balance on their production.

AUTHOR CONTRIBUTIONS

SF wrote the manuscript, NL prepared the figures and tables, NL and RL analyzed the data and contributed to manuscript preparation.

FUNDING

The reviewed studies were partly supported from the Region of Haute Normandie, France, Fonds Français Alimentation et Santé, Fondation Charles Nicolle and Nutriset, France.

REFERENCES

Kojima M, Hosoda H, Date Y, Nakazato M, Matsuo H, Kangawa K. Ghrelin is a growth-hormone-releasing acylated peptide from stomach. *Nature* (1999) 402(6762):656–60. doi:10.1038/45230

Nakazato M, Murakami N, Date Y, Kojima M, Matsuo H, Kangawa K, et al. A role for ghrelin in the central regulation of feeding. *Nature* (2001) 409(6817):194–8. doi:10.1038/35051587

Asakawa A, Inui A, Kaga T, Yuzuriha H, Nagata T, Ueno N, et al. Ghrelin is an appetite-stimulatory signal from stomach with structural resemblance to motilin. *Gastroenterology* (2001) 120(2):337–45. doi:10.1053/gast.2001.22158

Tschöp M, Smiley DL, Heiman ML. Ghrelin induces adiposity in rodents. *Nature* (2000) 407(6806):908–13. doi:10.1038/35038090

Davenport AP, Bonner TI, Foord SM, Harmar AJ, Neubig RR, Pin J-P, et al. International Union of Pharmacology. LVI. Ghrelin receptor nomenclature, distribution, and function. *Pharmacol Rev* (2005) 57(4):541–6. doi:10.1124/pr.57.4.1

Bednarek MA, Feighner SD, Pong SS, McKee KK, Hreniuk DL, Silva MV, et al. Structure-function studies on the new growth hormone-releasing peptide, ghrelin: minimal sequence of ghrelin necessary for activation of growth hormone secretagogue receptor 1a. *J Med Chem* (2000) 43(23):4370–6. doi:10.1021/jm0001727

Hosoda H, Kojima M, Matsuo H, Kangawa K. Ghrelin and des-acyl ghrelin: two major forms of rat ghrelin peptide in gastrointestinal tissue. *Biochem Biophys Res Commun* (2000) 279(3):909–13. doi:10.1006/bbrc.2000.4039

Asakawa A, Inui A, Kaga T, Katsuura G, Fujimiya M, Fujino MA, et al. Antagonism of ghrelin receptor reduces food intake and body weight gain in mice. *Gut* (2003) 52(7):947–52. doi:10.1136/gut.52.7.947

De Vriese C, Gregoire F, Lema-Kisoka R, Waelbroeck M, Robberecht P, Delporte C. Ghrelin degradation by serum and tissue homogenates: identification of the cleavage sites. *Endocrinology* (2004) 145(11):4997–5005. doi:10.1210/en.2004-0569

Satou M, Nishi Y, Yoh J, Hattori Y, Sugimoto H. Identification and characterization of acyl-protein thioesterase 1/lysophospholipase I as a ghrelin deacylation/lysophospholipid hydrolyzing enzyme in fetal bovine serum and conditioned medium. *Endocrinology* (2010) 151(10):4765–75. doi:10.1210/ en.2010-0412

Tong J, Dave N, Mugundu GM, Davis HW, Gaylinn BD, Thorner MO, et al. The pharmacokinetics of acyl, des-acyl, and total ghrelin in healthy human subjects. *Eur J Endocrinol* (2013) 168(6):821–8. doi:10.1530/eje-13-0072

Depoortere I. Targeting the ghrelin receptor to regulate food intake. *Regul Pept* (2009) 156(1–3):13–23. doi:10.1016/j.regpep.2009.04.002

Takagi K, Legrand R, Asakawa A, Amitani H, François M, Tennoune N, et al. Anti-ghrelin immunoglobulins modulate ghrelin stability and its orexigenic effect in obese mice and humans. *Nat Commun* (2013) 4:2685. doi:10.1038/ ncomms3685

François M, Barde S, Legrand R, Lucas N, Azhar S, el Dhaybi M, et al. High- fat diet increases ghrelin-expressing cells in stomach, contributing to obesity. *Nutrition* (2016) 32(6):709–15. doi:10.1016/j.nut.2015.12.034

François M, Takagi K, Legrand R, Lucas N, Beutheu Youmba S, Bôle-Feysot C, et al. Increased ghrelin but low ghrelin-reactive immunoglobulins in a rat model of methotrexate chemotherapy-induced anorexia. *Front Nutr* (2016) 3:23. doi:10.3389/fnut.2016.00023

Lucas N, Legrand R, Breton J, Déchelotte P, Fetissov S. Increased affinity of ghrelin-reactive immunoglobulins in obese Zucker rats. *Nutrition* (2016). doi:10.1016/j.nut.2016.11.007

Legrand R, Lucas N, Breton J, Azhar S, do Rego J-C, Déchelotte P, et al. Ghrelin treatment prevents development of activity based anorexia in mice. *Eur Neuropsychopharmacol* (2016) 26(6):948–58. doi:10.1016/j. euroneuro.2016.03.010

Legrand R, Takagi K, Fetissov SO. Immunoglobulin G preparation from plasma samples and analysis of its affinity kinetic binding to peptide hor- mones. *Protoc Exch* (2014). doi:10.1038/protex.2014.004

Fetissov SO, Hamze Sinno M, Coëffier M, Bole-Feysot C, Ducrotté P, Hökfelt T, et al. Autoantibodies against appetite-regulating peptide hormones and neuropeptides: putative modulation by gut microflora. *Nutrition* (2008) 24(4):348–59. doi:10.1016/j.nut.2007.12.006

Terashi M, Asakawa A, Harada T, Ushikai M, Coquerel Q, Sinno MH, et al. Ghrelin reactive autoantibodies in restrictive anorexia nervosa. *Nutrition* (2011) 27(4):407–13. doi:10.1016/j.nut.2011.01.002

François M, Schaefer JM, Bole-Feysot C, Déchelotte P, Verhulst FC, Fetissov SO. Ghrelin-reactive immunoglobulins and anxiety, depression and stress-induced cortisol response in adolescents. The TRAILS study. *Prog Neuropsychopharmacol Biol Psychiatry* (2015) 59(0):1–7. doi:10.1016/j. pnpbp.2014.12.011

Tennoune N, Legrand R, Ouelaa W, Breton J, Lucas N, Bole-Feysot C, et al. Sex-related effects of nutritional supplementation of *Escherichia coli*: relevance to eating disorders. *Nutrition* (2015) 31(3):498–507. doi:10.1016/j. nut.2014.11.003

Tlaskalova-Hogenova H, Mandel L, Stepankova R, Bartova J, Barot R, Leclerc M, et al. Autoimmunity: from physiology to pathology. Natural antibodies, mucosal immunity and development of B cell repertoire. *Folia Biol (Praha)* (1992) 38(3–4):202–15.

Avrameas S. Natural autoantibodies: from 'horror autotoxicus' to 'gnothi seauton'. *Immunol Today* (1991) 12(5):154–9. doi:10.1016/S0167-5699(05) 80045-3

Gallas S, Fetissov SO. Ghrelin, appetite and gastric electrical stimulation. *Peptides* (2011) 32(11):2283–9. doi:10.1016/j.peptides.2011.05.027

Gallas S, Sinno MH, Boukhettala N, Coëffier M, Dourmap N, Gourcerol G, et al. Gastric electrical stimulation increases ghrelin production and inhibits catecholaminergic brainstem neurons in rats. *Eur J Neurosci* (2011) 33(2):276–84. doi:10.1111/j.1460-9568.2010.07474.x

Kau AL, Ahern PP, Griffin NW, Goodman AL, Gordon JI. Human nutrition, the gut microbiome and the immune system. *Nature* (2011) 474(7351):327–36. doi:10.1038/nature10213

Hardet R, Chevalier B, Dupaty L, Naimi Y, Riou G, Drouot L, et al. Oral-tolerization prevents immune responses and improves transgene persistence following gene transfer mediated by adeno-associated viral vector. *Mol Ther* (2016) 24(1):87–95. doi:10.1038/mt.2015.146

Oldstone MB. Molecular mimicry, microbial infection, and autoimmune disease: evolution of the concept. *Curr Top Microbiol Immunol* (2005) 296:1–17.

Tennoune N, Chan P, Breton J, Legrand R, Chabane YN, Akkermann K, et al. Bacterial ClpB heat-shock protein, an antigen-mimetic of the anorexigenic peptide [alpha]-MSH, at the origin of eating disorders. *Transl Psychiatry* (2014) 4:e458. doi:10.1038/tp.2014.98

Stawerska R, Czkwianianc E, Matusiak A, Smyczynska J, Hilczer M, Chmiela M, et al. Prevalence of autoantibodies against some selected growth and appetite-regulating neuropeptides in serum of short children exposed to *Candida albicans* colonization and/or *Helicobacter pylori* infection: the molecular mimicry phenomenon. *Neuro Endocrinol Lett* (2015) 36(5):458–64.

Stawerska R, Czkwianianc E, Matusiak A, Smyczynska J, Hilczer M, Chmiela M, et al. Assessment of ghrelin, leptin, orexin A and alpha-MSH serum concentrations and the levels of the autoantibodies against the aforementioned peptides in relation to *Helicobacter pylori* infections and *Candida albicans* colonization in children with short stature. *Pediatr Endocrinol Diabetes Metab* (2016) 21(3):102–10. doi:10.18544/PEDM-21.03.0031

Nwokolo CU, Freshwater DA, O'Hare P, Randeva HS. Plasma ghrelin following cure of *Helicobacter pylori*. *Gut* (2003) 52(5):637–40. doi:10.1136/ gut. 52.5.637

Sebriakova M, Little JA. A method for the determination of plasma insulin antibodies and its application in normal and diabetic subjects. *Diabetes* (1973) 22(1):30–40. doi:10.2337/diab.22.1.30

Fetissov SO, Hamze Sinno M, Coquerel Q, Do Rego JC, Coëffier M, Gilbert D, et al. Emerging role of autoantibodies against appetite-regulating neuropeptides in eating disorders. *Nutrition* (2008) 24(9):854–9. doi:10.1016/j. nut.2008.06.021

Holst B, Brandt E, Bach A, Heding A, Schwartz TW. Nonpeptide and peptide growth hormone secretagogues act both as ghrelin receptor agonist and as positive or negative allosteric modulators of ghrelin signaling. *Mol Endocrinol* (2005) 19(9):2400–11. doi:10.1210/me.2005-0059

Lucas N, Legrand R, Akkermann K, Harro J, Bole-Feysot C, Breton J, et al. Anti-α-melanocyte-stimulating hormone autoantibodies in patients with eating disorders and melanocortin 4 receptor signaling. *Eur Neuropsychopharmacol* (2014) 24:S704–5. doi:10.1016/S0924-977X(14)71136-8

Lucas N, Legrand R, Ouelaa W, Breton J, Tennoune N, Bole-Feysot C, et al. Effects of rabbit anti-α-melanocyte-stimulating hormone (α-MSH) immuno- globulins on α-MSH signaling related to food intake control. *Neuropeptides* (2014) 48:21–7. doi:10.1016/j.npep.2013.10.017

Asakawa A, Inui A, Fujimiya M, Sakamaki R, Shinfuku N, Ueta Y, et al. Stomach regulates energy balance via acylated ghrelin and desacyl ghrelin. *Gut* (2005) 54(1):18–24. doi:10.1136/gut.2004.038737

Fernandez G, Cabral A, Cornejo MP, De Francesco PN, Garcia-Romero G, Reynaldo M, et al. Des-acyl ghrelin directly targets the arcuate nucleus in a ghrelin-receptor independent manner and impairs the orexigenic effect of ghrelin. *J Neuroendocrinol* (2016) 28(2). doi:10.1111/jne.12349

Filigheddu N, Gnocchi VF, Coscia M, Cappelli M, Porporato PE, Taulli R, et al. Ghrelin and des-acyl ghrelin promote differentiation and fusion of C2C12 skeletal muscle cells. *Mol Biol Cell* (2007) 18(3):986–94. doi:10.1091/ mbc. E06-05-0402

Cummings DE. Ghrelin and the short- and long-term regulation of appetite and body weight. *Physiol Behav* (2006) 89(1):71–84. doi:10.1016/j. physbeh.2006.05.022

Druce MR, Wren AM, Park AJ, Milton JE, Patterson M, Frost G, et al. Ghrelin increases food intake in obese as well as lean subjects. *Int J Obes Relat Metab Disord* (2005) 29(9):1130–6. doi:10.1038/sj.ijo.0803001

Zigman JM, Bouret SG, Andrews ZB. Obesity impairs the action of the neuroendocrine ghrelin system. *Trends Endocrinol Metab* (2016) 27(1):54–63. doi:10.1016/j.tem.2015.09.010

Tschöp M, Weyer C, Tataranni PA, Devanarayan V, Ravussin E, Heiman ML. Circulating ghrelin levels are decreased in human obesity. *Diabetes* (2001) 50(4):707–9. doi:10.2337/diabetes.50.4.707

Shiiya T, Nakazato M, Mizuta M, Date Y, Mondal MS, Tanaka M, et al. Plasma ghrelin levels in lean and obese humans and the effect of glucose on ghrelin secretion. *J Clin Endocrinol Metab* (2002) 87(1):240–4. doi:10.1210/ jcem.87.1.8129

Barazzoni R, Zanetti M, Ferreira C, Vinci P, Pirulli A, Mucci M, et al. Relationships between desacylated and acylated ghrelin and insulin sensitivity in the metabolic syndrome. *J Clin Endocrinol Metab* (2007) 92(10):3935–40. doi:10.1210/jc.2006-2527

Pacifico L, Poggiogalle E, Costantino F, Anania C, Ferraro F, Chiarelli F, et al. Acylated and nonacylated ghrelin levels and their associations with insulin resistance in obese and normal weight children with meta- bolic syndrome. *Eur J Endocrinol* (2009) 161(6):861–70. doi:10.1530/eje- 09-0375

Cummings DE, Clement K, Purnell JQ, Vaisse C, Foster KE, Frayo RS. Elevated plasma ghrelin levels in Prader Willi syndrome. *Nat Med* (2002) 8:643–4. doi:10.1038/nm0702-643

Ariyasu H, Takaya K, Hosoda H, Iwakura H, Ebihara K, Mori K, et al. Delayed short-term secretory regulation of ghrelin in obese animals: evidenced by a specific RIA for the active form of ghrelin. *Endocrinology* (2002) 143(9):3341- 50. doi:10.1210/en.2002-220225

Beck B, Richy S, Stricker-Krongrad A. Ghrelin and body weight regulation in the obese Zucker rat in relation to feeding state and dark/light cycle. *Exp Biol Med* (2003) 228(10):1124–31.

Crisp G, Nyunt O, Musthaffa Y, Seim I, Chopin L, Harris M, et al. Ghrelin-reactive autoantibodies are elevated in children with Prader-Willi syndrome compared to unaffected sibling controls. *55th Annual Conference of European Society for Paediatric Endocrinology*. Paris, France: ESPE Abstracts (2016).

Otto B, Tschöp M, Frühauf E, Heldwein W, Fichter M, Otto C, et al. Postprandial ghrelin release in anorectic patients before and after weight gain. *Psychoneuroendocrinology* (2005) 30(6):577–81. doi:10.1016/j.psyneuen.2005.01.009

Germain N, Galusca B, Grouselle D, Frere D, Tolle V, Zizzari P, et al. Ghrelin/obestatin ratio in two populations with low body weight: constitutional thinness and anorexia nervosa. *Psychoneuroendocrinology* (2009) 34(3): 413–9. doi:10.1016/j.psyneuen.2008.10.001

Méquinion M, Langlet F, Zgheib S, Dickson S, Dehouck B, Chauveau C, et al. Ghrelin: central and peripheral implications in anorexia nervosa. *Front Endocrinol* (2013) 4:15. doi:10.3389/fendo.2013.00015

François M, Barde S, Achamrah N, Breton J, do Rego J-C, Coëffier M, et al. The number of preproghrelin mRNA expressing cells is increased in mice with activity-based anorexia. *Neuropeptides* (2015) 51:17–23. doi:10.1016/j.npep.2015.04.003

Fetissov SO. Role of the gut microbiota in host appetite control: bacterial growth to animal feeding behaviour. *Nat Rev Endocrinol* (2017) 13:11–25. doi:10.1038/nrendo.2016.150

11

Sweet Taste Receptor Serves to Activate Glucose- and Leptin-Responsive Neurons in the Hypothalamic Arcuate Nucleus and Participates in Glucose Responsiveness

Daisuke Kohno [1,2]*, ***Miho Koike*** [1], ***Yuzo Ninomiya*** [3,4], ***Itaru Kojima*** [5], ***Tadahiro Kitamura*** [2] ***and Toshihiko Yada*** [6]

[1] Advanced Scientific Research Leaders Development Unit, Gunma University, Maebashi, Japan, [2] Metabolic Signal Research Center, Institute for Molecular and Cellular Regulation, Gunma University, Maebashi, Japan, [3] Division of Sensory Physiology, Research and Development Center for Taste and Odor Sensing, Kyushu University, Fukuoka, Japan, [4] Monell Chemical Senses Center, Philadelphia, PA, USA, [5] Department of Cell Biology, Institute for Molecular and Cellular Regulation, Gunma University, Maebashi, Japan, [6] Division of Integrative Physiology, Department of Physiology, School of Medicine, Jichi Medical University, Shimotsuke, Japan

***Correspondence:**
Daisuke Kohno
daisuke.kohno@gunma-u.ac.jp

The hypothalamic feeding center plays an important role in energy homeostasis. In the feeding center, whole-body energy signals including hormones and nutrients are sensed, processed, and integrated. As a result, food intake and energy expenditure are regulated. Two types of glucose-sensing neurons exist in the hypothalamic arcuate nucleus (ARC): glucose-excited neurons and glucose-inhibited neurons. While some molecules are known to be related to glucose sensing in the hypothalamus, the mechanisms underlying glucose sensing in the hypothalamus are not fully understood. The sweet taste receptor is a heterodimer of taste type 1 receptor 2 (T1R2) and taste type 1 receptor 3 (T1R3) and senses sweet tastes. T1R2 and T1R3 are distributed in multiple organs including the tongue, pancreas, adipose tissue, and hypothalamus. However, the role of sweet taste receptors in the ARC remains to be clarified. To examine the role of sweet taste receptors in the ARC, cytosolic Ca^{2+} concentration ($[Ca^{2+}]_i$) in isolated single ARC neurons were measured using Fura-2 fluorescent imaging. An artificial sweetener, sucralose at 10^{-5}–10^{-2} M dose dependently increased $[Ca^{2+}]_i$ in 12–16% of ARC neurons. The sucralose-induced $[Ca^{2+}]_i$ increase was suppressed by a sweet taste receptor inhibitor, gurmarin. The sucralose-induced $[Ca^{2+}]_i$ increase was inhibited under an extracellular Ca^{2+}-free condition and in the presence of an L-type Ca^{2+} channel blocker, nitrendipine. Sucralose-responding neurons were activated by high-concentration of glucose. This response to glucose was markedly suppressed by gurmarin. More than half of sucralose-responding neurons were activated by leptin but not ghrelin. Percentages of proopiomelanocortin (POMC) neurons among sucralose-responding neurons and sweet taste receptor expressing neurons were low, suggesting that majority of sucralose-responding neurons are non-POMC neurons. These data suggest that sweet taste receptor-mediated cellular activation mainly occurs on non-POMC leptin-responding neurons and contributes to glucose responding. Endogenous sweet molecules including glucose may regulate energy homeostasis through sweet taste receptors on glucose-and leptin-responsive neurons in the ARC.

Keywords: feeding, sweet taste receptor, sucralose, glucose, leptin, POMC

INTRODUCTION

The feeding center in the hypothalamus plays an important role in energy homeostasis. Neurons in the feeding center are activated or suppressed by the molecules reflecting peripheral energy status, including hormones such as ghrelin, leptin and insulin, and nutrients such as glucose, free fatty acids, and amino acids. These neuronal responses are integrated by intracellular signaling and the brain circuit; as a result, feeding and metabolism are controlled (Williams and Elmquist, 2012). Therefore, nutrient sensing is important for the control of energy balance.

There are two types of glucose-sensing neurons in the hypothalamic arcuate nucleus (ARC; Routh et al., 2014). One is the glucose-excited (or glucose-responsive) neurons, which are activated by high concentrations of glucose and inhibited by low concentrations of glucose. They are thought to be satiety neurons. The other is glucose-inhibited (glucose-sensitive) neurons, which are activated by low concentrations of glucose and inhibited by high concentrations of glucose. Glucose-inhibited neurons are thought to be orexigenic neurons. Regarding the mechanism of glucose-sensing in the hypothalamic neurons, several molecules have been proposed, which include Na^+, K^+ ATPase, AMP-activated protein kinase, ATP-sensitive K^+ channel, and glut2 (Oomura et al., 1974; Ibrahim et al., 2003; Bady et al., 2006; O'Malley et al., 2006; Claret et al., 2007; Routh et al., 2014; Kurita et al., 2015). However, the precise mechanisms underlying glucose-sensing in the hypothalamus are not fully understood.

Glucose-receptor hypothesis was first proposed some decades ago, and recent progress has suggested the sweet taste receptor as the candidate molecule for glucose receptor (Kojima et al., 2015). The sweet taste receptor is a heterodimer of taste type 1 receptor 2 (T1R2) and taste type 1 receptor 3 (T1R3), and this receptor senses multiple sweet taste molecules. In the body, there are variety of sweet taste molecules including carbohydrate, amino acids, polypeptides, proteins, glycosides, and glycerol. T1R2 and T1R3 are distributed throughout multiple organs including the tongue, intestine, pancreas, brain, testis, and lung (Ren et al., 2009; Li, 2013). Recent studies have shown that sweet taste receptors in the pancreatic β cells are necessary for the first phase of glucose response (Nakagawa et al., 2009, 2015). In the brain, the sweet taste receptor is abundantly expressed in the hypothalamus including ARC and the expression level of sweet taste receptor in the hypothalamus is affected by metabolic conditions (Ren et al., 2009; Herrera Moro Chao et al., 2016). However, the role of the sweet taste receptor in the regulation of ARC cellular activities is not understood. Here, we explored the potential contribution of sweet taste receptor to glucose-responses in ARC neurons that could be implicated in energy homeostasis.

MATERIALS AND METHODS

Materials

Sucralose, leptin, and nitrendipine were purchased from Sigma (Sigma-Aldrich, St. Louis, MO). ω-Contoxin GIVA and ghrelin were purchased from Peptide Institute (Osaka, Japan). All of the other chemicals were purchased from Wako Pure Chemical Industries (Osaka, Japan).

Animals

All mouse care and experimental procedures were approved by the Institutional Animal Care and Experimentation Committee at Gunma University. Mice were kept at room temperature (20–24°C) with a 12 h light/dark cycle. All mice used in this study were backcrossed to C57B6J more than eight generations. Regular chow (CLEA Rodent diet CE-2; CLEA Japan, Tokyo, Japan) and water were provided *ad libitum*. POMC-GFP mice were kindly provided by Dr. Jeffrey Friedman (Pinto et al., 2004).

Preparation of Single Neurons from ARC

Single neurons were prepared according to procedures reported previously (Kohno et al., 2003, 2007) with slight modifications. Briefly, mice were anesthetized with 10% pentobarbital (10 μl/g) injected intraperitoneally (IP) and decapitated. Their brains were taken out and brain slices containing the entire ARC were prepared. The entire ARC was excised from the left and right sides. The dissected tissues were washed with 10 mM HEPES-buffered Krebs-Ringer bicarbonate buffer (HKRB) containing 1 mM glucose. They were then incubated in HKRB supplemented with 20 U/ml papain (Sigma-Aldrich, P4762), 0.015 mg/ml DNase II (Sigma-Aldrich, D-4138), and 0.75 mg/ml BSA (Sigma-Aldrich, A2153) for 16 min at 36°C. This was followed by gentle mechanical trituration. Then, the cell suspension was centrifuged at 100 × g for 5 min. The pellet was resuspended in HKRB and distributed onto coverslips. The cells were kept in moisture-saturated dishes for up to 4 h at RT.

Measurements of $[Ca^{2+}]_i$ in Single ARC Neurons

Cytosolic Ca^{2+} concentration ($[Ca^{2+}]_i$) was measured by ratiometric fura-2 microfluorometry in combination with digital imaging, as previously reported (Kohno et al., 2003, 2007). Briefly, after incubation with 2 μM fura-2/AM (Dojindo, Kumamoto, Japan, F016) for 45 min, the cells were mounted in a chamber and superfused with HKRB at 1 ml/min at 33°C.

Fluorescence images due to excitation at 340 and 380 nm were detected every 10 s with a cooled charge-coupled device camera (ORCA-R2 C10600, Hamamatsu Photonics, Hamamatsu, Japan), and the ratio image was produced by an Aquacosmos (Hamamatsu Photonics). The data were obtained from single cells identified as neurons by previously reported procedures (Kohno et al., 2003, 2007); briefly, they have a relatively large diameter (≥10 μm), and their cell bodies are clear and round on phase-contrast microscopy. Cells with astrocyte-like flat morphology were excluded. The data were obtained from cells that met these criteria for neurons.

Criteria for $[Ca^{2+}]_i$ Responses and Expression of Results

Agents were administered in the superfusion solution. When increases in $[Ca^{2+}]_i$ took place within 5 min after adding agents and their amplitudes were 0.25 or larger, they were considered to have responded. In the studies using inhibitor and blockers, when the amplitude of $[Ca^{2+}]_i$ responses with drug treatment was 40% or smaller than that of $[Ca^{2+}]_i$ responses without drugs, inhibition was judged to have occurred. Each experiment was based on data prepared from at least 3 mice. A total of 896 neurons were examined.

Immunohistochemistry

Mice were anesthetized with 10% pentobarbital (10 ml/kg, IP). Then, mice were perfused transcardially with saline and 10% formalin (Wako, 062-01661). Brains were taken out and post-fixed overnight at 4°C. Then, they were transferred to phosphate-buffered saline (PBS, pH 7.4) containing 20% sucrose. The brains were frozen and kept at −80°C until sectioning. Coronal sections were cut at 25 μm using a cryostat (1:5 series). Sections were collected in, transferred to a cryoprotectant solution, and stored at −30°C.

Double immunostaining of T1R2 and POMC were performed as follows. Sections were rinsed in PBS and then blocked with 3% normal donkey serum (NDS; Abcam, Cambridge, UK, ab7475) diluted in PBS containing 0.25% Triton X-100 for 30 min. Next, sections were incubated in goat anti-T1R2 antibody (Santa Cruz Biotechnology, Dallas, TX, SC-22456, 1:50) and rabbit anti-POMC antibody (Phoenix Pharmaceuticals, H-029-30, 1:500) diluted in blocking solution overnight. After rinsing in PBS, sections were incubated with Alexa 488 donkey-anti-goat IgG (Thermo Fisher Scientific, A-11055, 1:400) and Alexa 594 goat-anti-rabbit IgG (Thermo Fisher Scientific, A-21207, 1:400) diluted in 3% NDS for 40 min.

Double immunostaining of T1R3 and POMC were performed as follows. Sections were rinsed in PBS and then blocked with 1.5% normal goat serum (NGS; Rockland Immunochemicals, Gilbertsville, PA, D204-00-0050) diluted in PBS containing 0.25% Triton X-100 for 30 min. Next, sections were treated with streptavidin solution and biotin solution (Vector laboratories, Burlingame, CA, SP-2002) for 15 min, respectively. They were then incubated in rabbit anti-T1R3 antibody (Abcam, ab65423, 1:1000) diluted in Can Get Signal immunostain solution A (Toyobo, Osaka, Japan, NKB-501) overnight. Sections were rinsed in PBS and incubated with biotinylated goat anti-rabbit IgG (Vector Laboratories, VA-1000, 1:400) for 40 min and incubated with ABC reagent (Vector Laboratories) for 40 min. Sections were rinsed in 0.1 mM Tris-HCl buffer (pH 7.5) containing 0.15 mM NaCl and 0.05% Tween 20, and they were blocked with 0.05% blocking reagent (PerkinElmer, Waltham, MA). They were then treated with biotinyl tyramide (PerkinElmer, NEL700001KT, 1:50) for 5 min. After rinsing in 0.1 mM Tris-HCl buffer (pH 7.5) containing 0.15 mM NaCl and 0.05% Tween 20, sections were incubated with streptavidin-Alexa 488 conjugate (Thermo Fisher Scientific, Waltham, MA, S-11223, 1:500) diluted in blocking reagent for 40 min. After a rinse in PBS, sections were incubated with anti-POMC antibody (1:500) diluted in Can Get Signal immunostain solution A overnight. After rinsing in PBS, sections were incubated with Alexa 594 goat-anti-rabbit IgG (Thermo Fisher Scientific, A-21207, 1:400) diluted in 1.5% NGS for 40 min.

Slices were mounted on slides and coverslipped with mounting medium (Vector Laboratories, H-1200). Fluorescence images were acquired with a BZ-9000 (Keyence, Tokyo, Japan). Confocal florescence images were acquired with a confocal laser-scanning microscope (FV10i, Olympus, Tokyo, Japan).

Intracerebroventricular (ICV) Administration of Sucralose and c-Fos and POMC Immunohistochemistry

ICV administration was performed as reported previously (Sasaki et al., 2010) with slight modification. Mice were anesthetized with 10% pentobarbital (7 μl/g, ip) and 5% xylazine (10 μg/g, ip) and guide cannula (C315G, Plastics One, Roanoke, VA) was implanted to the right lateral ventricle, and secured to the skull with dental cement (QUICK RESIN, SHOFU, Kyoto, Japan) and adhesion bond (Loctite 454, Henkel, Dusseldorf, Germany). The cannula tip was located 0.2 mm caudal and 1.0 mm right to bregma and 2.5 mm below the skull. More than 1 week after the surgery, mice that had recovered to 90% of their preoperative weight were used for injection. PBS or 0.085 mg sucralose diluted in PBS (0.5 μl) were injected. Thirty min after injection, mice were perfused transcardially with saline and 10% formalin.

Double immunostaining of c-Fos and POMC were performed as follows. Sections were rinsed in PBS, and then treated with 0.3% H_2O_2 diluted in PBS for 15 min. Sections were then blocked with 1% BSA and 2% NGS diluted in PBS containing 0.25% Triton X-100 for 30 min. Next, sections were incubated in rabbit anti-c-Fos antiserum (Merck Millipore, PC38, 1:25,000) diluted in blocking solution overnight. After rinsing in PBS, sections were incubated with biotinylated goat anti-rabbit IgG (Vector Laboratories, VA-1000, 1:400) for 40 min and incubated with ABC reagent (Vector Laboratories) for 40 min. Sections were rinsed in PBS and 0.175M sodium acetate buffer (pH 5.6), and color was developed with a nickel-diaminobenzidine solution (10 g/liter nickel ammonium sulfate, 0.2 g/liter DAB, and 0.006% H_2O_2 in sodium acetate buffer). After rinsing in PBS, sections were treated with 0.3% H_2O_2 diluted in PBS for 15 min. Sections were then blocked with blocking solution. Next, sections were incubated in anti-POMC antibody (1:4000) diluted in blocking solution overnight. After rinsing in PBS, sections were incubated with biotinylated goat anti-rabbit IgG (1:400) for 40 min and incubated with ABC reagent (Vector Laboratories) for 40 min. Sections were rinsed in PBS and 0.1 mM Tris-HCl buffer (pH 7.5) containing 0.15 mM NaCl, and color was developed with a diaminobenzidine solution.

Statistical Analysis

Data are presented as mean ± SEM. Statistical analyses were performed using IBM SPSS Statistics 23. Unpaired Student's *t*-test was used to evaluate differences, with values of $P < 0.05$ considered significant.

RESULTS

Sucralose Dose-Dependently Increased $[Ca^{2+}]_i$ in ARC Neurons

To observe the effect of sweet taste molecules on ARC neurons, an artificial sweetener, sucralose, in a concentration range from 10^{-6} to 10^{-2} M was administered to single ARC neurons. Sucralose at 10^{-6} M increased $[Ca^{2+}]_i$ in 1 of 56 neurons (2%); at 10^{-5} M in 16 of 136 neurons (12%); at 10^{-4} M in 40 of 248 neurons (16%); at 10^{-3} M in 33 of 229 neurons (14%); and at 10^{-2} M in 35 of 229 neurons (15%), showing a concentration-dependent effect (**Figures 1A,B**). In a neuron presented in **Figure 1A**, sucralose at 10^{-5} M induced a small $[Ca^{2+}]_i$ increase, and at 10^{-4} M a sustained $[Ca^{2+}]_i$ increase with a larger amplitude. Peak fura-2 ratio amplitudes of sucralose-response were concentration dependent. Peak fura-2 ratio amplitudes of response to sucralose at 10^{-5}, 10^{-4}, 10^{-3}, and 10^{-2} M were significantly higher than the peak amplitude of basal fura-2 oscillation level (**Figure 1C**).

Sucralose-Induced $[Ca^{2+}]_i$ Increases Were Inhibited by Sweet Taste Receptor Inhibitors, under Ca^{2+}-Free Condition, and by L-Type Calcium Channel Blocker

The second administration of sucralose induced repeated $[Ca^{2+}]_i$ increases in 16 of the 20 single-ARC neurons (80%; **Figures 2A,F**). The second addition of sucralose in each neuron was performed in the presence of drugs or in the absence of Ca^{2+}. In the presence of sweet taste receptor inhibitor, gurmarin (Imoto et al., 1991; Shigemura et al., 2008), at 3 μg/ml suppressed sucralose-induced $[Ca^{2+}]_i$ increase in 8 of 10 neurons (80%; **Figures 2B,F**). Peak amplitudes of sucralose-induced $[Ca^{2+}]_i$ increase in the presence of gurmarin were significantly decreased compared with those of control (**Figure 2G**). These data suggest that the sucralose-induced $[Ca^{2+}]_i$ increases in ARC neurons are mediated by the sweet taste receptor. Under extracellular Ca^{2+}-free condition (added with no Ca^{2+} and 0.1 M EGTA), the $[Ca^{2+}]_i$ increase in response to sucralose was abolished in all of 12 neurons (100%; **Figures 2C,F**). The sucralose-induced $[Ca^{2+}]_i$ increase was suppressed by an L-type Ca^{2+} channel blocker, nitrendipine, at 2 μM in 6 of 10 neurons (60%; **Figures 2D,F**) and peak amplitudes of sucralose-induced $[Ca^{2+}]_i$ increase in the presence of nitrendipine were significantly decreased (**Figure 2G**). In contrast, an N-type Ca^{2+} channel blocker, ω-conotoxin GIVA at 500 nM, failed to affect the sucralose-induced $[Ca^{2+}]_i$ increase in most [7 of 8 (80%)] of the sucralose-responding neurons (**Figures 2E–G**). These data suggest that the sucralose-induced $[Ca^{2+}]_i$ increase in ARC neurons depends on sweet taste receptor and extracellular Ca^{2+} influx, especially through the L-type Ca^{2+} channel.

Activation in Response to High-Concentration of Glucose is Mediated by Sweet Taste Receptor

The relationship between sucralose-response and glucose response was examined. Among 22 neurons that responded to sucralose at 10^{-4} M, 12 neurons (55%) exhibited $[Ca^{2+}]_i$ increases in response to elevating the glucose concentration from 1 to 10 mM, the response used to judge the glucose-excited neurons (**Figures 3A,C**). On the other hand, among 22 neurons that increased $[Ca^{2+}]_i$ in response to elevating glucose, 12 neurons (55%) exhibited $[Ca^{2+}]_i$ increases in response to sucralose at 10^{-4} M (**Figures 3A–C**). Notably, there were no sucralose-responding neurons in glucose-inhibited neurons that decreased $[Ca^{2+}]_i$ in response to elevating the glucose

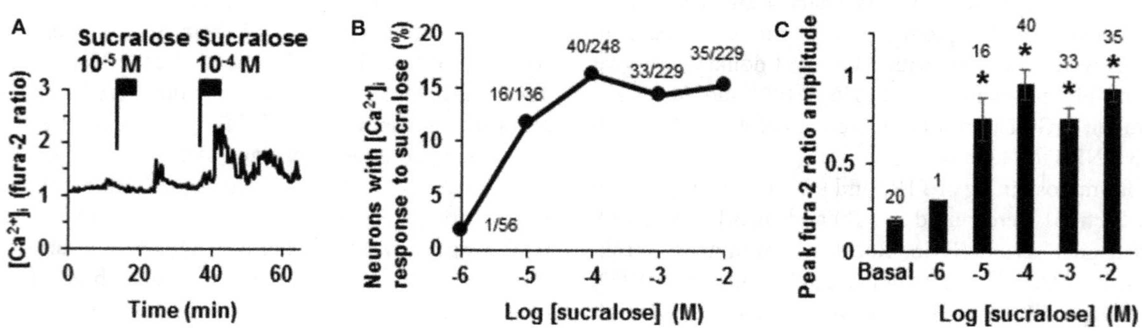

FIGURE 1 | Increase of cytosolic calcium concentration ($[Ca^{2+}]_i$) in ARC neurons after the administration of sucralose. (A) Sequential addition of sucralose at 10^{-5} and 10^{-4} M increased $[Ca^{2+}]_i$ in an ARC neuron. **(B)** Response is expressed as the percentage of neurons that exhibited $[Ca^{2+}]_i$ increases in response to sucralose. The numbers above each point indicate the number of neurons that responded over the number of neurons examined. **(C)** Peak amplitudes of basal oscillation and sucralose-induced $[Ca^{2+}]_i$ increases are expressed. The numbers above each point indicate the number of neurons examined. Mean ± SEM. Unpaired Student's *t*-test was performed to compare peak amplitudes with basal oscillation peak. $^*p < 0.001$.

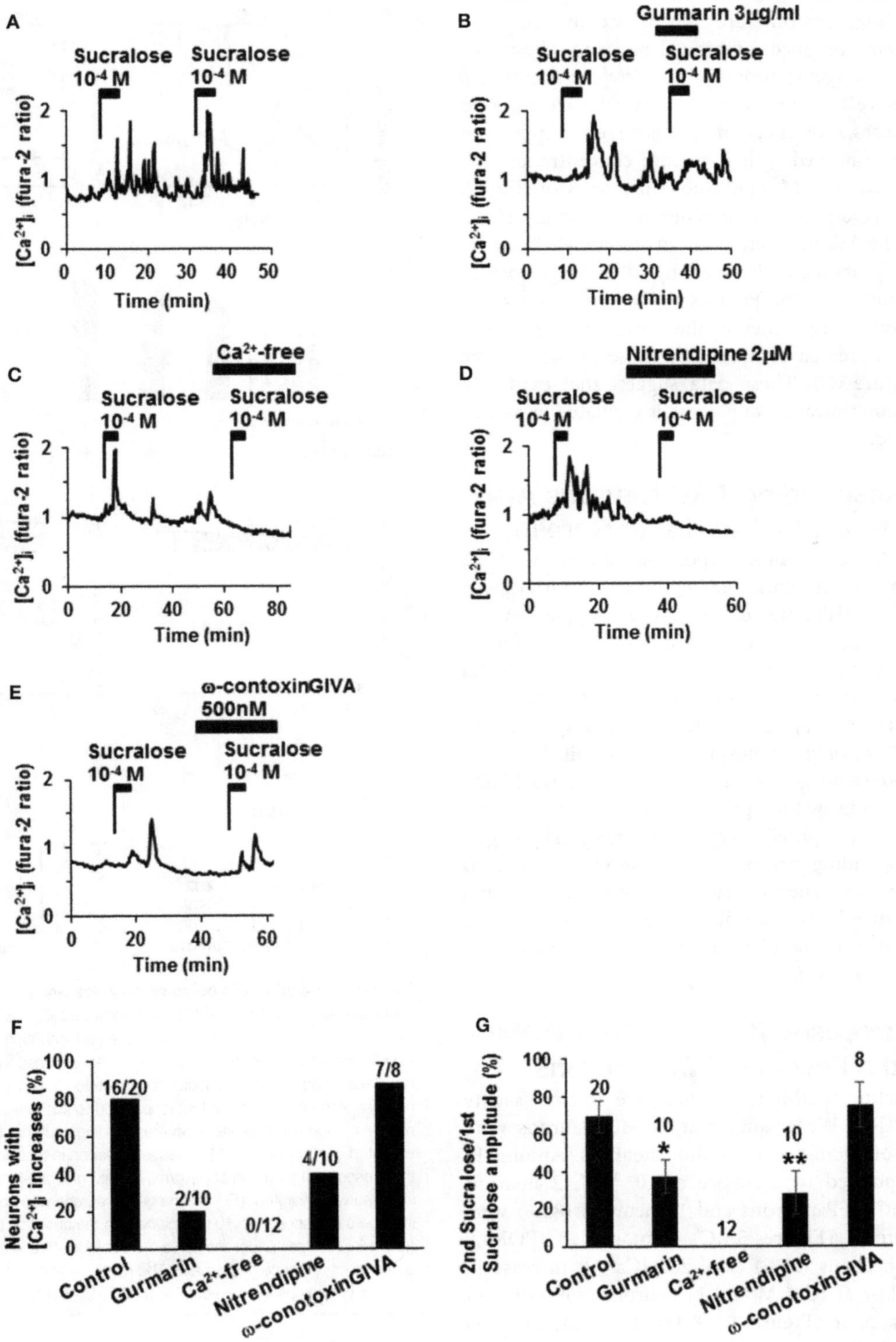

FIGURE 2 | Mechanisms underlying sucralose-induced $[Ca^{2+}]_i$ increases. (A) Administration of sucralose at 10^{-4} M twice induced repeated $[Ca^{2+}]_i$ increases in an ARC neuron. **(B)** Sucralose-induced $[Ca^{2+}]_i$ increases in an ARC neuron were suppressed by gurmarin, an inhibitor of the sweet taste receptor. **(C)** Sucralose-induced $[Ca^{2+}]_i$increases were abolished under a Ca^{2+}-free condition. Sucralose-induced $[Ca^{2+}]_i$ increases were markedly inhibited by nitrendipine, a blocker of L-type Ca^{2+} channel, at 2 μM **(D)**, while it was unaltered by ω-conotoxin GVIA, a blocker of N-type Ca^{2+} channel, at 500 nM **(E)**. **(F)** Incidence of response under control and test conditions is expressed as the percentage of cells that exhibited $[Ca^{2+}]_i$ responses to the second addition of sucralose in each cell. The numbers above each bar indicate the number of neurons that responded over the number of neurons examined. **(G)** The amplitude of sucralose-induced $[Ca^{2+}]_i$ increases under control and test conditions is expressed. The numbers above each point indicate the number of neurons examined. Unpaired Student's *t*-test was performed to compare amplitudes with control. $^*P < 0.05$, $^{**}P < 0.01$.

concentration. These data indicate that more than half of sucralose-responding neurons are glucose-excited neurons, while none of them are glucose-inhibited neurons. These data emphasize the anorexigenic property of sucralose-responding neurons. To explore the contribution of sweet taste receptor to glucose responses, the effect of gurmarin on response to high-glucose was examined. When glucose concentration was increased from 1 to 10 mM, continuous increases of $[Ca^{2+}]_i$ were observed in 11 out of 11 glucose-excited neurons (100%; **Figures 3D,F**). The administration of gurmarin at 3 μg/ml suppressed $[Ca^{2+}]_i$ increases induced by 10 mM glucose in 8 out of 12 neurons (67%; **Figures 3E,F**). Area under the curve of fura-2 ratio amplitudes in the presence of gurmarin was significantly decreased compared to those in the absence of gurmarin (**Figure 3G**). These data suggest that excitation induced by high-concentration of glucose is mediated in part by sweet taste receptor.

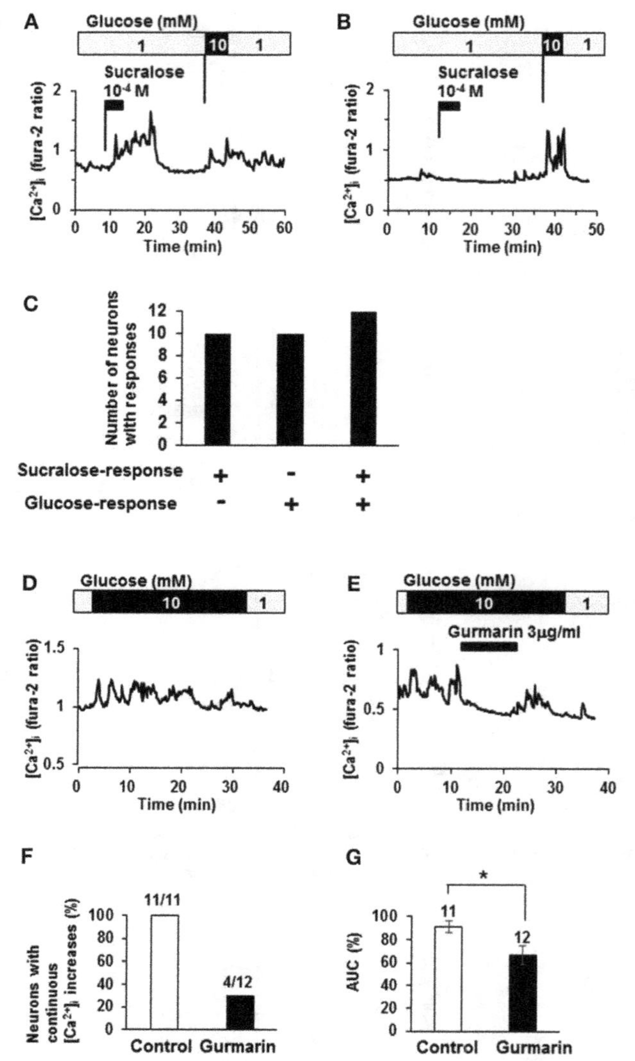

FIGURE 3 | Relationship between sucralose-response and glucose-sensing. (A) An ARC neuron exhibited $[Ca^{2+}]_i$ increases in response to sucralose and raising glucose concentration from 1 to 10 mM. **(B)** An ARC neuron did not exhibit $[Ca^{2+}]_i$ increase in response to sucralose but did in response to raising glucose concentration from 1 to 10 mM. **(C)** The number of the ARC neurons that responded to sucralose and/or glucose at 10 mM. + responding neurons, − non-responding neurons. **(D)** An ARC neuron exhibited continuous $[Ca^{2+}]_i$ increase in response to 10 mM glucose. **(E)** In the presence of gurmarin at 3 μg/ml, 10 mM glucose-induced $[Ca^{2+}]_i$ increase was inhibited. **(F)** Percentage of neurons with continuous $[Ca^{2+}]_i$ increases in response to 10 mM glucose in the absence or presence of gurmarin. **(G)** Area under the curve (AUC) of fura-2 ratio amplitude in the absence or presence of gurmarin. The numbers above bar indicate the number of neurons examined. $^*P < 0.05$ (Unpaired *t*-test).

Sucralose-Responding ARC Neurons Also Responded to Leptin but Not to Ghrelin

To further characterize sucralose-responding neurons in ARC, responsiveness to a satiety hormone, leptin, and an orexigenic hormone, ghrelin, (Nakazato et al., 2001; Coppari et al., 2005; Kohno et al., 2007) was examined. Among 25 neurons that responded to sucralose at 10^{-4} M, 13 neurons (52%) exhibited $[Ca^{2+}]_i$ increases in response to leptin at 10^{-10} M (**Figures 4A,B**). Among 11 neurons that responded to sucralose at 10^{-4} M, only 2 neurons (18%) exhibited $[Ca_{2+}]_i$ increases in response to ghrelin at 10^{-10} M (**Figures 4C,D**). The high overlapping with leptin-responding neurons and low overlapping with ghrelin-responding neurons suggest that sucralose-responding neurons are primarily the neurons implicated in negative energy balance. However, it should be noted that sucralose-responding neurons also include considerable number of non-leptin-responding neurons and ghrelin-responding neurons.

Sucralose Increased $[Ca^{2+}]_i$ in Non-POMC Neurons and a Few of POMC Neurons

Proopiomelanocortin (POMC) neurons are major satiety neurons in the ARC. We examined if POMC neurons were large population of sucralose-responding neurons. Among 14 neurons that responded to sucralose at 10^{-4} M, 2 neurons (14%) were POMC-GFP neurons and 12 neurons (86%) were non-POMC neurons (**Figures 5A,C**). Among 13 POMC-GFP neurons, 2 neurons (15%) exhibited $[Ca^{2+}]_i$ increase in response to sucralose at 10^{-4} M and 11 neurons (85%) did not exhibit $[Ca^{2+}]_i$ increase (**Figures 5A,B,D**). Thus, the majority of sucralose-responding neurons are non-POMC neurons, and only a small part of the POMC neurons responded to sucralose.

Expression of Sweet Taste Receptor on POMC Neurons

Colocalization of T1R2 or T1R3 on POMC neurons was examined. T1R2-immunoreactivity was observed on 31.7 ± 3.0 % (n = 3 brains) of POMC-immunoreactive (IR) neurons (**Figures 6A–D**). Among T1R2-IR neurons in the ARC, 20.7 ± 4.7 % (n = 3 brains) were POMC-IR neurons (**Figures 6A–C,E**). T1R3-immunoreactivity was observed on 17.8 ± 2.8 % (n = 3 brains) of POMC-IR neurons (**Figures 7A–D**). Among T1R3-IR neurons in the ARC, 20.5 ± 4.6 % (n = 3 brains) were POMC-IR neurons (**Figures 7A–C,E**). The colocalization was confirmed by confocal microscopy (**Figures 6F–H, 7F–H**). These

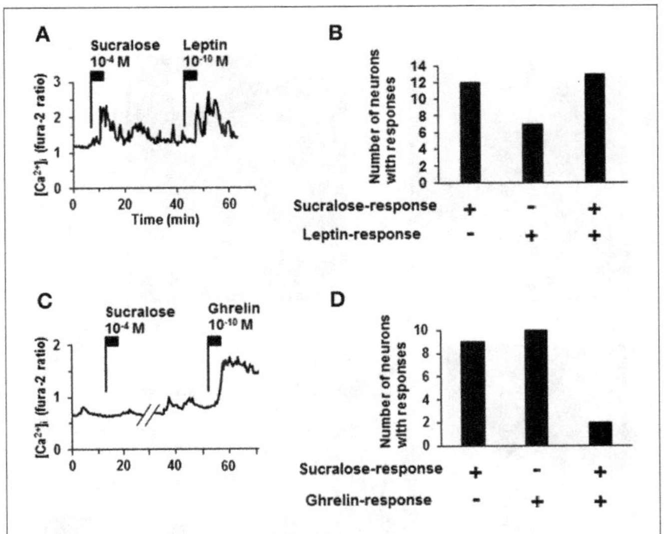

FIGURE 4 | Relationship of sucralose-response to leptin- and ghrelin-response. (A) An ARC neuron exhibited $[Ca^{2+}]_i$ increase in response to both sucralose at 10^{-4} M and leptin at 10^{-10} M. **(B)** The number of responding neurons to sucralose and/or leptin. **(C)** An ARC neurons exhibited $[Ca^{2+}]_i$ increase in response to ghrelin at 10^{-10} M but not to sucralose at 10^{-4} M. **(D)** The number of the ARC neurons that responded to sucralose and/or ghrelin. + responding neurons, – non-responding neurons.

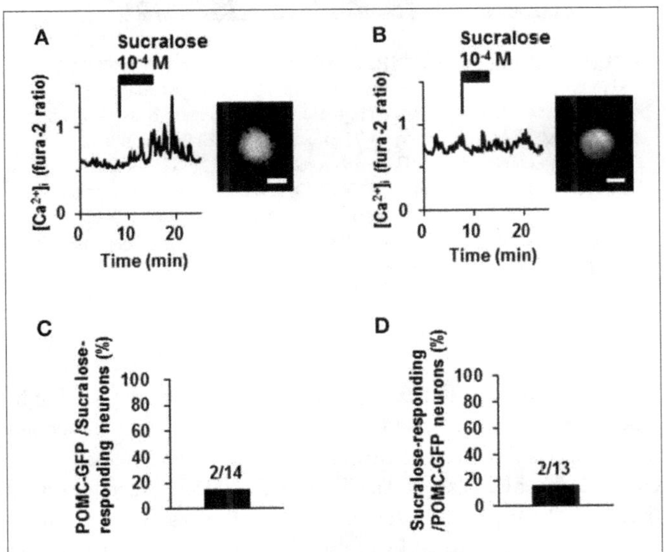

FIGURE 5 | Effect of sucralose on POMC-GFP neurons. (A) A neuron with POMC-GFP fluorescent (right) exhibited $[Ca^{2+}]_i$ increase in response to sucralose (left). **(B)** Another neuron with POMC-GFP fluorescent (right) did not increase $[Ca^{2+}]_i$ in response to sucralose (left). **(C)** Percentage of POMC-GFP neurons among sucralose-responding neurons in ARC. **(D)** Percentage of sucralose-responding neurons among POMC-GFP neurons. The numbers above bar indicate the number of neurons examined. Scale bar 10 μm.

data indicate that the sweet taste receptor is expressed on ARC neurons including a part of the POMC neurons, but non-POMC neurons are major property of sweet taste receptor expressing ARC neurons.

Expression of c-Fos after ICV Administration of Sucralose

Using c-Fos protein as a marker of neuronal activation, activation of ARC neurons following ICV administration of 0.085 mg of sucralose was observed. The number of c-Fos-IR ARC neurons were significantly increased in sucralose-administered mice [266.7 ± 50.5 % (n = 3 brains)] compared to PBS-administered mice [105.7 ± 12.1 % (n = 3 brains); **Figures 8A–E**]. The number of ARC neurons that were IR to both c-Fos and POMC trended to be increased in sucralose-administered mice [33.3 ± 4.3% (n = 3 brains)] compared to PBS-administered mice [18.7 ± 3.9 % (n = 3 brains); $P = 0.07$; **Figure 8F**]. The percentage of POMC-IR neurons among c-Fos-IR neurons (**Figure 8G**) and the percentage of c-Fos-IR neurons among POMC-IR neurons (**Figure 8H**) were not altered after sucralose administration. These data indicate that the sucralose in the brain activates ARC neurons, which partly contain POMC neurons.

DISCUSSION

In this study, we found that an artificial sweetener, sucralose, at 10^{-5}–10^{-2} M increases $[Ca^{2+}]_i$ in ~15% of ARC neurons through the sweet taste receptor-mediated pathway. Sucralose-induced $[Ca^{2+}]_i$ increases were dependent on the extracellular Ca^{2+} influx at least partly through the L-type Ca^{2+} channel. A large part of sucralose-responding ARC neurons were high-glucose- and leptin-responsive neurons. In addition, response to high concentration of glucose was contributed by sweet taste receptor. Low percentage of POMC neurons were included in sucralose responding neurons, c-Fos expressing neurons, and sweet taste receptor-expressing neurons in the ARC. These findings indicate that sweet taste receptor mediated neuronal activation occurs mainly in high-glucose-and leptin- responsive non-POMC neurons in the ARC, which may contribute to the neuronal activation in response to high-glucose. These mechanisms could be implicated in feeding regulation and energy homeostasis.

There are variety of natural and artificial sweet taste molecules in the body and in food, including carbohydrates, numerous amino acids, metabolites, peptides, glycoside, and artificial sweeteners. Carbohydrates are common natural sweet taste molecules and work as an energy source after being catabolized in each cell. Sucralose is barely catabolized and is thereby non-nutritive. In addition, the sweetness intensity of sucralose is much higher than sucrose (Knight, 1994). To purely observe the effect of the sweet taste molecules and to exclude their nutritive effects, sucralose was used in this study. Indeed, most effects of sucralose were suppressed by the inhibitor of the sweet taste receptor, suggesting that sucralose works as a sweet taste molecule but not as fuel for cellular metabolism.

We found that sucralose at 10^{-5}–10^{-2} M induces $[Ca^{2+}]_i$ increases in ARC neurons. Similarly, it is reported that sucralose at 10^{-3}–5×10^{-2} M induces $[Ca^{2+}]_i$ increases in MIN6 cells, a mouse pancreatic β-cell line (Nakagawa et al., 2009). Additionally, sucralose at 2×10^{-4}–5×10^{-3} M induces GLP-1 secretion from NCI-H716 cells, a human enteroendocrine L cell

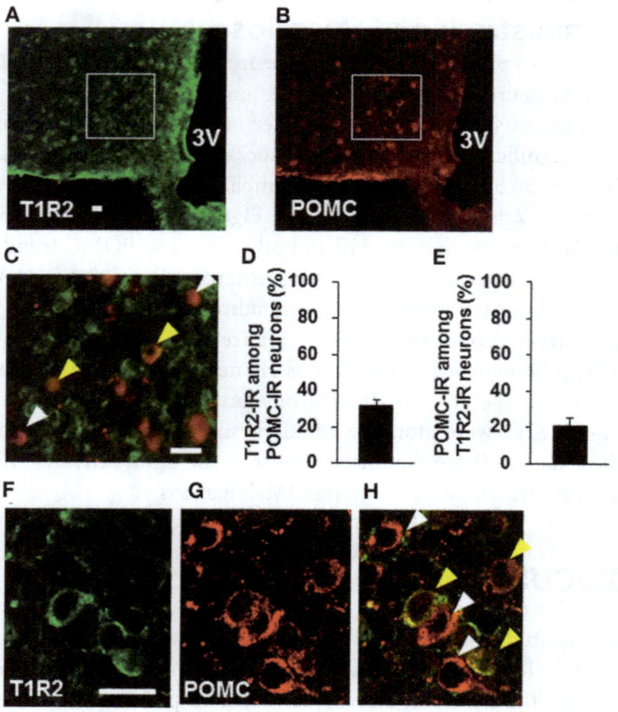

FIGURE 6 | Distribution of T1R2 on POMC neurons in the ARC. T1R2 **(A)** and POMC **(B)** immunofluorescent images and their merged image with high magnification **(C)**. **(D)** Percentage of T1R2-imunoreactive (IR) neurons among POMC-IR neurons in the ARC ($n = 3$ brains). **(E)** Percentage of POMC-IR neurons among T1R2-IR neurons in the ARC ($n = 3$ brains). Confocal images of T1R2 **(F)** and POMC **(G)** immunofluorescent and their merged image **(H)**. White arrowhead indicates non-colocalizing POMC-IR neuron, and yellow arrowhead indicates a colocalizing neuron. Scale bar; 20 μm. Graphs show mean ± SEM.

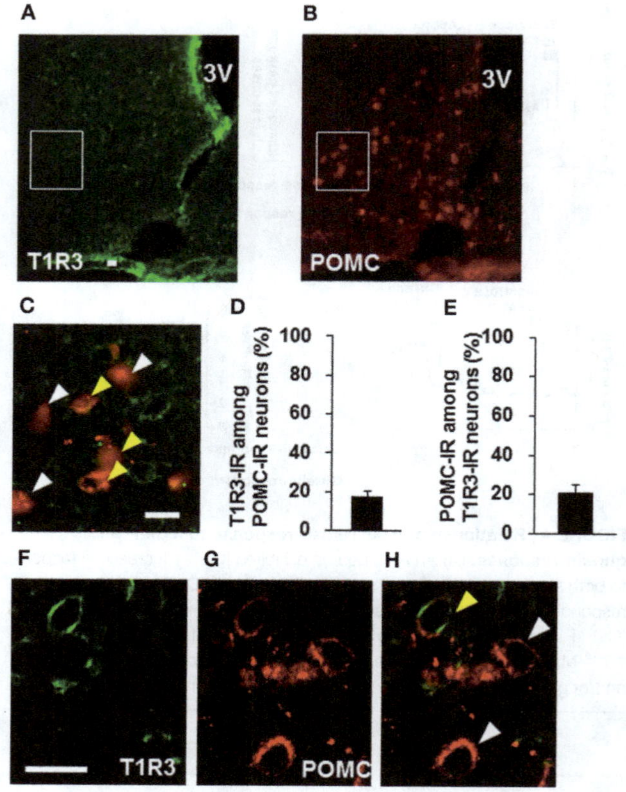

FIGURE 7 | Distribution of T1R3 on POMC neurons in the ARC. T1R3 **(A)** and POMC **(B)** immunofluorescent images and their merged image with high-magnification **(C)**. **(D)** Percentage of T1R3-imunoreactive (IR) neurons among POMC-IR neurons in the ARC ($n = 3$ brains). **(E)** Percentage of POMC-IR neurons among T1R3-IR neurons in the ARC ($n = 3$ brains). Confocal images of T1R3 **(F)** and POMC **(G)** immunofluorescent and their merged image **(H)**. White arrowhead indicates non-colocalizing POMC-IR neuron, and yellow arrowhead indicates a colocalizing neuron. Scale bar; 20 μm. Graphs show mean ± SEM.

line (Jang et al., 2007). These data support the assumption that sucralose may induce the excitement of cellular activity in a sweet taste receptor-dependent manner. Higher sensitivity of ARC neurons to sucralose could be related to the lower concentration of sweet taste molecules, such as glucose, in the brain compared to the periphery. Glucose concentration in the brain is estimated to be lower than that in blood (Routh et al., 2014).

Sucralose-induced $[Ca^{2+}]_i$ increases in ARC neurons were dependent on extracellular Ca^{2+} influx, especially through L-type Ca^{2+} channel. Of note, sucralose-induced intracellular signaling could just be a part of the signals that may be induced at the downstream of sweet taste receptors. In pancreatic β-cells and intestinal GLP-1-secreting cells, a variety of sweeteners induce diverse patterns of intracellular signals (Nakagawa et al., 2013; Ohtsu et al., 2014).

In this study, we found sweet taste receptor contributes to the response to high-concentration of glucose. This is similar to role of sweet taste receptor in the pancreatic beta cells where sweet taste receptors serve as glucose receptors (Nakagawa et al., 2009; Hamano et al., 2015; Kojima et al., 2015). RNA expression levels of T1R2 and T1R3 are altered in response to the change of glucose concentration and obesity (Ren et al., 2009; Herrera Moro Chao et al., 2016). Glucose-sensing mediated by sweet taste receptor could be affected by whole body energy status. High-glucose responses are also contributed by some other molecules including AMP-activated protein kinase and ATP-sensitive K^+ channel (Ibrahim et al., 2003; Claret et al., 2007). In fact, we found that in 33% of glucose-excited neurons, the responses to high-glucose were not altered by the inhibitor of sweet taste receptor, suggesting that high-glucose responses are mediated by sweet taste receptor and other signaling mechanisms. These distinct mechanisms are segregated but could interact with each other. Further studies are required to clarify the precise mechanisms of high-glucose response.

While high-glucose response was suppressed by sweet taste receptor inhibitor in 67% of glucose-excited neurons, sucralose response was observed only in 55% of glucose-responding neurons. This 12% of the difference could be due to the differences between glucose and sucralose as a ligand of sweet taste receptor. The characteristics of sweet taste receptor that can induce multiple downstream signaling cascades depending on ligands (Nakagawa et al., 2013) may have caused the difference

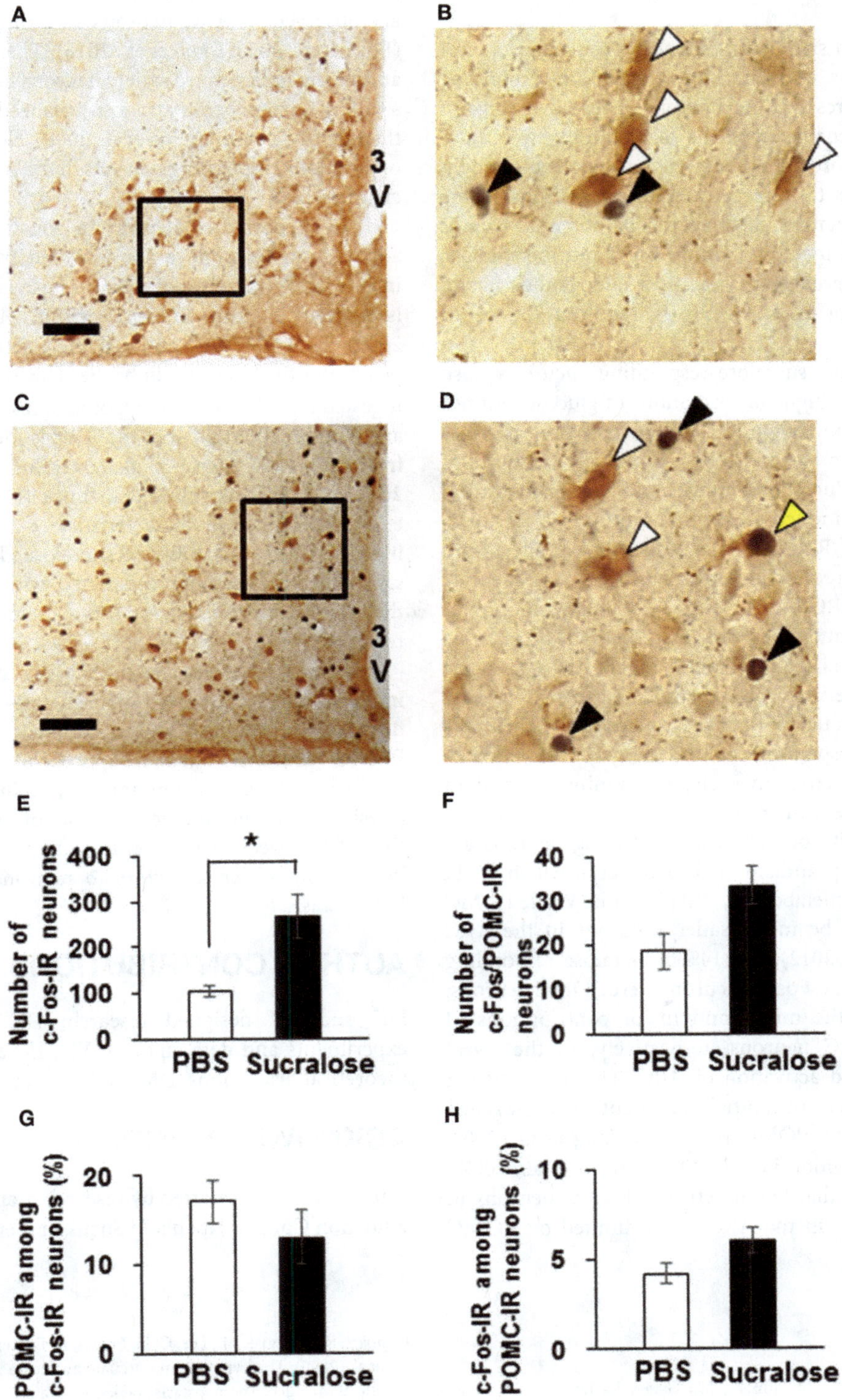

FIGURE 8 | Expression of c-Fos on POMC neurons after intracerebroventricular (ICV) administration of sucralose. Mice ($n = 3$) were given a single ICV administration of PBS **(A,B)** or 0.085 mg of sucralose **(C,D)** and killed 30 min later. c-Fos-IR neurons (black) and POMC-IR neurons (brown) were detected in the ARC. Scale bar 100 μm. Black arrowhead, c-Fos-IR neuron, white arrowhead, POMC-IR neurons, yellow arrowhead, neuron immunoreactive to both c-Fos and POMC. **(E)** The number of c-Fos-IR ARC neurons 30 min after ICV administration of PBS or 0.085 mg of sucralose. **(F)** The number of ARC neurons that are immunoreactive to both c-Fos and POMC 30 min after ICV administration of PBS or 0.085 mg of sucralose. **(G)** Percentage of POMC-IR neurons among c-Fos-IR neurons. **(H)** Percentage of c-Fos-IR neurons among POMC-IR neurons. Graphs show mean ± SEM. $^*P < 0.05$ (Unpaired t-test).

between glucose and sucralose in inducing sweet taste receptor-mediated responses.

In this study, 45% of sucralose-responding neurons were not glucose-excited neurons, and also 18% of sucralose-responding neurons were ghrelin-responding neurons. These data suggest that wide variety of neurons could be regulated by sweet taste receptor. Not only glucose but other sweet taste molecules might also be ligands of sweet taste receptor on these neurons. There are several other sweet molecules that can be potential ligands of sweet taste receptor, including amino acids and metabolites, such as glycerol. Comprehensive search of endogenous ligand of sweet taste receptor in the ARC is required for better understanding.

More than half of sucralose-responding neurons also responded to leptin and high concentrations of glucose, but not ghrelin. The concentration of ghrelin in blood rises preprandially while glucose and leptin levels rise post-prandially (Cummings et al., 2001). Ghrelin induces food intake and high-concentration of glucose and leptin induce satiety (Cummings et al., 2001; Nakazato et al., 2001; Routh et al., 2014). These effects are largely mediated by direct actions of ghrelin on neuropeptide Y/AgRP neurons in ARC and by direct excitatory actions of glucose and leptin on satiety neurons including POMC neurons in ARC (Nakazato et al., 2001; Kohno et al., 2003; Coppari et al., 2005). Therefore, the role of ARC neurons in feeding regulation can be suspected by their responsiveness to these key molecules. Sucralose-responding neurons largely responded to both leptin and high-glucose. Inversely, only a minor fraction of sucralose-responding neurons responded to ghrelin. These data implies that the majority of sucralose-responding neurons are those functioning post-prandially or in fed states, which could control feeding, energy metabolism, and glycemia. While POMC neurons are known to be major satiety neurons in the ARC (Williams and Elmquist, 2012), only 14% of sucralose-responding neurons and only 13% of c-Fos-IR neurons were POMC neurons. These results suggest the minor and major contributions of POMC and non-POMC neurons, respectively, to the sweet taste receptor-medicated activation of ARC. This is consistent with previous reports that substantial fraction of glucose-excited neurons in ARC are non-POMC neurons (Wang et al., 2004; Claret et al., 2007; Fioramonti et al., 2007; Parton et al., 2007). While it is well-known that leptin activates POMC neurons in the ARC, leptin's action in the ARC is not limited on POMC neurons. Leptin receptor and leptin-induced immediate signals are observed in ARC neurons including non-POMC neurons (Elias et al., 2000; Lima et al., 2016). There could be unidentified and/or uncharacterized satiety neurons in the ARC. For example, a satiety hormone, nesfatin-1, is localized in ARC neurons other than POMC neurons (Foo et al., 2008). Neurochemical properties of sucralose-responding neurons in the ARC remain to be further characterized.

It is reported that only a small percentage of orally administrated sucralose are absorbed from the intestinal tract in rats, and that most of intravenously administrated sucralose is excreted in urine and feces within 24 h in rats (Sims et al., 2000). It is not yet known if the portion of blood sucralose penetrates the blood-brain barrier (BBB), and the effect of orally ingested sucralose on the hypothalamus is unknown (Schiffman and Rother, 2013). BBB in the ARC is morphologically different from other area (Shaver et al., 1992; Rodríguez et al., 2010; Ciofi, 2011) and is compromised in mice from obese mother (Kim et al., 2016). These characteristics of BBB in the ARC might increase the permeability of sucralose. To clarify the potential side effect of sucralose consumed with foods and to explore the therapeutic application of sucralose, further studies are required.

In this study, we found that the sweet taste receptor is implicated in activation of high-glucose- and leptin- responsive neurons in the ARC, the majority of which are non-POMC neurons. Further, approaches including genetically modified mouse and non-antibody staining could uncover the physiological role and localization of sweet taste receptor in the ARC. Sweet taste receptors may play an important role in coupling systemic factors to neuronal activity and energy homeostasis.

AUTHOR CONTRIBUTIONS

DK and TY designed research; DK and MK performed experiments and data analysis; YN, IK, and TK contributed to theoretical discussions. DK and TY wrote the paper.

ACKNOWLEDGMENTS

This work was supported by research grants for DK from Nestlé Nutrition Council Japan and Suzuken memorial foundation.

REFERENCES

Bady, I., Marty, N., Dallaporta, M., Emery, M., Gyger, J., Tarussio, D., et al. (2006). Evidence from glut2-null mice that glucose is a critical physiological regulator of feeding. *Diabetes* 55, 988–995. doi: 10.2337/diabetes.55.04.06.db05-1386

Ciofi, P. (2011). The arcuate nucleus as a circumventricular organ in the mouse. *Neurosci. Lett.* 487, 187–190. doi: 10.1016/j.neulet.2010.10.019

Claret, M., Smith, M. A., Batterham, R. L., Selman, C., Choudhury, A. I., Fryer, L. G., et al. (2007). AMPK is essential for energy homeostasis regulation and glucose sensing by POMC and AgRP neurons. *J. Clin. Invest.* 117, 2325–2336. doi: 10.1172/JCI31516

Coppari, R., Ichinose, M., Lee, C. E., Pullen, A. E., Kenny, C. D., McGovern, R. A., et al. (2005). The hypothalamic arcuate nucleus: a key site for mediating leptin's effects on glucose homeostasis and locomotor activity. *Cell Metab.* 1, 63–72. doi: 10.1016/j.cmet.2004.12.004

Cummings, D. E., Purnell, J. Q., Frayo, R. S., Schmidova, K., Wisse, B. E., and Weigle, D. S. (2001). A preprandial rise in plasma ghrelin levels suggests a role in meal initiation in humans. *Diabetes* 50, 1714–1719. doi: 10.2337/diabetes.50.8.1714

Elias, C. F., Kelly, J. F., Lee, C. E., Ahima, R. S., Drucker, D. J., Saper, C. B., et al. (2000). Chemical characterization of leptin-activated neurons in the rat brain. *J. Comp. Neurol.* 423, 261–281. doi: 10.1002/1096-9861(20000724)423:2<261::AID-CNE6>3.0.CO;2-6

Fioramonti, X., Contié, S., Song, Z., Routh, V. H., Lorsignol, A., and Pénicaud, L. (2007). Characterization of glucosensing neuron subpopulations in the arcuate nucleus: integration in neuropeptide Y and pro-opio melanocortin networks? *Diabetes* 56, 1219–1227. doi: 10.2337/db06-0567

Foo, K. S., Brismar, H., and Broberger, C. (2008). Distribution and neuropeptide coexistence of nucleobindin-2 mRNA/nesfatin-like immunoreactivity in the rat CNS. *Neuroscience* 156, 563–579. doi: 10.1016/j.neuroscience.2008.07.054

Hamano, K., Nakagawa, Y., Ohtsu, Y., Li, L., Medina, J., Tanaka, Y., et al. (2015). Lactisole inhibits the glucose-sensing receptor T1R3 expressed in mouse pancreatic beta-cells. *J. Endocrinol.* 226, 57–66. doi: 10.1530/JOE-15-0102

Herrera Moro Chao, D., Argmann, C., Van Eijk, M., Boot, R. G., Ottenhoff, R., Van Roomen, C., et al. (2016). Impact of obesity on taste receptor expression in extra-oral tissues: emphasis on hypothalamus and brainstem. *Sci. Rep.* 6:29094. doi: 10.1038/srep29094

Ibrahim, N., Bosch, M. A., Smart, J. L., Qiu, J., Rubinstein, M., Ronnekleiv, O. K., et al. (2003). Hypothalamic proopiomelanocortin neurons are glucose responsive and express K(ATP) channels. *Endocrinology* 144, 1331–1340. doi: 10.1210/en.2002-221033

Imoto, T., Miyasaka, A., Ishima, R., and Akasaka, K. (1991). A novel peptide isolated from the leaves of Gymnema sylvestre–I. Characterization and its suppressive effect on the neural responses to sweet taste stimuli in the rat. *Comp. Biochem. Physiol. A Comp. Physiol.* 100, 309–314. doi: 10.1016/0300-9629(91)90475-R

Jang, H. J., Kokrashvili, Z., Theodorakis, M. J., Carlson, O. D., Kim, B. J., Zhou, J., et al. (2007). Gut-expressed gustducin and taste receptors regulate secretion of glucagon-like peptide-1. *Proc. Natl. Acad. Sci. U.S.A.* 104, 15069–15074. doi: 10.1073/pnas.0706890104

Kim, D. W., Glendining, K. A., Grattan, D. R., and Jasoni, C. L. (2016). Maternal obesity in the mouse compromises the blood-brain barrier in the arcuate nucleus of offspring. *Endocrinology* 157, 2229–2242. doi: 10.1210/en.2016-1014

Knight, I. (1994). The development and applications of sucralose, a new high-intensity sweetener. *Can. J. Physiol. Pharmacol.* 72, 435–439. doi: 10.1139/y94-063

Kohno, D., Gao, H. Z., Muroya, S., Kikuyama, S., and Yada, T. (2003). Ghrelin directly interacts with neuropeptide-Y-containing neurons in the rat arcuate nucleus: Ca2+ signaling via protein kinase A and N-type channel-dependent mechanisms and cross-talk with leptin and orexin. *Diabetes* 52, 948–956. doi: 10.2337/diabetes.52.4.948

Kohno, D., Nakata, M., Maekawa, F., Fujiwara, K., Maejima, Y., Kuramochi, M., et al. (2007). Leptin suppresses ghrelin-induced activation of neuropeptide Y neurons in the arcuate nucleus via phosphatidylinositol 3-kinase- and phosphodiesterase 3-mediated pathway. *Endocrinology* 148, 2251–2263. doi: 10.1210/en.2006-1240

Kojima, I., Nakagawa, Y., Ohtsu, Y., Hamano, K., Medina, J., and Nagasawa, M. (2015). Return of the glucoreceptor: glucose activates the glucose-sensing receptor T1R3 and facilitates metabolism in pancreatic beta-cells. *J. Diabetes Investig.* 6, 256–263. doi: 10.1111/jdi.12304

Kurita, H., Xu, K. Y., Maejima, Y., Nakata, M., Dezaki, K., Santoso, P., et al. (2015). Arcuate Na+,K+-ATPase senses systemic energy states and regulates feeding behavior through glucose-inhibited neurons. *Am. J. Physiol. Endocrinol. Metab.* 309, E320–E333. doi: 10.1152/ajpendo.00446.2014

Li, F. (2013). Taste perception: from the tongue to the testis. *Mol. Hum. Reprod.* 19, 349–360. doi: 10.1093/molehr/gat009

Lima, L. B., Metzger, M., Furigo, I. C., and Donato, J. Jr. (2016). Leptin receptor-positive and leptin receptor-negative proopiomelanocortin neurons innervate an identical set of brain structures. *Brain Res.* 1646, 366–376. doi: 10.1016/j.brainres.2016.06.024

Nakagawa, Y., Nagasawa, M., Medina, J., and Kojima, I. (2015). Glucose evokes rapid Ca2+ and cyclic AMP signals by activating the cell-surface glucose-sensing receptor in pancreatic β-cells. *PLoS ONE* 10:e0144053. doi: 10.1371/journal.pone.0144053

Nakagawa, Y., Nagasawa, M., Mogami, H., Lohse, M., Ninomiya, Y., and Kojima, I. (2013). Multimodal function of the sweet taste receptor expressed in pancreatic beta-cells: generation of diverse patterns of intracellular signals by sweet agonists. *Endocr. J.* 60, 1191–1206. doi: 10.1507/endocrj.EJ13-0282

Nakagawa, Y., Nagasawa, M., Yamada, S., Hara, A., Mogami, H., Nikolaev, V. O., et al. (2009). Sweet taste receptor expressed in pancreatic beta-cells activates the calcium and cyclic AMP signaling systems and stimulates insulin secretion. *PLoS ONE* 4:e5106. doi: 10.1371/journal.pone.0005106

Nakazato, M., Murakami, N., Date, Y., Kojima, M., Matsuo, H., Kangawa, K., et al. (2001). A role for ghrelin in the central regulation of feeding. *Nature* 409, 194–198. doi: 10.1038/35051587

Ohtsu, Y., Nakagawa, Y., Nagasawa, M., Takeda, S., Arakawa, H., and Kojima, I. (2014). Diverse signaling systems activated by the sweet taste receptor in human GLP-1-secreting cells. *Mol. Cell. Endocrinol.* 394, 70–79. doi: 10.1016/j.mce.2014.07.004

O'Malley, D., Reimann, F., Simpson, A. K., and Gribble, F. M. (2006). Sodium-coupled glucose cotransporters contribute to hypothalamic glucose sensing. *Diabetes* 55, 3381–3386. doi: 10.2337/db06-0531

Oomura, Y., Ooyama, H., Sugimori, M., Nakamura, T., and Yamada, Y. (1974). Glucose inhibition of the glucose-sensitive neurone in the rat lateral hypothalamus. *Nature* 247, 284–286. doi: 10.1038/247284a0

Parton, L. E., Ye, C. P., Coppari, R., Enriori, P. J., Choi, B., Zhang, C. Y., et al. (2007). Glucose sensing by POMC neurons regulates glucose homeostasis and is impaired in obesity. *Nature* 449, 228–232. doi: 10.1038/nature06098

Pinto, S., Roseberry, A. G., Liu, H., Diano, S., Shanabrough, M., Cai, X., et al. (2004). Rapid rewiring of arcuate nucleus feeding circuits by leptin. *Science* 304, 110–115. doi: 10.1126/science.1089459

Ren, X., Zhou, L., Terwilliger, R., Newton, S. S., and De Araujo, I. E. (2009). Sweet taste signaling functions as a hypothalamic glucose sensor. *Front. Integr. Neurosci.* 3:12. doi: 10.3389/neuro.07.012.2009

Rodríguez, E. M., Blázquez, J. L., and Guerra, M. (2010). The design of barriers in the hypothalamus allows the median eminence and the arcuate nucleus to enjoy private milieus: the former opens to the portal blood and the latter to the cerebrospinal fluid. *Peptides* 31, 757–776. doi: 10.1016/j.peptides.2010.01.003

Routh, V. H., Hao, L., Santiago, A. M., Sheng, Z., and Zhou, C. (2014). Hypothalamic glucose sensing: making ends meet. *Front. Syst. Neurosci.* 8:236. doi: 10.3389/fnsys.2014.00236

Sasaki, T., Kim, H. J., Kobayashi, M., Kitamura, Y. I., Yokota-Hashimoto, H., Shiuchi, T., et al. (2010). Induction of hypothalamic Sirt1 leads to cessation of feeding via agouti-related peptide. *Endocrinology* 151, 2556–2566. doi: 10.1210/en.2009-1319

Schiffman, S. S., and Rother, K. I. (2013). Sucralose, a synthetic organochlorine sweetener: overview of biological issues. *J. Toxicol. Environ. Health B Crit. Rev.* 16, 399–451. doi: 10.1080/10937404.2013.842523

Shaver, S. W., Pang, J. J., Wainman, D. S., Wall, K. M., and Gross, P. M. (1992). Morphology and function of capillary networks in subregions of the rat tuber cinereum. *Cell Tissue Res.* 267, 437–448. doi: 10.1007/BF00319366

Shigemura, N., Nakao, K., Yasuo, T., Murata, Y., Yasumatsu, K., Nakashima, A., et al. (2008). Gurmarin sensitivity of sweet taste responses is associated with co-expression patterns of T1r2, T1r3, and gustducin. *Biochem. Biophys. Res. Commun.* 367, 356–363. doi: 10.1016/j.bbrc.2007.12.146

Sims, J., Roberts, A., Daniel, J. W., and Renwick, A. G. (2000). The metabolic fate of sucralose in rats. *Food Chem. Toxicol.* 38(Suppl. 2), S115–S121. doi: 10.1016/S0278-6915(00)00034-X

Wang, R., Liu, X., Hentges, S. T., Dunn-Meynell, A. A., Levin, B. E., Wang, W., et al. (2004). The regulation of glucose-excited neurons in the hypothalamic arcuate nucleus by glucose and feeding-relevant peptides. *Diabetes* 53, 1959–1965. doi: 10.2337/diabetes.53.8.1959

Williams, K. W., and Elmquist, J. K. (2012). From neuroanatomy to behavior: central integration of peripheral signals regulating feeding behavior. *Nat. Neurosci.* 15, 1350–1355. doi: 10.1038/nn.3217

12

Hypothalamic Integration of Metabolic, Endocrine and Circadian Signals in Fish: Involvement in the Control of Food Intake

*María J. Delgado[1], José M. Cerdá-Reverter[2] and José L. Soengas[3]**

[1] Departamento de Fisiología (Fisiología Animal II), Facultad de Biología, Universidad Complutense de Madrid, Madrid, Spain, [2] Departamento de Fisiología de Peces y Biotecnología, Instituto de Acuicultura Torre de la Sal, Consejo Superior de Investigaciones Científicas, Castellón, Spain, [3] Laboratorio de Fisioloxía Animal, Departamento de Bioloxía Funcional e Ciencias da Saúde, Facultade de Bioloxía, Universidade de Vigo, Vigo, Spain

***Correspondence:**
José L. Soengas
jsoengas@uvigo.es

The regulation of food intake in fish is a complex process carried out through several different mechanisms in the central nervous system (CNS) with hypothalamus being the main regulatory center. As in mammals, a complex hypothalamic circuit including two populations of neurons: one co-expressing neuropeptide Y (NPY) and Agouti-related peptide (AgRP) and the second one population co-expressing pro-opiomelanocortin (POMC) and cocaine- and amphetamine-regulated transcript (CART) is involved in the integration of information relating to food intake control. The production and release of these peptides control food intake, and the production results from the integration of information of different nature such as levels of nutrients and hormones as well as circadian signals. The present review summarizes the knowledge and recent findings about the presence and functioning of these mechanisms in fish and their differences vs. the known mammalian model.

Keywords: food intake, fish, hypothalamus, review, nutrient sensing, circadian rhythm, leptin, ghrelin

INTRODUCTION

Food intake is regulated through positive and negative loops acting at different locations and at different times (Langhans and Scharrer, 1992; Langhans, 1999). The positive loop (starting of food intake) results from the relationship among prior experience with nutrient availability, status of the animal and sensory qualities of the food. The negative loop relates to metabolic and gastrointestinal inputs displaying changes prior and after absorption (Langhans, 1999). Three regulatory levels have been suggested following this model: (i) short-term regulatory factors: those influenced by the size of a single meal, (ii) mid-term regulatory factors: those operating through several days; and (iii) long-term regulatory factors: those operating through longer time periods (weeks, months, and years) reflecting energy balance of the animal. These levels of regulation create a feedback loop that continuously modulate the immediate signal input from sense organs and internal sensors, which together with prior learning integrate information from the energy reserves of the body. The control determining the feeding behavior and food intake is elicited by the central nervous system (CNS) through various pathways, and hypothalamus is the main center involved in such regulation (Schwartz et al., 2000; Berthoud, 2002).

In fish is difficult to establish which factors act in the mid- or long-term, since most available data come from short-term studies. The basic mechanisms involved in regulation of food intake in fish appear to be similar to those of mammals with differences implying the existence of specific mechanisms in fish (Kulczykowska and Sánchez-Vázquez, 2010; Hoskins and Volkoff, 2012; Volkoff, 2016). In the following sections, we review the existing knowledge about hypothalamic integration in fish of metabolic, endocrine, and circadian information to elicit a coordinated feeding response, as summarized in **Figure 1**.

HYPOTHALAMIC NEUROPEPTIDES INVOLVED IN THE CONTROL OF FOOD INTAKE

The integration of information involved in the control of food intake takes place in mammals through a circuit mainly localized in hypothalamic areas including arcuate (ARC), ventromedial, paraventricular, and lateral hypothalamus (Berthoud and Morrison, 2008; Zheng and Berthoud, 2008). These circuits include two populations of neurons (Mobbs et al., 2005; Blouet and Schwartz, 2010; Waterson and Horvath, 2015). The first population co-expresses neuropeptide Y (NPY) and agouti-related peptide (AgRP) and the second population co-expresses pro-opiomelanocortin (POMC) and cocaine- and amphetamine-regulated transcript (CART). Moreover, these two populations of neurons inhibit each other resulting in signaling to other higher-order neurons. The production and release of these peptides control food intake, and this occurs through integration of signals of metabolic, endocrine, and circadian nature. Other peptides such as orexins are involved in food intake modulation but they are not involved in this main integrative core.

Avaliable studies in fish (mostly through asssessment of mRNA abundance) demonstrated expression of these neuropeptides in hypothalamus. Neurons expressing NPY, AgRP, CART, and POMC in fish respond to energy challenge suggesting that the main hypothalamic pathways coordinating a response to regulate energy homeostasis are conserved throughout vertebrate evolution (Volkoff et al., 2005).

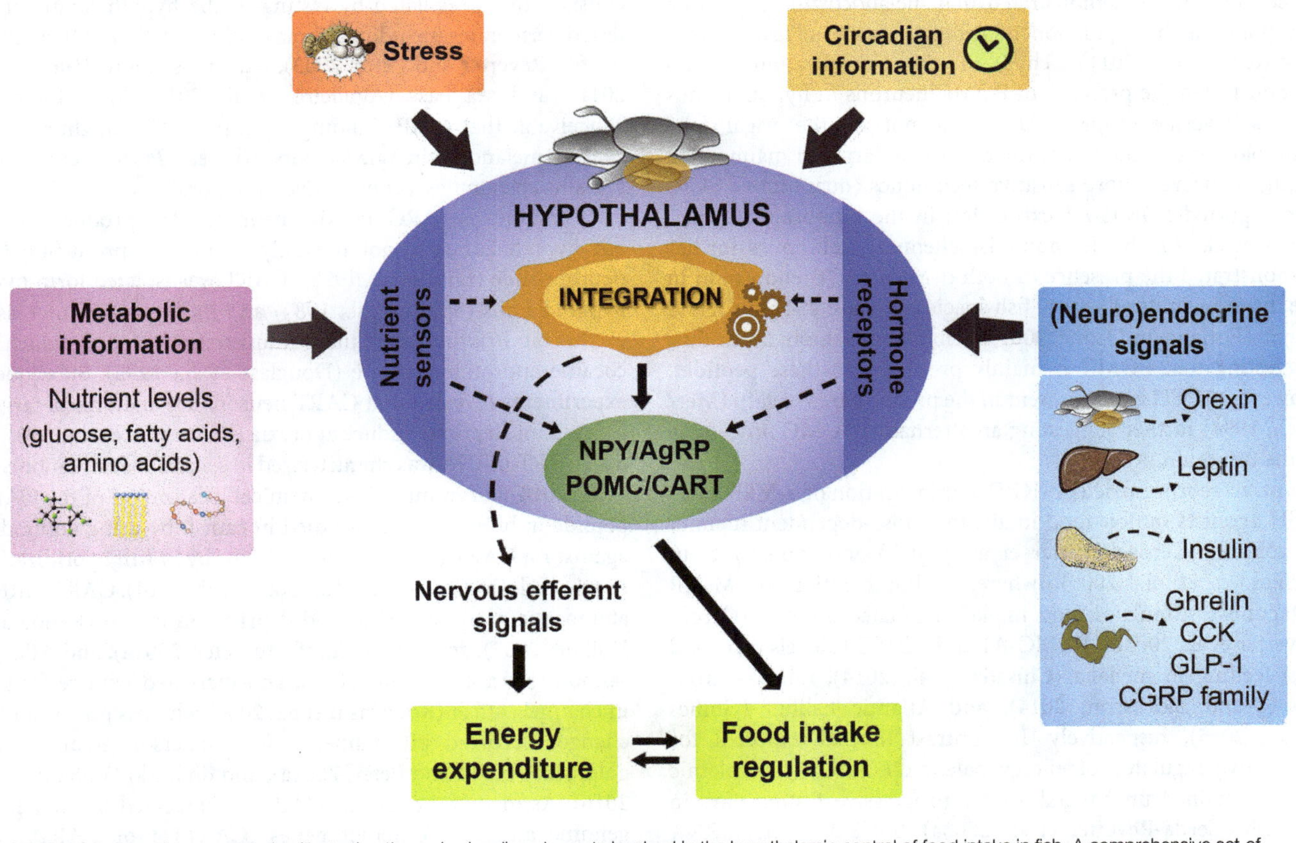

FIGURE 1 | Schematic representation illustrating the main signaling elements involved in the hypothalamic control of food intake in fish. A comprehensive set of central and peripheral neuroendocrine messengers in a coordinated way with the metabolic information provided by nutrient levels constitute the main signaling that regulates hypothalamic neurocircuits involved in the regulation of food intake. The detailed description of such main functional neuropeptidergic circuits is shown in the text. The hypothalamus also integrates the stress response in the generation of the adaptive changes in food intake and energy expenditure according to the exposure to stressful conditions. Finally, the role of hypothalamus in the internal coordination of circadian rhythmicity related to feeding behavior is also described in the text. AgRP, agouti-related peptide; CART, cocaine- and amphetamine-related transcript; CCK, cholecystokinin; CGRP, calcitonin gene-related peptide; GLP-1, glucagon-like peptide 1; POMC, pro-opiomelanocortin; NPY, neuropeptide Y.

CART/POMC

Melanocortins integrate a key system in the regulation of food intake in vertebrates. These peptides, exhibiting melanotropic (melanin stimulation) and corticotropic (corticosteroid stimulation) activity encoded in the common precursor POMC. Two discrete groups of neurons in ARC and the caudal region of the nucleus of the tractus solitarius of the medulla produce POMC, mainly processed into α-melanocyte-stimulating hormone (α-MSH) and β-endorphin. Melanocortin signaling is transduced by five different G-coupled receptors (MC1R-MC5R) but only two are conspicuously expressed in the mammalian brain, i.e., MC3R and MC4R. Central activation of these receptors appears to mediate melanocortin effects on energy balance since both MC3R knockout rat and MC4R knockout mice display severe alterations in energy homeostasis (obesity, increased food intake and linear growth in MC4R; hypophagia, increased fat mass and food efficiency but reduced lean mass in MC3R). Accordingly, central administration of MC3/4Rs agonists results in a dose-dependent reduction in food intake in mice but MC4R-deficient mice do not respond to anorectic effects of agonists, suggesting that α-MSH inhibits feeding primarily by activating MC4R (reviewed by Anderson et al., 2016).

Several studies demonstrated that melanocortin system is a key point in the regulation of energy balance in fish (Cerdá-Reverter et al., 2011). Thus, *in situ* hybridization studies demonstrated the presence of POMC neurons in hypothalamus (Cerdá-Reverter et al., 2003a) but not in the vagal lobe (homolog of the nucleus of the tractus solitarius in mammalian brain). However, more sensitive techniques (quantitative PCR) also reported POMC-A1 expression in the hindbrain (Conde-Sieira et al., 2010b). Immunohistochemical techniques further demonstrated the presence of both α-MSH and β-endorphin in the hypothalamus of several fish species, including zebrafish and tilapia (Forlano and Cone, 2007; Chabbi and Ganesh, 2016) thus suggesting that POMC is mainly processed to these peptides. However, ACTH is also present in the preoptic area of carp (Metz et al., 1994) further suggesting an alternative POMC processing in the fish brain.

Intracerebroventricular (ICV) administration of α-MSH or α-MSH agonists inhibit food intake in a dose-dependent manner in goldfish (Cerdá-Reverter et al., 2003b) and rainbow trout (Schjolden et al., 2009), whereas administration of MC4R antagonists stimulates food intake in satiated animals (Cerdá-Reverter et al., 2003b). POMC-A1 and POMC-C levels increased post-feeding in medaka (Chisada et al., 2014), rainbow trout (Gong and Björnsson, 2014), and Atlantic halibut (Gomes et al., 2015), respectively. In contrast to that expected for a negative regulator of energy balance, POMC hypothalamic levels remained unchanged after 7 progressive fasting days in goldfish (Cerdá-Reverter et al., 2003a), but POMC-A1 mRNA decreased 50% after 28 fasting days in rainbow trout (Leder and Silverstein, 2006). Surprisingly, another study demonstrated that hypothalamic POMC A1, A2 and B levels increased after 118 fasting days in the latter species (Jørgensen et al., 2016). The lack of a consistent POMC regulation by energy balance also occurred in mammalian species. Thus, sheep with about 40% of total body-weight loss did not exhibit changes in POMC mRNA levels (Henry et al., 2001). A similar situation occurred in ewes that lost about 30% body fat (Henry et al., 2000). The constrasting effects of POMC-encoded peptides could explain the paradoxical absence of POMC regulation by energy balance. Thus, central injections of β-endorphin, the C-terminal peptide of POMC, stimulate appetite in the goldfish (De Pedro et al., 1995). It is then plausible that the effects of nutritional status might regulate post-transcriptional POMC-derived peptide levels by selective regulation of prohormone convertases. Under negative energy balance situations, when animals display an enhanced feeding drive, POMC might be processed into β-endorphin. In contrast, a positive energy balance may preferentially drive the processing of POMC into production of the food intake inhibitor α-MSH.

The melanocortin activity may be also modulated by receptor signaling. Accordingly, energy balance, in the absence of an agonist regulation, could up/down regulate the neuronal receptor density in feeding-related areas of the CNS. Studies in the sea bass suggest that hypothalamic MC4R expression remains unchanged after long-term fasting precluding this regulatory pathway (Sánchez et al., 2009). Alternatively, the melanocortin system also exhibits endogenous antagonists competing by binding and activation of the melanocortin receptors. AgRP1 is consistently upregulated by fasting in the hypothalamus of all tested vertebrates including zebrafish (Song et al., 2003), goldfish (Cerdá-Reverter and Peter, 2003), Atlantic salmon (Valen et al., 2011), and sea bass (Agulleiro et al., 2014). It is therefore conceivable that AgRP1 binding to central MCRs might regulate central melanocortinergic activity whereas POMC expression remains constant as a constitutive inhibitor.

In mammals, ARC POMC neurons also produce CART but hypothalamus is not the only brain area producing this neuropeptide (Elias et al., 1998). CART was isolated form ovine hypothalamus (Spiess et al., 1981) and its expression increased in the rat *striatum* after the administration of drugs such as cocaine and amphetamine (Douglass et al., 1995). Subsequent experiments revealed that CART neurons are anatomical targets for systemic leptin to induce anorexia (Kristensen et al., 1998). In fish, CART mRNA was characterized in several species (Subhedar et al., 2014) but immunohistochemical localization of the CART peptide in brain was only studied in catfish by using antibodies against rat CART (Singru et al., 2007) or by *in situ* hybridization in zebrafish (Nishio et al., 2012; Akash et al., 2014). CART mRNA abundance decreased with food deprivation in cod (Kehoe and Volkoff, 2007), goldfish (Volkoff and Peter, 2001a), and Atlantic salmon (Murashita et al., 2009), and increased with re-feeding in channel catfish (Kobayashi et al., 2008) whereas post-prandial changes occurred in channel catfish (Peterson et al., 2012), goldfish (Volkoff and Peter, 2001a), and dourado (Volkoff et al., 2016). As many other genes, CART is duplicated in the teleost genome and four different genes (CART1-4 or CART1, 2a, 2b, 4) encoding CART peptides are reported in zebrafish (Nishio et al., 2012) or up to seven genes in Senegalese sole (Bonacic et al., 2015). All of them are expressed in zebrafish CNS but only CART2 and 4 are produced in the hypothalamus (Akash et al., 2014). Unfortunately, CART/POMC colocalization in the neurons of the tuberal hypothalamus has not been assessed in fish yet. Both CART2 and CART4 are downregulated by fasting in ventrocaudal telencephalon (CART2) and ventral hypothalamus (CART2 and CART4) (Akash et al., 2014), as expected for a negative regulator of the energy balance and thus further suggesting their involvement in the regulation of energy balance in fish. Accordingly, ICV administration of CART peptides inhibit food intake in goldfish (Volkoff and Peter, 2000).

AgRP/NPY

Atypically, melanocortin signaling is not exclusively regulated by the binding of endogenous agonists (see above), since naturally occurring antagonists, agouti-signaling protein (ASIP) and AgRP, compete with melanocortin peptides by binding to MCRs. ASIP and AgRP molecules exhibit a cysteine-rich C-terminal domain essential for the structural and biological properties of the peptide. A basic domain and a proline-rich area precede the cysteine knot in ASIP; AgRP sequences lacks both regions but, in contrast, exhibits a processing site prior to the cysteine domain where the propeptide is cleaved (reviewed by Cerdá-Reverter et al., 2011). In mammalian species, ASIP produced in the ventral skin regulates pigment pattern and binds MC1R and MC4R with similar affinity (Cerdá-Reverter et al., 2005). In contrast, AgRP is mainly expressed in the same NPY-producing neurons in the ARC. In fact, 95% of NPY neurons co-express AgRP (Hahn et al., 1998). AgRP/NPY neurons also produce GABA (Horvath et al., 1997) and regulate the activity of hypothalamic POMC/CART neurons. In addition, the GABAergic innervation from AgRP/NPY neurons to the parabrachial nucleus in the brainstem is able to regulate feeding behavior (Wu et al., 2009). Hypothalamic AgRP sharply increases with fasting, and overexpression in transgenic mice induces overfeeding and obesity but also enhances linear growth (Ollmann et al., 1997). The selective ablation of NPY/AgRP neurons induces a rapid decrease in food intake leading to starvation (Luquet et al., 2005).

Fish exhibit two copies of AgRP named AgRP1 and AgRP2. Few studies to date have precisely localized AgRP1 mRNA in brain regions of teleost fish (Cerdá-Reverter and Peter, 2003; Song and Cone, 2007) whereas others reported AgRP-ir in fish brain (Forlano and Cone, 2007; Agulleiro et al., 2014). All studies identified AgRP1 production within the posterior region of the ventral hypothalamus of the goldfish, zebrafish and sea bass. In the zebrafish, AgRP1 and α-MSH projections strikingly match the nuclei that express MC4R (Cerdá-Reverter et al., 2003b) and MC5R mRNA (Cerdá-Reverter et al., 2003c) in the goldfish. In fact, binding studies with zebrafish receptors demonstrated that AgRP1 acts as a competitive antagonist at MC3R, MC4R, and MC5R, all of them expressed in the brain (Song and Cone, 2007). Pharmacological studies in sea bass have shown that AgRP1 works as an inverse agonist at constitutively activated MC4R (Sánchez et al., 2009). In addition, ASIP1 overexpression working at central MC4R in transgenic zebrafish model results in enhanced feeding, feed efficiency, weight and linear growth but not in obesity (Guillot et al., 2016), in a similar way to the AgRP1 transgenic zebrafish (Song and Cone, 2007). Studies in zebrafish using first developmental stages demonstrated that AgRP1 knockdown results in reduced growth suggesting that AgRP1 suppression of MC4R activity is essential for larval growth (Zhang et al., 2012). Therefore, melanocortin system seems to impose a constitutive break to feeding and growth in fish probably through constitutive activity of MC4R. AgRP1 overexpression is the soundest response to fasting reported in fish, and its hypothalamic expression is essential to counteract MC4R negative effects on energy balance by inverse agonism on the receptor thus driving fish to feeding and concomitantly enhancing fish growth both dependently and independently on feeding levels (Guillot et al., 2016). In fact, AgRP1 mRNA abundance in hypothalamus increased in food deprived zebrafish (Song et al., 2003), goldfish (Cerdá-Reverter and Peter, 2003), sea bass (Agulleiro et al., 2013), and carp (Zhong et al., 2013) but not in Atlantic salmon (Murashita et al., 2009). Post-feeding did not induce changes in AgRP1 hypothalamic mRNA abundance in medaka (Chisada et al., 2014), but the increase in food intake in the GH-transgenic carp is associated with increased values of AgRP1 mRNA (Zhong et al., 2013).

There are no studies on NPY/AgRP colocalization in hypothalamic neurons in fish brain. The NPY family of peptides consists of 36-amino-acid peptides exhibiting carboxy terminal (C-terminal) amidation (Cerdá-Reverter and Larhammar, 2000). The family comprises three different peptides, the NPY, tyrosine-tyrosine peptide, (PYY), and the pancreatic polypeptide (PP). Tetrapod species produce all three peptides, whereas non-tetrapod vertebrates have only NPY and PYY. Teleost fish synthesize two different versions of NPY and PYY but not PP (Sundström et al., 2008). Brain distribution of NPY peptides was reported in detail only in the sea bass by *in situ* hybridization (Cerdá-Reverter et al., 2000a,b), and only NPY1 expressed in the rostral hypothalamus, where the AgRP1 neurons are localized in this species. Concomitant coexpression in the rostral hypothalamus suggests that both NPY1 and AgRP1 colocalize also in the tuberal hypothalamus, ventral telencephalon and preoptic area of fish.

NPY is the most potent orexigenic factor in vertebrates (Stanley and Leibowitz, 1985) and many studies shown this effect after ICV administration in several fish (López-Patiño et al., 1999; Aldegunde and Mancebo, 2006; Kiris et al., 2007; Yokobori et al., 2012). The mRNA abundance of NPY decreased after meal in goldfish (Kehoe and Volkoff, 2007), zebrafish (Tian et al., 2015), and grass carp (Zhou et al., 2013), though responses were contradictory in other species, such as orange-spotted grouper (Tang et al., 2013), rainbow trout (Gong and Björnsson, 2014), and zebrafish (Chen et al., 2016). Food deprivation in rainbow trout also resulted in decreased mRNA abundance of NPY (Gong et al., 2016b) but also after NPY intraperitoneal (IP) injections in flounder (Li et al., 2016). Accordingly, brain expression is upregulated by fasting in several fish species (Matsuda et al., 2012b) but the number of NPY immunoreactive neurons increase in the hypothalamus and posterior tuberculum after seven days fasting in the goldfish but not in the thalamus (Yokobori et al., 2012). Peripheral leptin is also able to regulate hypothalamic NPY expression since IP injection of recombinant leptin inhibits AgRP1/NPY but upregulates POMC/CART expression in goldfish (Yan et al., 2016). In addition, NPY was suggested to link the reproductive system and the central circuitry regulating energy balance in sea bass (Cerdá-Reverter et al., 1999).

HYPOTHALAMIC INTEGRATION OF METABOLIC INFORMATION

The detection of nutrient levels in hypothalamus modulates different neurocircuits related to food intake regulation, metabolite homeostasis, energy expenditure, and status of body reserves (Morton et al., 2006; Blouet and Schwartz, 2010). The neurons coexpressing NPY/AgRP or POMC/CART are included in these circuits, and respond with decreased or increased peptide expression, respectively, to rises in circulating levels of glucose, fatty acids, or amino acids (Mobbs et al., 2005; Blouet and Schwartz, 2010; Efeyan et al., 2015). Thus, POMC/CART neurons depolarize while NPY/AgRP hyperpolarize in response to the increase in nutrient levels (Levin et al., 2004; Fioramonti et al., 2007).

The sensing of a particular nutrient may involve the direct binding of the sensed molecule to the sensor, or occur by an indirect mechanism relying on the detection of a related molecule that reflects nutrient abundance (Efeyan et al., 2015). Different organisms detect extracellular and intracellular levels of sugars, amino acids, and fatty acids. We provide a picture of the current knowledge of the systems already characterized in fish, i.e., those involved in the sensing of glucose and fatty acids (Soengas, 2014).

As for amino acids, in mammals the increase in the levels of branched-chain amino acids (BCAA) such as leucine result in decreased food intake. This effect is mediated by activation of central amino acid sensing through changes in target of rapamycin (mTOR) and/or AMP-activated protein-kinase (AMPK), and BCAA metabolism (Heeley and Blouet, 2016; Morrison et al., 2016). Furthermore, the deficiency in essential amino acids elicit an increase in food intake through central amino acids sensors mediated by general control non-depressable 2 (GCN2) and eukaryotic initiation factor 2α (eiF2α) (Fromentin et al., 2012; Maurin et al., 2014). Considering that most fish are carnivorous (strongly dependent on dietary protein/amino acid), the presence of amino acid sensors in central areas involved in the regulation of food intake like hypothalamus is likely. However, no studies are available in fish about the presence and functioning in central areas of amino acid sensors. The only available information relates to the effect of different protein levels and/or composition on food intake with contradictory responses observed (Figueiredo-Silva et al., 2012b; Wacyk et al., 2012; Tan et al., 2016).

A summary of the main findings achieved as well as the hypothetical pathways involved in nutrient sensing in fish hypothalamus is shown in **Figure 2**.

Glucosensors and Control of Food Intake

Glucosensing Mechanisms

Hypothalamic POMC/CART neurons increase and NPY/AgRP neurons decrease their firing rate in response to increased levels of glucose in mammals (Levin et al., 2004; Marty et al., 2007). This process is glucosensing. The best characterized glucosensing mechanism is that dependent on glucokinase (GK), and is similar to that existing in β-cells of endocrine pancreas (Blouet and Schwartz, 2010; Efeyan et al., 2015). Glucose is transported into the cell by glucose facilitative carrier type 2 (GLUT2) and then phosphorylated by GK. Once phosphorylated, glucose is metabolized through glycolysis then increasing intracellular ATP/ADP ratio leading to the closure of the ATP-dependent inward rectified potassium channel ($K^{+}{}_{ATP}$), membrane depolarization, calcium entry through L-type voltage-dependent calcium channel, and increased neuronal activity (Marty et al., 2007; De Backer et al., 2016). However, since not all glucosensing neurons rely on this mechanism (Fioramonti et al., 2004; De Backer et al., 2016), evidence for the existence of alternative glucosensing mechanisms obtained in several studies. Thus, high glucose concentrations stimulate the expression of liver X receptor (LXR) (Mitro et al., 2007) resulting in an inhibition of gluconeogenesis (Anthonisen et al., 2010; Archer et al., 2014). The stimulation by glucose of sweet taste receptors (similar to those in lingual taste cells) depending on a heterodimer of type 1 taste receptor subunits (T1Rs) formed by T1R2 + T1R3 and the G protein α-gustducin activates an intracellular signaling cascade (Ren et al., 2009). The expression of sodium/glucose co-transporter 1 (SGLT-1) increases in response to enhanced glucose levels (Díez-Sampedro et al., 2003; González et al., 2009; Herrera Moro Chao et al., 2016). Finally, another mechanism relies on mitochondrial production of reactive oxygen species leading to increased expression of uncoupling protein 2 in response to increased glucose levels (Blouet and Schwartz, 2010). In addition, several of these systems appear to be inter-connected. Thus, for instance, T1R3 and α-gustducin are necessary for increased SGLT-1 induction by dietary carbohydrates (Wauson et al., 2013).

In fish, recent studies demonstrated the presence and functioning of components of a GK-dependent glucosensing mechanism in brain areas of different species (Polakof et al., 2011d, 2012; Soengas, 2014). The response in rainbow trout hypothalamus after IP, ICV or dietary treatments inducing changes in the levels of glucose is shown in **Table 1**. Moreover, recent studies (Otero-Rodiño et al., 2015, 2016) provided evidence in rainbow trout for the presence and response to changes in circulating levels of glucose of glucosensing mechanisms in hypothalamus dependent on mitochondrial activity, LXR, and sweet taste receptor. No other studies attempted to elucidate the presence of glucosensing mechanisms in fish though glucose-sensing properties have been recently described in medaka hypothalamus (Hasebe et al., 2016).

Glucose and Food Intake Control

The detection of changes in glucose levels induces several regulatory responses allowing the animal to control glycemia, and one of these responses is food intake regulation (Marty et al., 2007). Thus, hypo- and hyperglycemia are known to increase and decrease food intake in mammals (Baird et al., 1997; Sanders et al., 2006) and birds (Seino and Miki, 2003), respectively.

Several studies carried out in fish suggest that changes in glucose levels may also modulate food intake response (Polakof et al., 2011d; Soengas, 2014), as summarized in **Table 1**. In

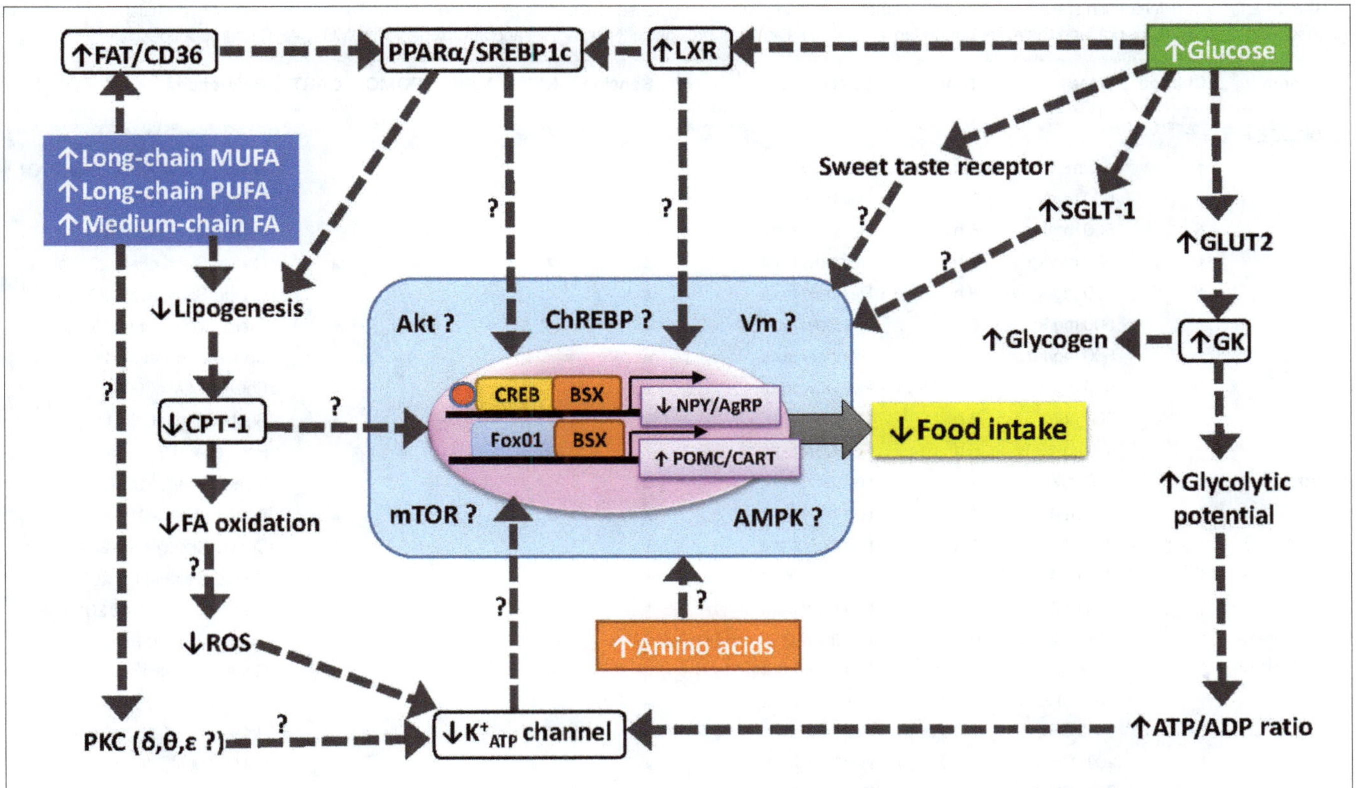

FIGURE 2 | Schematic drawing with a hypothetical model of food intake regulation through different nutrient sensing mechanisms in fish hypothalamus. The increase in levels of specific fatty acids is sensed through several mechanisms including (1) inhibition of CPT-1 to import FA-CoA into the mitochondria for oxidation, (2) increased binding to FAT/CD36 resulting in the modulation of PPARα and SREBP1c, (3) the translocation and activation of specific isoforms of PKC, and (4) the enhanced ROS production in mitochondria by electron leakage. The increase in levels of glucose is sensed through increased GK activity, activation of LXR and modulation o sweet taste receptors. The integration of different sensing mechanisms result in changes in the expression of neuropeptides controlling food intake (NPY/AgRP and CART/POMC) through unknown mechanisms.↑, increase; ↓, decrease; ?, unknown; AgRP, agouti-related peptide; Akt, protein kinase B; AMPK, AMP-activated protein kinase; BSX, brain homeobox transcription factor; CART, cocaine- and amphetamine-related transcript; ChREBP, carbohydrate-responsive element-binding protein; CPT-1, carnitine palmitoyl transferase type 1; CREB, cAMP response-element binding protein FA, fatty acid; FAT/CD36, fatty acid translocase; FoxO1, forkhead box protein O1; K^+_{ATP}, inward rectifier ATP-dependent K^+ channel; GK, glucokinase (hexokinase IV); GLUT2, facilitative glucose carrier type 2; LXR, liver X receptor; mTOR, target of rapamycin; MUFA, monounsaturated fatty acid; NPY, neuropeptide Y; POMC, pro-opio melanocortin; PPARα, peroxisome proliferator-activated receptor type α; PUFA, polyunsaturated fatty acid; SGLT-1, sodium/glucose co-transporter 1; SREBP1c, sterol regulatory element-binding protein type 1c; PKC, protein kinase C; ROS, reactive oxygen species; Vm, membrane potential.

general, fish fed with high-carbohydrate diets, or with glucose levels raised through IP or ICV treatments, displayed a decreased food intake, as demonstrated studies carried out in rainbow trout, goldfish, and tilapia. However, in some studies no changes occurred in food intake, as in sea bass or gilthead sea bream. Furthermore, fish fed a diet without carbohydrates or with low glucose levels resultant of IP or ICV treatments, increased food intake (Polakof et al., 2008a,b).

The mRNA of NPY, AgRP, POMC, and CART was detected in brain of different fish species in areas analogous to those of mammals (Cerdá-Reverter and Canosa, 2009), and changes in mRNA abundance related to food intake control (Volkoff et al., 2009). The presence in the same areas of rainbow trout brain of a marker of glucosesning such as GK protein (Polakof et al., 2009) and mRNA of neuropeptides involved in food intake control suggest that both findings are related. There are however few studies in fish assessing changes in hypothalamic neuropeptide mRNA abundance under conditions of altered glucose levels (**Table 1**). In rainbow trout NPY mRNA abundance decreased in hypothalamus after glucose treatment (Conde-Sieira et al., 2010b, 2012b; Aguilar et al., 2011; Otero-Rodiño et al., 2015) or after fish were fed with a high carbohydrate diet (Narnaware and Peter, 2002; Figueiredo-Silva et al., 2012b). Moreover, increased CART mRNA levels were observed in hypothalamus after experimental rising of glucose levels in catfish (Subhedar et al., 2011) and rainbow trout (Conde-Sieira et al., 2010b, 2012b; Otero-Rodiño et al., 2015), or in rainbow trout fed with a diet enriched with carbohydrates (Figueiredo-Silva et al., 2012b). Hypothalamic POMC-A1 mRNA abundance also increased in rainbow trout after hyperglycaemic treatment (Conde-Sieira et al., 2010b; Otero-Rodiño et al., 2015). Thus, increased glucose levels elicit increased anorectic potential whereas decreased glucose levels elicit increased orexigenic potential in agreement with the changes in food intake reported in the same species (Polakof et al., 2008a,b).

TABLE 1 | Effects in different fish species of different treatments eliciting changes in glucose levels (change) on food intake (FI), the response of hypothalamic glucosensing systems (sensing), and the mRNA abundance in hypothalamus of orexigenic (NPY, AgRP) and anorexigenic (POMC, CART) neuropeptides.

Treatment	Change	Dose	Time	Species	FI	Sensing	NPY	AgRP	POMC	CART	References
GLUCOSE											
Oral	↑	1 g/mL	4 h	Rainbow trout	↓						Soengas and Aldegunde, 2004
IP	↑	500 mg/kg	3 h	Rainbow trout	▼						Ruibal et al., 2002
	↑	500 mg/kg	6 h	Rainbow trout		▲					Polakof et al., 2007a
	↑	500 mg/kg	6 h	Rainbow trout		▲	▼		▲	▲	Conde-Sieira et al., 2010b
	↑	500 mg/kg	6 h	Rainbow trout		▲					Conde-Sieira et al., 2012b
	↑	500 mg/kg	6 h	Rainbow trout		▲	≈	≈	↑	↑	Otero-Rodiño et al., 2015
	↑	500 mg/kg	2–5 days	Rainbow trout	↓	▲					Conde-Sieira et al., 2010a
	↑	500 mg/kg	1–10 days	Rainbow trout	↓	▲					Polakof et al., 2008a
ICV		100 ng/g	2 h	Catfish						▲	Subhedar et al., 2011
		4 μg/g	6 h	Rainbow trout		↑					Polakof and Soengas, 2008
In vitro	↑	2–8 mM	1 h	Rainbow trout		▲					Polakof et al., 2007b
	↑	2–8 mM	1 h	Rainbow trout		▲	▼		▲	▲	Aguilar et al., 2011
	↑	2–8 mM	1 h	Rainbow trout		↑	↓		≈	↑	Conde-Sieira et al., 2011
	↑	2–8 mM	1 h	Rainbow trout		↑	↓		≈	≈	Conde-Sieira et al., 2012a
	↑	2–8 mM	6 h	Rainbow trout		↑					Otero-Rodiño et al., 2016
Carbohydrate-enriched diet	↑	35–55% CHO	0.5 h	Goldfish	↓		↓				Narnaware and Peter, 2002
	↑	31% CHO	1–6 h	Rainbow trout			≈			↑	Figueiredo-Silva et al., 2012b
	↑	20% CHO	1–24 h	Rainbow trout		▲					Polakof et al., 2008c
	↑	20% CHO	1–10 days	Rainbow trout	↓	▲					Polakof et al., 2008b
	↑	20% CHO	1–10 days	Rainbow trout		▲					Polakof et al., 2008c
	↑	23% CHO	28 days	Rainbow trout	↓						Krogdahl et al., 2004
	↑	31% CHO	42 days	Rainbow trout	↓						Figueiredo-Silva et al., 2012b
	↑	31% CHO	42 days	Rainbow trout	↓						Figueiredo-Silva et al., 2013
	↑	27–46% CHO	48 days	Tilapia	↓						Saravanan et al., 2012
	↑	26% CHO	48 days	Tilapia	↓						Figueiredo-Silva et al., 2013
	≈	33% CHO	70 days	Gilthead sea bream	≈						Rocha et al., 2016
	↑	19% CHO	73 days	Sea bass	≈						Castro et al., 2015
	↑	30–40% CHO	84 days	Rainbow trout	↓						Suárez et al., 2002
	↑	38% CHO	126 days	Rainbow trout	↓						Kaushik et al., 1989
Carbohydrate-free diet	↓	<0.3% CHO	1–10 days	Rainbow trout	↑	↓					Polakof et al., 2008b
	↓	<0.3% CHO	1–10 days	Rainbow trout		▼					Polakof et al., 2008c
	↓	<0.1% CHO	28 days	Rainbow trout	↑						Sánchez-Muros et al., 1998
	↓	0.2% CHO	70 days	Rainbow trout	↑						Capilla et al., 2003

↑, Increase; ▲, strong increase; ↓, decrease; ▼, strong decrease; ≈, no changes; IP, intraperitoneal; ICV, intracerebroventricular; CHO, carbohydrate.

Fatty Acid Sensors and Control of Food Intake

Fatty Acid Sensing Mechanisms

Evidence in mammals supports that specialized neurons in hypothalamus detect changes in circulating levels of long-chain fatty acid (LCFA), but not short- (SCFA) or medium-chain fatty acid (MCFA) contributing to neural control of energy homeostasis (Migrenne et al., 2007; Gao et al., 2013; Duca and Yue, 2014; Efeyan et al., 2015). The most accepted mechanism is of metabolic nature. Thus, increased LCFA levels in plasma induced an increase in malonyl-CoA levels and subsequent inhibition of carnitinepalmitoyltransferase 1 (CPT-1) to import FA-CoA into the mitochondria for oxidation (López et al., 2005, 2007). Other fatty acid sensing mechanisms are present in hypothalamus. Thus, the increased binding to fatty acid translocase (FAT/CD36) induced by increased levels of LCFA results in the modulation of transcription factors like sterol regulatory element-binding protein type 1c (SREBP1c), and peroxisome proliferator-activated receptor type α (PPARα) (Le Foll et al., 2009). The translocation and activation of specific isoforms of protein kinase C (PKC) in response to enhanced LCFA levels results in PI3K inhibition (Benoit et al., 2009; Blouet and Schwartz, 2010). The enhanced production of reactive oxygen species in mitochondria in response to raised levels of LCFA results in K^{+}_{ATP} inhibition (Blouet and Schwartz, 2010). Finally, the activity of lipoprotein lipase related to increased levels of LCFA (Picard et al., 2013). The 18 carbon monounsaturated fatty acid oleate (C18:1 n-9) is the most studied LCFA in mammals involved in the activation of fatty acid sensing systems (López et al., 2007; Blouet and Schwartz, 2010; Duca and Yue,

2014). Fatty acid unsaturation appears to be important since the saturated fatty acid palmitate (C16:0) does not activate hypothalamic fatty acid sensing systems (Ross et al., 2010; Schwinkendorf et al., 2011; Greco et al., 2014). Moreover, the presence of more than one double bond, such as for linoleate (C18:2 n-6) or docosahexanoate (C22:6 n-3), does not activate fatty acid sensing systems in mammals (Gomez-Pinilla and Ying, 2010; Ross et al., 2010; Schwinkendorf et al., 2011; Greco et al., 2014).

In fish, lipids are main nutrients involved in metabolically sustaining relevant physiological processes (Tocher, 2003; Polakof et al., 2010). Thus, it is reasonable that lipids are involved in food intake control. In recent years, the presence and function of fatty acid sensing systems in the hypothalamus was characterized in fish (Librán-Pérez et al., 2012, 2013, 2014a,b, 2015a,b), as summarized in **Table 2**. IP (Librán-Pérez et al., 2012), ICV (Librán-Pérez et al., 2014a), and *in vitro* (Librán-Pérez et al., 2013) administration in rainbow trout of oleate or the MCFA octanoate (C8:0) induced a response in hypothalamus compatible with fatty acid sensing. This included reduced potential of lipogenesis and fatty acid oxidation, decreased potential of $K^{+}{}_{ATP}$, and modulation of FAT/CD36 with subsequent changes in the expression of transcription factors (Librán-Pérez et al., 2012, 2013, 2014a). This response is comparable with that of mammals with the main difference of the capacity of fish to respond to increased levels of an MCFA like octanoate (Hu et al., 2011). This could relate to the finding that body lipids in teleosts contain considerable amounts of MCFA (Davis et al., 1999; Trushenski, 2009) and that in rainbow trout there is no preferential oxidation of MCFA compared with LCFA (Figueiredo-Silva et al., 2012a), in contrast with the mammalian situation (Ooyama et al., 2009).

All vertebrate species have dietary requirements for specific polyunsaturated fatty acid (PUFA), and diets for marine fish are particularly rich in long chain PUFA (Sargent et al., 2002). The brain of marine fish displays high levels of n-3 PUFA, mainly in α-linolenate (C18:3 n-3), eicosapentanoate (C20:5 n-3), and docosahexanoate (Tocher et al., 1992; Betancor et al., 2014). Therefore, it is reasonable to hypothesize that fish hypothalamic FA sensing systems, particularly in marine species, could differ from those of mammals in the ability to sense PUFA. Accordingly, a recent study in Senegalese sole (Conde-Sieira et al., 2015) demonstrated that its fatty acid sensing systems were activated not only by oleate but also by an n-3 PUFA such as α-linolenate. However, in the same study authors showed that another PUFA such as eicosapentanoate did not alter fatty acid sensing systems suggesting that the response might be specific to certain PUFA.

If fatty acid sensing systems activated when levels of specific fatty acid rise, what happens in those systems when levels of fatty acids fall? It is not possible to decrease the levels of a particular fatty acid. The only available studies in mammals used pharmacological treatments inhibiting lipolysis to induce a general decline in levels of all circulating fatty acids, which coincided with decreased activity of fatty acid sensing systems (Oh et al., 2012, 2014). A similar experimental approach in rainbow trout resulted in an inhibition of fatty acid sensing mechanisms in hypothalamus associated with the activation of the hypothalamus-pituitary-interrenal (HPI) axis (Librán-Pérez et al., 2014b).

Fatty Acids and Control of Food Intake

Feeding fish with diets enriched in lipids result in a decrease in food intake as observed in different species (**Table 2**). A comparable lower food intake also occurred in fish containing high fat stores (Shearer et al., 1997; Silverstein et al., 1999; Johansen et al., 2002, 2003). Considering the qualitative and quantitative importance of fatty acids within the lipid pool in fish diets and tissue composition, it is not surprising that the available studies are focussed on fatty acids.

In recent studies in rainbow trout, increased levels of oleate or octanoate *in vivo*, either after IP (Librán-Pérez et al., 2012) or ICV (Librán-Pérez et al., 2014a) treatments, resulted in decreased food intake, with more potent effects for octanoate. Moreover, also in rainbow trout fed diets with different lipid composition, the fish with the highest levels of fatty acid in plasma were those in which a decreased food intake occurred (Luo et al., 2014). Therefore, the inhibition of food intake reported in fish by feeding lipids is probably due to the action of central fatty acid sensors. This is also supported by the finding that the treatment of rainbow trout with C75 (fatty acid synthase inhibitor) resulted in a reduced food intake counteracted by TOFA (acetyl-CoA carboxylase inhibitor) (Librán-Pérez et al., 2012). In Senegalese sole, a decreased food intake occurred after IP treatment with oleate as well as different types of fatty acids including saturated fatty acids like stearate, and two types of PUFA such as α-linolenate and eicosapentanoate (Conde-Sieira et al., 2015). When levels of circulating fatty acids decreased through non-specific pharmacological treatment, a sound increase in food intake occurred in rainbow trout (Librán-Pérez et al., 2014b).

In mammals, enhanced levels of LCFA resulted in a decrease in mRNA abundance of AgRP and NPY as well as an increase of CART and POMC (López et al., 2005). However, few studies assessed in fish hypothalamus mRNA abundance of neuropeptides in response to changes in levels of fatty acids in circulation (**Table 2**). In rainbow trout the treatment with oleate or octanoate either IP (Librán-Pérez et al., 2012), ICV (Librán-Pérez et al., 2014a), or *in vitro* (Librán-Pérez et al., 2013) resulted in a decrease in mRNA abundance of NPY and an increase of CART and POMC-A1. The decrease in NPY is comparable to that described in rat hypothalamus after oleate ICV treatment (Blouet and Schwartz, 2010). Changes in mRNA abundance of neuropeptides suggest an enhancement of anorexigenic potential, which is in agreement with the decrease observed in food intake of rainbow trout after oleate or octanoate treatment (Librán-Pérez et al., 2012, 2014a). It is important to emphasize that the response to octanoate is unique to fish since in mammals octanoate is not inducing any change in mRNA abundance of neuropeptides (Hu et al., 2011). In Senegalese sole, the increase in circulating levels of oleate also resulted in decreased mRNA abundance of AgRP-2 and increased values of CART-2b again favoring increased anorectic potential (Conde-Sieira et al., 2015). In the same species the IP treatment with PUFA such as α-linolenate or eicosapentanoate

TABLE 2 | Effects in different fish species of different treatments eliciting changes in fatty acid levels (change) on food intake (FI), the response in hypothalamus of fatty acid sensing systems (sensing), and the mRNA abundance in hypothalamus of orexigenic (NPY, AgRP) and anorexigenic (POMC, CART) neuropeptides.

Treatment	Change	Dose	Time	Species	FI	Sensing	NPY	AgRP	POMC	CART	References
OLEATE											
IP	↑	300 μg/kg	3 h	Senegalese sole		▲	≈	▼	≈	▲	Conde-Sieira et al., 2015
	↑	60–300 μg/kg	6 h	Rainbow trout		▲	▼		▲	↓	Librán-Pérez et al., 2012
	↑	300 μg/kg	6 h	Rainbow trout		↑	≈		≈	≈	Librán-Pérez et al., 2015a
	↑	60–300 μg/kg	6–24 h	Rainbow trout	▼						Librán-Pérez et al., 2012
	↑	300 μg/kg	6–24 h	Rainbow trout	↓						Librán-Pérez et al., 2015a
	↑	300 μg/kg	4–48 h	Senegalese sole	↓						Conde-Sieira et al., 2015
ICV	↑	10 nmol/g	2–6 h	Rainbow trout		↑	↓	↓	▲	↑	Velasco et al., 2016a
	↑	10 nmol/g	6 h	Rainbow trout		↑	▼		▲	↑	Librán-Pérez et al., 2014a
	↑	10 nmol/g	6–24 h	Rainbow trout	▼						Librán-Pérez et al., 2014a
	↑	10 nmol/g	6–48 h	Rainbow trout	▼						Velasco et al., 2016a
In vitro	↑	1–100 μM	1 h	Rainbow trout		▲	▼		▲	▲	Librán-Pérez et al., 2013
Stearate (IP)	↑	300 μg/kg	3 h	Senegalese sole		≈	≈	≈	≈	↓	Conde-Sieira et al., 2015
	↑	300 μg/kg	4–48 h	Senegalese sole	≈						Conde-Sieira et al., 2015
α-Linolenate (IP)	↑	300 μg/kg	3 h	Senegalese sole		▲	≈	▼	≈	↑	Conde-Sieira et al., 2015
	↑	300 μg/kg	4–48 h	Senegalese sole	↓						Conde-Sieira et al., 2015
Eicosapentanoate (IP)	↑	300 μg/kg	3 h	Senegalese sole		≈	≈	≈	≈	▲	Conde-Sieira et al., 2015
	↑	300 μg/kg	4–48 h	Senegalese sole	↓						Conde-Sieira et al., 2015
OCTANOATE											
IP	↑	60–300 μg/kg	6 h	Rainbow trout		▲	≈		≈	↓	Librán-Pérez et al., 2012
	↑	300 μg/kg	6 h	Rainbow trout		↑	≈		≈	≈	Librán-Pérez et al., 2015a
	↑	60–300 μg/kg	6–24 h	Rainbow trout	▼						Librán-Pérez et al., 2012
	↑	60–300 μg/kg	6–24 h	Rainbow trout	↓						Librán-Pérez et al., 2015a
ICV	↑	10 nmol/g	2–6 h	Rainbow trout		↑	↓		▲	≈	Librán-Pérez et al., 2014a
	↑	10 nmol/g	6–24 h	Rainbow trout	▼						Librán-Pérez et al., 2014a
In vitro	↑	1–100 μM	1 h	Rainbow trout		▲	≈		▲	▲	Librán-Pérez et al., 2013
Lipid- enriched diet	↑	20% Lipid	1–6 h	Rainbow trout				↓		≈	Figueiredo-Silva et al., 2012b
	↑	25–34% Lipid	1–10 days	Rainbow trout	≈						Geurden et al., 2006
	↑	21% Lipid	21 days	Rainbow trout	≈						Luo et al., 2014
	↑	19% Lipid	28 days	Rainbow trout	≈	↑	↑	≈	▲	▲	Librán-Pérez et al., 2015b
	↑	30–40% Lipid	40 days	Rainbow trout	↓						Forsman and Ruohonen, 2009
	↑	19–27% Lipid	42 days	Rainbow trout	↓						Saravanan et al., 2013
	↑	20% Lipid	42 days	Rainbow trout	↓						Figueiredo-Silva et al., 2012b
	↑	20% Lipid	42 days	Rainbow trout	↑						Figueiredo-Silva et al., 2013
	↑	21% Lipid	48 days	Tilapia	≈						Figueiredo-Silva et al., 2013
	↑	18% Lipid	50 days	Rainbow trout	↓						Peragón et al., 2000
	↑	35% Lipid	56 days	Polka-dot grouper	↓						Williams et al., 2006
	↑	34% Lipid	56 days	Atlantic salmon	↓		≈	≈	≈	↑	Hevroy et al., 2012
	↑	21% Lipid	56 days	Grass carp	↓						Li et al., 2016
	↑	30% Lipid	63–84 days	Rainbow trout	↓						Gélineau et al., 2001
	↑	21% Lipid	105 days	Rainbow trout	≈						Figueiredo-Silva et al., 2012a
SDW WAG994 (IP)	↓	60 mg/kg	6 h	Rainbow trout		↓	≈		▼	▼	Librán-Pérez et al., 2014b
	↓	60 mg/kg	24–48 h	Rainbow trout	↑						Librán-Pérez et al., 2014b
Insulin (IP; het.)	↓	2 mg/kg	6 h	Rainbow trout		↑	≈		≈	↓	Librán-Pérez et al., 2015a
	↓	2 mg/kg	6–24 h	Rainbow trout	▼						Librán-Pérez et al., 2015a
Ghrelin (ICV; hom.)	↑	2 ng/g	2–6 h	Rainbow trout		↓	↑	↑	↓	↓	Velasco et al., 2016a
	↑	2 ng/g	6–48 h	Rainbow trout	↑						Velasco et al., 2016a

↑, Increase; ▲, strong increase; ↓, decrease; ▼, strong decrease; ≈, no changes; IP, intraperitoneal; ICV, intracerebroventricular; hom., homologous hormone; het. Heterologous hormone.

(Conde-Sieira et al., 2015) increased anorectic potential based on decreased mRNA abundance of AgRP-2 (α-linolenate) and increased mRNA abundance of CART-2b (α-linolenate and eicosapentanoate). The decrease in circulating levels of fatty acid induced in rainbow trout by pharmacological treatment resulted in a fall of anorexigenic potential based on decreased mRNA abundance of POMC-A1 and CART (Librán-Pérez et al., 2014b).

Integration of Nutrient Sensing Information

The precise mechanisms connecting changes in glucose or fatty acid sensing systems and the mRNA abundance of orexigenic and anorexigenic factors are mostly unknown. Changes in neuropeptide expression have been associated with the modulation of brain homeobox transcription factor (BSX), forkhead box01 (Fox01), and phosphorylated cAMP response-element binding protein (pCREB) (Diéguez et al., 2011). The actions of these factors would result in the enhancement of CART and POMC, and the inhibition of NPY and AgRP, ultimately leading to decreased food intake (López et al., 2007; Diéguez et al., 2011). How these transcription factors relate to the activity of the different nutrient sensing systems? Several possibilities were suggested in mammals including (1) direct action of malonyl CoA or CPT1c, (2) indirect action through inhibition of CPT-1, (3) modulation by protein kinase B (Akt), AMPK, carbohydrate-responsive element-binding protein (ChREBP), or mTOR, or (4) involvement of ceramides (López et al., 2007; Diéguez et al., 2011; Gao et al., 2013).

In fish, a preliminary study in rainbow trout (Librán-Pérez et al., 2015b) showed that the cell signaling pathways that are dependent on Akt, AMPK, and mTOR activated in hypothalamus of fish fed a lipid-enriched diet. In the same species, a recent study (Velasco et al., 2016b) pointed to a possible role of ceramides in connecting hypothalamic fatty acid sensing systems and neuropeptide mRNA abundance with food intake control. Besides these studies, there is no further evidence in fish about the integration of the metabolic information of different nutrient (glucose, fatty acids, amino acids) sensing systems into a unique pathway regulating transcription factors involved in the production of neuropeptides controlling food intake. A summary of hypothetical relationships is shown in **Figure 2**.

HYPOTHALAMIC INTEGRATION OF ENDOCRINE INFORMATION

The hypothalamic neurons producing neuropeptides that control food intake in response to changes in the levels of nutrients are also responsive, through binding to appropriate receptors, to the effect of hormones (Levin et al., 2004; Blouet and Schwartz, 2010). These include hormones providing information regarding metabolic stores or energy *status* such as leptin and insulin, and gastrointestinal hormones providing information regarding absence/presence of food and its composition, including ghrelin and cholecystokinin (CCK), among others (Blouet and Schwartz, 2010). The same hormones modulate the activity of fatty acid- and glucose-sensing systems and mRNA abundance of neuropeptides related to the control of food intake in hypothalamus, as summarized in **Table 2** (fatty acid) and **Table 3** (glucose).

Insulin

Insulin and insulin receptors are present in fish hypothalamus (Gutiérrez and Plisetskaya, 1994; Leibush et al., 1996; Caruso et al., 2008). The effects of insulin treatment on food intake in fish are however contradictory. Thus, in rainbow trout IP administration of insulin either resulted in inhibition (Librán-Pérez et al., 2015a) or activation (Polakof et al., 2008a; Conde-Sieira et al., 2010b) of food intake, whereas ICV treatment did not affect food intake in catfish (Silverstein and Plisetskaya, 2000) but induced a decrease in rainbow trout (Soengas and Aldegunde, 2004). The anorectic effects in rainbow trout agree with the increased anorexigenic potential (increased CART and decreased NPY mRNA abundance) observed in hypothalamus after insulin treatment (Librán-Pérez et al., 2015a). Moreover, insulin administration in rainbow trout inhibits the glucosensing system dependent on GK (Polakof et al., 2007a, 2008a; Conde-Sieira et al., 2010b) whereas no clear effects were noted on fatty acid sensing systems (Librán-Pérez et al., 2015a).

Leptin

Multiple forms of leptin exist in fishes, with the major form, leptin A, being the most likely candidate for food intake regulation and energy signaling (Gorissen and Flik, 2014). The treatment with either fish or recombinant human leptin in fish usually results in an anorectic response (De Pedro et al., 2006; Murashita et al., 2008; Kling et al., 2009; Vivas et al., 2011; Won et al., 2012; Gong et al., 2016a). This anorexigenic action of leptin appears to be mediated by brain leptin receptors, particularly in the hypothalamus (Kurokawa et al., 2008; Tinoco et al., 2012; Angotzi et al., 2016), where leptin exerts its anorectic action through regulation of neuropeptide expression. Accordingly, the leptin receptor-deficient medaka shows increased food intake accompanied by increased NPYa and AgRP mRNA abundance, and decreased POMC1 mRNA abundance (Chisada et al., 2014). Moreover, ICV injection of leptin reduced NPY mRNA levels in hypothalamus and telencephalon of goldfish (Volkoff et al., 2003), and in the whole brain of grass carp (Li et al., 2010). Peripheral treatment with recombinant salmon leptin A1 in rainbow trout induced a hypothalamic transient reduction and elevation of NPY and POMC-A1 mRNA levels, respectively (Murashita et al., 2011). Moreover, central injection of leptin increased CART-I mRNA levels in hypothalamus of goldfish (Volkoff and Peter, 2001a), and POMC-A1, A2 and B, and CART mRNA levels in rainbow trout (Gong et al., 2016a). On the other hand, the leptin anorectic effects also related in rainbow trout to the activation of central glucosensing systems (Aguilar et al., 2010, 2011).

The action of leptin on food intake regulation depends on the time of hormone administration, indicating a circadian dependence of leptin anorexigenic effects (Vivas et al., 2011). In this sense, leptin-aI and leptin-aII mRNAs in hypothalamus

TABLE 3 | Effects in different fish species of different hormone (either homologous: hom., or heterologous: het.) treatments eliciting changes in glucose levels (change) on food intake (FI), the response of hypothalamic glucosensing systems (sensing), and the mRNA abundance in hypothalamus of orexigenic (NPY, AgRP) and anorexigenic (POMC, CART) neuropeptides.

Treatment	Change	Dose	Time	Species	FI	Sensing	NPY	AgRP	POMC	CART	References
INSULIN											
IP	↓	4 mg/kg (het.)	6 h	Rainbow trout		▼					Polakof et al., 2007a
	↓	4 mg/kg (het.)	6 h	Rainbow trout		↓	≈		≈	≈	Conde-Sieira et al., 2010b
	↓	4 mg/kg (het.)	2–5 days	Rainbow trout	↑	↓					Conde-Sieira et al., 2010a
	↓	4 mg/kg (het.)	1–10 days	Rainbow trout	↑	↓					Polakof et al., 2008a
ICV		104 ng/fish (het.)	2 h	Catfish						↑	Subhedar et al., 2011
		20 ng/g (het.)	1–24 h	Catfish	≈						Silverstein and Plisetskaya, 2000
		90 ng/g (het.)	26–50 h	Rainbow trout	↓						Soengas and Aldegunde, 2004
GLP-1											
IP	≈	50–200 ng/g (het.)	1 h	Channel catfish	≈		≈		≈		Schroeter et al., 2015
	↑	100 µg/kg (het.)	2 h	Rainbow trout		▲	↑		▲	≈	Polakof et al., 2011b
		50–300 ng/g (het.)	4 h	Coho salmon	▼						White et al., 2016
ICV	↑	20 ng/g (het.)	1 h	Rainbow trout		≈	≈		↓	≈	Polakof et al., 2011b
		5–50 ng/g (hom.)	1 h	Catfish	▼						Silverstein et al., 2001
In vitro		0.1–10 nM (het.)	1 h	Rainbow trout		↑	↓		↑	↑	Polakof et al., 2011b
LEPTIN											
IP		120 ng/g (hom.)	1–8 h	Rainbow trout	▼		▼		▲	↑	Murashita et al., 2008
	↓	0.1–3.3 µg/g (het.)	2–8 h	Goldfish	▼						De Pedro et al., 2006
	↑	1 µg/g (het.)	8 h	Goldfish	▼						Vivas et al., 2011
ICV		50 ng/g (het.)	1 h	Goldfish	▼						Volkoff and Peter, 2001a
		1–100 ng/g (het.)	1 h	Goldfish	↓						Volkoff et al., 2003
		40 ng/g (het.)	1 h	Catfish	≈						Silverstein and Plisetskaya, 2000
		10 ng/g (het.)	2 h	Catfish						↑	Subhedar et al., 2011
		0.5–5 ng/g (hom.)	2 h	Rainbow trout	▼		↑		▲	↑	Gong et al., 2016a
		50 ng/g (het.)	2–6 h	Goldfish			↓			↑	Volkoff and Peter, 2001a
	↑	50 ng/g (het.)	6 h	Rainbow trout		▲					Aguilar et al., 2010
	↑	50 ng/g (het.)	6–24 h	Rainbow trout	▼						Aguilar et al., 2010
In vitro	↑	10–50 nM (het.)	1–3 h	Rainbow trout		▲	▼		≈	≈	Aguilar et al., 2011
GHRELIN											
IP		100 ng/g (het.)	0.5 h	Cavefish	▲					≈	Penney and Volkoff, 2014
	≈	200 ng/g (hom.)	1 h	Rainbow trout	↓						Jönsson et al., 2010
	≈	50–200 ng/g (hom.)	1 h	Channel catfish	▼		≈		≈		Schroeter et al., 2015
		100 µg/kg (het.)	2 h	Rainbow trout		▲	≈		≈	≈	Polakof et al., 2011c
		16 pmol/g (hom.)	1–6 h	Goldfish			≈				Miura et al., 2006
		475 ng/g (hom.)	7 days	Brown trout	▲		≈				Tinoco et al., 2014a
ICV		1 pmol/g (hom.)	1 h	Goldfish	▲						Miura et al., 2006
	≈	20 ng/g (het.)	2 h	Rainbow trout		≈	≈		≈	≈	Polakof et al., 2011c
		1 pmol/g (hom.)	1–6 h	Goldfish			↑				Miura et al., 2006
In vitro		0.1–10 nM (het.)	1 h	Rainbow trout		↑	↑		≈	↓	Polakof et al., 2011c
CCK											
IP		100 ng/g (het.)	0.5 h	Goldfish	▼						Himick and Peter, 1994
		50 ng/g (het.)	0.5 h	Cavefish	▼						Penney and Volkoff, 2014
		50–200 ng/g (het.)	1 h	Channel catfish	≈		≈		↓		Schroeter et al., 2015
	↑	50 µg/kg (het.)	2 h	Rainbow trout		≈					Polakof et al., 2011a
		50–500 ng/g (het.)	4 h	Coho salmon	▼					↓	White et al., 2016
ICV		50 ng/g (het.)	0.5 h	Goldfish	▼						Himick and Peter, 1994
		50–100 pmol/g (het.)	1 h	Goldfish	↓				▲		Kang et al., 2010
		10 ng/g (het.)	1 h	Catfish	▼						Silverstein and Plisetskaya, 2000
	↑	10 ng/g (het.)	2 h	Rainbow trout		↑					Polakof et al., 2011a

↑, Increase; ▲, strong increase; ↓, decrease; ▼, strong decrease; ≈, no changes; IP, intraperitoneal; ICV, intracerebroventricular.

of goldfish show 24-h rhythms under light–dark cycle and scheduled feeding conditions (Tinoco et al., 2014b). Post-prandial increases of hypothalamic and liver leptin-aI expression (Huising et al., 2006; Moen and Finn, 2013; Zhang et al., 2013) are in agreement with the anorexigenic role of this hormone in fish. As expected for an anorexigenic hormone, feeding changes and nutritional status modifies the leptin system in fish, but different responses occurred depending on the feeding regime and species. Thus, leptin genes expression or circulating leptin levels rise with food restriction or starvation, when energy stores decline, and decrease during refeeding in some species (Gorissen and Flik, 2014; Johansson and Björnsson, 2015), but not in others (Huising et al., 2006; Tinoco et al., 2012). These, and other recent studies (Chisada et al., 2014; Londraville et al., 2014; Salmerón et al., 2015; Jørgensen et al., 2016) support that leptin in fish should not be considered as a lipostat signal in contrast to mammals. In this way, zebrafish knockout for leptin suggest the involvement of leptin in glucose homeostasis but not in adipostasis (Michel et al., 2016). Nevertheless, the existence of different leptin paralogs in fish differentially involved in the regulation on energy resources in a species/tissue dependent manner might explain the variety of results.

Gastrointestinal Hormones

Ghrelin

Ghrelin is a peptide mainly synthesized in the stomach or its equivalent in stomachless fish species (Kaiya et al., 2008), although its gene expression is also detected in other peripheral locations and in brain (Kojima et al., 1994; Unniappan et al., 2002; Feng et al., 2013). Some studies point to the endocrine cells in the digestive mucosa as the peripheral primary synthesizing site of ghrelin in fish (Jönsson, 2013). Ghrelin is also widely expressed in fish brain, particularly in hypothalamus (Jönsson and Holmgren, 2012; Sánchez-Bretaño et al., 2015b). Ghrelin requires a post-translational acylation (catalyzed by ghrelin O-acyltransferase, GOAT) before binding to its receptor (Yang et al., 2008). Due to tetraploidization experienced by some fish species, two paralog genes of ghrelin receptor and four or eight receptor subtypes are present in some fish (Kaiya et al., 2013). The wide distribution of transcripts of these receptors, and particularly its presence in gastrointestinal tract, liver, brain sensory areas, and pituitary may indicate multiple targets for the regulation of energy balance by this hormone (Jönsson, 2013). Particularly, the GHS-R1a subtype (specifically involved in energy balance, Kaiya et al., 2010) exhibits a dense expression in discrete hypothalamic nucleus, such as the *lateral recessus nucleus*, in support of the orexigenic role of the ghrelinergic system (Sánchez-Bretaño et al., 2015b).

Ghrelin stimulates feeding in all mammalian species studied so far, primarily through increased release of NPY and AgRP (Patton and Mistlberger, 2013). However, this generalized orexigenic effect is not so evident in fish. Ghrelin is an orexigenic peptide in many fishes (Miura et al., 2006; Kaiya et al., 2008; Picha et al., 2009; Kang et al., 2011; Jönsson, 2013; Penney and Volkoff, 2014; Tinoco et al., 2014a). However, this peptide exerts anorexigenic actions in tilapia (Peddu et al., 2009) and both anorexigenic (Jönsson et al., 2010) and orexigenic (Velasco et al., 2016a,b) effects in rainbow trout. The orexigenic action of ghrelin in goldfish is mediated by hypothalamic activation of NPY (Miura et al., 2006) and orexin-A (Miura et al., 2007; Nisembaum et al., 2014b) mRNA via vagus nerve (Matsuda et al., 2006b), as peripheral administration of ghrelin does not modify NPY mRNA expression in goldfish hypothalamus (Nisembaum et al., 2014b). Interestingly, the expression of ghs-r1 ghrelin receptor (Sánchez-Bretaño et al., 2015b) and GOAT (Blanco et al., 2016b) in hypothalamic nuclei that also express orexin-A and NPY in goldfish reinforces the suggested mechanism for the orexigenic action of ghrelin in this teleost. On the other hand, the post-feeding decrease of circulating ghrelin levels (Unniappan et al., 2004) and the preprandial rise of circulating acyl-ghrelin and GOAT (Blanco et al., 2016a) support the role of this peptide as a meal initiator in goldfish. In agreement with this action of ghrelin, the hypothalamic mRNA expression of GH secretagogue receptors (sbGHSR-1a and sbGHSR-1b) was higher in fasted than in fed seabream (Zhang et al., 2008).

In addition to the effects of ghrelin on the feeding regulatory neurons in hypothalamus, some studies suggest that the effects of ghrelin on food intake are also mediated by gastrointestinal motility in the periphery, as in zebrafish (Olsson et al., 2008). However, this is not the rule in fish, since ghrelin does not modify intestinal motility in other teleost (Kitazawa et al., 2012). Localization studies agree with this lack of ghrelin effect on gut motility since ghrelin receptor expressing cells are not present in the muscle layer of gut (Sánchez-Bretaño et al., 2015b).

Feeding and nutritional status are the main factors involved in the regulation of ghrelinergic system in mammals, but this is controversial in fish. Different responses to food deprivation occurred depending on the species, tissue, and duration of food deprivation. Accordingly, different effects are found on ghrelin release, its expression in different central and peripheral tissues, and GOAT activity (Unniappan et al., 2004; Jönsson et al., 2007; Fox et al., 2009; Hevrøy et al., 2011; Blanco et al., 2016b).

The effect of ghrelin treatment on central nutrient sensing systems was assessed in rainbow trout, and glucosensing systems appear to be activated by ghrelin treatment (Polakof et al., 2011c), an effect opposed to that addressed in mammals (Wang et al., 2008). In agreement with the well-known effect in mammals, fatty acid sensing systems are inhibited in rainbow trout by ICV ghrelin treatment (Velasco et al., 2016a,b). These changes agree with the increased mRNA abundance of AgRP/NPY and decreased mRNA abundance of POMC-A1/CART observed simultaneously (Velasco et al., 2016a,b).

CCK

CCK is a member of the CCK-gastrin family that exerts a key role in digestive physiology of vertebrates, including fish (Olsson and Holmgren, 2011). Partial and complete mRNA sequences of CCK are available for a number of fish species, and CCK-like-ir is present in gut and nervous system of several teleost species (Jönsson et al., 1987; Micale et al., 2012, 2014; Ji et al., 2015). CCK-like peptides are potent anorexigenic signals in fish (Himick and Peter, 1994; Volkoff et al., 2005; Rubio et al., 2008; MacDonald and Volkoff, 2009;

White et al., 2016). Moreover, these hormones are involved in many digestive functions and glucose homeostasis (Rajjo et al., 1988; Aldman and Holmgren, 1995; Einarsson et al., 1997; Polakof et al., 2011a; Tinoco et al., 2014b). CCK-8 may be involved in the seasonal changes of food intake experienced by salmonids (White et al., 2016), and starvation challenge experiments support the anorexigenic action of CCK-8 in fish. The expression levels of CCK mRNA decreased in brain and intestine after starvation in different fish species (Murashita et al., 2006; Feng et al., 2012; Ji et al., 2015), while CCK is released after feeding in intestine (Aldman and Holmgren, 1995). The mechanisms underlying the anorexigenic effect of CCK-like peptides are unknown, but the lack of effect after peripheral administration in channel catfish (Schroeter et al., 2015) suggests that anorexigenic action occur at the central level. Interactions with other feeding regulators, as the hypothalamic expression of amylin, have been described in goldfish (Thavanathan and Volkoff, 2006), but the mechanisms involved appear to be different when comparing peripheral and central administration (Hoskins and Volkoff, 2012). Accordingly, a differential distribution pattern of CCK receptors subtypes is present in goldfish with high expression of CCKAR subtype in the intestine, whereas the CCKBR subtype predominantly expressed in hypothalamus and vagal lobe (Tinoco et al., 2015). Finally, CCK-8 treatment activated glucosensing capacity in hypothalamus and hindbrain of rainbow trout (Polakof et al., 2011a).

Other Gastrointestinal Hormones

Glucagon-like peptide 1 (GLP-1) appears to be anorectic in fish (Silverstein et al., 2001; White et al., 2016). In rainbow trout GLP-1 treatment activated hypothalamic glucosensing systems (Polakof et al., 2011b) in parallel with altered mRNA abundance of several neuropeptides including increased values for CART and POMC-A1 and decreased values for NPY (Polakof et al., 2011b).

Other gastrointestinal peptides also show anorexigenic properties in fish including those peptides belonging to the calcitonin gene-related peptide family, such as the calcitonin gene-related peptide (CGRP), intermedin (or adrenomedulin) and amylin (or islet amyloid polypeptide). These peptides act through a calcitonin receptor-like receptor and show a broad distribution in brain and peripheral tissues in fish (Ogoshi et al., 2003; Martínez-Álvarez et al., 2008). CGRP mRNA is widely expressed in the central and peripheral nervous system, intermedin-ir is present in brain, pituitary and most peripheral tissues, including endocrine pancreas (López et al., 1999). Amylin is present in Brockmann bodies, thus suggesting that once produced in the periphery transported into brain where it has central actions (Westermark et al., 2002). ICV injections of these three peptides in goldfish induced a decrease in food intake (Martínez-Álvarez et al., 2009) mediated at the central level through unknown mechanisms. The presence of CGRP fibers innervating ventromedial hypothalamic nucleus (Batten and Cambre, 1989) support a direct effect on hypothalamus probably in a paracrine or autocrine manner (Martínez-Álvarez et al., 2009).

HYPOTHALAMIC INTEGRATION OF CIRCADIAN INFORMATION

Hypothalamus and Peripheral Circadian Clocks

Feeding shows a rhythmic pattern in a widespread of fish (Madrid et al., 2001), occurring periodically through the 24-h light/dark cycle, but tidal, lunar and seasonal feeding rhythms are also been described in some species (López-Olmeda and Sánchez-Vázquez, 2010). These feeding rhythms, as many other aspects of energy metabolism and homeostatic balance, are coordinated by the phylogenetically well-conserved circadian system, which generates an internal timing that allow animals to anticipate cyclic environmental and endogenous variations, and then, prepare the physiology for upcoming challenges. In the functional organization of circadian system, multiple endogenous clocks, synchronized by environmental and endogenous cues, generate an internal rhythmicity close to 24 h (Albrecht, 2012). The hypothalamus plays a key role in the circadian timekeeping system of vertebrates, acting as an integrative neuronal network. In mammals, a bilateral structure in the anterior hypothalamus, the suprachiasmatic nucleus (SCN), is an autonomously rhythmic nucleus that drives overt circadian rhythms in behavior and physiology, including food intake (Partch et al., 2014). The SCN is formed by clusters of interconnected neurons with individual molecular clock mechanisms inside each cell that function as an autonomous oscillator, and the intercelular coupling among these individual cells is critical for the coordination of endogenous rhythmicity and the outputs to downstream tissues (Evans and Gorman, 2016). Additional neuronal clocks are also present in ARC, ventromedial hypothalamus, and the dorsomedial hypothalamus, and in a variety of peripheral tissues, including liver, adipose tissue, adrenal and muscle (Dibner et al., 2010). In mammals, it is widely accepted that the internal coordination of circadian rhythmicity is established by the temporal signals provided by the master SCN to other hypothalamic nuclei and peripheral organs through a wide variety of direct and indirect pathways that form a network of oscillators. Fish hypothalamus also contains circadian oscillators (Velarde et al., 2009; Patiño et al., 2011; Vatine et al., 2011; Idda et al., 2012; Martín-Robles et al., 2012; Nisembaum et al., 2012; Vera et al., 2013), but no master clock has been yet identified. In contrast, the functional relevance of endogenous clocks in a variety of fish tissues supports the existence of a multiple network of endogenous oscillators in the brain (hypothalamus, diencephalon, pineal, retina, optic tectum, pituitary) and peripheral (liver, gut, gonads, head kidney) locations (Isorna et al., 2017). A summary of the main components in the fish circadian organization is shown in **Figure 3**.

The key molecules that establish the functional core of self-sustained circadian oscillators clocks are highly conserved from invertebrates to mammals, including fish (Partch et al., 2014), although important differences are found in fish regarding the additional number of copies of the clock genes resulting from the 3R teleost-specific genome duplication. The generation of

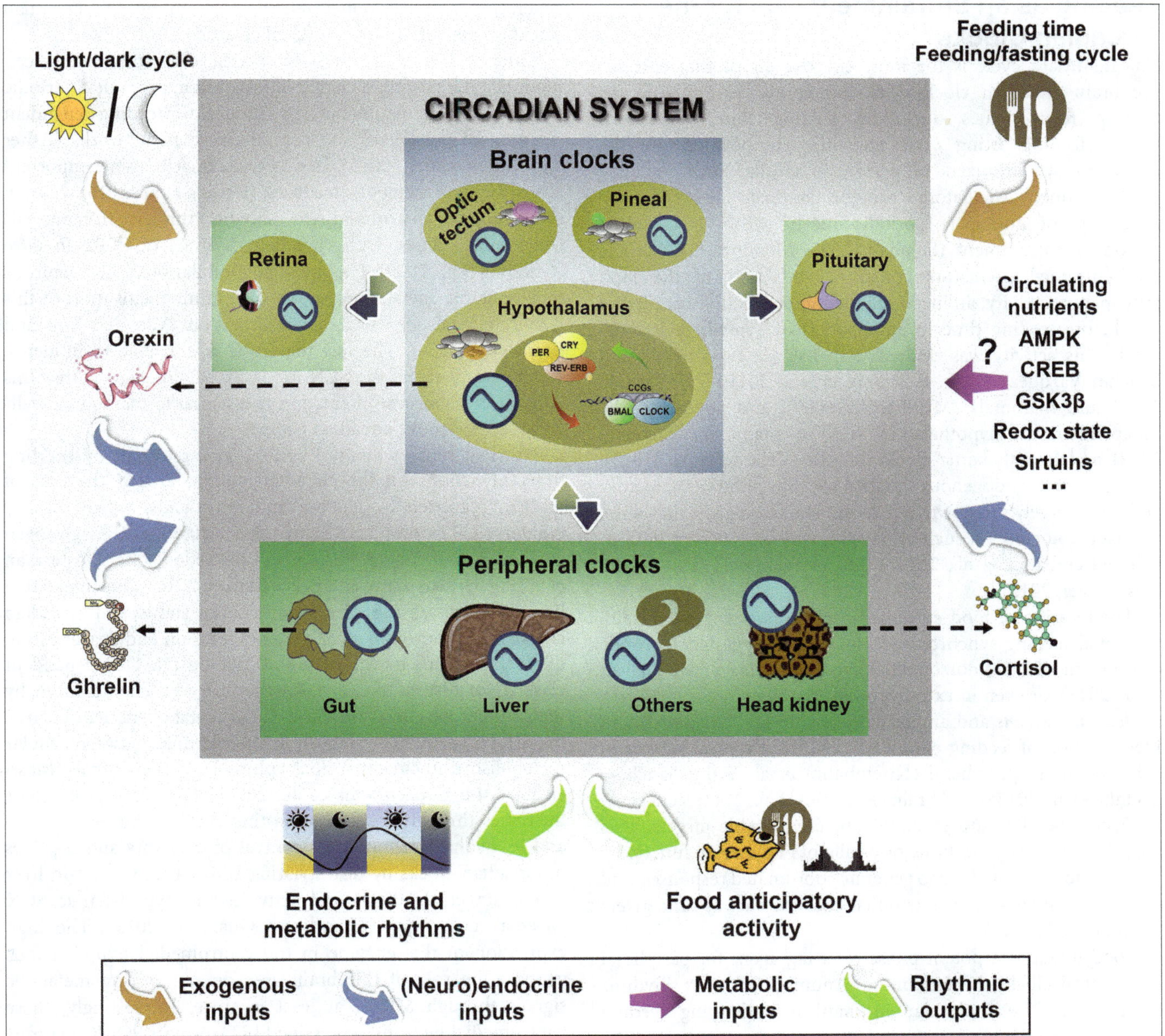

FIGURE 3 | Hallmarks of functional organization of circadian system in fish emphasizing the main external and endogenous inputs that synchronizes brain and peripheral clocks to generate rhythmic outputs, and particularly, the daily food anticipatory activity and food intake. In fish, the lack of a master clock in the functional circadian system organization shapes a more flexible model with different intercommunicated clocks located in many tissues throughout the organism. As external inputs, the light/dark cycle is one of the best characterized, but other time cues (such as feeding time and feeding/fasting cycle) are the dominant exogenous synchronizers of peripheral clocks. The possible role of circulating nutrients and some central and peripheral regulatory signals (such as orexin, ghrelin or cortisol) is discussed in the text. ?, Unknown; AMPK, AMP-activated protein kinase; CREB, cAMP response-element binding protein; GSK3β, Glycogen synthase kinase 3 beta. Clock genes: PER, CRY, REV-ERB, BMAL, CLOCK, CCG. Circadian oscillator: .

cellular circadian oscillations is based on autoregulatory 24-h transcriptional/translational feedback loops of a set of clock genes (Ko and Takahashi, 2006). The proteins BMAL1, CLOCK and its analog NPAS2 act as transcriptional activators via E-box sequences driving the expression of clock controlled genes, some of them encoding other core clock protein repressors (PER and CRY). These PER and CRY proteins form complexes that are translocated into the nucleus where they shut down their own expression by removing the CLOCK(NPAS2)/BMAL1 complexes, defining a main negative loop. Some reinforcing loops are formed by the orphan nuclear receptors from the REV-ERBα-β and RORα-β families, to modulate the rhythmic transcription of *Bmal1*, *Npas* and *Clock* (Guillaumond et al., 2005; Schibler et al., 2015). Recent studies demonstrated that such oscillations in clock genes expression paralleled critical events of chromatin remodeling (Coomans et al., 2015; Masri et al., 2015).

Feeding as an Entrainment Cue for the Circadian Clocks

The light/dark cycle is the most effective signal that entrains the brain circadian clocks (Schibler et al., 2015). However, feeding related cues, including feeding time, nutritional inputs, feeding/fasting cycle and diet composition are the dominant synchronizers of peripheral clocks. Such so-called food-entrained oscillators provide animals the adaptive advantage of anticipate periodic meals within a circadian period of entrainment (Stephan, 2002; Mendoza, 2006). The food-entrained oscillators constitute the basis of the food anticipatory activity, an increase in locomotor activity occurring just before feeding time in anticipation of a predictable daily meal. This activity was evidenced in fish (López-Olmeda and Sánchez-Vázquez, 2010; Feliciano et al., 2011; Vera et al., 2013) and mammals (Mistlberger, 2009), and appears to be independent on hypothalamic SCN in mammals (Stephan, 2002) and hypothalamic clocks in fish (Velarde et al., 2009). To date, the endogenous control of the food anticipatory activity is largely unknown, but recent studies suggest that some orexigenic hormones, such as ghrelin, may be involved both in fish (Nisembaum et al., 2014b) and in mammals (Patton and Mistlberger, 2013).

The location of food-entrained oscillators is not yet certain. Neuronal feeding-synchronized clocks are suggested to reside in ventromedial and dorsomedial hypothalamus (Acosta-Galvan et al., 2011), or even in extrahypothalamic brain areas including *nucleus accumbens* and amygdala in mammals. The search and identification of feeding entrained clocks is a topical subject in fish, and both, peripheral (Nisembaum et al., 2012; Sánchez-Bretaño et al., 2015a) and brain (Feliciano et al., 2011; Vera et al., 2013; Sánchez-Bretaño et al., 2015b) are possible targets. This complex variety of locations of oscillators requires a functional organization among them to generate coordinated responses, and recent data suggest that nutritional cues may act as time givers (Dattolo et al., 2016).

Food intake is a potent phase-resetting agent for peripheral and central clocks, by entraining a number of overt rhythms in animals. The molecular mechanism underlying feeding entrainment remains largely unknown. In mammals, feeding modifies the phase of molecular oscillations in ARC and dorsomedial hypothalamic nuclei independently on the hypothalamic SCN (Feillet et al., 2008). In fish, a daily feeding schedule synchronizes rhythmicity of central (hypothalamus and optic tectum) and peripheral (gut and liver) clock genes (Feliciano et al., 2011; Nisembaum et al., 2012; Vera et al., 2013). The nature of the endogenous signals associated with feeding that may be capable of resetting peripheral clocks is not fully characterized yet, but metabolites, nutrient sensors, hormones, and possibly neuronal signals transmitted from nutrient-sensing areas to peripheral organs are good candidates.

Metabolic Signals and Circadian Clocks

The circadian system controls the expression of essential genes in numerous metabolic pathways (Ribas-Latre and Eckel-Mahan, 2016), but, in turns, it can be synchronized by its own effectors, generating a bidirectional relationship among the circadian clocks and metabolic signals (Challet, 2013).

Little is known about how specific diet components can modulate the circadian clocks, although it appears that periodic availability of circulating nutrients induces the feeding dependent resetting of peripheral and central circadian networks (Asher and Sassone-Corsi, 2015). In this context, ARC is an important target for such metabolic feedback (Uchida et al., 2016). Certain populations of neurons in ARC show rhythmicity in mammals (Ellis et al., 2008), with circadian rhythms of PER2 *in vitro* (Guilding et al., 2009). The circadian modulation of ARC neurons by circulating metabolites support the timing activation of this center for sensory metabolic information (Van den Top and Spanswick, 2006). The fact that ARC is also able to influence the functionality of the SCN (Yi et al., 2006), suggest that this ARC-SCN reciprocal interaction is essential to maintain a well-balanced metabolic circadian pattern.

Nutrient sensors evolved as time-giving signals by exerting different actions on the circadian clocks. This is the case of AMPK, regulated by glucose and fatty acids, which directly regulates CRYs proteins (Lamia et al., 2009), CREB, glycogen synthase kinase 3 beta, PPARs, and the redox state (Oosterman et al., 2015; Ribas-Latre and Eckel-Mahan, 2016). One interesting link between sensing of cellular energy status and circadian clocks is the control of clock genes expression and deacetylation of clock proteins by the sirtuins (SIRT), a (NAD^+)-dependent class III of histone deacetylases that are well characterized by their numerous effects on intracellular metabolism. Particularly, the SIRT1 and SIRT6 establish functional links between cellular metabolism and circadian clocks physiology in mammals (Masri et al., 2014; Orozco-Solis et al., 2015). The activity of SIRT1 fluctuates through the feeding/fasting cycle (Cakir et al., 2009) and is involved in the cyclic control of cofactors and peptides of circadian clocks by deacetylating BMAL1 and PER2 in liver (Nakahata et al., 2008) and activates the hypothalamic SCN pacemaker in mice (Chang and Guarente, 2013). The high expression of this enzyme in the ventromedial hypothalamus support the role of this brain area on monitoring metabolic signals through SIRT1, at least in mice. Interestingly, these ventromedial neurons expressing SIRT1 project POMC neurons in the ARC, and innervate the outer shell of SCN, providing a basis to integrate and communicate metabolic signals in the hypothalamus (Orozco-Solis et al., 2015). SIRT6 appears to be involved in the cyclic synthesis of lipids and carbohydrates (Masri et al., 2014), which may reflect differential responses to distinct nutritional intakes. Whether these molecular sensors modulate brain and peripheral clocks in fish remains to be elucidated. Preliminary studies in rainbow trout assessed changes in mRNA abundance of SIRT-1 in parallel with the functioning of fatty acid sensing systems (Velasco et al., 2016a,b). The clearly adaptive significance of circadian clocks entrainment by nutrient status is supported in fishes by the feeding-related rhythms driven by the circadian system in digestive enzymes (Vera et al., 2007; Montoya et al., 2010; Nisembaum et al., 2014b). Furthermore, changes described in parameters related to glucose, fatty acid, and amino acid metabolism in brain (Polakof et al., 2007c) and peripheral tissues (Polakof et al., 2007d;

Hernández-Pérez et al., 2015) also support the involvement of nutrient status.

Endocrine Signals in the Entrainment of Circadian Clocks

It is widely accepted that daily endocrine rhythms are outputs of the circadian system, but recent reports suggest that several hormones may act as inputs in the timing signalization of hypothalamic and peripheral clocks (Challet, 2015; Coomans et al., 2015).

Ghrelin may prove to be an endocrine signal that participates in the integration of gastrointestinal signals by the central clocks. The rhythmic expression of ghrelin transcript in hypothalamus, pituitary and gut (Sánchez-Bretaño et al., 2015b), and the periprandial variations in plasma of goldfish (Blanco et al., 2016a), and in hypothalamus of tilapia, zebrafish and goldfish (Peddu et al., 2009; Blanco et al., 2016b) indicate that ghrelin may work as an output of food-entrained oscillators. Ghrelin receptors are widely expressed in fish brain (Chen et al., 2008; Sánchez-Bretaño et al., 2015b), including those hypothalamic areas involved in the integration of food intake control, as well as the preoptic region and the anterior periventricular nucleus (Kaiya et al., 2010; Sánchez-Bretaño et al., 2015b). The expression of clock genes in these hypothalamic areas (Mazurais et al., 2000; Sánchez-Bretaño et al., 2015c) and the induction of *per* genes by ghrelin (Nisembaum et al., 2014b) support the role of ghrelin as an input of food-entrained clocks. *In vivo* (Nisembaum et al., 2014b) and *in vitro* (Sánchez-Bretaño et al., 2016b) studies carried out in goldfish reinforce the role of ghrelin in the feeding and metabolism-related signaling in hypothalamic and liver clocks. Furthermore, some reports indicate that this hormone may also participate in the regulation of food anticipatory activity in goldfish, as it modifies locomotor activity (Matsuda et al., 2006a), and this locomotor activity is blocked by a ghrelin antagonist (Nisembaum et al., 2014b).

The orexin/hypocretin system is involved in the coordination of rhythmic daily functions, such as feeding and energy balance in fish (Matsuda et al., 2012a). Taking in mind the orexigenic role of this regulator and its stimulatory effect on daily activity rhythms in the absence of other inputs (Nisembaum et al., 2014a), the possible role of orexin system in the physiology of certain brain areas involved in food intake and circadian regulation is intriguing. Orexin fibers found in some central oscillators, such as the pineal and the SCN, and other brain regions related to the regulation of activity/rest cycles (Wong et al., 2011; López et al., 2014). As a rule, orexins exert excitatory effects on various brain nuclei with the exception of a direct hyperpolarisation of clock cells in SCN during the night (Belle et al., 2014).

The orexin system is under the control of the molecular clock, as orexin neurons projecting into the pineal show circadian daily rhythmicity driven by the clock (Appelbaum et al., 2010), and daily variations in the hypothalamic expression of orexin in goldfish related to clock genes oscillations (Hoskins and Volkoff, 2012). Nevertheless, recent studies suggest that this peptidergic system also acts as an input to the clockworks. Particularly, this peptide seems to play an important role in food intake anticipation in fish, as its central administration up-regulates *per* genes in hypothalamus (central) and foregut (peripheral) clocks (Nisembaum et al., 2014a). The induction of *per* genes by orexin, as produced ghrelin, questions the existence of synergy between both orexigenic regulators in their actions on the food-entrained clocks.

Glucocorticoids display strong daily rhythms in vertebrates including fish. Cortisol daily rhythms are clear outputs of the circadian system, which are synchronized by the feeding-fasting cycle and feeding time in fish (Isorna et al., 2017). However, little is known about the possible role of glucocorticoids as inputs to the circadian system in fish. Recent reports in goldfish show that cortisol induces *per1a* and *per1b* expression, and represses the positive elements (*bmal1a* and *clock*) in liver clockwork (Sánchez-Bretaño et al., 2016a). Interestingly, such actions of cortisol on the liver, one of the most sensitive peripheral clockwork, link the entrainment of food-entrained clocks by both, metabolic signals and hormones.

HYPOTHALAMIC INTEGRATION OF OTHER FACTORS

Stress

The endocrine stress response in fish is mediated by both the hypothalamic-sympathetic chromaffin cell and the HPI axes. The activation of both systems restores homeostasis by mobilizing fuel to make energy available to cope with increased metabolic demand (Wenderlar Bonga, 1997; Mommsen et al., 1999). A disruption of the feeding behavior is a common feature of the behavioral response to stress in fish (Bernier and Peter, 2001; Bernier, 2006). The activation of HPI in response to stress involves the synthesis of corticotrophin relasing factor (CRF) in the neurons of the preotic area of the CNS that, in turn, stimulates release of adrenocorticotropic hormone (ACTH) from the corticotrophic cells in the adenohypophysis. ACTH binds to the MC2R in the surface of the interrenal cells of the head kidney to stimulate glucocorticoid release into the blood (Wenderlar Bonga, 1997; Mommsen et al., 1999). Cortisol, the main glucocorticoid in fish mediates many effects of stressors on metabolic and behavioral processes (Barton, 2002; Bernier, 2006; Aluru and Vijayan, 2009).

In the fish brain, CRF is abundantly expressed within the dorsal telencephalic structures but also in the preoptic area and tuberal hypothalamus of zebrafish (Alderman and Bernier, 2007). ICV administration induces a dose-dependent reduction in food intake levels in goldfish (De Pedro et al., 1993; Bernier, 2006) that is reverted by the injection of receptor antagonist (De Pedro et al., 1997; Bernier and Peter, 2001). Goldfish treated with glucocorticoid antagonists or inhibitors of cortisol synthesis, display increased CRF mRNA brain levels and reduced feeding, which again can be reverted by CRF receptor antagonist (Bernier and Peter, 2001). It is suggested that CRF is a major physiological transductor of stress effects on food intake in fish (Bernier, 2006). In addition, CRF seems also to regulate social effects since its increased expression is responsible of the reduced feeding levels in subordinate fish (Doyon et al., 2003).

Recent studies demonstrated that MC4R is able to bind ACTH in the presence of the melanocortin receptor accessory protein 2 in zebrafish. In addition, ACTH administration inhibits food intake in zebrafish but only in animals carrying a functional copy of MC4R (Agulleiro et al., 2013). Together with the ACTH production in carp brain (Metz et al., 1994) this suggests that ACTH can also transduce stress information into feeding circuitry downstream of the melanocortin system. In addition, MC4R is highly expressed in the magnocellular neurons of the preoptic area where CRF is synthesized thus suggesting that central melanocortins could modulate the activity of the CRF neurons (Cerdá-Reverter et al., 2003a; Sánchez et al., 2009). Stress conditions not only regulate CRF and melanocortinergic pathways in fish as the activity of many other central systems vary with stressful conditions and/or increased glucocorticoid signaling. Changes in the activity of central monoaminergic systems including serotoninergic and dopaminergic systems occurred after stressful conditions. These central monoaminergic systems can play a key role in the integration of information during the exposition to the stressor but also in organizing the coordinated stress response (Lanfumey et al., 2008). Studies in rainbow trout demonstrated that the severity of the stressors were able to produce a rated stress response, but serotonin central levels were not accordingly gradated suggesting that some other systems must be integrating the magnitude of the stress response (Gesto et al., 2015). Chronic treatment with fluoxetine (inhibitor of serotonin recapture) is able to reduce whole body cortisol levels and display anxiolytic effects in zebrafish (Egan et al., 2009) but, on the contrary, acute stress induced a rapid increase of serotoninergic and dopaminergic activity in the forebrain of rainbow trout (Gesto et al., 2013). Accordingly, both dopamine (Leal et al., 2009) and serotonin (Ortega et al., 2013) inhibit food intake in fish supporting both dopaminergic and serotoninergic pathways as neuroanatomical substrates for the integration of stress effects on behavioral pathways regulating food intake.

The reduced food intake observed in response to stress in fish could also relate to changes in the ability of nutrient sensing systems to modulate food intake. In rainbow trout chronic stress induced a readjustment in the activity of hypothalamic glucosensing mechanisms (Conde-Sieira et al., 2010a; Otero-Rodiño et al., 2015). The readjustment resulted in an inability of the fish to compensate with changes in food intake those of circulating glucose levels as observed in non-stressed fish. The response of hypothalamic mRNA abundance of CART, POMC, and NPY to glucose changed under stress conditions (Conde-Sieira et al., 2010a; Otero-Rodiño et al., 2015). CRF might be involved in the mechanism through which stress influences food intake control (Evans et al., 2004; McCrimmon et al., 2006). Accordingly, CRF treatment of rainbow trout hypothalamus *in vitro* readjusted glucosensing mechanisms (Conde-Sieira et al., 2011) in a way similar to that observed under stress conditions (Conde-Sieira et al., 2010a).

Orexins

The orexins/hypocretins are neuropeptides belonging to the incretin gene family of peptides and are involved in many physiological processes in fish, including feeding (Hoskins and Volkoff, 2012), locomotion/rest cycles (Volkoff, 2012; Nakamachi et al., 2014; Nisembaum et al., 2014a) and reproduction (Wong et al., 2011). The cDNA sequences encoding for preproorexin in fish contains orexin A and orexin B, with a high degree of homology with other orexins in vertebrates (Kaslin et al., 2004). Orexins are present in numerous fish species with a broad distribution. Thus, orexin ir-cell bodies, preproorexin mRNA, and orexin proteins are abundant in hypothalamus and preoptic area of most species so far studied (Volkoff, 2015), areas associated with the control of food intake in fish.

Orexins stimulate food intake in all fishes investigated so far. Earlier studies demonstrated this effect in goldfish (Volkoff et al., 1999; Facciolo et al., 2011; Matsuda et al., 2012a), and zebrafish (Novak et al., 2005; Yokobori et al., 2012). Currently, it is generally accepted that orexins are potent orexigenic regulators in fish (Hoskins and Volkoff, 2012; Matsuda et al., 2012a; Penney and Volkoff, 2014). The stimulation of appetite by orexin injections in many of the species studied is consistent with increases in preproorexin brain mRNA expression levels displayed after different periods of food deprivation (Novak et al., 2005; Abott and Volkoff, 2011; Volkoff, 2014). In goldfish, the presence of orexin-like-ir in the hypothalamic *nucleus recessus lateralis* is induced by fasting condition (Nakamachi et al., 2006). These stimulations of the hypothalamic orexin system by fasting suggest that this peptide play a role in long-term regulation of feeding in fish. Thus, short-term periprandial changes in the expression of orexin occurred in fishes. Orexin expression in the brain increases 1 h before the scheduled mealtime in Mexican blind cavefish (Wall and Volkoff, 2013); and hypothalamic preproorexin expression peaks around mealtime, and decreases after feeding in Atlantic cod (Xu and Volkoff, 2007) and orange-spotted grouper (Yan et al., 2011). These results suggest that orexin may be a signal preceding food supply under scheduled feeding conditions. Recently, it has been shown that orexin-A enhances locomotor activity in goldfish (Nakamachi et al., 2014), and synchronizes locomotor activity in goldfish maintained under 24 L and fasting conditions (Nisembaum et al., 2014a), which allowed authors to suggest that orexin might mediate the locomotor activity entrainment by food schedule in this teleost.

Orexin system is a good target to investigate possible interactions among food intake regulators. Central administration of orexin increases the expression of hypothalamic NPY in goldfish (Volkoff and Peter, 2001b; Nisembaum et al., 2014a), and in the orange spotted grouper (Yan et al., 2011). Desensitizing the orexin system by treatment with high doses of orexin A results in a decrease in NPY-induced feeding (Volkoff and Peter, 2001b), while the blocking of NPY receptors reduces feeding induced by orexin A (Kojima et al., 2009). In addition, ICV co-administration of orexin-A and NPY results in a synergistic orexigenic effect in goldfish (Volkoff and Peter, 2001b; Volkoff et al., 2003). Thus, a functional interdependence may exist between orexin-A and NPY in the stimulation of food intake. On the other hand, ICV orexin-A treatment stimulates ghrelin mRNA 1 h post-injection in goldfish foregut. This agrees with the increase of diencephalic ghrelin induced by orexin-A in this teleost (Miura et al., 2007), and demonstrates that the interaction between these two peptides takes place not only into the hypothalamus, but also suggests a brain-gut communication (Unniappan et al., 2004; Nakamachi et al., 2006). Neuroanatomical evidences support the interactions above described among orexin-A and other appetite-regulating peptides, as NPY and ghrelin (Volkoff et al., 2003; Miura et al., 2007). Recent studies suggested a role of tyrosine hydroxylase in the regulation of food intake and locomotor activity in vertebrates (Wall and Volkoff, 2013). The increased mRNA expression levels of this enzyme induced by fasting or orexin in cavefish may suggest the involvement of catecholamines in the actions of orexin (Abott and Volkoff, 2011).

Melanin-Concentrating Hormone (MCH)

Melanin-concentrating hormone (MCH) characterized in chum salmon as a circulating-cyclic heptadecapeptide involved in color change (Kawauchi et al., 1983). MCH is mainly produced within the tuberal hypothalamus, stored in the pituitary neural lobe, and released under adaptation to a light-colored background (Cerdá-Reverter and Canosa, 2009). MCH is a potent orexigenic factor inducing weight gain in mammals (Qu et al., 1996). In fish, however, contradictory results were obtained, such as in goldfish (Matsuda et al., 2006c). Data reported in barfin flounder showed increased hypothalamic MCH expression after food deprivation (Takahasi et al., 2004) and enhanced somatic growth after white background adaptation (Yamanome et al., 2005). Transgenic medaka overexpressing MCH exhibit lightened body color, but development, growth, feeding behavior and reproduction do not remarkably differ from non-transgenic siblings (Kinoshita et al., 2001).

CONCLUSIONS

We aimed with this review to show readers the existing information about the way in which fish hypothalamus integrates information of metabolic, endocrine, and circadian nature to elicit a coordinated food intake response. Compared with the mammalian models, the available studies in fish are more limited resulting in the lack of knowledge in several important aspects of hypothalamic integration. Thus, we have almost no idea about how mechanisms governing food intake operate in the long-term since the available information in fish refers to mechanisms operating at short-term periods. The absence of knowledge is also relevant in terms of characterizing the hypothalamic specific nuclei involved in the process of integration of information as well as in the relationship among cells in those nuclei. In this way, almost all available studies in fish assessed the whole hypothalamus, and this may result in differences in the amount and type of neurons assessed. The large diversity of fish species is not sufficiently covered in the available studies, which in some cases (metabolic control) rely on a handful of species. The possible presence and functioning of amino acid sensing systems in fish, as well as the elucidation of signaling pathways linking activity of sensors with the effectors controlling homeostasis are also open questions demanding further research.

Even in the short-term mechanisms comparable to those known in mammals regarding the existence of neurons involved, presence of nutrient sensing systems and modulatory effects of hormones, the specific responses obtained are not identical to those observed in mammals. In some cases, these differences may relate to the limited available studies in fish precluding us to formulate clear hypothesis. Moreover, other factors might be involved, and we can only speculate about some of them. For instance, the activation of fatty acid sensing systems in mammalian hypothalamus relates to the thermogenic capacity of brown adipose tissue (Contreras et al., 2016), i.e., one of the mechanisms involved in thermoregulation that is not present in fish. Accordingly, the reduced energy expenditure in fish may relate to differential food intake regulation as suggested in a recent review (Van de Pol et al., 2017). A second reason might relate to the gene duplication present in actinopterygians resulting in multiple isoforms of neuropeptides, transporters, enzymes, etc. Accordingly, different subfunctions or different functions may attribute to different isoforms in fish, and this might explain some of the differential effects of hormones when comparing fish and mammals, but this has been evaluated only in a few cases. A third reason may relate to the fact that since fish live in a great variety of habitats they also display many species-specific adaptations such as those related to feeding behavior. Fish eating habits (carnivores, omnivores or herbivores) may be responsible of specific differences in gastrointestinal morphology and hormone functions, and this could be responsible (at least in part) of the differences observed when comparing responses among fish species. Finally, many fish species, including several of the models studied such as rainbow trout, are carnivorous, which is in contrast with the mammalian models studied so far (almost all of them omnivorus/herbivorous species). Accordingly, several of the differences in food intake regulation might relate to this fact. However, this is probably not so simple since the scarce data available in carnivorous mammals (Batchelor et al., 2011) also display differential responses compared with carnivorous fish.

The research carried out in the field in recent years provided evidence for several of the mechanisms involved, though certainly more research is needed, especially to ascertain the interactions among different regulatory mechanisms as well as to establish what are the intracellular common mechanisms through which the information is integrated to elicit a food intake response. Ongoing research in our groups, as well as in many others, will provide responses in the near future.

AUTHOR CONTRIBUTIONS

All authors listed, have made substantial, direct and intellectual contribution to the work, and approved it for publication.

FUNDING

The authors acknowledge grants from Spanish Agencia Estatal de Investigación (AEI) and European Fund of Regional Development (FEDER) to MD (AGL2016-74857-C3-2-R), JC (AGL2016-74857-C3-3-R), and JS (AGL2016-74857-C3-1-R).

ACKNOWLEDGMENTS

The authors acknowledge all present and past members of their research groups for their scientific and personal inputs throughout years of hard work.

REFERENCES

Abott, M., and Volkoff, H. (2011). Thyrotropin releasing hormone (TRH) in goldfish (*Carassius auratus*): role in the regulation of feeding and locomotor behaviors and interactions with the orexin system and cocaine- and amphetamine regulated transcript (CART). *Horm. Behav.* 59, 236–245. doi: 10.1016/j.yhbeh.2010.12.008

Acosta-Galvan, G., Yi, C. X., van der Vliet, J., Jhamandas, J. H., Panula, P., Angeles-Castellanos, M., et al. (2011). Interaction between hypothalamic dorsomedial nucleus and the suprachiasmatic nucleus determines intensity of food anticipatory behavior. *Proc. Natl. Acad. Sci. U.S.A.* 108, 5813–5818. doi: 10.1073/pnas.1015551108

Aguilar, A. J., Conde-Sieira, M., López-Patiño, M. A., Míguez, J. M., and Soengas, J. L. (2011). *In vitro* leptin treatment of rainbow trout hypothalamus and hindbrain affects glucosensing and gene expression of neuropeptides involved in food intake regulation. *Peptides* 32, 232–240. doi: 10.1016/j.peptides.2010.11.007

Aguilar, A. J., Conde-Sieira, M., Polakof, S., Míguez, J. M., and Soengas, J. L. (2010). Central leptin treatment modulates brain glucosensing function and peripheral energy metabolism of rainbow trout. *Peptides* 31, 1044–1054. doi: 10.1016/j.peptides.2010.02.026

Agulleiro, M. J., Cortés, R., Fernández-Durán, B., Guillot, R., Navarro, S., Meimaridou, E., et al. (2013). Melanocortin 4 receptor becomes an ACTH receptor by coexpression of melanocortin receptor accessory protein 2. *Mol. Endocrinol.* 27, 1934–1945. doi: 10.1210/me.2013-1099

Agulleiro, M. J., Cortés, R., Leal, E., Ríos, D., Sánchez, E., and Cerdá-Reverter, J. M. (2014). Characterization, tissue distribution and regulation by fasting of the agouti family of peptides in the sea bass (*Dicentrarchus labrax*). *Gen. Comp. Endocrinol.* 205, 251–259. doi: 10.1016/j.ygcen.2014.02.009

Akash, G., Kaniganti, T., Tiwari, N. K., Subhedar, N. K., and Ghose, A. (2014). Differential distribution and energy status-dependent regulation of the four CART neuropeptide genes in the zebrafish brain. *J. Comp. Neurol.* 522, 2266–2285. doi: 10.1002/cne.23532

Albrecht, U. (2012). Timing to perfection: the biology of central and peripheral circadian clocks. *Neuron* 74, 246–260. doi: 10.1016/j.neuron.2012.04.006

Aldegunde, M., and Mancebo, M. (2006). Effects of neuropeptide Y on food intake and brain biogenic amines in the rainbow trout (*Oncorhynchus mykiss*). *Peptides.* 27, 719–727. doi: 10.1016/j.peptides.2005.09.014

Alderman, S. L., and Bernier, N. J. (2007). Localization of corticotropin-releasing factor, urotensin I, and CRF-binding protein gene expression in the brain of the zebrafish, Danio rerio. *J. Comp. Neurol.* 502, 783–793. doi: 10.1002/cne.21332

Aldman, G., and Holmgren, S. (1995). Intraduodenal fat and amino acids activate gallbladder motility in the rainbow trout, *Oncorhynchus mykiss*. *Gen. Comp. Endocrinol.* 100, 27–32. doi: 10.1006/gcen.1995.1128

Aluru, N., and Vijayan, M. M. (2009). Stress transcriptomics in fish: a role for genomic cortisol signaling. *Gen. Comp. Endocrinol.* 164, 142–150. doi: 10.1016/j.ygcen.2009.03.020

Anderson, E. J., Çakir, I., Carrington, S. J., Cone, R. D., Ghamari-Langroudi, M., Gillyard, T., et al. (2016). 60 YEARS OF POMC: regulation of feeding and energy homeostasis by α-MSH. *J. Mol. Endocrinol.* 56, T157–T174. doi: 10.1530/jme-16-0014

Angotzi, A. R., Stefansson, S. O., Nilsen, T. O., Øvrebø, J. I., Andersson, E., Taranger, G. L., et al. (2016). Identification of a novel leptin receptor duplicate in Atlantic salmon: expression analyses in different life stages and in response to feeding status. *Gen. Comp. Endocrinol.* 235, 108–119. doi: 10.1016/j.ygcen.2016.06.004

Anthonisen, E. H., Berven, L., Holm, S., Nygård, M., Nebb, H. I., and Grønning-Wang, L. M. (2010). Nuclear receptor liver X receptor is O-GlcNAc-modified in response to glucose. *J. Biol. Chem.* 285, 1607–1615. doi: 10.1074/jbc.M109.082685

Appelbaum, L., Wang, G., Yokogawa, T., Skariah, G. M., Smith, S. J., Mourrain, P., et al. (2010). Circadian and homeostatic regulation of structural synaptic plasticity in hypocretin neurons. *Neuron* 68, 87–98. doi: 10.1016/j.neuron.2010.09.006

Archer, A., Laurencikiene, J., Ahmed, O., Steffensen, K. R., Parini, P., Gustafsson, J.-A., et al. (2014). Skeletal muscle as a target of LXR agonist after long-term treatment: focus on lipid homeostasis. *Am. J. Physiol. Endocrinol. Metab.* 306, E494–E502. doi: 10.1152/ajpendo.00410.2013

Asher, G., and Sassone-Corsi, P. (2015). Time for food: the intimate interplay between nutrition, metabolism, and the circadian clock. *Cell* 161, 84–92. doi: 10.1016/j.cell.2015.03.015

Baird, J.-P., Grill, H. J., and Kaplan, J. M. (1997). Intake suppression after hepatic portal glucose infusion: all-or-none effect and its temporal threshold. *Am. J. Physiol. Regul. Integr. Comp. Physiol.* 272, R1454–R1460.

Barton, B. A. (2002). Stress in fishes: a diversity of responses with particular reference to changes in circulating corticosteroids. *Integr. Comp. Biol.* 42, 517–525. doi: 10.1093/icb/42.3.517

Batchelor, D. J., Al-Rammahi, M., Moran, A. W., Brand, J. G., Li, X., Haskins, M., et al. (2011). Sodium/glucose cotransporter-1, sweet receptor, and disaccharidase expression in the intestine of the domestic dog and cat: two species of different dietary habit. *Am. J. Physiol. Regul. Integr. Comp. Physiol.* 300, R67–R75. doi: 10.1152/ajpregu.00262.2010

Batten, T. F. C., and Cambre, M. L. (1989). Calcitonin gene-related peptide-like immunoreactive fibres innervating the hypothalamic inferior lobes of teleost fishes. *Neurosci. Lett.* 98, 1–7. doi: 10.1016/0304-3940(89)90363-7

Belle, M. D. C., Hughes, A. T. L., Bechtold, D. A., Cunningham, P., Pierucci, M., Burdakov, D., et al. (2014). Acute suppressive and long-term phase modulation actions of orexin on the mammalian circadian clock. *J. Neurosci.* 34, 3607–3621. doi: 10.1523/jneurosci.3388-13.2014

Benoit, S. C., Kemp, C. J., Elias, C. F., Abplanalp, W., Herman, J. P., Migrenne, S., et al. (2009). Palmitic acid mediates hypothalamic insulin resistance by altering PKC-O subcellular localization in rodents. *J. Clin. Invest.* 119, 2577–2589. doi: 10.1172/JCI36714

Bernier, N. J. (2006). The corticotrophin-releasing factor system as mediator of the appetite-suppressing effects of stress in fish. *Gen. Comp. Endocrinol.* 144, 45–55 doi: 10.1016/j.ygcen.2005.11.016

Bernier, N. J., and Peter, R. E. (2001). The hypothalamic-pituitary-interrenal axis and the control of food intake in teleost fish. *Comp. Biochem. Physiol.* 129, 639–644. doi: 10.1016/S1096-4959(01)00360-8

Berthoud, H. R. (2002). Multiple neural systems controlling food intake and body weight. *Neurosci. Biobehav. Rev.* 26, 393–428. doi: 10.1016/S0149-7634(02)00014-3

Berthoud, H.-R., and Morrison, C. (2008). The brain, appetite, and obesity. *Annu. Rev. Psychol.* 59, 55–92. doi: 10.1146/annurev.psych.59.103006.093551

Betancor, M. B., Howarth, F. J. E., Glencross, B. D., and Tocher, D. R. (2014). Influence of dietary docosahexanoic acid in combination with other long-chain polyunsaturated fatty acids on expression of biosynthesis genes and phospholipid fatty acid compositions in tissues of post-smolt Atlantic salmon (*Salmo salar*). *Comp. Biochem. Physiol. B.* 172, 74–89. doi: 10.1016/j.cbpb.2014.04.007

Blanco, A. M., Gómez-Boronat, M., Redondo, I., Valenciano, A. I., and Delgado, M. J. (2016a). Periprandial changes and effects of short- and long-term fasting on ghrelin, GOAT, and ghrelin receptors in goldfish (*Carassius auratus*). *J. Comp. Physiol. B* 186, 727–738. doi: 10.1007/s00360-016-0986-0

Blanco, A. M., Sánchez-Bretaño, A., Delgado, M. J., and Valenciano, A. I. (2016b). Brain mapping of ghrelin O-acyltransferase in goldfish (*Carassius auratus*): novel roles for the ghrelinergic system in fish? Anat. *Rec.* 299, 748–758. doi: 10.1002/ar.23346

Blouet, C., and Schwartz, G. J. (2010). Hypothalamic nutrient sensing in the control of energy homeostasis. *Behav. Brain Res.* 209, 1–12. doi: 10.1016/j.bbr.2009.12.024

Bonacic, K., Martínez, A., Martín-Robles, A. J., Muñoz-Cueto, J. A., and Morais, S. (2015). Characterization of seven cocaine- and amphetamine-regulated transcripts (CARTs) differentially expressed in the brain and peripheral tissues of *Solea senegalensis* (Kaup). *Gen. Comp. Endocrinol.* 224, 260–272. doi: 10.1016/j.ygcen.2015.08.017

Cakir, I., Perello, M., Lansari, O., Messier, N. J., Vaslet, C. A., and Nillni, E. A. (2009). Hypothalamic Sirt1 regulates food intake in a rodent model system. *PLoS ONE* 4:e8322. doi: 10.1371/journal.pone.0008322

Capilla, E., Médale, F., Navarro, I., Panserat, S., Vachot, C., Kaushik, S., et al. (2003). Muscle insulin binding and plasma levels in relation to liver glucokinase activity, glucose metabolism and dietary carbohydrates in rainbow trout. *Reg. Peptides* 110, 123–132. doi: 10.1016/S0167-0115(02)00212-4

Caruso, M. A., Kittilson, J. D., Raine, J., and Sheridan, M. A. (2008). Rainbow trout (*Oncorhynchus mykiss*) possess two insulin-encoding mRNAs that are differentially expressed. *Gen. Comp. Endocrinol.* 155, 695–704. doi: 10.1016/j.ygcen.2007.09.006

Castro, C., Corraze, G., Pérez-Jimenez, A., Larroquet, L., Cluzeaud, M., Panserat, S., et al. (2015). Dietary carbohydrate and lipid source affect cholesterol metabolism of European sea bass (*Dicentrarchus labrax*) juveniles. *Br. J. Nutr.* 114, 1584–1593. doi: 10.1017/S0007114515003360

Cerdá-Reverter, J. M., Agulleiro, M. J., Guillot, R., Sánchez, E., Ceinos, R., and Rotllant, J. (2011). Fish melanocortin system. *Eur. J. Pharm.* 660, 53–60. doi: 10.1016/j.ejphar.2010.10.108

Cerdá-Reverter, J. M., Anglade, I., Martínez-Rodríguez, G., Mazurais, D., Muñoz-Cueto, J. A., Carrillo, M., et al. (2000b). Characterization of neuropeptide Y expression in the brain of a perciform fish, the sea bass (*Dicentrarchus labrax*). *J. Chem. Neuroanat.* 19, 197–210. doi: 10.1016/S0891-0618(00)00063-6

Cerdá-Reverter, J. M., and Canosa, L. F. (2009). "Neuroendocrine systems of the fish brain," in *Fish Neuroendocrinology*, eds N. J. Bernier, G. J. Van der Kraak, A. P. Farrell, and C. J. Brauner (Amsterdam: Elsevier), 3–74.

Cerdá-Reverter, J. M., Haitina, T., Schioth, H. B., and Peter, R. E. (2005). Gene structure of the goldfish agouti-signaling protein: a putative role in the dorsal-ventral pigment pattern of fish. *Endocrinology* 146, 1597–1610. doi: 10.1210/en.2004-1346

Cerdá-Reverter, J. M., and Larhammar, D. (2000). Neuropeptide Y family of peptides: structure, anatomical expression, function and molecular evolution. *Biochem. Cell Biol.* 78, 371–392. doi: 10.1139/o00-004

Cerdá-Reverter, J. M., Martínez-Rodríguez, G., Zanuy, S., Carrillo, M., and Larhammar, D. (2000a). Molecular evolution of the neuropeptide Y (NPY) family of peptides: cloning of three NPY-related peptides from the sea bass (*Dicentrarchus labrax*). *Regul. Pept.* 95, 25–34. doi: 10.1016/S0167-0115(00)00132-4

Cerdá-Reverter, J. M., Ling, M. K., Schiöth, H. B., and Peter, R. E. (2003c). Molecular cloning, characterization and brain mapping of the melanocortin 5 receptor in the goldfish. *J. Neurochem.* 87, 1354–1367. doi: 10.1046/j.1471-4159.2003.02107.x

Cerdá-Reverter, J. M., and Peter, R. E. (2003). Endogenous melanocortin antagonist in fish: structure, brain mapping, and regulation by fasting of the goldfish agouti-related protein gene. *Endocrinology* 144, 3552–4561. doi: 10.1210/en.2003-0453

Cerdá-Reverter, J. M., Ringholm, A., Schiöth, H. B., and Peter, R. E. (2003b). Molecular cloning, pharmacological characterization, and brain mapping of the melanocortin 4 receptor in the goldfish: involvement in the control of food intake. *Endocrinology* 144, 2336–2349. doi: 10.1210/en.2002-0213

Cerdá-Reverter, J. M., Schiöth, H. B., and Peter, R. E. (2003a). The central melanocortin system regulates food intake in goldfish. *Regul. Peptides* 115, 101–113. doi: 10.1016/S0167-0115(03)00144-7

Cerdá-Reverter, J. M., Sorbera, L. A., Carrillo, M., and Zanuy, S. (1999). Energetic dependence of NPY-induced LH secretion in a teleost fish (*Dicentrarchus labrax*). *Am. J. Physiol. Regul. Integr. Comp. Physiol.* 277, R1627–R1634.

Chabbi, A., and Ganesh, C. B. (2016). Neuroanatomical evidence for the involvement of β-endorphin during reproductive stress response in the fish *Oreochromis mossambicus*. *J. Chem. Neuroanat.* 77, 161–168. doi: 10.1016/j.jchemneu.2016.07.002

Challet, E. (2013). Circadian clocks, food intake, and metabolism. *Prog. Mol. Biol. Transl. Sci.* 119, 105–135. doi: 10.1016/B978-0-12-396971-2.00005-1

Challet, E. (2015). Keeping circadian time with hormones. *Diabetes Obes. Metab.* 17(Suppl. 1), 76–83. doi: 10.1111/dom.12516

Chang, H.-C., and Guarente, L. (2013). SIRT1 mediates central circadian control in the SCN by a mechanism that decays with aging. *Cell* 153, 1448–1460. doi: 10.1016/j.cell.2013.05.027

Chen, H., Huang, H., Chen, X., Deng, S., Zhu, C., Huang, H., et al. (2016). Structural and functional characterization of neuromedin S in the teleost fish, zebrafish (*Danio rerio*). *Comp. Biochem. Physiol. B.* 191, 76–83. doi: 10.1016/j.cbpb.2015.09.007

Chen, T., Tang, Z., Yan, A., Li, W., and Lin, H. (2008). Molecular cloning and mRNA expression analysis of two GH secretagogue receptor transcripts in orange-spotted grouper (*Epinephelus coioides*). *J. Endocrinol.* 199, 253–265. doi: 10.1677/JOE-08-0325

Chisada, S.-I., Kurokawa, T., Murashita, K., Rønnestad, I., Taniguchi, Y., Toyoda, A., et al. (2014). Leptin receptor-deficient (knockout) medaka, *Oryzias latipes*, show chronical up-regulated levels of orexigenic neuropeptides, elevated food intake and stage specific effects on growth and fat allocation. *Gen. Comp. Endocrinol.* 195, 9–20. doi: 10.1016/j.ygcen.2013.10.008

Conde-Sieira, M., Aguilar, A. J., López-Patiño, M. A., Míguez, J. M., and Soengas, J. L. (2010a). Stress alters food intake and glucosensing response in hypothalamus, hindbrain, liver, and Brockmann bodies of rainbow trout. *Physiol. Behav.* 101, 483–493. doi: 10.1016/j.physbeh.2010.07.016

Conde-Sieira, M., Agulleiro, M. J., Aguilar, A. J., Míguez, J. M., Cerdá-Reverter, J. M., and Soengas, J. L. (2010b). Effect of different glycaemic conditions on gene expression of neuropeptides involved in control of food intake in rainbow trout; interaction with stress. *J. Exp. Biol.* 213, 3858–3865. doi: 10.1242/jeb.048439

Conde-Sieira, M., Bonacic, K., Velasco, C., Valente, L. M. P., Morais, S., and Soengas, J. L. (2015). Hypothalamic fatty acid sensing in Senegalese sole (*Solea senegalensis*): response to long-chain saturated, monounsaturated, and polyunsaturated (n-3) fatty acids. *Am. J. Physiol. Regul. Integr. Comp. Physiol.* 309, R1521–R1531. doi: 10.1152/ajpregu.00386.2015

Conde-Sieira, M., Librán-Pérez, M., López Patiño, M. A., Míguez, J. M., and Soengas, J. L. (2011). CRF treatment indices a readjustment in glucosensing capacity in the hypothalamus and hindbrain of rainbow trout. *J. Exp. Biol.* 214, 3887–3894. doi: 10.1242/jeb.061564

Conde-Sieira, M., Librán-Pérez, M., López Patiño, M. A., Soengas, J. L., and Míguez, J. M. (2012a). Melatonin treatment alters glucosensing capacity and mRNA expression levels of peptides related to food intake control in rainbow trout hypothalamus. *Gen. Comp. Endocrinol.* 178, 131–138. doi: 10.1016/j.ygcen.2012.04.011

Conde-Sieira, M., López-Patiño, M. A., Míguez, J. M., and Soengas, J. L. (2012b). Glucosensing capacity in rainbow trout liver displays day-night variations possibly related to melatonin action. *J. Exp. Biol.* 215, 3112–3119. doi: 10.1242/jeb.069740

Contreras, C., Nogueiras, R., Diéguez, C., Medina-Gómez, G., and López, M. (2016). Hypothalamus and thermogenesis: heating the BAT, browning the WAT. *Mol. Cell Endocrinol.* 438, 107–115. doi: 10.1016/j.mce.2016.08.002

Coomans, C. E., Lucassen, E. A., Kooijman, S., Fifel, K., Deboer, D., Rensen, P. C. N., et al. (2015). Plasticity of circadian clocks and consequences for metabolism. *Diab. Obes. Metab.* 17(Suppl. 1), 65–75. doi: 10.1111/dom.12513

Dattolo, T., Coomans, C. P., Van diepen, H. C., Patton, D. F., Power, S., Antle, M. C., et al. (2016). A neural activity in the suprachiasmatic circadian clock of nocturnal mice anticipating a daytime meal. *Neuroscience* 315, 91–103. doi: 10.1016/j.neuroscience.2015.12.014

Davis, D. A., Lazo, J. P., and Arnold, C. R. (1999). Response of juvenile red drum (*Sciaenops ocellatus*) to practical diets supplemented with medium chain triglycerides. *Fish Physiol. Biochem.* 21, 235–247. doi: 10.1023/A:1007836612376

De Backer, I., Hussain, S. S., Bloom, S. R., and Gardiner, J. V. (2016). Insights into the role of neuronal glucokinase. *Am. J. Physiol. Endocrinol. Metab.* 311, E42–E55. doi: 10.1152/ajpendo.00034.2016

De Pedro, N., Alonso-Gomez, A. L., Gancedo, B., Delgado, M. J., and Alonso-Bedate, M. (1993). Role of corticotropin-releasing factor (CRF) as a food intake regulator in goldfish. *Physiol. Behav.* 53, 517–520. doi: 10.1016/0031-9384(93)90146-7

De Pedro, N., Alonso-Gomez, A. L., Gancedo, B., Valenciano, A. I., Delgado, M. J., and Alonso-Bedate, M. (1997). Effect of α-helical-CRF (9-41) on feeding in goldfish: involvement of cortisol and catecholamines. *Behav. Neurosci.* 111, 398–403. doi: 10.1037/0735-7044.111.2.398

De Pedro, N., Delgado, M. J., and Alonso-Bedate, M. (1995). Central administration of β-endorphin increases food intake in goldfish: pretreatment with the opioid antagonist naloxone. *Regul. Peptides* 55, 189–195. doi: 10.1016/0167-0115(95)92305-V

De Pedro, N., Martínez-Álvarez, R., and Delgado, M. J. (2006). Acute and chronic leptin reduces food intake and body weight in goldfish (*Carassius auratus*). *J. Endocrinol.* 188, 513–520. doi: 10.1677/joe.1.06349

Dibner, C., Schibler, U., and Albrecht, U. (2010). The mammalian circadian timing system: organization and coordination of central and peripheral clocks. *Annu. Rev. Physiol.* 72, 517–549. doi: 10.1146/annurev-physiol-021909-135821

Diéguez, C., Vazquez, M. J., Romero, A., López, M., and Nogueiras, R. (2011). Hypothalamic control of lipid metabolism: focus on leptin, ghrelin and melanocortins. *Neuroendocrinology* 94, 1–11. doi: 10.1159/000328122

Díez-Sampedro, A., Hirayama, B. A., Osswald, C., Gorboulev, V., Baumgarten, K., Volk, C., et al. (2003). A glucose sensor hiding in a family of transporters. *Proc. Natl. Acad. Sci. U.S.A.* 100, 11753–11758. doi: 10.1073/pnas.1733027100

Douglass, J., McKinzie, A. A., and Couceyro, P. (1995). PCR differential display identifies a rat brain mRNA that is transcriptionally regulated by cocaine and amphetamine. *J. Neurosci.* 15, 2471–2481.

Doyon, C., Gilmour, K. M., Trudeau, V. L., and Moon, T. W. (2003). Corticotropin-releasing factor and neuropeptide Y mRNA levels are elevated in the preoptic area of socially subordinate rainbow trout. *Gen. Comp. Endocrinol.* 133, 260–271. doi: 10.1016/S0016-6480(03)00195-3

Duca, F. A., and Yue, J. T. Y. (2014). Fatty acid sensing in the gut and the hypothalamus: *in vivo* and *in vitro* perspectives. *Mol. Cell Endocrinol.* 397, 23–33. doi: 10.1016/j.mce.2014.09.022

Efeyan, A., Comb, W. C., and Sabatini, D. M. (2015). Nutrient sensing mechanisms and pathways. *Nature* 517, 302–310. doi: 10.1038/nature14190

Egan, R. J., Bergner, C. L., Hart, P. C., Cachat, J. M., Canavello, P. R., Elegante, M. F., et al. (2009). Understanding behavioral and physiological phenotypes of stress and anxiety in zebrafish. *Behav. Brain Res.* 205, 38–44. doi: 10.1016/j.bbr.2009.06.022

Einarsson, S., Davies, P. S., and Talbot, C. (1997). Effect of exogenous cholecystokinin on the discharge of the gallbladder and the secretion of trypsin and chymotrypsin from the pancreas of the Atlantic salmon, *Salmo salar* L. *Comp. Biochem. Physiol. C.* 117, 63–67. doi: 10.1016/s0742-8413(96)00226-5

Elias, C. F., Lee, C., Kelly, J., Aschkenasi, C., Ahima, R. S., Couceyro, P. R., et al. (1998). Leptin activates hypothalamic CART neurons projecting to the spinal cord. *Neuron* 21, 1375–1385. doi: 10.1016/S0896-6273(00)80656-X

Ellis, C., Moar, K. M., Logie, T. J., Ross, A. W., Morgan, P. J., and Mercer, J. G. (2008). Diurnal profiles of hypothalamic energy balance gene expression with photoperiod manipulation in the Siberian hamster, *Phodopus sungorus*. *Am. J. Physiol. Regul. Integr. Comp. Physiol.* 294, R1148–R1153. doi: 10.1152/ajpregu.00825.2007

Evans, J. A., and Gorman, M. R. (2016). In synch but not in step: circadian clock circuits regulating plasticity in daily rhythms. *Neuroscience* 320, 259–280. doi: 10.1016/j.neuroscience.2016.01.072

Evans, M. L., McCrimmon, R. J., Flanagan, D. E., Keshavarz, T., Fan, X., McNay, E., et al. (2004). Hypothalamic ATP-sensitive K^+ channels play a key role in sensing hypoglycemia and triggering counter-regulatory epinephrine and glucagon responses. *Diabetes* 53, 2542–2551. doi: 10.2337/diabetes.53.10.2542

Facciolo, R. M., Crudo, M., Zizza, M., Giusi, G., and Canonaco, M. (2011). Feeding behaviors and ORXR-β-GABAAR subunit interactions in *Carassius auratus*. *Neurotoxicol. Teratol.* 33, 641–650. doi: 10.1016/j.ntt.2011.09.008

Feillet, C. A., Mendoza, J., Albrecht, U., Pevet, P., and Challet, E. (2008). Forebrain oscillators ticking with different clock hands. *Mol. Cell Neurosci.* 37, 209–221. doi: 10.1016/j.mcn.2007.09.010

Feliciano, A., Vivas, Y., De Pedro, N., Delgado, M. J., Velarde, E., and Isorna, E. (2011). Feeding time synchronizes clock gene rhythmic expression in brain and liver of goldfish (*Carassius auratus*). *J. Biol. Rhythms* 26, 24–33. doi: 10.1177/0748730410388600

Feng, K., Zhang, G.-R., Wei, K.-J., and Xiong, B.-X. (2013). Molecular cloning, tissue distribution, and ontogenetic expression of ghrelin and regulation of expression by fasting and refeeding in the grass carp (*Ctenopharyngodon idellus*). *J. Exp. Zool.* 319, 202–212. doi: 10.1002/jez.1784

Feng, K., Zhang, G. R., Wei, K. J., Xiong, B. X., Liang, T., and Ping, H. C. (2012). Molecular characterization of cholecystokinin in grass carp (*Ctenopharyngodon idellus*): cloning, localization, developmental profile, and effect of fasting and refeeding on expression in the brain and intestine. *Fish Physiol. Biochem.* 38, 1825–1834. doi: 10.1007/s10695-012-9679-0

Figueiredo-Silva, A. C., Saravanan, S., Schrama, J. W., Kaushik, S., and Geurden, I. (2012b). Macronutrient-induced differences in food intake relate with hepatic oxidative metabolism and hypothalamic regulatory neuropeptides in rainbow trout (*Oncorhynchus mykiss*). *Physiol. Behav.* 106, 499–505. doi: 10.1016/j.physbeh.2012.03.027

Figueiredo-Silva, A. C., Saravanan, S., Schrama, J. W., Panserat, S., Kaushik, S., and Geurden, I. (2013). A comparative study of the metabolic response in rainbow trout and Nile tilapia to changes in dietary macronutrient composition. *Br. J. Nutr.* 109, 816–826. doi: 10.1017/S000711451200205X

Figueiredo-Silva, A. C., Kaushik, S., Terrier, F., Schrama, J. W., Médale, F., and Geurden, I. (2012a). Link between lipid metabolism and voluntary food intake in rainbow trout fed coconut oil rich in medium-chain TAG. *Br. J. Nutr.* 107, 1714–1725. doi: 10.1017/S0007114511004739

Fioramonti, X., Conti,é, S., Song, Z., Routh, V. H., Lorsignol, A., and Pénicaud, L. (2007). Characterization of glucosensing neuron subpopulations in the arcuate nucleus. Integration in neuropeptide Y and pro-opio melanocortin networs? *Diabetes* 56, 1219–1227. doi: 10.2337/db06-0567

Fioramonti, X., Lorsignol, A., Taupignon, A., and Pénicaud, L. (2004). A new ATP-sensitive K^+ channel-independent mechanism is involved in glucose-excited neurons of mouse arcuate nucleus. *Diabetes* 53, 2767–2775. doi: 10.2337/diabetes.53.11.2767

Forlano, P. M., and Cone, R. D. (2007). Conserved neurochemical pathways involved in hypothalamic control of energy homeostasis. *J. Comp. Neurol.* 505, 235–248. doi: 10.1002/cne.21447

Forsman, A., and Ruohonen, K. (2009). Dynamics of protein and lipid intake regulation of rainbow trout studied with a wide lipid range of encapsulated diets and self-feeders. *Physiol. Behav.* 96, 85–90. doi: 10.1016/j.physbeh.2008.08.018

Fox, B. K., Breves, J. P., Hirano, T., and Grau, E. G. (2009). Effects of short- and long-term fasting on plasma and stomach ghrelin, and the growth hormone/insulin-like growth factor I axis in the tilapia, *Oreochromis mossambicus*. *Domest. Anim. Endocrinol.* 37, 1–11. doi: 10.1016/j.domaniend.2009.01.001

Fromentin, G., Darcel, N., Chaumontet, C., Marsset-Baglieri, A., Nadkarni, N., and Tomé, D. (2012). Peripheral and central mechanisms involved in the control of food intake by dietary amino acids and proteins. *Nutr. Res. Rev.* 25, 29–39. doi: 10.1017/S0954422411000175

Gao, S., Moran, T. H., Lopaschuk, G. D., and Butler, A. A. (2013). Hypothalamic malonyl-CoA and the control of food intake. *Physiol. Behav.* 122, 17–24. doi: 10.1016/j.physbeh.2013.07.014

Gélineau, A., Corraze, G., Boujard, T., Larroquet, L., and Kaushik, S. (2001). Relation between dietary lipid level and voluntary feed intake, growth, nutrient gain, lipid deposition and hepatic lipogenesis in rainbow trout. *Reprod. Nutr. Dev.* 41, 487–503. doi: 10.1051/rnd:2001103

Gesto, M., López-Patiño, M. A., Hernández, J., Soengas, J. L., and Míguez, J. M. (2013). The response of brain serotonergic and dopaminergic systems to an acute stressor in rainbow trout: a time course study. *J. Exp. Biol.* 216, 4435–4442. doi: 10.1242/jeb.091751

Gesto, M., López-Patiño, M. A., Hernández, J., Soengas, J. L., and Míguez, J. M. (2015). Gradation of the stress response in rainbow trout exposed to stressors of different severity: the role of brain serotonergic and dopaminergic systems. *J. Neuroendocrinol.* 27, 131–141. doi: 10.1111/jne.12248

Geurden, I., Gondouin, E., Rimbach, M., Koppe, W., Kaushik, S., and Boujard, T. (2006). The evaluation of energy intake adjustments and preferences in juvenile rainbow trout fed increasing amounts of lipid. *Physiol. Behav.* 88, 325–332. doi: 10.1016/j.physbeh.2006.03.033

Gomes, A. S., Olderbakk Jordal, A.-E., Olsen, K., Harboe, T., Power, D. M., and Ronnestad, I. (2015). Neuroendocrine control of appetite in Atlantic halibut (*Hippoglossus hippoglossus*): changes during metamorphosis and effects of feeding. *Comp. Biochem. Physiol. A.* 183, 116–125. doi: 10.1016/j.cbpa.2015.01.009

Gomez-Pinilla, F., and Ying, Z. (2010). Differential effects of exercise and dietary docosahexanoic acid on molecular systems associated with control of allostasis in the hypothalamus and hippocampus. *Neuroscience* 168, 130–137. doi: 10.1016/j.neuroscience.2010.02.070

Gong, N., and Björnsson, B. T. (2014). Leptin signaling in the rainbow trout central nervous system is modulated by a truncated leptin receptor isoform. *Endocrinology* 155, 2445–2455. doi: 10.1210/en.2013-2131

Gong, N., Johansson, M., and Björnsson, B. T. (2016b). Impaired central leptin signaling and sensitivity in rainbow trout with high muscle adiposity. *Gen. Comp. Endocrinol.* 235, 48–56. doi: 10.1016/j.ygcen.2016.06.013

Gong, N., Jönsson, E., and Björnsson, B. T. (2016a). Acute anorexigenic action of leptin in rainbow trout is mediated by the hypothalamic Pi3k pathway. *J. Mol. Endocrinol.* 56, 227–238. doi: 10.1530/JME-15-0279

González, J. A., Reimann, F., and Burdakov, D. (2009). Dissociation between sensing and metabolism of glucose in sugar sensing neurones. *J. Physiol.* 587, 41–48. doi: 10.1113/jphysiol.2008.163410

Gorissen, M., and Flik, G. (2014). Leptin in teleostean fish, towards the origins of leptin physiology. *J. Chem. Neuroanat.* 61–62, 200–206. doi: 10.1016/j.jchemneu.2014.06.005

Greco, J. A., Oosterman, J. E., and Belsham, D. D. (2014). Differential effects of omega-3 fatty acid docosahexanoic acid and palmitate on the circadian transcriptional profile of clock genes in immortalized hypothalamic neurons. *Am. J. Physiol. Regul. Integr. Comp. Physiol.* 307, R1049–R1060. doi: 10.1152/ajpregu.00100.2014

Guilding, C., Hughes, A. T., Brown, T. M., Namvar, S., and Piggins, H. D. (2009). A riot of rhythms: neuronal and glial circadian oscillators in the mediobasal hypothalamus. *Mol. Brain.* 2:28. doi: 10.1186/1756-6606-2-28

Guillaumond, F., Dardente, H., Giguère, V., and Cermakian, N. (2005). Differential control of Bmal1 circadian transcription by REV-ERB and ROR nuclear receptors. *J. Biol. Rhythms* 20, 391–400. doi: 10.1177/07487304052 77232

Guillot, R., Cortés, R., Navarro, S., Mischitelli, M., García-Herranz, V., Sánchez, E., et al. (2016). Behind melanocortin antagonist overexpression in the zebrafish brain: a behavioral and transcriptomic approach. *Horm Behav.* 82, 87–100. doi: 10.1016/j.yhbeh.2016.04.011

Gutiérrez, J., and Plisetskaya, E. M. (1994). "Peptide receptor assay: insulin receptors" in *Biochemistry and Molecular Biology of Fishes, Vol. 3*, eds P. W. Hochachka and T. P. Mommsen (Amsterdam: Elsevier), 429–444.

Hahn, T. M., Breininger, J. F., Baskin, D. G., and Schwartz, M. W. (1998). Coexpression of Agrp and NPY in fasting-activated hypothalamic neurons. *Nat. Neurosci.* 1, 271–272. doi: 10.1038/1082

Hasebe, M., Kanda, S., and Oka, Y. (2016). Female specific glucose-sensitivity of GhRH neurons leads to sexually dimorphic inhibition of reproduction in medaka. *Endocrinology* 157, 4318–4329. doi: 10.1210/en.2016-1352

Heeley, N., and Blouet, C. (2016). Central amino acid sensing in the control of feeding behavior. *Front. Endocrinol.* 7:148. doi: 10.3389/fendo.2016.00148

Henry, B. A., Rao, A., Ikenasio, B. A., Mountjoy, K. G., Tilbrook, A. J., and Clarke, I. J. (2001). Differential expression of cocaine- and amphetamine-regulated transcript and agouti-related protein in chronically food-restricted sheep. *Brain. Res.* 918, 40–50. doi: 10.1016/S0006-8993(01)02918-3

Henry, B. A., Tilbrook, A. J., Dunshea, F. R., Rao, A., Blache, D., Martin, G. B., et al. (2000). Long-term alterations in adiposity affect expression of melanin concentrating hormone and enkephalin but not proopiomelanocortin in the hypothalamus of ovarectomized ewes. *Endocrinology* 141, 1506–1514. doi: 10.1210/endo.141.4.7434

Hernández-Pérez, J., Míguez, J. M., Librán-Pérez, M., Otero-Rodiño, C., Naderi, F., Soengas, J. L., et al. (2015). Daily rhythms in activity and mRNA abundance of enzymes involved in glucose and lipid metabolism in liver of rainbow trout, *Oncorhynchus mykiss*. Influence of light and food availability. *Chronobiol. Int.* 32, 1391–1408. doi: 10.3109/07420528.2015.1100633

Herrera Moro Chao, D., Argmann, C., Van Eijk, M., Boot, R. G., Ottenhoff, R., Van Roomen, C., et al. (2016). Impact of obesity on taste receptor expression in extra-oral tissues: emphasis on hypothalamus and brainstem. *Sci. Rep.* 6:29094. doi: 10.1038/srep29094

Hevrøy, E. M., Azpeleta, C., Shimizu, M., Lanzén, A., Kaiya, H., Espe, M., et al. (2011). Effects of short-term starvation on ghrelin, GH-IGF system, and IGF-binding proteins in Atlantic salmon. *Fish Physiol. Biochem.* 37, 217–232. doi: 10.1007/s10695-010-9434-3

Hevroy, E. M., Waagbo, R., Torstensen, B. E., Takle, H., Stubhaug, I., Jorgensen, S. M., et al. (2012). Ghrelin is involved in voluntary anorexia in Atlantic salmon raised at elevated sea temperatures. *Gen. Comp. Endocrinol.* 175, 118–134. doi: 10.1016/j.ygcen.2011.10.007

Himick, B. A., and Peter, R. E. (1994). CCK/gastrin-like immunoreactivity in brain and gut, and CCK suppression of feeding in goldfish. *Am. J. Physiol. Regul. Integr. Comp. Physiol.* 267, R841–R851.

Horvath, T. L., Bechmann, I., Naftolin, F., Kalra, S. P., and Leranth, C. (1997). Heterogeneity in the neuropeptide Y-containing neurons of the rat arcuate nucleus: GABAergic and non-GABAergic subpopulations. *Brain Res.* 756, 283–286. doi: 10.1016/S0006-8993(97)00184-4

Hoskins, L. J., and Volkoff, H. (2012). The comparative endocrinology of feeding in fish: insights and challenges. *Gen. Comp. Endocrinol.* 176, 327–335. doi: 10.1016/j.ygcen.2011.12.025

Hu, Z., Cha, S. H., Chohnan, S., and Lane, M. D. (2011). Hypothalamic malonyl-CoA as a mediator of feeding behavior. *Proc. Natl. Acad. Sci. U.S.A.* 100, 12624–12629. doi: 10.1073/pnas.1834402100

Huising, M. O., Geven, E. J. W., Kruiswijk, C. P., Nabuurs, S. B., Stolte, E. H., Spanings, F. A. T., et al. (2006). Increased leptin expression in common carp (*Cyprinus carpio*) after food intake but not after fasting or feeding to satiation. *Endocrinology* 147, 5786–5797. doi: 10.1210/en.2006-0824

Idda, M. L., Bertolucci, C., Vallone, D., Gothilf, Y., Sánchez-Vázquez, F. J., and Foulkes, N. S. (2012). Circadian clocks: lessons from fish. *Prog. Brain Res.* 199, 41–57. doi: 10.1016/B978-0-444-59427-3.00003-4

Isorna, E., de Pedro, N., Valenciano, A. I., Alonso-Gómez, A. L., and Delgado, M. J. (2017). Interplay between the endocrine and circadian systems in fishes. *J. Endocrinol.* 232, R141–R159. doi: 10.1530/joe-16-0330

Ji, W., Ping, H.-C., Wei, K.-J., Zhang, G.-R., Shi, Z.-C., Yang, R. B., et al. (2015). Ghrelin, neuropeptide Y (NPY) and cholecystokinin (CCK) in blunt snout bream (*Megalobrama amblycephala*): cDNA cloning, tissue distribution and mRNA expression changes responding to fasting and refeeding. *Gen. Comp. Endocrinol.* 223, 108–119. doi: 10.1016/j.ygcen.2015.08.009

Johansen, S. J. S., Ekli, M., and Jobling, M. (2002). Is there lipostatic regulation of feed intake in Atlantic salmon *Salmo salar* L.? *Aquacult. Res.* 33, 515–524. doi: 10.1046/j.1365-2109.2002.00736.x

Johansen, S. J. S., Sveier, H., and Jobling, M. (2003). Lipostatic regulation of feed intake in Atlantic salmon *Salmo salar* L. defending adiposity at the expense of growth? *Aquacult. Res.* 34, 317–331. doi: 10.1046/j.1365-2109.2003. 00821.x

Johansson, M., and Björnsson, B. T. (2015). Elevated plasma leptin levels of fasted rainbow trout decrease rapidly in response to feed intake. *Gen. Comp. Endocrinol.* 214, 24–29. doi: 10.1016/j.ygcen.2015.02.020

Jönsson, A. C., Holmgren, S., and Holstein, B. (1987). Gastrin/CCK-like immunoreactivity in endocrine cells and nerves in the gastrointestinal tract of the cod, Gadus morhua, and the effect of peptides of the gastrin/CCK family on cod gastrointestinal smooth muscle. *Gen. Comp. Endocrinol.* 66, 190–202. doi: 10.1016/0016-6480(87)90267-X

Jönsson, E. (2013). The role of ghrelin in energy balance regulation in fish. *Gen. Comp. Endocrinol.* 187, 79–85. doi: 10.1016/j.ygcen.2013.03.013

Jönsson, E., Forsman, A., Einarsdottir, I. E., Kaiya, H., Ruohonen, K., and Björnsson, B. T. (2007). Plasma ghrelin levels in rainbow trout in response to fasting, feeding and food composition, and effects of ghrelin on voluntary food intake. *Comp. Biochem. Physiol. A* 147, 1116–1124. doi: 10.1016/j.cbpa.2007.03.024

Jönsson, E., and Holmgren, S. (2012). "The endocrine system of the gut," in *Encyclopedia of Fish Physiology: From Gene to Environment*, ed A. P. Farrell (Amsterdam: Elsevier), 1341–1347.

Jönsson, E., Kaiya, H., and Björnsson, B. T. (2010). Ghrelin decreases food intake in juvenile rainbow trout (*Oncorhynchus mykiss*) through the central anorexigenic corticotropin-releasing factor system. *Gen. Comp. Endocrinol.* 166, 39–46. doi: 10.1016/j.ygcen.2009.11.001

Jørgensen, E. H., Bernier, N. J., Maule, A. G., and Vijayan, M. M. (2016). Effect of long-term fasting and a subsequent meal on mRNA abundances of hypothalamic appetite regulators, central and peripheral leptin expression and plasma leptin levels in rainbow trout. *Peptides* 86, 162–170. doi: 10.1016/j.peptides.2015.08.010

Kaiya, H., Kangawa, K., and Miyazato, M. (2013). Ghrelin receptors in nonmammalian vertebrates. *Front. Endocrinol.* 4:81. doi: 10.3389/fendo. 2013.00081

Kaiya, H., Miura, T., Matsuda, K., Miyazato, M., and Kangawa, K. (2010). Two functional growth hormone secretagogue receptor (ghrelin receptor) type 1a and 2a in goldfish, *Carassius auratus*. *Mol. Cell. Endocrinol.* 327, 25–39. doi: 10.1016/j.mce.2010.06.004

Kaiya, H., Miyazato, M., Kangawa, K., Peter, R. E., and Unniappan, S. (2008). Ghrelin: a multifunctional hormone in non-mammalian vertebrates. *Comp. Biochem. Physiol. A.* 149, 109–128. doi: 10.1016/j.cbpa.2007. 12.004

Kang, K. S., Yahashi, S., Azuma, M., and Matsuda, K. (2010). The anorexigenic effect of cholecystokinin octapeptide in a goldfish model is mediated by the vagal afferent and subsequently through the melanocortin- and corticotropin-releasing hormone-signaling pathways. *Peptides* 31, 2130–2134. doi: 10.1016/j.peptides.2010.07.019

Kang, K. S., Yahashi, S., and Matsuda, K. (2011). Central and peripheral effects of ghrelin on energy balance, food intake and lipid metabolism in teleost fish. *Peptides* 32, 2242–2247. doi: 10.1016/j.peptides.2011.05.006

Kaslin, J., Nystedt, J. M., Ostergard, M., Peitsaro, N., and Panula, P. (2004). The orexin/hypocretin system in zebrafish is connected to the aminergic and cholinergic systems. *J. Neurosci.* 24, 2678–2689. doi: 10.1523/JNEUROSCI.4908-03.2004

Kaushik, S., Médale, F., Fauconneau, B., and Blanc, D. (1989). Effect of digestible carbohydrates on protein - Energy utilization and on glucose metabolism in rainbow trout (*Salmo gairdneri* R). *Aquaculture* 79, 63–74. doi: 10.1016/0044-8486(89)90446-8

Kawauchi, H., Kawazoe, I., Tsubokawa, M., Kishida, M., and Baker, B. I. (1983). Characterization of melanin-concentrating hormone in chum salmon pituitaries. *Nature* 305, 321–323 doi: 10.1038/305321a0

Kehoe, A. S., and Volkoff, H. (2007). Cloning and characterization of neuropeptide Y (NPY) and cocaine and amphetamine regulated transcript (CART) in Atlantic cod (*Gadus morhua*). *Comp. Biochem. Physiol. A.* 146, 451–461. doi: 10.1016/j.cbpa.2006.12.026

Kinoshita, M., Morita, T., Toyohara, H., Hirata, T., Sakaguchi, M., Ono, M., et al. (2001). Transgenic medaka overexpressing a melanin-concentrating hormone exhibit lightened body color but no remarkably abnormality. *Mar. Biotechnol.* 3, 536–543. doi: 10.1007/s10126-001-0061-Y

Kiris, G. A., Kumlu, M., and Dikel, S. (2007). Stimulatory effects of neuropeptide Y on food intake and growth of *Oreochromis niloticus*. *Aquaculture* 264, 383–389. doi: 10.1016/j.aquaculture.2006.12.004

Kitazawa, T., Itoh, K., Yaosak, N., Maruyama, K., Matsuda, K., Teraoka, H., et al. (2012). Ghrelin does not affect gastrointestinal contractility in rainbow trout and goldfish *in vitro*. *Gen. Comp. Endocrinol.* 178, 539–545. doi: 10.1016/j.ygcen.2012.06.025

Kling, P., Ronnestad, I., Stefansson, S. O., Murashita, K., Kurokawa, T., and Björnsson, B. T. (2009). A homologous salmonid leptin radioimmunoassay indicates elevated plasma leptin levels during fasting of rainbow trout. *Gen. Comp. Endocrinol.* 162, 307–312. doi: 10.1016/j.ygcen.2009.04.003

Ko, C. H., and Takahashi, J. S. (2006). Molecular components of the mammalian circadian clock. *Hum. Mol. Genet.* 15, R271–R277. doi: 10.1093/hmg/ddl207

Kobayashi, Y., Peterson, B. C., and Waldbieser, G. C. (2008). Association of cocaine- and amplhetamine-regulated transcript (CART) messenger RNA level, food intake, and growth in channel catfish. *Comp. Biochem. Physiol. A.* 151, 219–225. doi: 10.1016/j.cbpa.2008.06.029

Kojima, K., Kamijo, M., Kageyama, H., Uchiyama, M., Shioda, S., and Matsuda, S. (2009). Neuronal relationship between orexin-A- and neuropeptide Y-induced orexigenic actions in goldfish. *Neuropeptides* 43, 63–71. doi: 10.1016/j.npep.2009.01.004

Kojima, M., Hosoda, H., Date, Y., Nakazato, M., Matsuo, H., and Kangawa, K. (1994). Ghrelin is a growth hormone- releasing acylated peptide from stomach. *Nature* 402, 656–660. doi: 10.1038/45230

Kristensen, P., Judge, M. E., Thim, L., Ribel, U., Christjansen, K. N., Wulff, B. S., et al. (1998). Hypothalamic CART is a new anorectic peptide regulated by leptin. *Nature.* 393, 72–76. doi: 10.1038/29993

Krogdahl, A., Sundby, A., and Olli, J. J. (2004). Atlantic salmon (*Salmo salar*) and rainbow trout (*Oncorhynchus mykiss*) digest and metabolize nutrients differently. Effects of water salinity and dietary starch level. *Aquaculture* 229, 335–360. doi: 10.1016/S0044-8486(03)00396-X

Kulczykowska, E., and Sánchez-Vázquez, F. J. (2010). Neurohormonal regulation of feed intake and response to nutrients in fish: aspects of feeding rhythm and stress. *Aquacul. Res.* 41, 654–657. doi: 10.1111/j.1365-2109.2009.02350.x

Kurokawa, T., Murashita, K., Suzuki, T., and Uji, S. (2008). Genomic characterization and tissue distribution of leptin receptor and leptin receptor overlapping transcript genes in the pufferfish, Takifugu rubripes. *Gen. Comp. Endocrinol.* 158, 108–114. doi: 10.1016/j.ygcen.2008.06.003

Lamia, K. A., Sachdeva, U. M., DiTacchio, L., Williams, E. C., Alvarez, J. G., Egan, D. F., et al. (2009). AMPK regulates the circadian clock by cryptochrome phosphorylation and degradation. *Science* 326, 437–440. doi: 10.1126/science.1172156

Lanfumey, L., Mongeau, R., Cohen-Salmon, C., and Hamon, M. (2008). Corticosteroid–serotonin interactions in the neurobiological mechanisms of stress-related disorders. *Neurosci. Biobehav. Rev.* 32, 1174–1184. doi: 10.1016/j.neubiorev.2008.04.006

Langhans, W. (1999). "Appetite regulation," in *Protein Metabolism and Nutrition*, eds G. E. Lobley, A. White, and J. C. MacRae (Wageningen: Wageningen Press), 225–251.

Langhans, W., and Scharrer, E. (1992). Metabolic control of eating. *World Rev. Nutr. Diet.* 70, 1–67. doi: 10.1159/000421670

Leal, E., Sánchez, E., Muriach, B., and Cerdá-Reverter, J. M. (2009). Sex steroid-induced inhibition of food intake in sea bass (Dicentrarchus labrax). *J. Comp. Physiol. B.* 179, 77–86. doi: 10.1007/s00360-008-0285-5

Leder, E. H., and Silverstein, J. T. (2006). The pro-opiomelanocortin genes in rainbow trout (*Oncorhynchus mykiss*): duplications, splice variants, and differential expression. *J Endocrinol.* 188, 355–363. doi: 10.1677/joe.1.06283

Le Foll, C., Irani, B. G., Magnan, C., Dunn-Meynell, A. A., and Levin, B. E. (2009). Characteristics and mechanisms of hypothalamic neuronal fatty acid sensing. *Am. J. Physiol. Regul. Integr. Comp. Physiol.* 297, R655–R664. doi: 10.1152/ajpregu.00223.2009

Leibush, B., Parrizas, I., Navarro, I., Lappova, M. A., Maestro, M., Encinas, M., et al. (1996). Insulin and insulin-like growth factor-I receptors in fish brain. *Regul. Peptides* 61, 155–161. doi: 10.1016/0167-0115(95)00154-9

Levin, B. E., Routh, V. H., Kang, L., Sanders, N. M., and Dunn-Meynell, A. A. (2004). Neuronal glucosensing. What do we know after 50 years? *Diabetes* 53, 2521–2528. doi: 10.2337/diabetes.53.10.2521

Li, A., Yuan, X., Liang, X.-F., Liu, L., Li, J., Li, B., et al. (2016). Adaptations of lipid metabolism and food intake in response to low and high fat diets in juvenile grass carp (*Ctenopharyngodon idellus*). *Aquaculture* 457, 43–49. doi: 10.1016/j.aquaculture.2016.01.014

Li, G.-G., Liang, X.-F., Xie, Q., Li, G., Yu, Y., and Lai, K. (2010). Gene structure, recombinant expression and functional characterization of grass carp leptin. *Gen. Comp. Endocrinol.* 166, 117–127. doi: 10.1016/j.ygcen.2009.10.009

Librán-Pérez, M., Geurden, I., Dias, K., Corraze, G., Panserat, S., and Soengas, J. L. (2015b). Feeding rainbow trout with a lipid-enriched diet: effects on fatty acid sensing, regulation of food intake and cellular signaling pathways. *J. Exp. Biol.* 218, 2610–2619. doi: 10.1242/jeb.123802

Librán-Pérez, M., López-Patiño, M. A., Míguez, J. M., and Soengas, J. L. (2013). Oleic acid and octanoic acid sensing capacity in rainbow trout *Oncorhynchus mykiss* is direct in hypothalamus and Brockmann bodies. *PLoS ONE* 8:e59507. doi: 10.1371/journal.pone.0059507

Librán-Pérez, M., Otero-Rodiño, C., López-Patiño, M. A., Míguez, J. M., and Soengas, J. L. (2014a). Central administration of oleate or octanoate activates hypothalamic fatty acid sensing and inhibits food intake in rainbow trout. *Physiol. Behav.* 129, 272–279. doi: 10.1016/j.physbeh.2014.02.061

Librán-Pérez, M., Polakof, S., López-Patiño, M. A., Míguez, J. M., and Soengas, J. L. (2012). Evidence of a metabolic fatty-acid sensing system in the hypothalamus and Brockmann bodies of rainbow trout: implications in food intake regulation. Am. J. Physiol. Regul. Integr. Comp. *Physiol.* 302, R1340–R1350. doi: 10.1152/ajpregu.00070.2012

Librán-Pérez, M., Velasco, C., López-Patiño, M. A., Míguez, J. M., and Soengas, J. L. (2014b). Counter-regulatory response to a fall in circulating fatty acid levels in rainbow trout. Possible involvement of the hypothalamus-pituitary-interrenal axis. *PLoS ONE* 9:e113291. doi: 10.1371/journal.pone.0113291

Librán-Pérez, M., Velasco, C., Otero-Rodiño, C., López-Patiño, M. A., Míguez, J. M., and Soengas, J. L. (2015a). Effects of insulin treatment on the response to oleate and octanoate of food intake and fatty acid-sensing systems in rainbow trout. *Domestic Anim. Endocrinol.* 53, 124–135. doi: 10.1016/j.domaniend.2015.06.004

Londraville, R. L., Macotela, Y., Duff, R. J., Easterling, M. R., Liu, Q., and Crespi, E. J. (2014). Comparative endocrinology of leptin: assessing function in a phylogenetic context. *Gen. Comp. Endocrinol.* 203, 146–157. doi: 10.1016/j.ygcen.2014.02.002

López, J., Cuesta, N., Cuttitta, F., and Martinez, A. (1999). Adrenomedullin in nonmammalian vertebrate pancreas: an immunocytochemical study. *Gen. Comp. Endocrinol.* 115, 309–322. doi: 10.1006/gcen.1999.7335

López, J. M., Sanz-Morello, B., and González, A. (2014). Organization of the orexin/hypocretin system in the brain of two basal actinopterygian fishes, the cladistians *Polypterus senegalus* and *Erpetoichthys calabaricus*. *Peptides* 61, 23–37. doi: 10.1016/j.peptides.2014.08.011

López, M., Lelliott, C. J., and Vidal-Puig, A. (2007). Hypothalamic fatty acid metabolism: a housekeeping pathway that regulates food intake. *BioEssays* 29, 248–261. doi: 10.1002/bies.20539

López, M., Tovar, S., Vázquez, M. J., Nogueiras, R., Señarís, R., and Diéguez, C. (2005). Sensing the fat: fatty acid metabolism in the hypothalamus and the melanocortin system. *Peptides* 26, 1753–1758. doi: 10.1016/j.peptides.2004.11.025

López-Olmeda, J. F., and Sánchez-Vázquez, F. J. (2010). "Feeding rhythms in fish: from behavioral to molecular approach," in *Biological Clock in Fish*, eds E. Kulczykowska, W. Popek, and B. G. Kapoor (Enfield: Science Pub CRC Press), 155–183.

López-Patiño, M. A., Guijarro, A. I., Isorna, E., Delgado, M. J., Alonso-Bedate, M., and De Pedro, N. (1999). Neuropeptide Y has a stimulatory action on feeding behavior in goldfish (*Carassius auratus*). *Eur. J. Pharmacol.* 377, 147–153.

Luo, L., Xue, M., Vachot, C., Geurden, I., and Kaushik, S. (2014). Dietary medium chain fatty acids from coconut oil have little effects on postprandial plasma metabolite profiles in rainbow trout (*Oncorhynchus mykiss*). *Aquaculture* 420–421, 24–31. doi: 10.1016/j.aquaculture.2013.10.024

Luquet, S., Perez, F. A., Hnasko, T. S., and Palmiter, R. D. (2005). NPY/AgRP neurons are essential for feeding in adult mice but can be ablated in neonates. *Science* 310, 683–685. doi: 10.1126/science.1115524

MacDonald, E., and Volkoff, H. (2009). Cloning, distribution and effects of season and nutritional status on the expression of neuropeptide Y (NPY), cocaine and amphetamine regulated transcript (CART) and cholecystokinin (CCK) in winter flounder (*Pseudopleuronectes americanus*). *Horm. Behav.* 56, 58–65. doi: 10.1016/j.yhbeh.2009.03.002

Madrid, J. A., Boujard, T., and Sánchez-Vázquez, F. J. (2001). "Feeding rhythms in fish," in *Food Intake in Fish*, eds D. F. Houlihan, T. Boujard, and M. Jobling (Oxford: Blackwell Science), 189–215.

Martínez-Álvarez, R. M., Volkoff, H., Muñoz-Cueto, J. A., and Delgado, M. J. (2008). Molecular characterization of calcitonin gene-related peptide (CGRP) related peptides (CGRP, amylin, adrenomedullin and adrenomedullin-2/intermedin) in goldfish (*Carassius auratus*): cloning and distribution. *Peptides* 29, 1534–1543. doi: 10.1016/j.peptides.2008.04.013

Martínez-Álvarez, R. M., Volkoff, H., Muñoz-Cueto, J. A., and Delgado, M. J. (2009). Effect of calcitonin gene-related peptide (CGRP), adrenomedullin and adrenomedullin-2/intermedin on food intake in goldfish (*Carassius auratus*). *Peptides* 30, 803–807. doi: 10.1016/j.peptides.2008.12.015

Martín-Robles, A. J., Whitmore, D., Sánchez-Vázquez, F. J., Pendón, C., and Muñoz-Cueto, J. A. (2012). Cloning, tissue expression pattern and daily rhythms of Period1, Period2, and Clock transcripts in the flatfish Senegalese sole, *Solea senegalensis*. *J. Comp. Physiol. B* 182, 673–685. doi: 10.1007/s00360-012-0653-z

Marty, N., Dallaporta, M., and Thorens, B. (2007). Brain glucose sensing, counteregulation, and energy homeostasis. *Physiology* 22, 241–251. doi: 10.1152/physiol.00010.2007

Masri, S., Orozco-Solis, R., Aguilar-Arnal, L., Cervantes, M., and Sassone-Corsi, P. (2015). Coupling circadian rhythms of metabolism and chromatin remodelling. *Diab. Obes. Metab.* 17(Suppl. 1), 17–22. doi: 10.1111/dom.12509

Masri, S., Rigor, P., Cervantes, M., Ceglia, N., Sebastian, C., Xiao, C., et al. (2014). Partitioning circadian transcription by SIRT6 leads to segregated control of cellular metabolism. *Cell* 158, 659–672. doi: 10.1016/j.cell.2014.06.050

Matsuda, K., Azuma, M., and Kang, K. S. (2012a). "Orexin system in teleost fish," in *Vitamins and Hormones*, ed L. Gerald (New York, NY: Academic Press), 341–361.

Matsuda, K., Miura, T., Kaiya, H., Maruyama, K., Shimakura, S. I., Uchiyama, M., et al. (2006b). Regulation of food intake by acyl and des-acyl-ghrelins in the goldfish. *Peptides* 27, 2321–2325. doi: 10.1016/j.peptides.2006.03.028

Matsuda, K., Miura, T., Kaiya, H., Maruyama, K., Uchiyama, M., Kangawa, K., et al. (2006a). Stimulatory effect of n-octanoylated ghrelin on locomotor activity in the goldfish, *Carassius auratus*. *Peptides* 27, 1335–1340. doi: 10.1016/j.peptides.2005.10.011

Matsuda, K., Sakashita, A., Yokobori, E., and Azuma, M. (2012b). Neuroendocrine control of feeding behavior and psychomotor activity by neuropeptide Y in fish. *Neuropeptides* 46, 275–283. doi: 10.1016/j.npep.2012.09.006

Matsuda, K., Shimakura, S. I., Maruyama, K., Miura, T., Uchiyama, M., Kawauchi, H., et al. (2006c). Central administration of melanin-concentrating hormone (MCH) suppresses food intake but not locomotor activity, in the goldfish, *Carassius auratus*. *Neurosci. Lett.* 399, 259–263. doi: 10.1016/j.neulet.2006.02.005

Maurin, A.-C., Benani, A., Lorsignol, A., Brenachot, X., Parry, L., Carraro, V., et al. (2014). Hypothalamic eIF2α signaling regulates food intake. *Cell Rep.* 6, 438–444. doi: 10.1016/j.celrep.2014.01.006

Mazurais, D., Le Dréan, G., Brierley, I., Anglade, I., Bromage, N., Williams, L. M., et al. (2000). Expression of clock gene in the brain of rainbow trout: comparison with the distribution of melatonin receptors. *J. Comp. Neurol.* 422, 612–620. doi: 10.1002/1096-9861(20000710)422:4<612::AID-CNE9>3.0.CO;2-Y

McCrimmon, R. J., Song, Z., Cheng, H., McNay, E. C., Weickart-Yeckel, C., Routh, V. H., et al. (2006). Corticotrophin-releasing factor receptors within the ventromedial hypothalamus regulate hypoglycemia-induced hormonal counterregulation. *J. Clin. Invest.* 116, 1723–1730. doi: 10.1172/JCI27775

Mendoza, J. (2006). Circadian clocks: setting time by food. *J. Neuroendocrinol.* 19, 127–137. doi: 10.1111/j.1365-2826.2006.01510.x

Metz, J. R., Huising, M. O., Meek, J., Taverne-Thiele, A. J., Wendelaar Bonga, S. E., and Flik, G. (1994). Localization, expression and control of adrenocorticotropic hormone in the nucleus preopticus and pituitary gland of common carp (*Cyprinus carpio* L.). *J. Endocrinol.* 182, 23–31. doi: 10.1677/joe.0.1820023

Micale, V., Campo, S., D'Ascola, A., Guerrera, C., Levanti, C., Germanà, A., et al. (2014). Cholecystokinin: how many functions? Observations in seabreams. *Gen. Comp. Endocrinol.* 205, 166–167. doi: 10.1016/j.ygcen.2014.02.019

Micale, V., Campo, S., D'Ascola, A., Guerrera, M. C., Levanti, M. B., German,à, A., et al. (2012). Cholecystokinin in white sea bream: molecular cloning, regional expression, and immunohistochemical localization in the gut after feeding and fasting. *PLoS ONE* 7:e52428. doi: 10.1371/journal.pone.0052428

Michel, M., Page-McCaw, P. S., Chen, W., and Cone, R. D. (2016). Leptin signaling regulates glucose homeostasis, but not adipostasis, in the zebrafish. *Proc. Natl. Acad. Sci. U.S.A.* 113, 3084–3089. doi: 10.1073/pnas.1513212113

Migrenne, S., Magnan, C., and Cruciani-Guglielmacci, C. (2007). Fatty acid sensing and nervous control of energy homeostasis. *Diabetes Metab.* 33, 177–182. doi: 10.1016/j.diabet.2007.01.006

Mistlberger, R. E. (2009). Food anticipatory circadian rhythms: concepts and methods. *Eur. J. Neurosci.* 30, 1718–1729. doi: 10.1111/j.1460-9568.2009.06965.x

Mitro, N., Mak, P. A., Vargas, L., Godio, C., Hampton, E., Molteni, V., et al. (2007). The nuclear receptor LXR is a glucose sensor. *Nature* 445, 219–223. doi: 10.1038/nature05449

Miura, T., Maruyama, K., Shimakura, S., Kaiya, H., Uchiyama, M., Kangawa, K., et al. (2006). Neuropeptide y mediates ghrelin-induced feeding in the goldfish, *Carassius auratus*. *Neurosci. Lett.* 407, 279–283. doi: 10.1016/j.neulet.2006.08.071

Miura, T., Maruyama, K., Shimakura, S., Kaiya, H., Uchiyama, M., Kangawa, K., et al. (2007). Regulation of food intake in the goldfish by interaction between ghrelin and orexin. *Peptides* 28, 1207–1213. doi: 10.1016/j.peptides.2007.03.023

Mobbs, C. V., Isoda, F., Makimura, H., Mastaitis, J., Mizuno, T., Shu, I.-W., et al. (2005). Impaired glucose signaling as a cause of obesity and the metabolic syndrome: the glucoadipostatic hypothesis. *Physiol. Behav.* 85, 2–23. doi: 10.1016/j.physbeh.2005.04.005

Moen, A. G., and Finn, R. N. (2013). Short-term, but not long-term feed restriction causes differential expression of leptins in Atlantic salmon. *Gen. Comp. Endocrinol.* 183, 83–88. doi: 10.1016/j.ygcen.2012.09.027

Mommsen, T. P., Vijayan, M. M., and Moon, T. W. (1999). Cortisol in teleosts: dynamics, mechanisms of action, and metabolic regulation. *Rev. Fish Biol. Fish.* 9, 211–268. doi: 10.1023/A:1008924418720

Montoya, A., López-Olmeda, J. F., Yúfera, M., Sánchez-Muros, M. J., and Sánchez-Vázquez, F. J. (2010). Feeding time synchronises daily rhythms of behaviour and digestive physiology in gilthead seabream (*Sparus auratus*). *Aquaculture* 306, 315–321. doi: 10.1016/j.aquaculture.2010.06.023

Morrison, C. D., Xi, X., White, C. L., Ye, J., and Martin, R. J. (2016). Amino acids inhibit *Agrp* gene expression via an mTOR-dependent mechanism. *Am. J. Physiol. Endocrinol. Metab.* 293, E165–E171. doi: 10.1152/ajpendo.00675.2006

Morton, G. J., Cummings, D. E., Baskin, D. G., Barsh, G. S., and Schwartz, M. W. (2006). Central nervous system control of food intake and body weight. *Nature* 443, 289–295. doi: 10.1038/nature05026

Murashita, K., Fukada, H., Hosokawa, H., and Masumoto, T. (2006). Cholecystokinin and peptide y in yellowtail (*Seriola quinqueradiata*): molecular cloning, real-time quantitative RT-PCR, and response to feeding and fasting. *Gen. Comp. Endocrinol.* 145, 287–297. doi: 10.1016/j.ygcen.2005.09.008

Murashita, K., Jordal, A.-E. O., Nilsen, T. O., Stefansson, S. O., Kurokawa, T., Björnsson, B. T. H., et al. (2011). Leptin reduces Atlantic salmon growth through the central pro-opiomelanocortin pathway. *Comp. Biochem. Physiol. A.* 158, 79–86. doi: 10.1016/j.cbpa.2010.09.001

Murashita, K., Kurokawa, T., Ebbesson, L. O. E., Stefansson, S. O., and Ronnestad, I. (2009). Characterization, tissue distribution, and regulation of agouti-related protein (AgRP), cocaine- and amphetamine-regulated transcript (CART) and neuropeptide Y (NPY) in Atlantic salmon (*Salmo salar*). *Gen. Comp. Endocrinol.* 162, 160–171. doi: 10.1016/j.ygcen.2009.03.015

Murashita, K., Uji, S., Yamamoto, T., Ronnestad, I., and Kurokawa, T. (2008). Production of recombinant leptin and its effects on food intake in rainbow trout (*Oncorhynchus mykiss*). *Comp. Biochem. Physiol. B.* 150, 377–384. doi: 10.1016/j.cbpb.2008.04.007

Nakahata, Y., Kaluzova, M., Grimaldi, B., Sahar, S., Hirayama, J., Chen, D., et al. (2008). The NAD$^+$–dependent deacetylase SIRT1 modulates CLOCK-mediated chromatin remodeling and circadian control. *Cell* 134, 329–340. doi: 10.1016/j.cell.2008.07.002

Nakamachi, T., Matsuda, K., Maruyama, K., Miura, T., Uchiyama, M., Funahashi, H., et al. (2006). Regulation by orexin of feeding behaviour and locomotor activity in the goldfish. *J. Neuroendocrinol.* 18, 290–297. doi: 10.1111/j.1365-2826.2006.01415.x

Nakamachi, T., Shibata, H., Sakashita, A., Iinuma, N., Wada, K., Konno, N., et al. (2014). Orexin A enhances locomotor activity and induces anxiogenic-like action in the goldfish, *Carassius auratus*. *Horm. Behav.* 66, 317–323. doi: 10.1016/j.yhbeh.2014.06.004

Narnaware, Y., and Peter, R. E. (2002). Influence of diet composition on food intake and neuropeptide Y (NPY) gene expression in goldfish brain. *Reg. Peptides* 103, 75–83. doi: 10.1016/S0167-0115(01)00342-1

Nisembaum, L. G., de Pedro, N., Delgado, M. J., and Isorna, E. (2014b). Crosstalking between the "gut-brain" hormone ghrelin and the circadian system in the goldfish. Effects on clock gene expression and food anticipatory activity. *Gen. Comp. Endocrinol.* 205, 287–295. doi: 10.1016/j.ygcen.2014.03.016

Nisembaum, L. G., de Pedro, N., Delgado, M. J., Sánchez-Bretaño, A., and Isorna, E. (2014a). Orexin as an input of circadian system in goldfish: effects on clock gene expression and locomotor activity rhythms. *Peptides* 52, 29–37. doi: 10.1016/j.peptides.2013.11.014

Nisembaum, L. G., Velarde, E., Tinoco, A. B., Azpeleta, C., de Pedro, N., Alonso-Gómez, A. L., et al. (2012). Light-dark cycle and feeding time differentially entrains the gut molecular clock of the goldfish (*Carassius auratus*). *Chronobiol. Int.* 29, 665–673. doi: 10.3109/07420528.2012.686947

Nishio, S., Gibert, Y., Berekelya, L., Bernard, L., Brunet, F., Guillot, E., et al. (2012). Fasting induces CART down-regulation in the zebrafish nervous system in a cannabinoid receptor 1-dependent manner. *Mol. Endocrinol.* 26, 1316–1326. doi: 10.1210/me.2011-1180

Novak, C. M., Jiang, X., Wang, C., Teske, J. A., Kotz, C. M., and Levine, J. A. (2005). Calorie restriction and physical activity in zebrafish (*Danio rerio*). *Neurosci. Lett.* 383, 99–104. doi: 10.1016/j.neulet.2005.03.048

Ogoshi, M., Inoue, K., and Takei, Y. (2003). Identification of a novel adrenomedullin gene family in teleost fish. *Biochem. Biophys. Res. Commun.* 311, 1072–1077. doi: 10.1016/j.bbrc.2003.10.111

Oh, Y. T., Kim, J., Kang, I., and Youn, J. H. (2014). Regulation of hypothalamic-pituitary-adrenal axis by circulating free fatty acids in male wistar rats: role of individual free fatty acids. *Endocrinology* 155, 923–931. doi: 10.1210/en.2013-1700

Oh, Y. T., Oh, K.-S., Kang, I., and Youn, J. H. (2012). A fall in plasma free fatty acid (FFA) level activates the hypothalamic-pituitary-adrenal axis independent of plasma glucose: evidence for brain sensing of circulating FFA. *Endocrinology* 153, 3587–3592. doi: 10.1210/en.2012-1330

Ollmann, M. M., Wilson, B. D., Yang, Y. K., Kerns, J. A., Chen, Y., Gantz, I., et al. (1997). Antagonism of central melanocortin receptors *in vitro* and *in vivo* by agouti-related protein. *Science* 278, 135–138. doi: 10.1126/science.278.5335.135

Olsson, C., Holbrook, J. D., Bompadre, G., Jönsson, E., Hoyle, C. H. V., Sanger, G. J., et al. (2008). Identification of genes for the ghrelin and motilin receptors and a novel related gene in fish, and stimulation of intestinal motility in zebrafish (*Danio rerio*) by ghrelin and motilin. *Gen. Comp. Endocrinol.* 155, 217–226. doi: 10.1016/j.ygcen.2007.05.016

Olsson, C., and Holmgren, S. (2011). Autonomic control of gut motility: a comparative view. *Auton. Neurosci.* 165, 80–101. doi: 10.1016/j.autneu.2010.07.002

Oosterman, J. E., Kalsbeek, A., la Fleur, S. E., and Belsham, D. D. (2015). Impact of nutrients on circadian rhythmicity. *Am. J. Physiol. Regul. Integr. Comp. Physiol.* 308, R337–R350. doi: 10.1152/ajpregu.00322.2014

Ooyama, Y., Kojima, K., Aoyama, T., and Takeuchi, H. (2009). Decrease of food intake in rats after ingestion of medium-chain triacylglycerol. *J. Nutr. Sci. Vitaminol.* 55, 423–427. doi: 10.3177/jnsv.55.423

Orozco-Solis, R., Ramadori, G., Coppari, R., and Sassone-Corsi, P. (2015). SIRT1 relays nutritional inputs to the circadian clock through the Sf1 neurons of the ventromedial hypothalamus. *Endocrinology* 156, 2174–2184. doi: 10.1210/en.2014-1805

Ortega, V. A., Lovejoy, D. A., and Bernier, N. J. (2013). Appetite-suppressing effects and interactions of centrally administered corticotropin-releasing factor, urotensin I and serotonin in rainbow trout (*Oncorhynchus mykiss*). *Front. Neurosci.* 7:196. doi: 10.3389/fnins.2013.00196

Otero-Rodiño, C., Librán-Pérez, M., Velasco, C., López-Patiño, M. A., Míguez, J. M., and Soengas, J. L. (2015). Evidence for the presence of glucosensor mechanisms not dependent on glucokinase in hypothalamus and hindbrain of rainbow trout (*Oncorhynchus mykiss*). *PLoS ONE* 10:e0128603. doi: 10.1371/journal.pone.0128603

Otero-Rodiño, C., Velasco, C., Álvarez-Otero, R., López-Patiño, M. A., Míguez, J. M., and Soengas, J. L. (2016). *In vitro* evidence supports the presence of glucokinase-independent glucosensing mechanisms in hypothalamus and hindbrain of rainbow trout. *J. Exp. Biol.* 219, 1750–1759. doi: 10.1242/jeb.137737

Partch, C. L., Green, C. B., and Takahashi, J. S. (2014). Molecular architecture of the mammalian circadian clock. *Trends Cell. Biol.* 24, 90–99. doi: 10.1016/j.tcb.2013.07.002

Patiño, M. A. L., Rodríguez-Illamola, A., Conde-Sieira, M., Soengas, J. L., and Míguez, J. M. (2011). Daily rhythmic expression patterns of clock1a, bmal1, and per1 genes in retina and hypothalamus of the rainbow trout, *Oncorhynchus mykiss*. *Chronobiol. Int.* 28, 381–389. doi: 10.3109/07420528.2011.566398

Patton, D. F., and Mistlberger, R. E. (2013). Circadian adaptations to meal timing; neuroendocrine mechanisms. *Front. Neurosci.* 7:185. doi: 10.3389/fnins.2013.00185

Peddu, S. C., Breves, J. P., Kaiya, H., Grau, E. G., and Riley, L. G. Jr. (2009). Pre- and postprandial effects on ghrelin signaling in the brain and on the GH/IGF-I axis in the Mozambique tilapia (*Oreochromis mossambicus*). *Gen. Comp. Endocrinol.* 161, 412–418. doi: 10.1016/j.ygcen.2009.02.008

Penney, C. C., and Volkoff, H. (2014). Peripheral injections of cholecystokinin, apelin, ghrelin and orexin in cavefish (*Astyanax fasciatus mexicanus*): effects on feeding and on the brain expression levels of tyrosine hydroxylase, mechanistic target of rapamycin and appetite-related hormones. *Gen. Comp. Endocrinol.* 196, 34–40. doi: 10.1016/j.ygcen.2013.11.015

Peragón, J., Barroso, J. B., García-Salguero, L., de la Higuera, M., and Lupiáñez, J. A. (2000). Dietary alterations in protein, carbohydrates and fat increase liver protein-turnover rate and decrease overall growth rate in the rainbow trout (*Oncorhynchus mykiss*). *Mol. Cell. Biochem.* 209, 97–104. doi: 10.1023/A:1007130906365

Peterson, B. C., Waldbieser, G. C., Riley, L. G. Jr., Upton, K. R., Kobayashi, Y., and Small, B. C. (2012). Pre- and postprandial changes in orexigenic and anorexigenic factors in channel catfish (*Ictalurus punctatus*). *Gen. Comp. Endocrinol.* 176, 231–239. doi: 10.1016/j.ygcen.2012.01.022

Picard, A., Rouch, C., Kassis, N., Moullé, V. S., Croizier, S., Denis, R. G., et al. (2013). Hippocampal lipoprotein lipase regulates energy balance in rodents. *Mol. Metab.* 3, 167–176. doi: 10.1016/j.molmet.2013.11.002

Picha, M. E., Strom, C. N., Riley, L. G., Walker, A. A., Won, E. T., Johnstone, W. M., et al. (2009). Plasma ghrelin and growth hormone regulation in response to metabolic state in hybrid striped bass: effects of feeding, ghrelin and insulin-like growth factor-I on *in vivo* and *in vitro* GH secretion. *Gen. Comp. Endocrinol.* 161, 365–372. doi: 10.1016/j.ygcen.2009.01.026

Polakof, S., Ceinos, R. M., Fernández-Durán, B., Míguez, J. M., and Soengas, J. L. (2007c). Daily changes in parameters of energy metabolism in brain of rainbow trout: dependence on feeding. *Comp. Biochem. Physiol. A.* 146, 265–273. doi: 10.1016/j.cbpa.2006.10.026

Polakof, S., Médale, F., Skiba-Cassy, S., Corraze, G., and Panserat, S. (2010). Molecular regulation of lipid metabolism in liver and muscle of rainbow trout subjected to acute and chronic insulin treatments. *Domestic Anim. Endocrinol.* 39, 26–33. doi: 10.1016/j.domaniend.2010.01.003

Polakof, S., Míguez, J. M., Moon, T. W., and Soengas, J. L. (2007a). Evidence for the presence of a glucosensor in hypothalamus, hindbrain, and Brockmann bodies of rainbow trout. *Am. J. Physiol. Regul. Integr. Comp. Physiol.* 292, R1657–R1666. doi: 10.1152/ajpregu.00525.2006

Polakof, S., Míguez, J. M., and Soengas, J. L. (2007b). *In vitro* evidences for glucosensing capacity and mechanisms in hypothalamus, hindbrain, and Brockmann bodies of rainbow trout. *Am. J. Physiol. Regul. Integr. Comp. Physiol.* 293, R1410–R1420. doi: 10.1152/ajpregu.00283.2007

Polakof, S., Míguez, J. M., and Soengas, J. L. (2007d). Daily changes in parameters of energy metabolism in liver, white muscle, and gills of rainbow trout: dependence on feeding. *Comp. Biochem. Physiol. A.* 147, 363–374. doi: 10.1016/j.cbpa.2007.01.009

Polakof, S., Míguez, J. M., and Soengas, J. L. (2008a). Changes in food intake and glucosensing function of hypothalamus and hindbrain in rainbow trout subjected to hyperglycemic or hypoglycemic conditions. *J. Comp. Physiol. A.* 194, 829–839. doi: 10.1007/s00359-008-0354-y

Polakof, S., Míguez, J. M., and Soengas, J. L. (2008b). Dietary carbohydrates induce changes in glucosensing capacity and food intake in rainbow trout. *Am. J. Physiol. Regul. Integr. Comp. Physiol.* 295, R478–R489. doi: 10.1152/ajpregu.00176.2008

Polakof, S., Míguez, J. M., and Soengas, J. L. (2011a). Cholecystokinin impact on rainbow trout glucose homeostasis: possible involvement of central glucosensors. *Reg. Peptides* 172, 23–29. doi: 10.1016/j.regpep.2011.08.002

Polakof, S., Míguez, J. M., and Soengas, J. L. (2011b). Evidence for a gut-brain axis used by glucagon-like peptide-1 to elicit hyperglycaemia in fish. *J. Neuroendocrinol.* 23, 508–518. doi: 10.1111/j.1365-2826.2011.02137.x

Polakof, S., Míguez, J. M., and Soengas, J. L. (2011c). Ghrelin effects on central glucosensing ad energy homeostasis-related peptides in rainbow trout. *Domestic Anim. Endocrinol.* 41, 126–136. doi: 10.1016/j.domaniend.2011.05.006

Polakof, S., Mommsen, T. P., and Soengas, J. L. (2011d). Glucosensing and glucose homeostasis: from fish to mammals. *Comp. Biochem. Physiol. B.* 160, 123–149. doi: 10.1016/j.cbpb.2011.07.006

Polakof, S., Panserat, S., Plagnes-Juan, E., and Soengas, J. L. (2008c). Altered dietary carbohydrates significantly affect gene expression of the major glucosensing components in Brockmannn bodies and hypothalamus of rainbow trout. *Am. J. Physiol. Regul. Integr. Comp. Physiol.* 295, R1077–R1088. doi: 10.1152/ajpregu.90476.2008

Polakof, S., Panserat, S., Soengas, J. L., and Moon, T. W. (2012). Glucose metabolism in fish: a review. *J. Comp. Physiol. B.* 182, 1015–1045. doi: 10.1007/s00360-012-0658-7

Polakof, S., Rodríguez-Alonso, M., and Soengas, J. L. (2009). Immunohistochemical localization of glucokinase in rainbow trout brain. *Comp. Biochem. Physiol. A.* 153, 352–358. doi: 10.1016/j.cbpa.2009.03.015

Polakof, S., and Soengas, J. L. (2008). Involvement of lactate in glucose metabolism and glucosensing function in selected tissues of rainbow trout. *J. Exp. Biol.* 211, 1075–1086. doi: 10.1242/jeb.014050

Qu, D., Ludwig, D. S., Gammeltoft, S., Piper, M., Pelleymounter, M. A., Cullen, M. J., et al. (1996). A role for melanin-concentrating hormone in the central regulation of feeding behaviour. *Nature.* 380, 243–247. doi: 10.1038/380243a0

Rajjo, I. M., Vigna, S. R., and Crim, J. W. (1988). Actions of cholecystokinin-related peptides on the gallbladder of bony fishes *in vitro*. *Comp. Biochem. Physiol. C.* 90, 267–273. doi: 10.1016/0742-8413(88)90132-6

Ren, X., Zhou, L., Terwiliger, R., Newton, S. S., and de Araujo, I. E. (2009). Sweet taste signaling functions as a hypothalamic glucose sensor. *Front. Integr. Neurosci.* 3:12. doi: 10.3389/neuro.07.012.2009

Ribas-Latre, A., and Eckel-Mahan, A. (2016). Interdependence of nutrient metabolism and the circadian clock system: importance for metabolic health. *Molec. Metab.* 5, 133–152. doi: 10.1016/j.molmet.2015.12.006

Rocha, F., Dias, J., Geurden, I., Dinis, M. T., Panserat, S., and Engrola, S. (2016). Dietary glucose stimulus at larval stage modifies the carbohydrate metabolic pathway in gilthead seabream (*Sparus aurata*) juveniles: an *in vivo* approach using ^{14}C-starch. *Comp. Biochem. Physiol. A.* 201, 189–199. doi: 10.1016/j.cbpa.2016.07.016

Ross, R. A., Rossetti, L., Lam, T. K. T., and Schwartz, G. J. (2010). Differential effects of hypothalamic long-chain fatty acid infusions on suppression of hepatic glucose production. *Am. J. Physiol. Endocrinol. Metab.* 299, E633–E639. doi: 10.1152/ajpendo.00190.2010

Rubio, V. C., Sánchez-Vázquez, F. J., and Madrid, J. A. (2008). Role of cholecystokinin and its antagonist proglumide on macronutrient selection in European sea bass *Dicentrarchus labrax*, L. *Physiol. Behav.* 93, 862–869. doi: 10.1016/j.physbeh.2007.12.001

Ruibal, C., Soengas, J. L., and Aldegunde, M. (2002). Brain serotonin and the control of food intake in rainbow trout (*Oncorhynchus mykiss*): effects of changes in plasma glucose levels. *J. Comp. Physiol. A.* 188, 479–484. doi: 10.1007/s00359-002-0320-z

Salmerón, C., Johansson, M., Asaad, M., Angotzi, A. R., Ronnestad, I., Stefansson, S. O., et al. (2015). Roles of leptin and ghrelin in adipogenesis and lipid metabolism of rainbow trout adipocytes *in vitro*. *Comp. Biochem. Physiol. A.* 188, 40–48. doi: 10.1016/j.cbpa.2015.06.017

Sánchez, E., Rubio, V. C., Thompson, D., Metz, J., Flik, G., Millhauser, G. L., et al. (2009). Phosphodiesterase inhibitor-dependent inverse agonism of agouti-related protein (AGRP) on melanocortin 4 receptor in sea bass (*Dicentrarchus labrax*). *Am. J. Physiol. Regul. Integr. Comp. Physiol.* 296, R1293–R1306. doi: 10.1152/ajpregu.90948.2008

Sánchez-Bretaño, A., Alonso-Gómez, A. L., Delgado, M. J., and Isorna, E. (2015a). The liver of goldfish as a component of the circadian system: integrating a network of signals. *Gen. Comp. Endocrinol.* 221, 213–216. doi: 10.1016/j.ygcen.2015.05.001

Sánchez-Bretaño, A., Alonso-Gómez, A. L., Delgado, M. J., and Isorna, E. (2016a). Clock genes expression rhythms in liver of goldfish in vivo and in vitro. Possible role of glucocorticoids as a synchronizer. *J. Comp. Physiol. B.* 186, 73–82.

Sánchez-Bretaño, A., Blanco, A. M., Unniappan, S., Kah, O., Gueguen, M. M., Bertucci, J. I., et al. (2015b). *In situ* localization and rhythmic expression of ghrelin and ghs-r1 ghrelin receptor in the brain and gastrointestinal tract of goldfish (*Carassius auratus*). *PLoS ONE* 10:e0141043. doi: 10.1371/journal.pone.0141043

Sánchez-Bretaño, A., Callejo, M., Montero, M., Alonso-Gómez, A. L., Delgado, M. J., and Isorna, E. (2016b). Performing a hepatic timing signal: glucocorticoids induce gper1a and gper1b expression and repress gclock1a and gbmal1a in the liver of goldfish. *J. Comp. Physiol. B* 186, 73–82. doi: 10.1007/s00360-015-0936-2

Sánchez-Bretaño, A., Gueguen, M. M., Cano-Nicolau, J., Kah, O., Alonso-Gómez, A. L., Delgado, M. J., et al. (2015c). Anatomical distribution and daily profile of gper1b gene expression in brain and peripheral structures of goldfish (*Carassius auratus*). *Chronobiol. Int.* 32, 889–902. doi: 10.3109/07420528.2015.1049615

Sánchez-Muros, M. J., García-Rejón, L., García-Salguero, L., de la Higuera, M., and Lupiáñez, J. A. (1998). Long-term nutritional effects on the pimary liver and kidney metabolism in rainbow trout. Adaptative response to starvation and high-protein, carbohydrate-free diet to glutamate dehydrogenase and alanine aminotransferase kinetics. *Int. J. Biochem.* 30, 55–63.

Sanders, N. M., Figlewicz, D. P., Taborsky, G. J. Jr., Wilkinson, C. W., Daumen, W., and Levin, B. E. (2006). Feeding and neuroendocrine responses after recurrent insulin-induced hypoglycemia. *Physiol. Behav.* 87, 700–706. doi: 10.1016/j.physbeh.2006.01.007

Saravanan, S., Geurden, I., Figueiredo-Silva, A. C., Kaushik, S., Haidar, M. N., Verreth, J. A. J., et al. (2012). Control of voluntary feed intake in fish: a role for dietary oxygen demand in Nile tilapia (*Oreochromis niloticus*) fed diets with different macronutrient profiles. *Br. J. Nutr.* 108, 1519–1529. doi: 10.1017/S0007114511006842

Saravanan, S., Geurden, I., Figueiredo-Silva, A. C., Kaushik, S., Verreth, J. A. J., and Schrama, J. W. (2013). Voluntary feed intake in rainbow trout is regulated by diet-induced diferences in oxygen use. *J. Nutr.* 143, 781–787. doi: 10.3945/jn.112.173062

Sargent, J. R., Tocher, D. R., and Bell, J. G. (2002). "The lipids," in *Fish Nutrition*, eds J. E. Halver and R. W. Hardy (San Diego, CA: Academic Press), 182–258.

Schibler, U., Gotic, I., Saini, C., Gos, P., Curie, T., Emmenegger, Y., et al. (2015). Clock-talk: interactions between central and peripheral circadian oscillators in mammals. *Old Spring Harb. Symp. Quant. Biol.* 80, 223–232. doi: 10.1101/sqb.2015.80.027490

Schjolden, J., Schiöth, H. B., Larhammar, D., Winberg, S., and Larson, E. T. (2009). Melanocortin peptides affect the motivation to feed in rainbow trout (*Oncorhynchus mykiss*). *Gen. Comp. Endocrinol.* 160, 134–138. doi: 10.1016/j.ygcen.2008.11.003

Schroeter, J. C., Fenn, C. M., and Small, B. C. (2015). Elucidating the roles of gut neuropeptides on channel catfish feed intake, glycemia, and hypothalamic NPY and POMC expression. *Comp. Biochem. Physiol. A.* 188, 168–174. doi: 10.1016/j.cbpa.2015.06.031

Schwartz, M. W., Woods, S. C., Porte, D. Jr., Seeley, R. J., and Baskin, D. G. (2000). Central nervous system control of food intake. *Nature* 404, 661–671. doi: 10.1038/35007534

Schwinkendorf, D. R., Tsatsos, N. G., Gosnell, B. A., and Mashek, D. G. (2011). Effects of central administration of distinct fatty acids on hypothalamic neuropeptide expression and energy metabolism. *Int. J. Obes.* 35, 336–344. doi: 10.1038/ijo.2010.159

Seino, S., and Miki, T. (2003). Physiological and pathophysiological roles of ATP-sensitive K^{+} channels. *Prog. Biophys. Mol. Biol.* 81, 133–176. doi: 10.1016/S0079-6107(02)00053-6

Shearer, K. D., Silverstein, J., and Plisetskaya, E. M. (1997). Role of adiposity in food intake control of juvenile chinook salmon (*Oncorhynchus tshawytscha*). *Comp. Biochem. Physiol. A.* 118, 1209–1215. doi: 10.1016/S0300-9629(97)86801-6

Silverstein, J. T., Bondareva, V. M., Leonard, J. B. K., and Plisetskaya, E. M. (2001). Neuropeptide regulation of feeding in catfish, *Ictalurus punctatus:* a role for glucagon-like peptide-1 (GLP-1)? *Comp. Biochem. Physiol. B.* 129, 623–631. doi: 10.1016/S1096-4959(01)00357-8

Silverstein, J. T., and Plisetskaya, E. M. (2000). The effects of NPY and insulin on food intake regulation in fish. *Am. Zool.* 40, 296–308. doi: 10.1093/icb/40.2.296

Silverstein, J. T., Shearer, K. D., Dickhoff, W. W., and Plisetskaya, E. M. (1999). Regulation of nutrient intake and energy balance in salmon. *Aquaculture* 177, 161–169. doi: 10.1016/S0044-8486(99)00076-9

Singru, P. S., Mazumdar, M., Sakharkar, A. J., Lechan, R. M., Thim, L., Clausen, J. T., et al. (2007). Immunohistochemical localization of cocaine- and amphetamine regulated transcript peptide in the brain of the catfish, *Clarias batrachus* (Linn.). *J. Comp. Neurol.* 502, 215–235. doi: 10.1002/cne.21295

Soengas, J. L. (2014). Contribution of glucose- and fatty acid sensing systems to the regulation of food intake in fish. *A review. Gen. Comp. Endocrinol.* 205, 36–48. doi: 10.1016/j.ygcen.2014.01.015

Soengas, J. L., and Aldegunde, M. (2004). Brain glucose and insulin: effects on food intake and brain biogenic amines of rainbow trout. *J. Comp. Physiol. A.* 190, 641–649. doi: 10.1007/s00359-004-0524-5

Song, Y., and Cone, R. D. (2007). Creation of a genetic model of obesity in a teleost. *FASEB J.* 21, 2042–2049. doi: 10.1096/fj.06-7503com

Song, Y., Golling, G., Thacker, T. L., and Cone, R. D. (2003). Agouti-related protein (AGRP) is conserved and regulated by metabolic state in the zebrafish, *Danio rerio*. *Endocrine* 22, 257–265. doi: 10.1385/ENDO:22:3:257

Spiess, J., Villarreal, J., and Vale, W. (1981). Isolation and sequence analysis of a somatostatin-like polypeptide from ovine hypothalamus. *Biochemistry* 20, 1982–1988. doi: 10.1021/bi00510a038

Stanley, B. G., and Leibowitz, S. F. (1985). Neuropeptide Y injected in the paraventricular hypothalamus: a powerful stimulant of feeding behavior. *Proc. Natl. Acad. Sci. U.S.A.* 82, 3940–3943. doi: 10.1073/pnas.82.11.3940

Stephan, F. K. (2002). The 'other' circadian system: food as a zeitgeber. *J. Biol. Rhythms* 17, 284–292. doi: 10.1177/074873002129002591

Suárez, M. D., Sanz, A., Bazoco, J., and García-Gallego, M. (2002). Metabolic effects of changes in the dietary protein:carbohydrate ratio in eel (*Anguilla anguilla*) and trout (*Oncorhynchus mykiss*). *Aquaculture Int.* 10, 143–156. doi: 10.1023/A:1021371104839

Subhedar, N. K., Nakhate, K. T., Upadhya, M. A., and Kokare, D. M. (2014). CART in the brain of vertebrates: circuits, functions and evolution. *Peptides* 54, 108–130 doi: 10.1016/j.peptides.2014.01.004

Subhedar, N., Varsagade, V. G., Singru, P. S., Thim, L., and Clausen, J. T. (2011). Cocaine- and amphetamine-regulated transcript peptide (CART) in the telencephalon of the catfish, *Clarias gariepinus*: distribution and response to fasting, 2-deoxy-D-glucose, glucose, insulin, and leptin treatments. *J. Comp. Neurol.* 519, 1281–1300. doi: 10.1002/cne.22569

Sundström, G., Larsson, T. A., Brenner, S., Venkatesh, B., and Larhammar, D. (2008). Evolution of neuropeptide y family: new genes by chromosome duplications in early vertebrate and in teleost fishes. *Gen. Comp. Endocrinol.* 155, 705–716. doi: 10.1016/j.ygcen.2007.08.016

Takahasi, A., Tsuchicha, K., Yamanome, T., Amano, M., Yasuda, A., Yamamori, K., et al. (2004). Possible involvement of melanin-concentrating hormone in food intake in a teleost fish, barfin flounder. *Peptides* 25, 1613–1622. doi: 10.1016/j.peptides.2004.02.022

Tan, X., Lin, H., Huang, Z., Zhou, C., Wang, A., Qi, C., et al. (2016). Effects of dietary leucine on growth performance, feed utilization, non-specific immune responses and gut morphology of juvenile golden pompano *Trachinotus ovatus*. *Aquaculture* 465, 100–107. doi: 10.1016/j.aquaculture.2016.08.034

Tang, Z., Sun, C., Yan, A., Wu, S., Qin, C., Zhang, Y., et al. (2013). Genes involved in fatty acid metabolism: molecular characterization and hypothalamic mRNA response to energy status and neuropeptide Y treatment in the orange-spotted grouper *Epinephelus coioides*. *Mol. Cell Endocrinol.* 376, 114–124. doi: 10.1016/j.mce.2013.06.020

Thavanathan, P., and Volkoff, H. (2006). Effects of amylin on feeding of goldfish: interactions with CCK. *Regul. Pept.* 133, 90–96. doi: 10.1016/j.regpep.2005.09.025

Tian, J., He, G., Mai, K., and Liu, C. (2015). Effects of postprandial starvation on mRNA expression of endocrine-, amino acid and peptide transporter-, and metabolic enzyme-related genes in zebrafish (*Danio rerio*). *Fish Physiol. Biochem.* 41, 773–787. doi: 10.1007/s10695-015-0045-x

Tinoco, A. B., Näslund, J., Delgado, M. J., De Pedro, N., Johnsson, J. I., and Jönsson, E. (2014a). Ghrelin increases food intake, swimming activity and growth in juvenile brown trout (*Salmo trutta*). *Physiol. Behav.* 124, 15–22. doi: 10.1016/j.physbeh.2013.10.034

Tinoco, A. B., Nisembaum, L. G., de Pedro, N., Delgado, M. J., and Isorna, E. (2014b). Leptin expression is rhythmic in brain and liver of goldfish (*Carassius auratus*). Role of feeding time. *Gen. Comp. Endocrinol.* 204, 239–247. doi: 10.1016/j.ygcen.2014.06.006

Tinoco, A. B., Nisembaum, L. G., Isorna, E., Delgado, M. J., and de Pedro, N. (2012). Leptins and leptin receptor expression in the goldfish (*Carassius auratus*). Regulation by food intake and fasting/overfeeding conditions. *Peptides* 34, 329–335. doi: 10.1016/j.peptides.2012.02.001

Tinoco, A. I., Valenciano, A. I., Gómez-Boronat, M., Blanco, A. M., Nisembaum, L. G., De Pedro, N., et al. (2015). Two cholecystokinin receptor subtypes are identified in goldfish, being the CCKAR involved in the regulation of intestinal motility. *Comp. Biochem. Physiol. A.* 187, 193–201. doi: 10.1016/j.cbpa.2015.05.027

Tocher, D. R. (2003). Metabolism and functions of lipids and fatty acids in teleost fish. *Rev. Fish. Sci.* 11, 107–184. doi: 10.1080/713610925

Tocher, D. R., Mourente, G., and Sargent, J. R. (1992). Metabolism of [1-^{14}C]Docosahexaenoate (22:6n-3), [1-^{14}C]Eicosapentaenoate (20:5n-3) and [1-^{14}C]Linolenate (18:3n-3) in brain cells from juvenile turbot *Scophthalmus maximus*. *Lipids* 27, 494–499. doi: 10.1007/BF02536129

Trushenski, J. T. (2009). Saturated lipid sources in feeds for sunshine bass: alterations in production performance and tissue fatty acid composition. *North Am. J. Aquac.* 71, 363–373. doi: 10.1577/A09-001.1

Uchida, H., Nakamura, T. J., Takasu, N. N., Todo, T., Sakai, T., and Nakamura, W. (2016). Cryptochrome-dependent circadian periods in the arcuate nucleus. *Neurosci. Lett.* 610, 123–128. doi: 10.1016/j.neulet.2015.10.071

Unniappan, S., Canosa, L. F., and Peter, R. E. (2004). Orexigenic actions of ghrelin in goldfish: feeding-induced changes in brain and gut mRNA expression and serum levels, and responses to central and peripheral injections. *Neuroendocrinology* 79, 100–108. doi: 10.1159/000076634

Unniappan, S., Lin, X., Cervini, L., Rivier, J., Kaiya, H., Kangawa, K., et al. (2002). Goldfish ghrelin: molecular characterization of the complementary deoxyribonucleic acid, partial gene structure and evidence for its stimulatory role in food intake. *Endocrinology* 143, 4143–4146. doi: 10.1210/en.2002-220644

Valen, R., Jordal, A. E., Murashita, K., and Rønnestad, I. (2011). Postprandial effects on appetite-related neuropeptide expression in the brain of Atlantic salmon, *Salmo salar*. *Gen. Comp. Endocrinol.* 171, 359–366. doi: 10.1016/j.ygcen.2011.02.027

Van den Top, M., and Spanswick, D. (2006). Integration of metabolic stimuli in the hypothalamic arcuate nucleus. *Prog Brain Res.* 153, 141–154. doi: 10.1016/S0079-6123(06)53008-0

Van de Pol, I., Flik, G., and Gorissen, M. (2017). Comparative physiology of energy metabolism: fishing for endocrine signals in the early vertebrate pool. *Front. Endocrinol.* 8:36. doi: 10.3389/fendo.2017.00036

Vatine, G., Vallone, D., Gothilf, Y., and Foulkes, N. S. (2011). It's time to swim! Zebrafish and the circadian clock. *FEBS Lett.* 585, 1485–1494. doi: 10.1016/j.febslet.2011.04.007

Velarde, E., Haque, R., Iuvone, P. M., Azpeleta, C., Alonso-Gómez, A. L., and Delgado, M. J. (2009). Circadian clock genes of goldfish, *Carassius auratus*: cDNA cloning and rhythmic expression of period and cryptochrome transcripts in retina, liver, and gut. *J. Biol. Rhythms* 24, 104–113. doi: 10.1177/0748730408329901

Velasco, C., Librán-Pérez, M., Otero-Rodiño, C., López-Patiño, M. A., Míguez, J. M., Cerdá-Reverter, J. M., et al. (2016a). Ghrelin modulates hypothalamic fatty acid-sensing and control of food intake in rainbow trout. *J. Endocrinol.* 228, 25–37. doi: 10.1530/JOE-15-0391

Velasco, C., Librán-Pérez, M., Otero-Rodiño, C., López-Patiño, M. A., Míguez, J. M., and Soengas, J. L. (2016b). Ceramides are involved in regulation of food intake in rainbow trout (*Oncorhynchus mykiss*). *Am. J. Physiol. Regul. Integr. Comp. Physiol.* 311, R658–R668. doi: 10.1152/ajpregu.00201.2016

Vera, L. M., De Pedro, N., Gómez-Milán, E., Delgado, M. J., Sánchez-Muros, M. J., Madrid, J. A., et al. (2007). Feeding entrainment of locomotor activity rhythms, digestive enzymes and neuroendocrine factors in goldfish. *Physiol. Behav.* 90, 518–524. doi: 10.1016/j.physbeh.2006.10.017

Vera, L. M., Negrini, P., Zagatti, C., Frigato, E., Sánchez-Vázquez, F. J., and Bertolucci, C. (2013). Light and feeding entrainment of the molecular circadian clock in a marine teleost (*Sparus aurata*). *Chronobiol. Int.* 30, 649–661. doi: 10.3109/07420528.2013.775143

Vivas, Y., Azpeleta, C., Feliciano, A., Velarde, E., Isorna, E., Delgado, M. J., et al. (2011). Time-dependent effects of leptin on food intake and locomotor activity in goldfish. *Peptides* 32, 989–995. doi: 10.1016/j.peptides.2011.01.028

Volkoff, H. (2012). "Sleep and orexins in nonmammalian vertebrates," in *Vitamins and Hormones*, ed L. Gerald (San Diego, CA: Academic Press), 315–339.

Volkoff, H. (2014). Appetite regulating peptides in red-bellied piranha, *Pygocentrus nattereri*: cloning, tissue distribution and effect of fasting on mRNA expression levels. *Peptides* 56, 116–124. doi: 10.1016/j.peptides.2014.03.022

Volkoff, H. (2015). Cloning and tissue distribution of appetite-regulating peptides in pirapitinga (*Piaractus brachypomus*). *J. Anim. Physiol. Anim. Nutr.* 99, 987–1001. doi: 10.1111/jpn.12318

Volkoff, H. (2016). The neuroendocrine regulation of food intake in fish: a review of current knowledge. *Front. Neurosci.* 10:540. doi: 10.3389/fnins.2016.00540

Volkoff, H., Bjorklund, J. M., and Peter, R. E. (1999). Stimulation of feeding behavior and food consumption in the goldfish, *Carassius auratus*, by orexin-A and orexin-B. *Brain Res.* 846, 204–209. doi: 10.1016/S0006-8993(99)02052-1

Volkoff, H., Canosa, L. F., Unniappan, S., Cerdá-Reverter, J. M., Bernier, N. J., Kelly, S. P., et al. (2005). Neuropeptides and the control of food intake in fish. *Gen. Comp. Endocrinol.* 142, 3–19. doi: 10.1016/j.ygcen.2004.11.001

Volkoff, H., Eykelbosh, A. J., and Peter, R. E. (2003). Role of leptin in the control of feeding of goldfish *Carassius auratus*: interactions with cholecystokinin, neuropeptide Y and orexin A, and modulation by fasting. *Brain Res.* 972, 90–109. doi: 10.1016/S0006-8993(03)02507-1

Volkoff, H., Hoskins, L. J., and Tuziak, S. M. (2009). Influence of intrinsic signals and environmental cue on the endocrine control of feeding in fish: potential application in aquaculture. *Gen. Comp. Endocrinol.* 167, 352–359. doi: 10.1016/j.ygcen.2009.09.001

Volkoff, H., and Peter, R. E. (2000). Effects of CART peptides on food consumption, feeding and associated behaviors in the goldfish, *Carassius auratus*: actions on neuropeptide Y- and orexin A-induced feeding. *Brain Res.* 887, 125–133. doi: 10.1016/S0006-8993(00)03001-8

Volkoff, H., and Peter, R. E. (2001a). Characterization of two forms of cocaine- and amphetamine-regulated transcript (CART) peptide precursors in goldfish: molecular cloning and distribution, modulation of expression by nutritional status, and interactions with leptin. *Endocrinology* 142, 5076–5088. doi: 10.1210/endo.142.12.8519

Volkoff, H., and Peter, R. E. (2001b). Interactions between orexin A, NPY and galanin in the control of food intake of the goldfish, *Carassius auratus*. *Regul. Pept.* 101, 59–72. doi: 10.1016/S0167-0115(01)00261-0

Volkoff, H., Sabioni, R. E., and Cyrino, J. E. P. (2016). Appetite regulating factors in dourado, *Salminus brasiliensis*: cDNA cloning and effects of fasting and feeding on gene expression. *Gen. Comp. Endocrinol.* 237, 34–42. doi: 10.1016/j.ygcen.2016.07.022

Wacyk, J., Powell, M., Rodnick, K. J., Overturf, K., Hill, R. A., and Hardy, R. (2012). Dietary protein source significantly alters growth performance, plasma variables and hepatic gene expression in rainbow trout (*Oncorhynchus mykiss*) fed amino acid balanced diets. *Aquaculture* 356–357, 223–234. doi: 10.1016/j.aquaculture.2012.05.013

Wall, A., and Volkoff, H. (2013). Effects of fasting and feeding on the brain mRNA expressions of orexin, tyrosine hydroxylase (TH), PYY and CCK in the Mexican blind cavefish (*Astyanax fasciatus mexicanus*). *Gen. Comp. Endocrinol.* 183, 44–52. doi: 10.1016/j.ygcen.2012.12.011

Wang, W. G., Chen, X., Jiang, H., and Jiang, Z. Y. (2008). Effects of ghrelin on glucose-sensing and gastric distension sensitive neurons in rat dorsal vagal complex. *Regul. Peptides* 146, 169–175. doi: 10.1016/j.regpep.2007.09.007

Waterson, M. J., and Horvath, T. L. (2015). Neuronal regulation of energy homeostasis: beyond the hypothalamus and feeding. *Cell Metab.* 22, 962–970. doi: 10.1016/j.cmet.2015.09.026

Wauson, E. M., Lorente-Rodríguez, A., and Cobb, M. H. (2013). Minireview: nutrient sensing by G protein-couple receptors. *Mol. Endocrinol.* 27, 1188–1197. doi: 10.1210/me.2013-1100

Wenderlar Bonga, S. (1997). The stress response in fish. *Physiol. Rev.* 77, 591–625.

Westermark, G. T., Falkmer, S., Steiner, D. F., Chan, S. J., Engstrom, U., and Westermark, P. (2002). Islet amyloid polypeptide is expressed in the pancreatic islet parenchyma of the teleostean fish, *Myoxocephalus (cottus) scorpius*. *Comp. Biochem. Physiol. B.* 133, 119–125. doi: 10.1016/S1096-4959(02)00113-6

White, S. L., Volkoff, H., and Devlin, R. H. (2016). Regulation of feeding behavior and food intake by appetite-regulating peptides in wild-type and growth hormone-transgenic coho salmon. *Hormone. Behav.* 84, 18–28. doi: 10.1016/j.yhbeh.2016.04.005

Williams, I., Williams, K. C., Smith, D. M., and Jones, M. (2006). Polka-dot grouper, *Cromileptes altivelis*, can utilize dietary fat efficiently. *Aquac. Nutr.* 12, 379–387. doi: 10.1111/j.1365-2095.2006.00437.x

Won, E. T., Baltzegar, D. A., Picha, M. E., and Borski, R. J. (2012). Cloning and characterization of leptin in a Perciform fish, the striped bass (*Morone saxatilis*): control of feeding and regulation by nutritional state. *Gen. Comp. Endocrinol.* 178, 98–107. doi: 10.1016/j.ygcen.2012.04.019

Wong, K. K., Ng, S. Y., Lee, L. T., Ng, H. K., and Chow, B. K. (2011). Orexins and their receptors from fish to mammals: a comparative approach. *Gen. Comp. Endocrinol.* 171, 124–130. doi: 10.1016/j.ygcen.2011.01.001

Wu, Q., Boyle, M. P., and Palmiter, R. D. (2009). Loss of GABAergic signaling by AgRP neurons to the parabrachial nucleus leads to starvation. *Cell.* 137, 1225–1234. doi: 10.1016/j.cell.2009.04.022

Xu, M., and Volkoff, H. (2007). Molecular characterization of prepro-orexin in Atlantic cod (*Gadus morhua*): cloning, localization, developmental profile and role in food intake regulation. *Mol. Cell. Endocrinol.* 271, 28–37. doi: 10.1016/j.mce.2007.03.003

Yamanome, T., Amano, M., and Takahasi, A. (2005). White background reduces the occurrence of staining, activates melanin-concentrating hormone and promotes somatic growth in barfin flounder. *Aquaculture* 244, 323–329. doi: 10.1016/j.aquaculture.2004.11.020

Yan, A. F., Chen, T., Chen, S., Ren, C. H., Hu, C. Q., Cai, Y. M., et al. (2016). Goldfish leptin-AI and leptin-AII: function and central mechanism in feeding control. *Int. J. Mol. Sci.* 17:783. doi: 10.3390/ijms17060783

Yan, A., Zhang, L., Tang, Z., Zhang, Y., Qin, C., Li, B., et al. (2011). Orange spotted grouper (*Epinephelus coioides*) orexin: molecular cloning, tissue expression, ontogeny, daily rhythm and regulation of NPY gene expression. *Peptides* 32, 1363–1370. doi: 10.1016/j.peptides.2011.05.004

Yang, J., Brown, M. S., Liang, G., Grishin, N. V., and Goldstein, J. L. (2008). Identification of the acyltransferase that octanoylates ghrelin, an appetite-stimulating peptide hormone. *Cell* 132, 387–396. doi: 10.1016/j.cell.2008.01.017

Yi, C. X., van der Vliet, J., Dai, J., Yin, G., Ru, L., and Buijs, R. M. (2006). Ventromedial arcuate nucleus communicates peripheral metabolic information to the suprachiasmatic nucleus. *Endocrinology* 147, 283–294. doi: 10.1210/en.2005-1051

Yokobori, E., Azuma, M., Nishiguchi, R., Kang, K. S., Kamijo, M., Uchiyama, M., et al. (2012). Neuropeptide Y stimulates food intake in the zebrafish, *Danio rerio*. *J. Neuroendocrinol.* 24, 766–773. doi: 10.1111/j.1365-2826.2012.02281.x

Zhang, C., Forlano, P. M., and Cone, R. D. (2012). AgRP and POMC neurons are hypophysiotropic and coordinately regulate multiple endocrine axes in a larval teleost. *Cell Metab.* 15, 256–264. doi: 10.1016/j.cmet.2011.12.014

Zhang, H., Chen, H., Zhang, Y., Li, S., Lu, D., Zhang, H., et al. (2013). Molecular cloning, characterization and expression profiles of multiple leptin genes and a leptin receptor gene in orange-spotted grouper (*Epinephelus coioides*). *Gen. Comp. Endocrinol.* 181, 295–305. doi: 10.1016/j.ygcen.2012.09.008

Zhang, Y., Liu, Y., Huang, X., Liu, X., Jiao, B., Meng, Z., et al. (2008). Two alternatively spliced GPR39 transcripts in seabream: molecular cloning, genomic organization, and regulation of gene expression by metabolic signals. *J. Endocrinol.* 199, 457–470. doi: 10.1677/JOE-07-0608

Zheng, H., and Berthoud, H.-R. (2008). Neural systems controlling the drive to eat: mind versus metabolism. *Physiology* 23, 75–83. doi: 10.1152/physiol.00047.2007

Zhong, C., Song, Y., Wang, Y., Zhang, T., Duan, M., Li, Y., et al. (2013). Increased food intake in growth hormone-transgenic common carp (*Cyprinus carpio* L.) may be mediated by upregulating Agouti-related protein (AgRP). *Gen. Comp. Endocrinol.* 192, 81–88. doi: 10.1016/j.ygcen.2013.03.024

Zhou, Y., Liang, X.-F., Yuan, X., Jie, L., He, Y., Fang, L., et al. (2013). Neuropeptide Y stimulates food intake and regulates metabolism in grass carp, *Ctenopharyngodon idellus*. *Aquaculture* 380–383, 52–61. doi: 10.1016/j.aquaculture.2012.11.033

13

Activity-Based Anorexia Reduces Body Weight without Inducing a Separate Food Intake Microstructure or Activity Phenotype in Female Rats—Mediation via an Activation of Distinct Brain Nuclei

Sophie Scharner[1], Philip Prinz[1], Miriam Goebel-Stengel[2], Peter Kobelt[1], Tobias Hofmann[1], Matthias Rose[1] and Andreas Stengel[1]*

[1] Division of Psychosomatic Medicine, Charité Center for Internal Medicine and Dermatology, Charité-Universitätsmedizin Berlin, Berlin, Germany, [2] Department of Internal Medicine and Institute of Neurogastroenterology, Martin-Luther-Krankenhaus Berlin, Berlin, Germany

Correspondence:
Andreas Stengel
andreas.stengel@charite.de

Anorexia nervosa (AN) is accompanied by severe somatic and psychosocial complications. However, the underlying pathogenesis is poorly understood, treatment is challenging and often hampered by high relapse. Therefore, more basic research is needed to better understand the disease. Since hyperactivity often plays a role in AN, we characterized an animal model to mimic AN using restricted feeding and hyperactivity. Female Sprague-Dawley rats were divided into four groups: no activity/*ad libitum* feeding (*ad libitum*, AL, $n = 9$), activity/*ad libitum* feeding (activity, AC, $n = 9$), no activity/restricted feeding (RF, $n = 12$) and activity/restricted feeding (activity-based anorexia, ABA, $n = 11$). During the first week all rats were fed *ad libitum*, ABA and AC had access to a running wheel for 24 h/day. From week two ABA and RF only had access to food from 9:00 to 10:30 a.m. Body weight was assessed daily, activity and food intake monitored electronically, brain activation assessed using Fos immunohistochemistry at the end of the experiment. While during the first week no body weight differences were observed ($p > 0.05$), after food restriction RF rats showed a body weight decrease: −13% vs. day eight ($p < 0.001$) and vs. AC (−22%, $p < 0.001$) and AL (−26%, $p < 0.001$) that gained body weight (+10% and +13%, respectively; $p < 0.001$). ABA showed an additional body weight loss (−9%) compared to RF ($p < 0.001$) reaching a body weight loss of −22% during the 2-week restricted feeding period ($p < 0.001$). Food intake was greatly reduced in RF (−38%) and ABA (−41%) compared to AL ($p < 0.001$). Interestingly, no difference in 1.5-h food intake microstructure was observed between RF and ABA ($p > 0.05$). Similarly, the daily physical activity was not different between AC and ABA ($p > 0.05$). The investigation of Fos expression in the brain showed neuronal activation in several brain nuclei such as the supraoptic nucleus, arcuate nucleus, locus coeruleus and nucleus of the solitary tract of ABA compared to AL rats. In conclusion,

ABA combining physical activity and restricted feeding likely represents a suited animal model for AN to study pathophysiological alterations and pharmacological treatment options. Nonetheless, cautious interpretation of the data is necessary since rats do not voluntarily reduce their body weight as observed in human AN.

Keywords: anorexia nervosa, body weight, brain-gut axis, eating disorder, Fos, psychosomatic, wheel running

INTRODUCTION

Anorexia nervosa (AN) is an eating disorder characterized by the desire to lose body weight or to maintain body weight at a lower level than normal for age and height. Moreover, patients suffer from an intense fear of gaining weight and a body image disturbance (American Psychiatric Association, 2013). AN has a high prevalence in adolescent girls and young women (Nagl et al., 2016); the lifetime prevalence for AN in European women was reported to be 0.9% (Preti et al., 2009), similar levels were reported for the United States (Hudson et al., 2007). The treatment of AN is challenging and mostly comprised of structured care and psychotherapy (Zipfel et al., 2014); however, treatment is hampered by a high relapse rate (Herzog et al., 1997; Zipfel et al., 2015). While only about half of the patients recover, one third improves but continues to have symptoms and 20% remain severely chronically ill (Steinhausen, 2002). Lastly, AN has a considerable weighted mortality rate (deaths per 1000 person-years) of 5.1 (Arcelus et al., 2011). It is to note that although AN is clinically well characterized, the pathogenesis underlying the disease is still not well established. Moreover, no specific pharmacological treatment is available. Therefore, more research is needed to better characterize the disease and to identify possible new treatment targets.

Progress in medical research is often achieved by establishing an animal model of a disease that can help to investigate the underlying pathophysiology. It was already in 1967 when Routtenberg and Kuznesof observed that rodents tend to self-starvation when exposed to a time-restricted feeding schedule and given the possibility of voluntary physical activity in a running wheel (Routtenberg and Kuznesof, 1967). As hyperactivity can be observed in a considerable subset (ranging from 31 to 80%) of patients with AN (Davis et al., 1997), animal models using physical activity mimic this condition. The combination of a restricted feeding schedule and the access to physical exercise using a running wheel has been used to mimic features of human AN; the model was termed activity-based anorexia (Casper et al., 2008).

Subsequently, the model has been largely characterized and several alterations observed such as an increased brain γ-aminobutyric acid (GABA) (Aoki et al., 2012) and endocannabinoid signaling (Casteels et al., 2014), disturbances in food-anticipatory dopamine and serotonin release (Verhagen et al., 2009) along with an involvement of several food intake-regulatory hormones, e.g., ghrelin (Legrand et al., 2016) and leptin (Hillebrand et al., 2005b) and lastly, an activation of the hypothalamus-pituitary-adrenal axis (Burden et al., 1993), changes that might play a role in human AN as well. These alterations are likely to be involved in several changes observed: besides a reduction in food intake and body weight also an intestinal barrier dysfunction (Jésus et al., 2014), a disruption of neural development in the hippocampus (Chowdhury et al., 2014) and an impairment of memory function (Paulukat et al., 2016), increased anxiety (Kinzig and Hargrave, 2010) and the development of stress ulcers (Doerries et al., 1991), features also observed (Kline, 1979; Ghadirian et al., 1993; Swinbourne and Touyz, 2007; Huber et al., 2015; Kjaersdam Telleus et al., 2015) or suspected in patients with AN. Taken together, activity-based anorexia—despite the major limitation of being an animal model merely mimicking features of a disease—is likely a suited tool to study aspects of the pathogenesis of human AN.

The aim of the present study was first to establish the model of activity-based anorexia in our laboratory investigating food intake, running wheel activity and body weight in female rats. Only female rats were used due to the higher prevalence of anorexia in females compared to males (Steinhausen and Jensen, 2015). Next, we investigated the food intake microstructure underlying the reduction in food intake in this animal model using an automated food intake monitoring system recently established for the use in rats (Teuffel et al., 2015). To further characterize possible underlying alterations in brain activity we used the neuronal expression marker Fos and performed a brain mapping in rats subjected to activity-based anorexia.

MATERIALS AND METHODS

Animals

Female Sprague-Dawley rats (Harlan-Winkelmann Co., Borchen, Germany) weighing 150–180 g upon their arrival were housed in groups under conditions of controlled illumination (12:12 h light/dark cycle, lights on/off: 06:00 a.m./06:00 p.m.) and temperature (21–23°C). Rats were fed with standard rat chow (ssniff Spezialdiäten GmbH, Soest, Germany) and tap water *ad libitum* unless otherwise specified. This study was carried out in accordance with the recommendation of the institutional guidelines; the protocol was approved by the state authority for animal research (#G 0117/14).

Activity-Based Anorexia

After an initial acclimatization period of 7 days, rats (total n = 44) were randomly assigned to one of four groups: (a) *ad libitum* group: no extra activity + *ad libitum* feeding schedule, (b) activity group: voluntary activity in a running wheel + *ad libitum* feeding schedule, (c) restricted feeding group: no extra activity + restricted feeding schedule, and (d) activity-based anorexia group: voluntary activity in a running wheel + restricted feeding schedule.

During the first week of the experiment, all rats were fed *ad libitum* and separated into single housing cages which were placed adjacent to each other to provide sight, acoustic and odor contact. Rats of the activity and activity-based anorexia group had access to a running wheel inside the cage for 24 h/day, while the sedentary groups (*ad libitum* and restricted feeding group) were housed without running wheel under otherwise identical conditions. All cages contained environmental enrichment and bedding material. Rats were acclimated to their new cages for 1 week and handled daily to become accustomed to the interaction with the investigator. This included daily removal of the rat from the cage to measure body weight. The daily routine was performed between 08:00 and 09:00 a.m.

Food restriction conditions started on day eight of the experiment. Rats of the restricted feeding as well as activity-based anorexia group received food from 09:00 to 10:30 a.m. (the 90-min feeding period during the light phase was based on Luyten et al., 2009; Wu et al., 2014), while the other two groups (*ad libitum* and activity group) continued to have access to food for 24 h/day. Body weight, food intake and activity were monitored over a period of 21 days. The experiment was discontinued and animals euthanized when the body weight loss exceeded 25%.

MEASUREMENTS

Monitoring of Body Weight

Rats were weighed daily between 08:00 and 09:00 a.m. Body weight and body weight changes were calculated for the whole 21-day experimental period (1 week of *ad libitum* food intake and 2 weeks of restricted feeding).

Monitoring of Food Intake and Food Intake Microstructure

The microstructural analysis of feeding behavior was conducted using the BioDAQ episodic food intake monitoring system for rats (BioDAQ, Research Diets, Inc., New Brunswick, NJ, USA) which allows the continuous monitoring of solid chow food intake in undisturbed rats as recently reported (Teuffel et al., 2015). The system contains a food hopper placed on an electronic microbalance, both are mounted on a regular rat single housing cage. Food intake parameters are measured continuously and can be extracted from the software (BioDAQ Monitoring Software 2.3.07); periods of interest can be chosen freely afterwards for data analysis. Every interaction of the rat with the food hopper is registered as a "bout." A meal is defined as food intake of at least 0.01 g, when feeding bouts occur after an interval of $\geq$15 min this is considered a new meal. Meal parameters extracted from the software include bout size, meal size, bout frequency, meal frequency, meal duration, time spent in meals and eating rate. The food intake microstructure was analyzed starting at 4 days after food restriction over a period of 4 days (expressed as mean value of 4 days/animal).

Monitoring of Physical Activity

Physical activity in the running wheel was assessed electronically using the software provided by the manufacturer (Campden Instruments Ltd., Loughborough, UK) and expressed as wheel rotations per day as described before (Wu et al., 2014). Here, the activity system was combined with the cages for automated food intake monitoring. Pilot studies did not indicate any deleterious interference between the two measurements (data not shown).

The estimation of energy consumption was based on an earlier study that determined oxygen consumption of rats running at a constant speed (Shepherd and Gollnick, 1976). A respiratory exchange ratio of 1.0 was assumed based on carbohydrates as largest component in the standard rat chow used (58% of calories from carbohydrates, manufacturer's information).

c-Fos Immunohistochemistry

At the end of the observation period, brain activation was assessed using c-Fos immunohistochemistry in *ad libitum* and activity-based anorexia rats (n = 3/group). In order to avoid signals from overfeeding and great distention of the stomach, food intake was restricted to 1.5 g in this last 1.5-h feeding period in the activity-based anorexia group. Directly after this feeding period, animals were perfused and brains processed for Fos immunohistochemistry as described before (Wang et al., 2011). Briefly, rats were deeply anesthetized by an intraperitoneal injection of 100 mg/kg ketamine (Ketanest™, Curamed, Karlsruhe, Germany) and 10 mg/kg xylazine (Rompun™2%, Bayer, Leverkusen, Germany). Transcardial perfusion was performed as described before (Stengel et al., 2009). After thoracotomy a cannula was inserted into the ascending aorta *via* the left heart ventricle. Perfusion consisted of a 1-min flush with sodium chloride (0.9%) followed by 500 ml of fixative (4% paraformaldehyde and 14% saturated picric acid in 0.1 M phosphate buffer, pH adjusted to 7.4). Afterwards, brains were removed and postfixed overnight in the same fixative at 4°C followed by a cryoprotection in 10% sucrose for 24 h. Lastly, brains were snap-frozen in dry ice-cooled 2-methylbutane (Carl Roth GmbH, Karlsruhe, Germany) and then stored at −80°C until further processing.

Rat brains from the two groups were processed in parallel to ensure similar conditions. Whole brains were cut into coronal sections (25 μm) from prefrontal forebrain to the caudal medulla using a cryostat (CryoStar NX70, Thermo Fisher Scientific, Waltham, MA, USA). Every third brain section was rinsed in phosphate-buffered saline (PBS) for 3 × 15 min. All incubations were performed using the free-floating technique at room temperature (except for the incubation with the primary antibody at 4°C) and followed by a 3 × 15 min washing step in PBS. The sections were first treated with 0.3% H_20_2 in PBS for 30 min to block endogenous peroxidase activity. After rinsing the sections, nonspecific binding was blocked by 2% normal goat serum (NGS, Jackson ImmunoResearch Laboratories Inc., West Grove, PA, USA) for another 30 min. Sections were washed again and incubated in rabbit polyclonal anti-cFos (1:20,000, Catalog No. ABE457, Merck Millipore, Darmstadt, Germany) as primary antibody (2 h at room temperature followed by overnight at 4°C). Sections were rinsed again and incubated with biotinylated secondary goat anti-rabbit IgG (1:1000, Catalog No. 111-065-144, Jackson ImmunoResearch) for 2 h. After rinsing, this was followed by the incubation with the avidin-biotin-peroxidase complex (ABC, 1:500, Vector Laboratories,

Burlingame, CA, USA) in 0.3% Triton-PBS for 1 h. Staining was visualized with diaminobenzidine tetrahydrochloride (DAB, Sigma-Aldrich, Darmstadt, Germany) and nickel ammonium sulfate (Fisher Scientific, Waltham, MA, USA). The color development was frequently checked with a light microscope and stopped after about 10 min. After staining, sections were mounted, air-dried, completely dehydrated through a gradient of ethanol, cleared in xylene and cover-slipped with Entellan™ new (Merck Millipore).

In a separate experiment, specificity of the cFos antibody was assessed by pre-absorption with synthetic SGFNADYEASSSRC (amino acids 4–17 of rat c-Fos, JPT Peptide Technologies GmbH, Berlin, Germany). The peptide (5 μg/ml) was incubated with the anti-c-Fos antibody diluted at 1:20,000 (Merck Millipore, antigen:antibody ratio of 100:1) for 2 h at room temperature followed by 22 h at 4°C. The solution was centrifuged for 15 min at 13,000 × g and the supernatant used for immunostaining as described above.

Immunoreactivity of brain sections was examined using a light microscope (Axiophot, Zeiss, Jena, Germany) and images were acquired using a connected camera (AxioCam HRc, Zeiss). The density of Fos positive cells in each brain section was determined semi-quantitatively using a 10x objective and described as −, no; +, low (∼1–10 cells); ++, medium (∼10–20 cells); and +++, high (>20 Fos positive cells in a 100 μm × 100 μm area of an ocular grid with a 10x objective) density of expression. Coordinates of the brain nuclei were identified according to the rat brain atlas (Paxinos and Watson, 2007). The investigator was blinded to the experimental group. The average density of Fos immunoreactive cells derived from the total number of sections analyzed for each nucleus was determined for each animal and used to calculate the mean density of expression per group.

Statistical Analysis

Distribution of the data was determined by the Kolmogorov-Smirnov test. Data are expressed as mean ± SEM and analyzed by one-way analysis of variance (ANOVA) followed by Tukey *post-hoc* test or two-way or three-way analysis of variance followed by the Holm-Sidak method. Differences were considered significant when $p < 0.05$ (SigmaStat 3.1., Systat Software, San Jose, CA, USA).

RESULTS

Activity-Based Anorexia Rats Show the Greatest Reduction in Body Weight

During the first week of the experiment (access to the running wheel in single housing cages for activity and activity-based anorexia group; regular single housing conditions for *ad libitum* and restricted feeding group) no body weight differences were observed between the four groups (**Figure 1**). After the start of food restriction, rats of the restricted feeding group as well as activity-based anorexia rats showed a body weight decrease, while the *ad libitum* and activity groups continued to gain body weight (**Figure 1**). At the end of the 14-day food restriction period, rats of the restricted feeding group showed a body weight decrease of −13% vs. day eight ($p < 0.001$) and vs. AC (−22%, $p < 0.001$) and AL (−26%, $p < 0.001$) that gained body weight (+10% and +13%, respectively; $p < 0.001$; **Figure 1**). Activity-based anorexia rats showed an additional body weight loss of −9% compared to rats of the restricted feeding group ($p < 0.001$; **Figure 1**) reaching an average body weight loss of −22% during the 14-day observation period. Three-way ANOVA showed a significant influence of time [$F_{(13, 504)} = 5.6, p < 0.001$], activity [$F_{(1, 504)} = 436.1, p < 0.001$] and feeding regimen [$F_{(1, 504)} = 9806.3, p < 0.001$] as well as an interaction of these three factors [$F_{(13, 504)} = 2.0, p = 0.02$].

It is to note that three out of 14 rats subjected to activity-based anorexia failed to lose body weight (or even gained body weight during the experimental period, data not shown) and were therefore excluded from further analyses (final $n = 11$).

Activity-Based Anorexia Rats Show a Similar Reduction in Food Intake As Observed in the Restricted Feeding Group

The food intake observed in the two *ad libitum* fed groups (*ad libitum* and activity group) did not differ from each other and was fairly stable over the 21-day observation period (**Figure 2**). While during the first 3 days of the habituation period—although during this time also fed *ad libitum*—the food intake was lower in the activity as well as activity-based anorexia group compared to the *ad libitum* and the restricted feeding groups ($p < 0.001$) giving rise to more time spent for physical activity and less for food intake, food intake was similar on days 6 and 7 (before food restriction) in all four groups (**Figure 2**). After food restriction to 1.5 h per day in the restricted feeding and activity-based anorexia group, food intake significantly dropped by −88% in these groups on the first day compared to the *ad libitum* group ($p < 0.001$) and slowly increased afterwards to reach the same level as observed in the *ad libitum* fed groups on the last day of the observation period (**Figure 2**). Overall, rats of the restricted feeding and activity-based anorexia group ate less (−38 and −41%, respectively) compared to the *ad libitum* group during the 14-day food restriction period (**Figure 2**). Three-way ANOVA indicated a significant impact of time [$F_{(20, 776)} = 24.5, p < 0.001$], activity [$F_{(1, 776)} = 68.3, p < 0.001$] and feeding regimen [$F_{(1, 776)} = 626.5, p < 0.001$] as well as an interaction of these three factors [$F_{(20, 776)} = 1.8, p = 0.02$]. Food intake during 1.5 h did not differ between the restricted feeding and activity-based anorexia group, while 24-h food intake did not differ between the *ad libitum* and activity group ($p > 0.05$; **Figure 3**).

Activity-Based Anorexia Rats Show a Similar Physical Activity As Observed in the Activity Group

Physical activity assessed using a running wheel slightly increased during the first week from ∼1500 to ∼2000 wheel rotations/day (**Figure 4**). During the food restriction period, physical activity more prominently increased reaching ∼3500 wheel rotations/day in both, the activity and activity-based anorexia groups (**Figure 4**), corresponding to ∼1300 m/day. No daily differences were observed either in the 1.5-h (data not

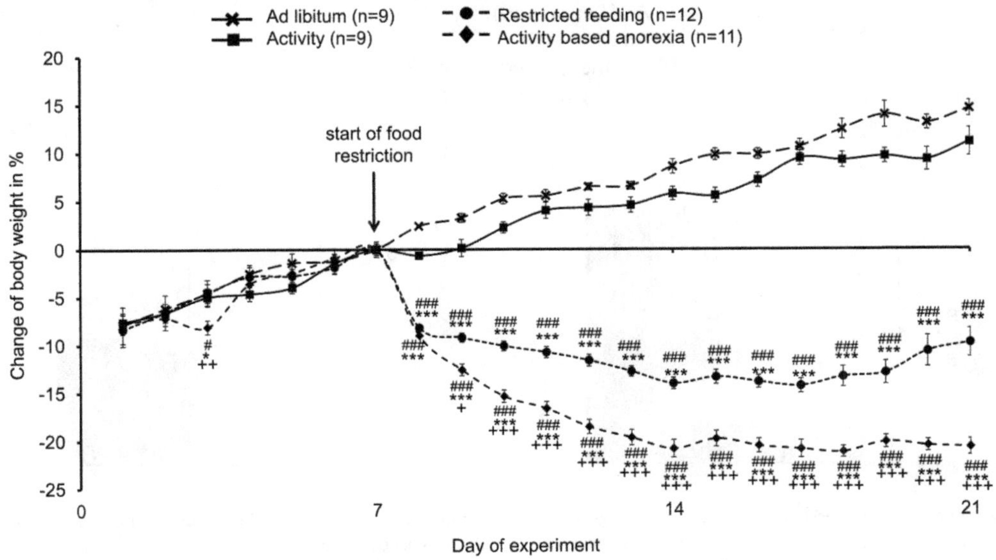

FIGURE 1 | Activity-based anorexia rats show the greatest body weight loss compared to all other groups. Animals had access to a running wheel for 24 h/day (activity and activity-based anorexia group) or were housed without wheel access under otherwise similar conditions (*ad libitum* and restricted feeding group). On day eight food intake was restricted to 1.5 h/day in the restricted feeding and activity-based anorexia group, while the activity and *ad libitum* group retained access to food for 24 h/day. Body weight changes are expressed in % changes from the day of food restriction. Data are expressed as mean ± SEM. *$p < 0.05$ and ***$p < 0.001$ vs. *ad libitum* group; #$p < 0.05$ and ###$p < 0.001$ vs. activity group; +$p < 0.05$, ++$p<0.01$ and +++$p < 0.001$ vs. restricted feeding group.

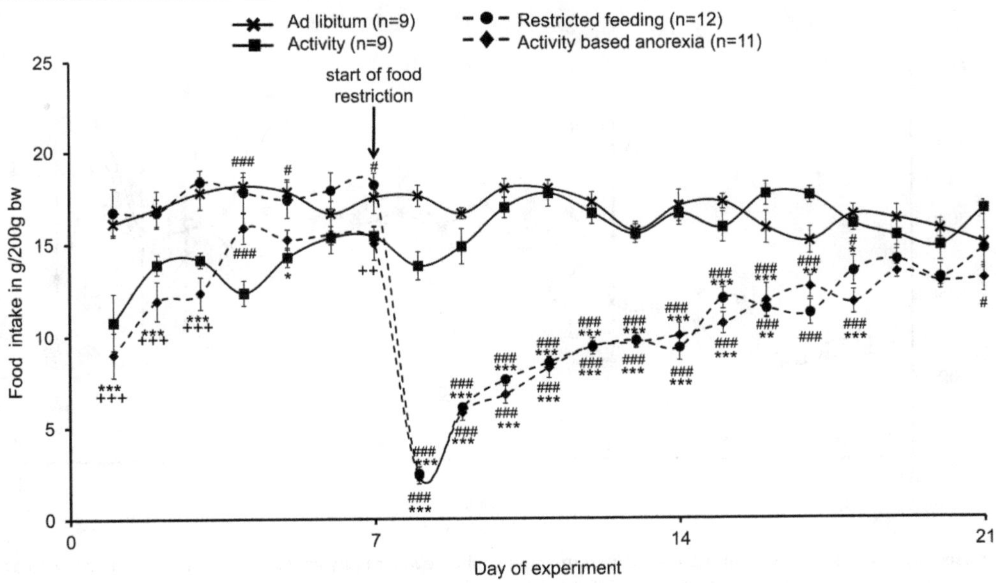

FIGURE 2 | Activity-based anorexia and restricted feeding group show a similar reduction in food intake over the whole observation period. Animals had access to a running wheel for 24 h/day (activity and activity-based anorexia group) or were housed without wheel access under otherwise similar conditions (*ad libitum* and restricted feeding group). On day eight food intake was restricted to 1.5 h/day in the restricted feeding and activity-based anorexia group, while the activity and *ad libitum* group retained access to food for 24 h/day. Food intake is calculated as g/200 g body weight; all data are expressed as mean ± SEM. *$p < 0.05$, **$p < 0.01$, and ***$p < 0.001$ vs. *ad libitum* group; #$p < 0.05$ and ###$p < 0.001$ vs. activity group; ++$p < 0.01$ and +++$p < 0.001$ vs. restricted feeding group.

shown) or 24-h wheel rotations between the activity and activity-based anorexia group ($p > 0.05$; **Figure 4**).

The daily energy expenditure including calculated resting energy expenditure and energy expenditure while running was ~35 kcal/200 g body weight at the beginning of the observation period (data not shown). This value slightly increased during the food restriction period in both the activity and activity-based anorexia group to ~38 kcal/200 g body weight (data not

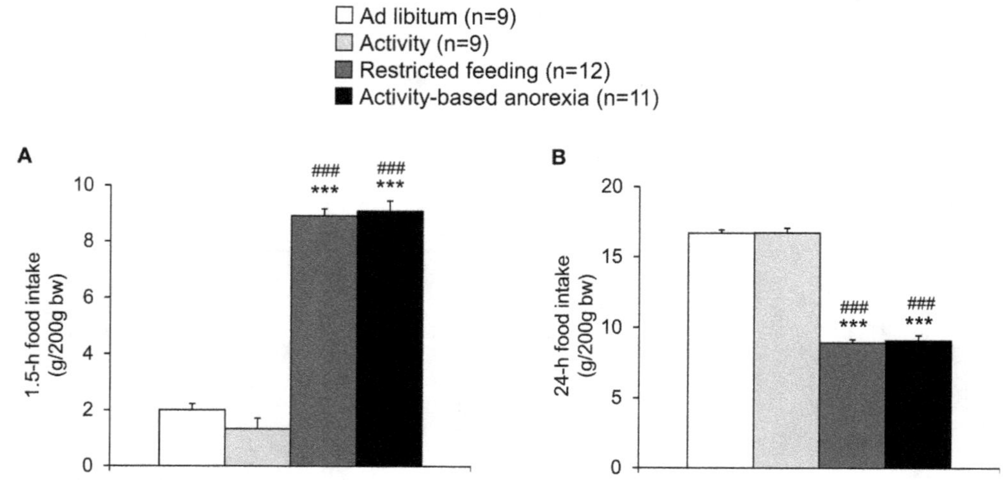

FIGURE 3 | Activity-based anorexia and restricted feeding group show a similar reduction in 1.5-h and 24-h food intake. Animals had access to a running wheel for 24 h/day (activity and activity-based anorexia group) or were housed without wheel access under otherwise similar conditions (*ad libitum* and restricted feeding group). On day eight food intake was restricted to 1.5 h/day in the restricted feeding and activity-based anorexia group, while the activity and *ad libitum* group retained access to food for 24 h/day. Food intake was monitored continuously using an automated food intake monitoring device and 1.5-h **(A)** as well as 24-h **(B)** food intake analyzed over a period of 4 days starting 4 days after food restriction (when a relatively stable food intake was observed). Data are expressed as mean ± SEM. $^{***}p < 0.001$ vs. *ad libitum* group and $^{\#\#\#}p < 0.001$ vs. activity group.

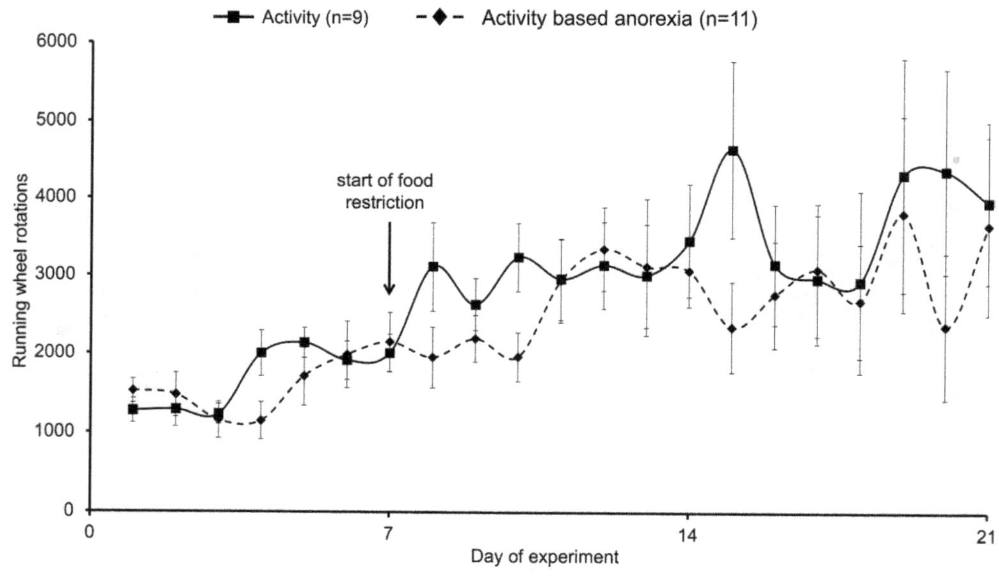

FIGURE 4 | Activity-based anorexia and activity group fed *ad libitum* show similar levels of physical activity. Animals had access to a running wheel for 24 h/day. On day eight food intake was restricted to 1.5 h/day in the activity-based anorexia group, while the activity group retained access to food for 24 h/day. Physical activity was monitored by measuring the wheel rotations per day. Data are expressed as mean ± SEM. $p > 0.05$.

shown). Two-way ANOVA indicated a significant impact of time [$F_{(20,\ 377)} = 3.6, p < 0.001$] and feeding regimen [$F_{(1,\ 377)} = 4.3, p = 0.04$].

Caloric deficit was calculated by subtracting energy expenditure from calculated caloric intake. All four groups showed a caloric surplus during the first 7 days of the experimental period (ranging from 9.6 to 21.4 kcal/day on day 7, data not shown). While this surplus remained visible in the *ad libitum* fed groups over the remaining 14-day observation period (14.2 ± 4.6 kcal in the *ad libitum* and 17.1 ± 2.3 kcal in the activity group), in the restricted feeding groups a caloric deficit was observed from the start of the food restriction (greatest levels on day 8: restricted feeding: −30.5 ± 1.4 kcal, activity-based anorexia: −29.6 ± 0.9 kcal) with a progressive decrease of caloric deficit reaching a surplus again on day 21 (restricted feeding: 10.4 ± 3.6 kcal, activity-based anorexia: 2.0 ± 0.9 kcal, data not shown). Three-way ANOVA indicated a significant impact of time [$F_{(20, 771)} = 22.3$, $p < 0.001$], activity [$F_{(1, 771)} = 125.8$, $p < 0.001$] and feeding regimen [$F_{(1, 771)} = 666.7$, $p < 0.001$] as well as an interaction of these three factors [($F_{(20, 771)} = 2.0$, $p < 0.01$].

Activity-Based Anorexia Rats Show a Similar Food Intake Microstructure Compared to the Restricted Feeding Group

After analysis of overall daily 24-h (in the *ad libitum* fed groups) and 1.5-h (in the restricted feeding groups) food intake, the underlying food intake microstructure was assessed using an automated food intake monitoring device. When analyzing the 1.5-h food intake microstructure no difference was observed between both restricted feeding groups (restricted feeding and activity-based anorexia, $p > 0.05$; **Figures 5A–G**). Similarly, the two *ad libitum* fed groups did not show a difference except for the bout size which was smaller in the activity compared to the *ad libitum* group ($p < 0.01$; **Figure 5A**). The two restricted feeding groups showed significantly higher levels for several parameters of the food intake microstructure such as meal size ($p < 0.001$; **Figure 5B**), bout frequency ($p < 0.001$; **Figure 5C**), meal duration ($p < 0.001$; **Figure 5E**), time spent in meals ($p < 0.001$; **Figure 5F**) and eating rate ($p < 0.001$; **Figure 5G**), while for meal frequency the difference was only observed when compared to the activity group ($p < 0.05$; **Figure 5D**).

Also when analyzing the 24-h food intake microstructure, no difference was observed between the two *ad libitum* fed groups (*ad libitum* and activity) or the two restricted feeding groups (restricted feeding and activity-based anorexia, $p > 0.05$; **Figures 6A–G**). While both restricted feeding groups showed higher levels in bout size ($p < 0.001$; **Figure 6A**), meal size ($p < 0.001$; **Figure 6B**), meal duration ($p < 0.001$; **Figure 6E**) and eating rate ($p < 0.001$; **Figure 6G**), values were lower for—as expected based on the feeding schedule—bout frequency ($p < 0.001$; **Figure 6C**), meal frequency ($p < 0.001$; **Figure 6D**) and time spent in meals ($p < 0.001$; **Figure 6F**).

Activity-Based Anorexia Robustly Activates Several Brain Nuclei in Different Areas of the Brain

To investigate neuronal activation of brain areas under conditions of activity-based anorexia we performed immunohistochemistry for the activity marker Fos. After pre-absorption of the Fos antibody with a synthetic Fos fragment no immunostaining was observed (data not shown) indicating the specificity of the antibody.

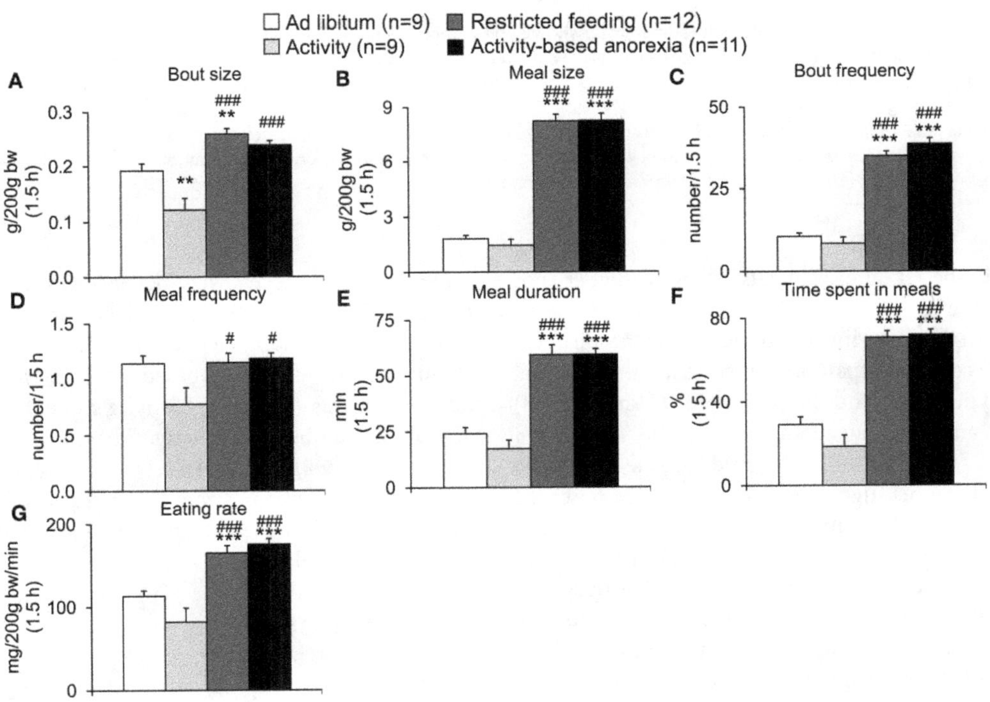

FIGURE 5 | Activity-based anorexia and restricted feeding group show similar changes in the 1.5-h food intake microstructure. Animals had access to a running wheel for 24 h/day (activity and activity-based anorexia group) or were housed without wheel access under otherwise similar conditions (*ad libitum* and restricted feeding group). On day eight food intake was restricted to 1.5 h/day (from 9:00 to 10:30 a.m.) in the restricted feeding and activity-based anorexia group, while the activity and *ad libitum* group retained access to food for 24 h/day. Food intake was monitored continuously using an automated food intake monitoring device and parameters of the food intake microstructure during the 1.5-h restricted feeding period, namely bout size **(A)**, meal size **(B)**, bout frequency **(C)**, meal frequency **(D)**, meal duration **(E)**, time spent in meals **(F)**, and eating rate **(G)** analyzed over a period of 4 days starting 4 days after food restriction (when a relatively stable food intake was observed). Data are expressed as mean ± SEM. $^{**}p < 0.01$ and $^{***}p < 0.001$ vs. *ad libitum* group; $^{\#}p < 0.05$ and $^{\#\#\#}p < 0.001$ vs. activity group.

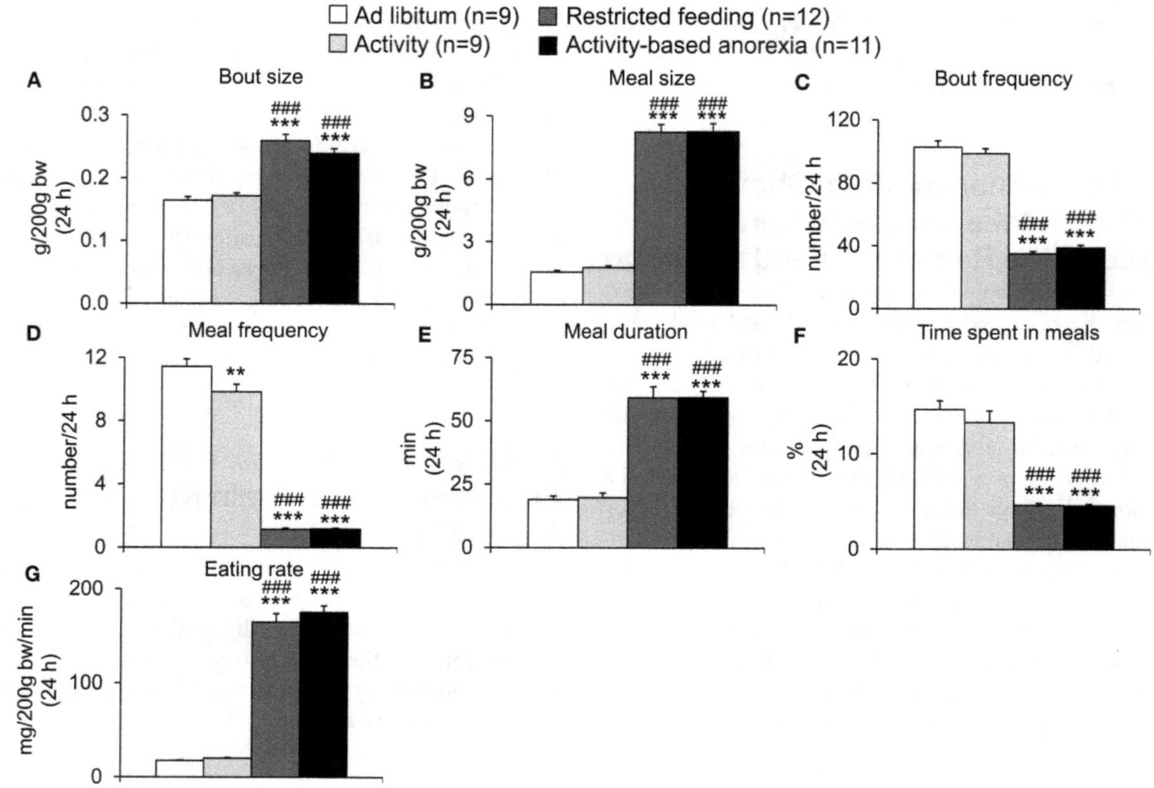

FIGURE 6 | Activity-based anorexia and restricted feeding group show similar changes in the 24-h food intake microstructure. Animals had access to a running wheel for 24 h/day (activity and activity-based anorexia group) or were housed without wheel access under otherwise similar conditions (*ad libitum* and restricted feeding group). On day eight food intake was restricted to 1.5 h/day (from 9:00 to 10:30 a.m.) in the restricted feeding and activity-based anorexia group, while the activity and *ad libitum* group retained access to food for 24 h/day. Food intake was monitored continuously using an automated food intake monitoring device and parameters of the 24-h food intake microstructure, namely bout size **(A)**, meal size **(B)**, bout frequency **(C)**, meal frequency **(D)**, meal duration **(E)**, time spent in meals **(F)**, and eating rate **(G)** analyzed over a period of 4 days starting 4 days after food restriction (when a relatively stable food intake was observed). Data are expressed as mean ± SEM. $^{**}p < 0.01$ and $^{***}p < 0.001$ vs. *ad libitum* group and $^{\#\#\#}p < 0.001$ vs. activity group.

Overall, activity-based anorexia rats showed higher Fos activation levels compared to *ad libitum* fed rats (**Table 1**). In the forebrain, higher activity was observed in the piriform cortex, cingulate cortex, somatomotor cortex, lateral septal nucleus, caudate putamen and hippocampus (**Figures 7A,B**) of activity-based anorexia rats compared to the *ad libitum* group, while no activation was observed in the amygdala (**Table 1**). In the thalamus higher Fos activation was observed in the paraventricular thalamic nucleus of activity-based anorexia rats compared to the *ad libitum* group, while in the lateral habenula similar numbers of Fos positive cells were detected using semiquantitative assessment (**Table 1**). Evaluation of hypothalamic nuclei showed more Fos signals in the suprachiasmatic nucleus, supraoptic nucleus (**Figures 7C,D**), anterior hypothalamic area, both magno- and parvocellular parts of the paraventricular nucleus (**Figures 7E,F**), lateral hypothalamic area (**Figures 7G,H**), dorsomedial hypothalamic nucleus (**Figures 7I,J**) and the medial part of the arcuate nucleus (**Figures 7K,L**) of activity-based anorexia rats compared to the *ad libitum* group, while similar levels were observed in the ventromedial hypothalamic nucleus (**Table 1**). In the midbrain similar levels were detected in the Edinger-Westphal nucleus (**Figures 8A,B**), while higher activation was observed in the dorsal raphe nuclei (**Figures 8C,D**) and locus coeruleus (**Figures 8E,F**) of activity-based anorexia compared to the *ad libitum* fed rats (**Table 1**). Lastly, also in the medulla a higher activation was observed in activity-based anorexia rats compared to the *ad libitum* group, namely in the raphe pallidus nucleus (**Figures 9A,B**), area postrema, rostral part of the nucleus of the solitary tract (**Figures 9C,D**) and the dorsal motor nucleus of the vagus nerve (**Table 1**).

DISCUSSION

In the present study we first established the activity-based anorexia model combining voluntary physical activity in a running wheel and a time-restricted feeding protocol and showed a body weight loss of −22% following 2 weeks of restricted feeding for 1.5 h per day and 24-h access to a running wheel. This body weight loss was greater (−9%) than that observed in the restricted feeding group, while rats of the *ad libitum* and activity group gained body weight. These data indicate the importance

TABLE 1 | Localization of Fos positive neurons in brains of rats fed *ad libitum* or under conditions of activity-based anorexia.

Area	Brain structure	*Ad libitum*	Activity based anorexia
Forebrain	Piriform cortex	++	+++
	Cingulate cortex	+	++
	Somatomotor cortex	+	+++
	Lateral septal nucleus	+ − ++	+++
	Caudate putamen	++	++ − +++
	Amygdala (central, medial and basolateral)	−	−
	Hippocampus	+ − ++	+++
Thalamus	Paraventricular thalamic nucleus, anterior part	+	++
	Lateral habenula	+ − ++	+ − ++
Hypothalamus	Suprachiasmatic nucleus	++	++ − +++
	Supraoptic nucleus	−	+++
	Anterior hypothalamic area	+	++
	Paraventricular nucleus	+	++
	Lateral hypothalamic area	++	+++
	Ventromedial hypothalamic nucleus	++	++
	Dorsomedial hypothalamic nucleus	−	++
	Arcuate nucleus, medial	+	+++
Midbrain	Edinger-Westphal nucleus	++	++
	Dorsal raphe nuclei	+	++
	Locus coeruleus	−	+
Medulla	Raphe pallidus nucleus	+	++
	Area postrema	−	+ − ++
	Nucleus of the solitary tract, rostral	−	+ − ++
	Dorsal motor nucleus of the vagus nerve	−	− − +

Data are expressed as mean derived from three rats/group. It is to note that rats in the activity-based anorexia group received a fixed amount of 1.5 g during the feeding period in order to avoid signals derived from overfilling of the stomach and/or nausea. Fos expression is expressed semi-quantitatively as +, low (~1–10 cells); ++, medium (~10–20 cells); and +++, high (>20 Fos positive cells in a 100 μm × 100 μm area of an ocular grid with a 10x objective) density of expression; −, no cells.

of food restriction for the present model. To gain further insight into the underlying changes, we next analyzed the food intake microstructure which greatly differed from the microstructure observed in the *ad libitum* fed groups (*ad libitum* and activity group) but was very similar to the one observed in the restricted feeding group. The increase in 1.5-h food intake observed in the two groups kept on the restricted feeding schedule was based on a larger meal size and an increase in eating rate. During these 1.5 h, rats spent 71% of the time in meals (eating and interacting with the food hopper). It is important to note that despite this great drive to eat, rats still exercised during this 1.5-h period.

Interestingly, daily activity was similar between the activity and activity-based anorexia group; however, daily activity increased over time in both groups. These data are in line with previous data from mice where daily activity also increased over time; however, in mice daily activity decreased during the last days of the 2.5-week observation period (Jésus et al., 2014). Whether this represents a species difference (rats vs. mice), sex difference (female vs. male) or is related to the slower weight loss in rats (−20% reached at day 15 vs. 11 in mice) warrants further investigation. At the same time we did not observe a decrease in food intake (which rather plateaued) which is different from the human situation where food intake decreases while activity increases with the progression of the disease (Davis et al., 1994). The relatively short observation period of 3 weeks likely contributes to/explains this difference. Taken together, the combination of both food restriction and activity is key in order to exert the pronounced weight loss observed in the activity-based anorexia group.

It is to note that in the present study three out of 14 rats did not develop activity-based anorexia and were therefore excluded from further analyses. This finding is in line with previous studies reporting that 20–30% of rats are not interested in running (Mondon et al., 1985) and do not develop activity-based anorexia (Carrera et al., 2014). These data well match the dropout rate described here (3 out of 14 = 21%). Interestingly, this finding also parallels human data where up to 80% of anorexic subjects display hyperactivity, whereas 20% do not (Davis et al., 1997). Whether a difference in leptin levels, hypothesized to play a role in the semi-starvation-induced hyperactivity in rats before (Exner et al., 2000), contributes to these differences will have to be further investigated. On the other hand, all rats of the restricted feeding group (12/12) show a reduction in body weight indicating that this effect cannot be eluded. However, the fact that rats of the activity-based anorexia group show a greater body weight loss than the restricted feeding group highlights the importance of the physical activity.

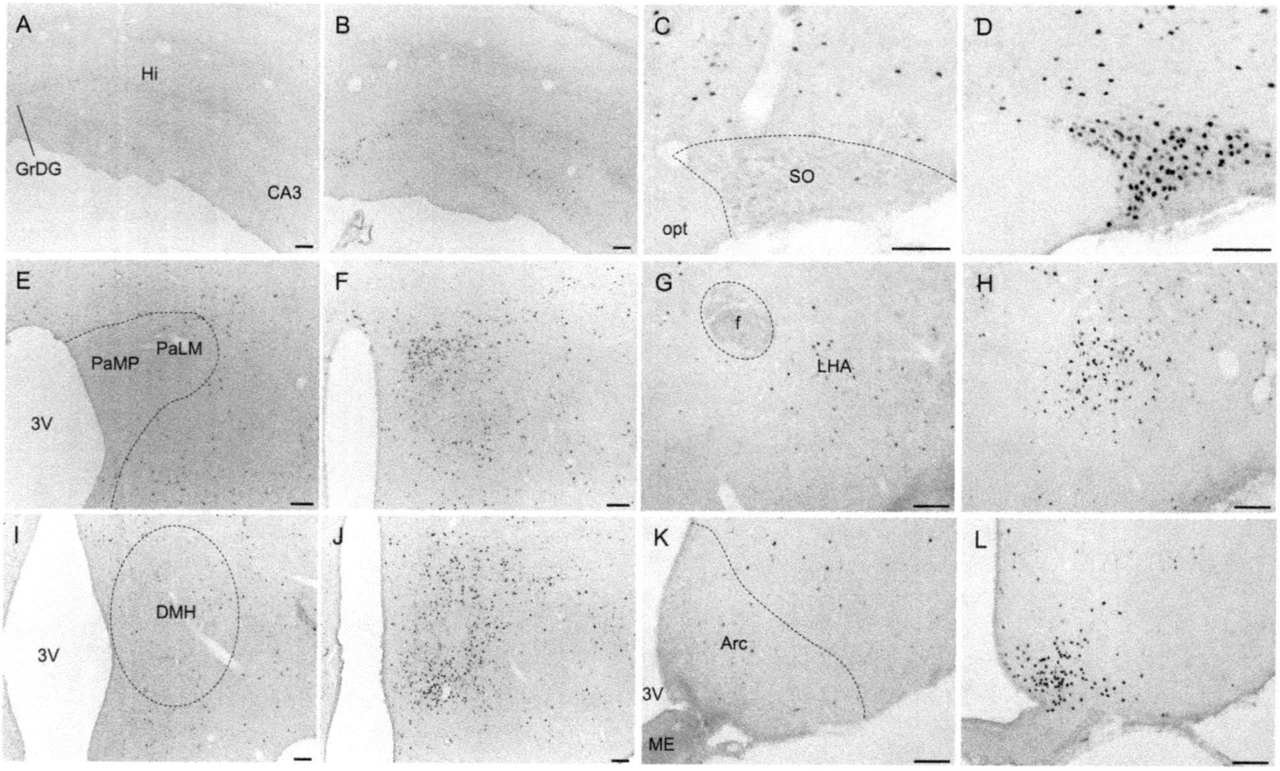

FIGURE 7 | Representative microphotographs of forebrain and hypothalamic structures in rats under *ad libitum* or activity-based anorexia conditions. Following the 21-day observation period rats received food for 1.5 h (activity-based anorexia) or were fed *ad libitum* and were transcardially perfused directly after this 1.5-h feeding period. It is to note that rats in the activity-based anorexia group received a fixed amount of 1.5 g during this feeding period in order to avoid signals derived from overfilling of the stomach and/or nausea. Brains were processed for Fos immunohistochemistry. Signals were observed in the hippocampus **(B)**, supraoptic nucleus **(D)**, magno- und parvocellular parts of the paraventricular nucleus **(F)**, lateral hypothalamic area **(H)**, dorsomedial hypothalamic nucleus **(J)** and medial part of the arcuate nucleus **(L)** of activity-based anorexia rats, while in the respective nuclei of the *ad libitum* group no **(C,I)** or few **(A,E,G,K)** signals were detected. The scale bars indicate 100 μm. Abbreviations: 3V, third ventricle; Arc, arcuate nucleus; CA3, field CA3 of the hippocampus; DMH, dorsomedial hypothalamic nucleus; f, fornix; GrDG, granular layer of the dentate gyrus; Hi, hippocampus; LHA, lateral hypothalamic area; ME, median eminence; opt, optic tract; PaLM, lateral magnocellular part of the paraventricular nucleus of the hypothalamus; PaMP, medial parvocellular part of the paraventricular nucleus of the hypothalamus; SO, supraoptic nucleus.

Despite the fact that the data mentioned above give rise to the use of the activity-based anorexia model as a suited tool to study pathophysiological alterations of AN, several limitations should be kept in mind. Although restriction of food and increased physical activity, two mean features of AN (Treasure et al., 2015) are used in this model, several other aspects such as genetic susceptibility (Clarke et al., 2012) or psychosocial and interpersonal factors (Zipfel et al., 2015) are not respected. Moreover, rats do not voluntarily reduce their body weight in contrast to human anorexic subjects. Whenever the rats' access to food is increased again, they start to regain body weight (Dixon et al., 2003; Ratnovsky and Neuman, 2011). Furthermore, the changes induced here are rather acute or subacute, while human AN is a chronic disease. Interestingly, after the initial sharp decline of food intake rats of the activity-based anorexia and restricted feeding group show a gradual increase of food intake reaching similar levels of daily food intake as observed in the *ad libitum* fed groups. Whether different dietary patterns as observed in human anorexia (Huse and Lucas, 1984; Elran-Barak et al., 2014) or a change of dietary patterns over time occurs in these rats as well will have to be further determined, preferably in a study with a longer monitoring time. Taken together, cautious interpretation of the data obtained in this model is necessary.

Several other anorexia models have been developed encompassing genetically engineered mouse models that share similarities with changes observed in AN; however, none of these reflect the multiple hormonal changes observed in AN (Méquinion et al., 2015). Lastly, other models use access to low caloric food or expose rats to various kinds of stressors (Méquinion et al., 2015). However, it is important to note that so far activity-based anorexia is considered the best animal model (Gutierrez, 2013) as it recapitulates two main features, physical activity and reduced food intake, of human AN.

To further characterize the activity-based anorexia rats we also investigated the activation of brain nuclei using the activity marker Fos (Sagar et al., 1988) and performed a whole brain mapping for activity-based anorexia and *ad libitum* fed rats. Neuronal activation was observed in brain areas involved in

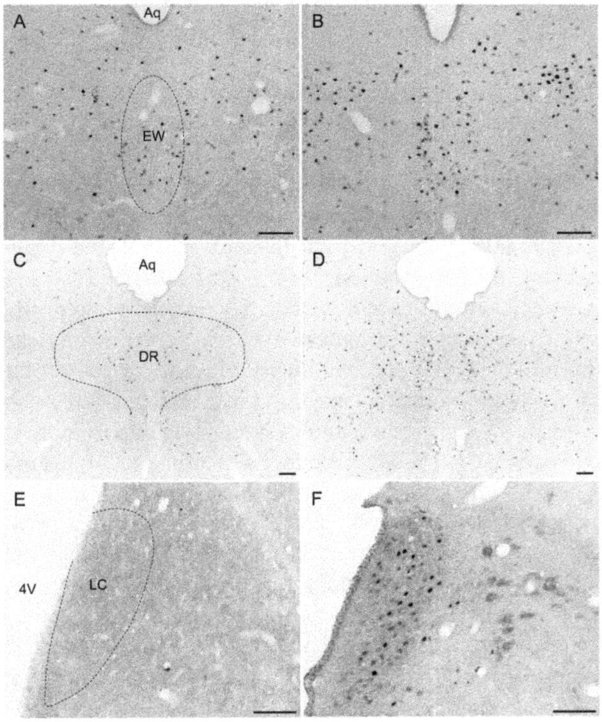

FIGURE 8 | Representative microphotographs of midbrain structures in rats under *ad libitum* or activity-based anorexia conditions. Following the 21-day observation period rats received food for 1.5 h (activity-based anorexia) or were fed *ad libitum* and were transcardially perfused directly after this 1.5-h feeding period. It is to note that rats in the activity-based anorexia group received a fixed amount of 1.5 g during this feeding period in order to avoid signals derived from overfilling of the stomach and/or nausea. Brains were processed for Fos immunohistochemistry. Signals were observed in the Edinger-Westphal nucleus **(B)**, dorsal raphe nuclei **(D)** and locus coeruleus **(F)** of the activity-based anorexia group, while in the respective nuclei of the *ad libitum* group no **(E)**, or few **(C)** signals were detected. It is to note that signals of similar density were observed in the Edinger-Westphal nucleus **(A)** of the *ad libitum* group. The scale bars indicate 100 μm. Abbreviations: 4V, fourth ventricle; Aq, aqueduct; DR, dorsal raphe nuclei; EW, Edinger-Westphal nucleus; LC, locus coeruleus.

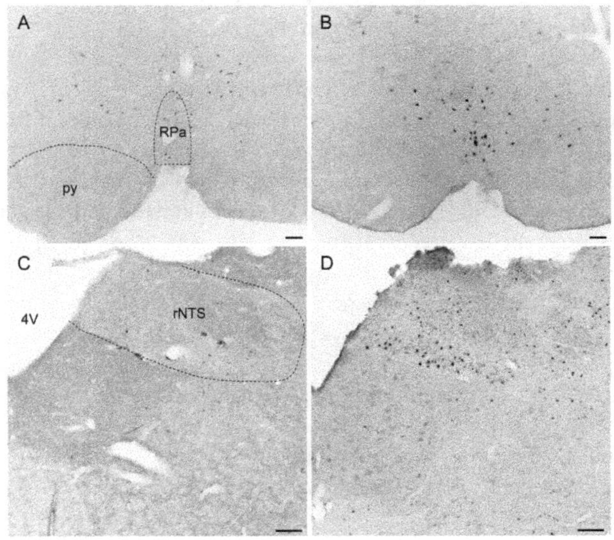

FIGURE 9 | Representative microphotographs of medulla structures in rats under *ad libitum* or activity-based anorexia conditions. Following the 21-day observation period rats received food for 1.5 h (activity-based anorexia) or were fed *ad libitum* and were transcardially perfused directly after this 1.5-h feeding period. It is to note that rats in the activity-based anorexia group received a fixed amount of 1.5 g during this feeding period to avoid signals derived from overfilling of the stomach and/or nausea. Signals were observed in the raphe pallidus nucleus **(B)** and the rostral part of the nucleus of the solitary tract **(D)** of the activity-based anorexia group, while in the respective nuclei of the *ad libitum* group no **(C)** or few **(A)** Fos positive neurons were detected. The scale bars indicate 100 μm. Abbreviations: 4V, fourth ventricle; py, pyramidal tract; rNTS, rostral part of the nucleus of the solitary tract; RPa, raphe pallidus nucleus.

the regulation of several functions such as motor activity, stress response, food intake and thermogenesis.

Analyzing brain areas involved in olfaction and the processing of olfactory stimuli (Roullet et al., 2005) an increased activation of neurons was observed in the piriform cortex, while in the lateral habenula similar Fos expression was observed in activity-based anorexia and *ad libitum* fed rats. This activation is likely associated with the increased interaction with food (as reflected in the increased number of bouts in activity-based anorexia rats compared to the *ad libitum* group) as well as the stimulated food intake during the 1.5-h feeding period. In line with this assumption, key areas of food intake regulation were activated as well, namely the lateral septal nucleus (Mitra et al., 2015), lateral hypothalamic area (Bernardis and Bellinger, 1993), the dorsomedial hypothalamic nucleus and the medial part of the Arc, both expressing the potent orexigenic transmitter neuropeptide Y (Wang et al., 2002; Bi et al., 2012) and lastly also the nucleus of the solitary tract (Stengel and Taché, 2011). Further corroborating the involvement of these nuclei in the orexigenic drive under conditions of activity-based anorexia, a previous study reported a robust upregulation of orexigenic agouti-related peptide and neuropeptide Y, whereas the anorexigenic transmitters pro-opiomelanocortin (POMC) and cocaine- and amphetamine-regulated transcript (CART) were reduced in the Arc of activity-based anorexia rats compared to sedentary food-restricted controls (de Rijke et al., 2005). Moreover, in the lateral hypothalamic area melanin-concentrating hormone mRNA expression was increased in activity-based anorexia rats (de Rijke et al., 2005). Associated with the orexigenic response, also brain nuclei involved in the regulation of gastrointestinal motility were activated, namely the lateral hypothalamic area (Gong et al., 2013), nucleus of the solitary tract and the dorsal motor nucleus of the vagus nerve (Stengel and Taché, 2011). This pronounced activation likely underlies the robust orexigenic response of activity-based anorexia rats observed during the 1.5-h feeding period. It is to note that—although food intake was restricted to 1.5 g in the last feeding period before brain processing for Fos immunohistochemistry to avoid unspecific gastric distention and nauseating signals—a moderate activation of the area postrema, known to be involved in the mediation of nausea (Horn, 2014), has been observed in the activity-based anorexia but not in the *ad libitum* fed group. Therefore, nauseating signals—at least to a certain extent—might play a role in this model as well and may modulate/limit food intake displayed during the restricted feeding period.

Besides the restriction of food intake, the stimulation of activity contributes to the weight loss observed in activity-based anorexia rats. Respective nuclei activated under these conditions and therefore likely implicated in the stimulation of activity encompass the somatomotor cortex (Elias et al., 2008) and caudate putamen (David et al., 2005). Interestingly, especially the dorsomedial hypothalamic nucleus has been implicated in the mediation of food-anticipatory activity under fixed-feeding conditions (Verhagen et al., 2011) as also observed in the present study. This activation likely also involves the suprachiasmatic nucleus working in a modulatory manner as part of an intrahypothalamic system (Acosta-Galvan et al., 2011). Moreover, the dorsomedial hypothalamic nucleus was implicated in the food-entrainable-related preprandial rise of body temperature, an effect that vanished after lesion of the nucleus (Gooley et al., 2006). This thermogenic response might also contribute to the observed decrease in body weight. However, it is important to note that activity-based anorexia was associated with a hypothermic response before (Hillebrand et al., 2005a) and an increase in ambient temperature was reported to reduce physical activity (Gutierrez et al., 2008). Future studies should further investigate these—likely very dynamic—changes of body temperature in activity-based anorexia rats.

Also stress mediated *via* the hypothalamic-pituitary-adrenal gland axis might play a role in the reduction of food intake and stimulation of physical activity. In the present study we observed a robust activation of lateral parvocellular neurons of the hypothalamic paraventricular nucleus of activity-based anorexia compared to *ad libitum* fed rats. This region is known for its predominant expression of corticotropin-releasing factor (CRF). Moreover, CRF mRNA expression was also reported to rise in the dorsomedial hypothalamic nucleus in rats with access to a running wheel (Kawaguchi et al., 2005). Interestingly, intracerebroventricular injection of the CRF antagonist, alpha-helical CRF attenuated the wheel-induced reduction of food intake and body weight (Kawaguchi et al., 2005) giving rise to a role of stimulated CRF signaling in activity-based anorexia. Lastly, this likely contributes to the increased circulating levels of corticosterone in rats (Burden et al., 1993) and cortisol in human anorexic subjects (Casper et al., 1979).

Lastly, also psychological parameters such as anxiety (Swinbourne and Touyz, 2007) and depressiveness (Debska et al., 2011) are often altered under conditions of AN. In the present study we observed an increased activation of the dorsal raphe nuclei and the raphe pallidus nucleus under conditions of activity-based anorexia, serotonergic nuclei that might play a role in the pathogenesis of depression (Michelsen et al., 2008). Interestingly, intraperitoneal injections of the serotonin agonist fenfluramine accelerated weight loss under conditions of activity-based anorexia compared to pair-fed controls giving rise to a mechanism other than reduced food intake (Atchley and Eckel, 2005). While the amygdala was not activated in the present study, the noradrenergic locus coeruleus showed a moderate activation in activity-based anorexia rats possibly leading to increased arousal (Aston-Jones and Waterhouse, 2016). Ascending projections might be involved in the observed activation of the paraventricular thalamic nucleus, the cingulate cortex and the hippocampus, brain structures involved in the processing of emotions and memory (Rolls, 2015). Interestingly, also the supraoptic nucleus as well as some magnocellular neurons of the paraventricular nucleus of the hypothalamus, two brain nuclei prominently expressing oxytocin, showed a robust activation in activity-based anorexia rats. It is important to note that oxytocin has been—besides its well-defined role during pregnancy—implicated in social memory, aggression and anxiety (Caldwell et al., 2016). Whether there is a direct link between anxiety or depressiveness and physical activity as suggested in humans (Holtkamp et al., 2004) warrants further investigation.

In summary, the activity-based anorexia model combines voluntary physical activity in a running wheel and time-restricted feeding to greatly reduce body weight. Interestingly, the food intake microstructure observed in activity-based anorexia rats did not differ from the one observed in the restricted feeding group arguing against a specific feeding phenotype. Also physical activity did not differ from the respective control group. Activity-based anorexia rats displayed an activation of distinct brain nuclei involved in the mediation of food intake, physical activity, thermoregulation as well as depression/anxiety and stress. Although these animal data have to be interpreted with caution, current data point toward the usefulness of the model to better understand pathophysiological alterations also occurring in AN.

AUTHOR CONTRIBUTIONS

SS performed the experiments and drafted the manuscript. PP performed the experiments and analyzed the data. MGS and PK performed the experiments and reviewed the manuscript. TH wrote and reviewed the manuscript. MR gave critical input throughout the study and reviewed the manuscript. AS planned the experiments, analyzed the data and wrote the manuscript.

ACKNOWLEDGMENTS

This work was supported by funding of the German Research Foundation STE 1765/3-1, Sonnenfeld Foundation and Charité University Funding UFF 89/441-176 (AS). We thank Petra Buße and Reinhard Lommel for their excellent technical assistance.

REFERENCES

Acosta-Galvan, G., Yi, C. X., Van Der Vliet, J., Jhamandas, J. H., Panula, P., Angeles-Castellanos, M., et al. (2011). Interaction between hypothalamic dorsomedial nucleus and the suprachiasmatic nucleus determines intensity of food anticipatory behavior. *Proc. Natl. Acad. Sci. U.S.A.* 108, 5813–5818. doi: 10.1073/pnas.1015551108

American Psychiatric Association (2013). *Diagnostic and Statistical Manual of Mental Disorders, 5th Edn (DSM-5)*. Washington, DC.

Aoki, C., Sabaliauskas, N., Chowdhury, T., Min, J. Y., Colacino, A. R., Laurino, K., et al. (2012). Adolescent female rats exhibiting activity-based anorexia express elevated levels of GABA(A) receptor alpha4 and delta subunits at the plasma membrane of hippocampal CA1 spines. *Synapse* 66, 391–407. doi: 10.1002/syn.21528

Arcelus, J., Mitchell, A. J., Wales, J., and Nielsen, S. (2011). Mortality rates in patients with anorexia nervosa and other eating disorders. A meta-analysis of 36 studies. *Arch. Gen. Psychiatry* 68, 724–731. doi: 10.1001/archgenpsychiatry.2011.74

Aston-Jones, G., and Waterhouse, B. (2016). Locus coeruleus: from global projection system to adaptive regulation of behavior. *Brain Res.* 1645, 75–78. doi: 10.1016/j.brainres.2016.03.001

Atchley, D. P., and Eckel, L. A. (2005). Fenfluramine treatment in female rats accelerates the weight loss associated with activity-based anorexia. *Pharmacol. Biochem. Behav.* 80, 273–279. doi: 10.1016/j.pbb.2004.11.006

Bernardis, L. L., and Bellinger, L. L. (1993). The lateral hypothalamic area revisited: neuroanatomy, body weight regulation, neuroendocrinology and metabolism. *Neurosci. Biobehav. Rev.* 17, 141–193. doi: 10.1016/S0149-7634(05)80149-6

Bi, S., Kim, Y. J., and Zheng, F. (2012). Dorsomedial hypothalamic NPY and energy balance control. *Neuropeptides* 46, 309–314. doi: 10.1016/j.npep.2012.09.002

Burden, V. R., White, B. D., Dean, R. G., and Martin, R. J. (1993). Activity of the hypothalamic-pituitary-adrenal axis is elevated in rats with activity-based anorexia. *J. Nutr.* 123, 1217–1225.

Caldwell, H. K., Aulino, E. A., Freeman, A. R., Miller, T. V., and Witchey, S. K. (2016). Oxytocin and behavior: lessons from knockout mice. *Dev. Neurobiol.* doi: 10.1002/dneu.22431. [Epub ahead of print].

Carrera, O., Fraga, Á., Pellón, R., and Gutiérrez, E. (2014). Rodent model of activity-based anorexia. *Curr. Protoc. Neurosci.* 67, 9.47.41–11. doi: 10.1002/0471142301.ns0947s67

Casper, R. C., Chatterton, R. T. Jr., and Davis, J. M. (1979). Alterations in serum cortisol and its binding characteristics in anorexia nervosa. *J. Clin. Endocrinol. Metab.* 49, 406–411. doi: 10.1210/jcem-49-3-406

Casper, R. C., Sullivan, E. L., and Tecott, L. (2008). Relevance of animal models to human eating disorders and obesity. *Psychopharmacology (Berl)* 199, 313–329. doi: 10.1007/s00213-008-1102-2

Casteels, C., Gérard, N., Van Kuyck, K., Pottel, L., Nuttin, B., Bormans, G., et al. (2014). Small animal PET imaging of the type 1 cannabinoid receptor in a rodent model for anorexia nervosa. *Eur. J. Nucl. Med. Mol. Imaging* 41, 308–321. doi: 10.1007/s00259-013-2522-8

Chowdhury, T. G., Ríos, M. B., Chan, T. E., Cassataro, D. S., Barbarich-Marsteller, N. C., and Aoki, C. (2014). Activity-based anorexia during adolescence disrupts normal development of the CA1 pyramidal cells in the ventral hippocampus of female rats. *Hippocampus* 24, 1421–1429. doi: 10.1002/hipo.22320

Clarke, T. K., Weiss, A. R., and Berrettini, W. H. (2012). The genetics of anorexia nervosa. *Clin. Pharmacol. Ther.* 91, 181–188. doi: 10.1038/clpt.2011.253

David, H. N., Ansseau, M., and Abraini, J. H. (2005). Dopamine-glutamate reciprocal modulation of release and motor responses in the rat caudate-putamen and nucleus accumbens of "intact" animals. *Brain Res. Brain Res. Rev.* 50, 336–360. doi: 10.1016/j.brainresrev.2005.09.002

Davis, C., Katzman, D. K., Kaptein, S., Kirsh, C., Brewer, H., Kalmbach, K., et al. (1997). The prevalence of high-level exercise in the eating disorders: etiological implications. *Compr. Psychiatry* 38, 321–326. doi: 10.1016/S0010-440X(97)90927-5

Davis, C., Kennedy, S. H., Ravelski, E., and Dionne, M. (1994). The role of physical activity in the development and maintenance of eating disorders. *Psychol. Med.* 24, 957–967. doi: 10.1017/S0033291700029044

Debska, E., Janas, A., Banczyk, W., and Janas-Kozik, M. (2011). Depression or depressiveness in patients diagnosed with anorexia nervosa and bulimia nervosa - pilot research. *Psychiatr. Danub.* 23, S87–S90.

de Rijke, C. E., Hillebrand, J. J., Verhagen, L. A., Roeling, T. A., and Adan, R. A. (2005). Hypothalamic neuropeptide expression following chronic food restriction in sedentary and wheel-running rats. *J. Mol. Endocrinol.* 35, 381–390. doi: 10.1677/jme.1.01808

Dixon, D. P., Ackert, A. M., and Eckel, L. A. (2003). Development of, and recovery from, activity-based anorexia in female rats. *Physiol. Behav.* 80, 273–279. doi: 10.1016/j.physbeh.2003.08.008

Doerries, L. E., Stanley, E. Z., and Aravich, P. F. (1991). Activity-based anorexia: relationship to gender and activity-stress ulcers. *Physiol. Behav.* 50, 945–949. doi: 10.1016/0031-9384(91)90419-O

Elias, C. F., Sita, L. V., Zambon, B. K., Oliveira, E. R., Vasconcelos, L. A., and Bittencourt, J. C. (2008). Melanin-concentrating hormone projections to areas involved in somatomotor responses. *J. Chem. Neuroanat.* 35, 188–201. doi: 10.1016/j.jchemneu.2007.10.002

Elran-Barak, R., Accurso, E. C., Goldschmidt, A. B., Sztainer, M., Byrne, C., and Le Grange, D. (2014). Eating patterns in youth with restricting and binge eating/purging type anorexia nervosa. *Int. J. Eat. Disord.* 47, 878–883. doi: 10.1002/eat.22289

Exner, C., Hebebrand, J., Remschmidt, H., Wewetzer, C., Ziegler, A., Herpertz, S., et al. (2000). Leptin suppresses semi-starvation induced hyperactivity in rats: implications for anorexia nervosa. *Mol. Psychiatry* 5, 476–481. doi: 10.1038/sj.mp.4000771

Ghadirian, A. M., Engelsmann, F., Leichner, P., and Marshall, M. (1993). Prevalence of psychosomatic and other medical illnesses in anorexic and bulimic patients. *Behav. Neurol.* 6, 123–127. doi: 10.1155/1993/356914

Gong, Y., Xu, L., Wang, H., Guo, F., Sun, X., and Gao, S. (2013). Involvements of the lateral hypothalamic area in gastric motility and its regulation by the lateral septum. *Gen. Comp. Endocrinol.* 194, 275–285. doi: 10.1016/j.ygcen.2013.09.022

Gooley, J. J., Schomer, A., and Saper, C. B. (2006). The dorsomedial hypothalamic nucleus is critical for the expression of food-entrainable circadian rhythms. *Nat. Neurosci.* 9, 398–407. doi: 10.1038/nn1651

Gutierrez, E. (2013). A rat in the labyrinth of anorexia nervosa: contributions of the activity-based anorexia rodent model to the understanding of anorexia nervosa. *Int. J. Eat. Disord.* 46, 289–301. doi: 10.1002/eat.22095

Gutierrez, E., Cerrato, M., Carrera, O., and Vazquez, R. (2008). Heat reversal of activity-based anorexia: implications for the treatment of anorexia nervosa. *Int. J. Eat. Disord.* 41, 594–601. doi: 10.1002/eat.20535

Herzog, W., Schellberg, D., and Deter, H. C. (1997). First recovery in anorexia nervosa patients in the long-term course: a discrete-time survival analysis. *J. Consult. Clin. Psychol.* 65, 169–177. doi: 10.1037/0022-006X.65.1.169

Hillebrand, J. J., de Rijke, C. E., Brakkee, J. H., Kas, M. J., and Adan, R. A. (2005a). Voluntary access to a warm plate reduces hyperactivity in activity-based anorexia. *Physiol. Behav.* 85, 151–157. doi: 10.1016/j.physbeh.2005.03.017

Hillebrand, J. J., Koeners, M. P., de Rijke, C. E., Kas, M. J., and Adan, R. A. (2005b). Leptin treatment in activity-based anorexia. *Biol. Psychiatry* 58, 165–171. doi: 10.1016/j.biopsych.2005.03.011

Holtkamp, K., Hebebrand, J., and Herpertz-Dahlmann, B. (2004). The contribution of anxiety and food restriction on physical activity levels in acute anorexia nervosa. *Int. J. Eat. Disord.* 36, 163–171. doi: 10.1002/eat.20035

Horn, C. C. (2014). The medical implications of gastrointestinal vagal afferent pathways in nausea and vomiting. *Curr. Pharm. Des.* 20, 2703–2712. doi: 10.2174/13816128113199990568

Huber, J., Salatsch, C., Ingenerf, K., Schmid, C., Maatouk, I., Weisbrod, M., et al. (2015). Characteristics of disorder-related autobiographical memory in acute anorexia nervosa patients. *Eur. Eat. Disord. Rev.* 23, 379–389. doi: 10.1002/erv.2379

Hudson, J. I., Hiripi, E., Pope, H. G. Jr., and Kessler, R. C. (2007). The prevalence and correlates of eating disorders in the National Comorbidity Survey Replication. *Biol. Psychiatry* 61, 348–358. doi: 10.1016/j.biopsych.2006.03.040

Huse, D. M., and Lucas, A. R. (1984). Dietary patterns in anorexia nervosa. *Am. J. Clin. Nutr.* 40, 251–254.

Jésus, P., Ouelaa, W., Francois, M., Riachy, L., Guérin, C., Aziz, M., et al. (2014). Alteration of intestinal barrier function during activity-based anorexia in mice. *Clin. Nutr.* 33, 1046–1053. doi: 10.1016/j.clnu.2013.11.006

Kawaguchi, M., Scott, K. A., Moran, T. H., and Bi, S. (2005). Dorsomedial hypothalamic corticotropin-releasing factor mediation of exercise-induced anorexia. *Am. J. Physiol. Regul. Integr. Comp. Physiol.* 288, R1800–R1805. doi: 10.1152/ajpregu.00805.2004

Kinzig, K. P., and Hargrave, S. L. (2010). Adolescent activity-based anorexia increases anxiety-like behavior in adulthood. *Physiol. Behav.* 101, 269–276. doi: 10.1016/j.physbeh.2010.05.010

Kjaersdam Telléus, G., Jepsen, J. R., Bentz, M., Christiansen, E., Jensen, S. O., Fagerlund, B., et al. (2015). Cognitive profile of children and adolescents with anorexia nervosa. *Eur. Eat. Disord. Rev.* 23, 34–42. doi: 10.1002/erv.2337

Kline, C. L. (1979). Anorexia nervosa: death from complications of ruptured gastric ulcer. *Can. J. Psychiatry* 24, 153–156.

Legrand, R., Lucas, N., Breton, J., Azhar, S., do Rego, J. C., Déchelotte, P., et al. (2016). Ghrelin treatment prevents development of activity based anorexia in mice. *Eur. Neuropsychopharmacol.* 26, 948–958. doi: 10.1016/j.euroneuro.2016.03.010

Luyten, L., Welkenhuysen, M., Van Kuyck, K., Fieuws, S., Das, J., Sciot, R., et al. (2009). The effects of electrical stimulation or an electrolytic lesion in the mediodorsal thalamus of the rat on survival, body weight, food intake and running activity in the activity-based anorexia model. *Brain Res. Bull.* 79, 116–122. doi: 10.1016/j.brainresbull.2009.01.001

Méquinion, M., Chauveau, C., and Viltart, O. (2015). The use of animal models to decipher physiological and neurobiological alterations of anorexia nervosa patients. *Front. Endocrinol.* (Lausanne*)* 6:68. doi: 10.3389/fendo.2015.00068

Michelsen, K. A., Prickaerts, J., and Steinbusch, H. W. (2008). The dorsal raphe nucleus and serotonin: implications for neuroplasticity linked to major depression and Alzheimer's disease. *Prog. Brain Res.* 172, 233–264. doi: 10.1016/S0079-6123(08)00912-6

Mitra, A., Lenglos, C., and Timofeeva, E. (2015). Inhibition in the lateral septum increases sucrose intake and decreases anorectic effects of stress. *Eur. J. Neurosci.* 41, 420–433. doi: 10.1111/ejn.12798

Mondon, C. E., Dolkas, C. B., Sims, C., and Reaven, G. M. (1985). Spontaneous running activity in male rats: effect of age. *J. Appl. Physiol. (1985)* 58, 1553–1557.

Nagl, M., Jacobi, C., Paul, M., Beesdo-Baum, K., Höfler, M., Lieb, R., et al. (2016). Prevalence, incidence, and natural course of anorexia and bulimia nervosa among adolescents and young adults. *Eur. Child. Adolesc. Psychiatry* 25, 903–918. doi: 10.1007/s00787-015-0808-z

Paulukat, L., Frintrop, L., Liesbrock, J., Heussen, N., Johann, S., Exner, C., et al. (2016). Memory impairment is associated with the loss of regular oestrous cycle and plasma oestradiol levels in an activity-based anorexia animal model. *World J. Biol. Psychiatry* 17, 274–284. doi: 10.3109/15622975.2016.1173725

Paxinos, G., and Watson, C. (2007). *The Rat Brain in Stereotaxic Coordinates.* San Diego, CA: Academic Press.

Preti, A., Girolamo, G. d., Vilagut, G., Alonso, J., Graaf, R. d., Bruffaerts, R., et al. (2009). The epidemiology of eating disorders in six European countries: results of the ESEMeD-WMH project. *J. Psychiatr. Res.* 43, 1125–1132. doi: 10.1016/j.jpsychires.2009.04.003

Ratnovsky, Y., and Neuman, P. (2011). The effect of pre-exposure and recovery type on activity-based anorexia in rats. *Appetite* 56, 567–576. doi: 10.1016/j.appet.2011.01.027

Rolls, E. T. (2015). Limbic systems for emotion and for memory, but no single limbic system. *Cortex* 62, 119–157. doi: 10.1016/j.cortex.2013.12.005

Roullet, F., Liénard, F., Datiche, F., and Cattarelli, M. (2005). Fos protein expression in olfactory-related brain areas after learning and after reactivation of a slowly acquired olfactory discrimination task in the rat. *Learn. Mem.* 12, 307–317. doi: 10.1101/lm.89605

Routtenberg, A., and Kuznesof, A. W. (1967). Self-starvation of rats living in activity wheels on a restricted feeding schedule. *J. Comp. Physiol. Psychol.* 64, 414–421. doi: 10.1037/h0025205

Sagar, S. M., Sharp, F. R., and Curran, T. (1988). Expression of c-fos protein in brain: metabolic mapping at the cellular level. *Science* 240, 1328–1331. doi: 10.1126/science.3131879

Shepherd, R. E., and Gollnick, P. D. (1976). Oxygen uptake of rats at different work intensities. *Pflugers Arch.* 362, 219–222. doi: 10.1007/BF00581173

Steinhausen, H. C. (2002). The outcome of anorexia nervosa in the 20th century. *Am. J. Psychiatry* 159, 1284–1293. doi: 10.1176/appi.ajp.159.8.1284

Steinhausen, H. C., and Jensen, C. M. (2015). Time trends in lifetime incidence rates of first-time diagnosed anorexia nervosa and bulimia nervosa across 16 years in a Danish nationwide psychiatric registry study. *Int. J. Eat. Disord.* 48, 845–850. doi: 10.1002/eat.22402

Stengel, A., Goebel, M., Wang, L., Rivier, J., Kobelt, P., Monnikes, H., et al. (2009). Central nesfatin-1 reduces dark-phase food intake and gastric emptying in rats: differential role of corticotropin-releasing factor2 receptor. *Endocrinology* 150, 4911–4919. doi: 10.1210/en.2009-0578

Stengel, A., and Taché, Y. (2011). "The physiological relationships between the brainstem, vagal stimulation and feeding," in *The International Handbook of Behavior, Diet and Nutrition*, Chapter 54, ed V. R. Preedy (London: Springer).

Swinbourne, J. M., and Touyz, S. W. (2007). The co-morbidity of eating disorders and anxiety disorders: a review. *Eur. Eat. Disord. Rev.* 15, 253–274. doi: 10.1002/erv.784

Teuffel, P., Wang, L., Prinz, P., Goebel-Stengel, M., Scharner, S., Kobelt, P., et al. (2015). Treatment with the ghrelin-O-acyltransferase (GOAT) inhibitor GO-CoA-Tat reduces food intake by reducing meal frequency in rats. *J. Physiol. Pharmacol.* 66, 493–503.

Treasure, J., Zipfel, S., Micali, N., Wade, T., Stice, E., Claudino, A., et al. (2015). Anorexia nervosa. *Nat. Rev. Dis. Primers* 1, 15074. doi: 10.1038/nrdp.2015.74

Verhagen, L. A., Luijendijk, M. C., de Groot, J. W., Van Dommelen, L. P., Klimstra, A. G., Adan, R. A., et al. (2011). Anticipation of meals during restricted feeding increases activity in the hypothalamus in rats. *Eur. J. Neurosci.* 34, 1485–1491. doi: 10.1111/j.1460-9568.2011.07880.x

Verhagen, L. A., Luijendijk, M. C., Korte-Bouws, G. A., Korte, S. M., and Adan, R. A. (2009). Dopamine and serotonin release in the nucleus accumbens during starvation-induced hyperactivity. *Eur. Neuropsychopharmacol.* 19, 309–316. doi: 10.1016/j.euroneuro.2008.12.008

Wang, L., Goebel-Stengel, M., Stengel, A., Wu, S. V., Ohning, G., and Taché, Y. (2011). Comparison of CRF-immunoreactive neurons distribution in mouse and rat brains and selective induction of Fos in rat hypothalamic CRF neurons by abdominal surgery. *Brain Res.* 1415, 34–46. doi: 10.1016/j.brainres.2011.07.024

Wang, L., Saint-Pierre, D. H., and Taché, Y. (2002). Peripheral ghrelin selectively increases Fos expression in neuropeptide Y - synthesizing neurons in mouse hypothalamic arcuate nucleus. *Neurosci. Lett.* 325, 47–51. doi: 10.1016/S0304-3940(02)00241-0

Wu, H., Van Kuyck, K., Tambuyzer, T., Luyten, L., Aerts, J. M., and Nuttin, B. (2014). Rethinking food anticipatory activity in the activity-based anorexia rat model. *Sci. Rep.* 4:3929. doi: 10.1038/srep03929

Zipfel, S., Giel, K. E., Bulik, C. M., Hay, P., and Schmidt, U. (2015). Anorexia nervosa: aetiology, assessment, and treatment. *Lancet Psychiatry* 2, 1099–1111. doi: 10.1016/S2215-0366(15)00356-9

Zipfel, S., Wild, B., Groß, G., Friederich, H. C., Teufel, M., Schellberg, D., et al. (2014). Focal psychodynamic therapy, cognitive behaviour therapy, and optimised treatment as usual in outpatients with anorexia nervosa (ANTOP study): randomised controlled trial. *Lancet* 383, 127–137. doi: 10.1016/S0140-6736(13)61746-8

14

Development and Function of the Blood-Brain Barrier in the Context of Metabolic Control

Roberta Haddad-Tóvolli, Nathalia R. V. Dragano, Albina F. S. Ramalho and Licio A. Velloso**

Laboratory of Cell Signaling and Obesity and Comorbidities Research Center, Faculty of Medical Sciences, University of Campinas, Campinas, Brazil

***Correspondence:**
Roberta Haddad-Tóvolli
robshtovolli@hotmail.com
Licio A. Velloso
lavelloso.unicamp@gmail.com.br

Under physiological conditions, the brain consumes over 20% of the whole body energy supply. The blood-brain barrier (BBB) allows dynamic interactions between blood capillaries and the neuronal network in order to provide an adequate control of molecules that are transported in and out of the brain. Alterations in the BBB structure and function affecting brain accessibility to nutrients and exit of toxins are found in a number of diseases, which in turn may disturb brain function and nutrient signaling. In this review we explore the major advances obtained in the understanding of the BBB development and how its structure impacts on function. Furthermore, we focus on the particularities of the barrier permeability in the hypothalamus, its role in metabolic control and the potential impact of hypothalamic BBB abnormities in metabolic related diseases.

Keywords: blood-brain barrier, neurovascular unit, development, hypothalamus, inflammation, obesity

INTRODUCTION

Blood vessels transport and deliver nutrients to warrant organism function. In the brain, they specialized into a dynamic structure that provides a protective and homeostatic interface between the central nervous system (CNS) and the remainder of the body. In this sense, the blood-brain barrier (BBB) controls the passage of selected substances into the brain, while transporting toxic products back into circulation. This efficient permeable boundary allows maintenance of the homeostasis of the CNS milieu and correct function of brain circuits.

The functionality of the BBB depends on a strict architecture. The combination of non-fenestrated brain endothelial cells (BECs) lining the walls of the CNS blood vessels, together with pericytes, neurons and glia constitute the neurovascular unit (NVU) and confer integrity to the BBB.

In the ventromedial hypothalamus, the barrier has specialized to allow the dynamic passage of hormones and nutrients from the blood to the energy-sensing arcuate nucleus of the hypothalamus (ARC) and the export of newly synthesized hormones to the pituitary. At the level of the median eminence (ME), the barrier is formed by fenestrated capillaries that allow faster transport of substances into the nutrient-sensing hypothalamic nuclei lying adjacent to it. However, ME tanycytes, specialized radial glia cells lining the walls of the third ventricle, form a physical barrier to control the correct transport of nutrients and metabolic hormones into the brain parenchyma (Weindl and Joynt, 1973; Ganong, 2000; Mullier et al., 2010; Rodríguez et al., 2010). The metabolic state, as well as the consumption of saturated fatty acids, can damage this barrier and alter the nutrient sensing of tanycytes (Lee et al., 2012; Haan et al., 2013; Langlet et al., 2013b). Changes in the development of the BBB in the hypothalamus, especially in the vicinity of the ME, may predispose to obesity (Lee et al., 2012; Kim et al., 2016).

BBB STRUCTURE AND FUNCTION

In the last decade, there has been exponential progress in the understanding of how BBB structure and function work both in health and pathological conditions (Daneman and Prat, 2015; Banks, 2016). The first evidence for the existence of a barrier controlling the passage of substances from the circulating blood to and from the CNS dates back to 1885 when the German researcher Paul Ehrlich carried out experiments injecting Trypan Blue dye into the bloodstream of mice. Surprisingly, he noted that the dye could penetrate several tissues but not the brain and spinal cord (Ehrlich, 1885; **Figure 3B**). Years later, further studies performed by Goldmann (1909, 1913), Ehrlich's student, indicated that injection of the same dye directly into the brain showed the opposite as observed previously: the brains turned blue, whereas the peripheral tissues did not (**Figure 3B**). The term "blood-brain-barrier" was introduced by Lewandowsky (1900), based on experiments demonstrating that neurotoxic substances, e.g., cholic acids or sodium ferrocyanide, exhibited neurological symptoms only after intraventricular applications but not when injected into the bloodstream. Only in the late 1960s, with the development of electron microscopy, Reese and Karnovsky (1967) were able to visualize for the first time, at ultrastructural level, that the brain endothelial cells present unique cell-to-cell junctions, constituting a structural barrier that creates an almost impermeable frontier between the blood and CNS (Ribatti et al., 2006).

Anatomically, the BBB is comprised by a thin monolayer of BECs that are in intimate contact with vascular cells (pericytes and vascular smooth muscle cells), glial cells (astrocytes, microglia) and neurons. The crosstalk and molecular signaling between them are collectively known as the neurovascular unit (NUV) (Obermeier et al., 2013; Chow and Gu, 2015; Banks, 2016) (**Figure 1**). This close connection between different cells types within the NUV allows the BBB to properly perform its fundamental physiological functions.

Next, we present the main features of the cellular components of the BBB:

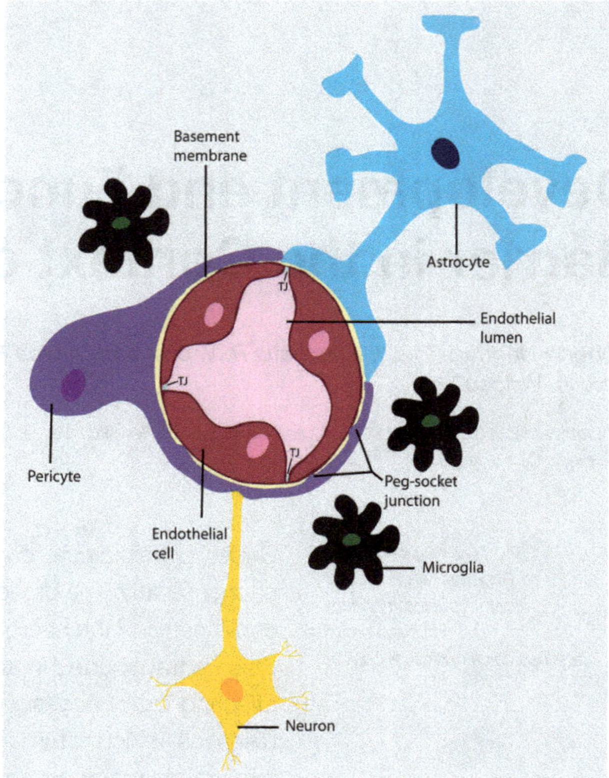

FIGURE 1 | Neurovascular unit (NVU). A layer of brain endothelial cells connected by tight junctions forms the blood-brain barrier. The intimate contact of these specialized endothelial cells with different cell types constitutes the NVU. A basement membrane embeds the brain endothelial cells, the pericytes, and astrocytes. In areas where the basement membrane is absent, brain endothelial cells and pericytes connect through peg-socket junctions. Astrocytes extend its end-feet and establish a close interaction with endothelial cells through transmembrane proteins, such as aquaporins. Astrocytes also connect with pericytes and neurons and together regulate BBB maintenance and function. The interaction of the cell components of the NVU with neurons and microglia can influence barrier function.

Brain Endothelial Cells

To sustain a more restrictive permeability, BECs enclose specific barrier properties, which differentiate them from peripheral endothelial cells (Andreone et al., 2015; Chow and Gu, 2015). One particular feature is the presence of junction complexes between adjacent BECs involving transmembrane proteins and multiple cytoplasmic adaptor proteins located on the apical and lateral sides of the plasma membrane.

The structural integrity of BBB is sustained mainly by tight junction (TJ) proteins and *adherens* junctions (AJ). Specifically, TJ are composed of claudin family members, occludin, junctional adhesion molecules (JAMs) and *zonulae occludens* (ZO-1, ZO-2, and ZO-3)—membrane-associated accessory proteins that connect the cytoplasmic tails of claudins and occludin to the actin cytoskeleton to sustain the TJ structure (Luissint et al., 2012; Tietz and Engelhardt, 2015).

The primary biological role of TJs is to establish a rigorous restriction of paracellular molecular diffusion, creating a high electrical resistance between the endothelial cells and ions and other polar solutes. Brain endothelial cell's AJs, ubiquitous in the vasculature, consist of cadherin proteins extended throughout the intercellular cleft that mediate cell-to-cell membrane adhesion and are anchored into the actin cytoskeleton by the scaffolding proteins alpha, beta and gamma catenin (Abbott et al., 2010; Blanchette and Daneman, 2015).

Although, the specific AJs function in the BBB is yet to be fully elucidated, it is known that they play an important role in the maintenance of TJs and the junctional complex by keeping the BECs together (Keaney and Campbell, 2015). In addition, brain endothelial cells display low rates of transcellular vesicular transport in comparison to peripheral endothelial cells, a process termed transcytosis (transport between the luminal and abluminal cell membranes). Still, transcytosis is the most common mechanism to selectively uptake macromolecules such as albumin, low-density lipoprotein and hormones, e.g., insulin and leptin (Holly and Perks, 2006; Xiao and Gan, 2013; Chow and Gu, 2015). As a result of this restrictive barrier, BECs express several transporters and receptor proteins, as Glut-1, that selectively allow the entry of nutrients, neurotransmitters and other essential macromolecules into the brain parenchyma, at the same time that ensure the elimination of potentially metabolic waste and neurotoxic substances from the CNS into the blood (Keller, 2013; Keaney and Campbell, 2015).

Another important feature of the BECs is the low expression levels of leukocyte adhesion molecules (LAMs) such as E-selectin and Icam1, compared with ECs in non-neuronal tissues (Andreone et al., 2015; Daneman and Prat, 2015). This characteristic greatly restrains the number of immune cells that enter the CNS. In general, the physical barrier properties mediated by the junctional complex and the reduced transcytosis along with a highly selective cellular transport system illustrates how the brain endothelium orchestrate the regulation of the brain microenvironment.

Pericytes

Pericytes were first characterized by Eberth (1871) and Rouget (1873) in the 1870's and initially named "Rouget cells." Later, Zimmermann (1923) introduced the term pericyte due to their location in close proximity to the endothelial cells. Anatomically, pericytes are located at the abluminal surface of microvessels, embedded in a common basement membrane with the BECs, and exhibit elongated cytoplasmic processes that wrap the endothelium around (Trost et al., 2016). The CNS vasculature has significantly higher pericyte density/coverage compared with peripheral tissues, which correlates with the particular endothelial barrier properties. It is estimated that the ratio of pericytes to endothelial cells in CNS is 1:1-1:3, while this ratio appears to be from 1:10-1:100 in striated muscles (Shepro and Morel, 1993; Millis et al., 2013). Despite being separated by the basal membrane, in areas lacking a basement membrane (BM) BM, pericytes and BECs make direct peg-and-socket contacts, in which pericyte cytoplasmic fingers (pegs) are inserted into endothelial invaginations (pockets) (Winkler et al., 2011). Several different transmembrane junctional proteins are present at these contact points, including N-cadherin, forming key AJs between the two cell types; connexin-43 (CX43), hemichannels that form gap junctions enabling the exchange of nutrients, secondary messengers and ions; adhesion plaques composed predominately of fibronectin that anchor pericytes to endothelial cells (Berger et al., 2005; Zlokovic, 2008; Armulik et al., 2011; Winkler et al., 2011).

Pericytes play essential roles in the regulation of several neurovascular functions. They are critical during angiogenesis, participating in vessel formation, remodeling and stabilization (see developmental section) (Armulik et al., 2011; Winkler et al., 2011). *In situ* and *In vivo* studies evidenced that pericytes are modulators of capillary diameter and blood flow in response to changes in neural activity (Peppiatt et al., 2006; Fernández-Klett et al., 2010; Hall et al., 2014). However, Hill et al. (2015) demonstrate that capillary pericytes are not contractile *in vivo*. Thus, the active regulation of the capillary blood flow by pericytes remains controversial presumably due to the lack of proper pericyte definition and identification (Trost et al., 2016).

Apart of their importance in BBB development (see BBB development section), pericytes are involved in the formation and maintenance of the highly selected permeability of the BBB in adulthood and aging (Armulik et al., 2010; Bell et al., 2010; Daneman et al., 2010a). Pericyte deficiency promotes severe BBB dysfunction as a result of increased vascular permeability (directly correlated with absolute pericyte coverage, increased rates of transcytosis and paracellular transport due to reduced expression of various TJ and AJ proteins). Pericytes also guide astrocytic foot processes to surrounding CNS blood vessels and mediate the polarization of astrocytic end-feet, highlighting the interdependence among components of the NVU (Armulik et al., 2010; Keaney and Campbell, 2015).

Increasing evidence has shown that pericytes may constitute multipotent stem/progenitor cells that could differentiate into mesenchymal cells and into non-mesenchymal cell types, including glial and neuronal lineages under different *in vitro* conditions (Bribair et al., 2013). Until now, there is still a lack of studies describing that such differentiation occurs in the brain (Dore-Duffy and Cleary, 2011; Trost et al., 2016). Moreover, pericytes can control several aspects of the CNS immune response (reviewed in Rustenhoven et al., 2016).

Astrocytes

Due to the position of astrocytes in the NUV (ensheathing almost 90% of brain microvasculature), many studies have focused on the role of astrocytes in the maturation and maintenance of BBB (Correale and Villa, 2009). Indeed, astrocytes can induce barrier properties in non-CNS endothelial cells *in vivo* (Janzer and Raff, 1987).

Astrocytes, the most abundant cells in the brain, are spongiform-shaped glial cells that extend many branching cellular processes, including astrocytic end-feet that cover brain endothelial cells. Specifically, astrocytic end-feets establish a close interaction with BECs through transmembrane proteins anchoring, such as the water channel Aquaporin-4 (Aqp4) and the potassium channel KIR4.1, critical for CNS water homeostasis regulation (Cabezas et al., 2014). Furthermore, astrocytes communicate between each other through gap junctions forming an extensive glial syncytium that is associated with well-coordinated responses within large groups of cells (Theis et al., 2005; Alvarez et al., 2013). Astrocytes perform several functions critical to CNS physiology, including the regulation of blood flow in response to changes in neuronal activity which results in enhanced delivery of oxygen and glucose to the active brain region; the maintenance of ion and neurotransmitters concentration within the extracellular space for proper synaptic transmission; the modulation of synaptic and neural activity by the release of gliotransmitters, such as glutamate, ATP, D-serine, and GABA; and are also able to respond to local levels of nutrients, glucose uptake from blood vessels and the storage of glycogen, which is hydrolyzed to release lactate into the extracellular space when glucose is scarce (Sofroniew and Vinters, 2010; Cabezas et al., 2014).

One of the essential roles attributed to astrocytes is to regulate the nutrient availability, such as glucose, and also the access of some peripheral hormones, including leptin, ghrelin and GLP-1.

Their privileged anatomical position, in close proximity to the blood vessels and neurons, allows them to act as important metabolic sensors. Actually, hypothalamic astrocytes express specific transporters and receptors that are involved in the control of energy homeostasis. The astrocytic end-feet that enclose capillaries express the glucose transporter GLUT-1 that transports glucose into the CNS. The uptaken glucose is stored in form of glycogen, which is mobilized to release lactate to the neurons when glucose is not abundant, as in periods of energy deficit (Argente-Arizón et al., 2015; Chowen et al., 2016). Astrocytes also express the glucose transporter GLUT-2 that is important for glucosensing process and in the homeostatic control of circulating glucose levels and food intake (Marty et al., 2005; Stolarczyk et al., 2010). GLUT-2 inactivation results in overeating, providing evidence that glucose detection by GLUT2 contributes to the control of food intake by the hypothalamus (Bady et al., 2006; Stolarczyk et al., 2010). Leptin receptors are expressed in hypothalamic astrocytes and their physiological relevance was recently demonstrated. The conditional deletion of the leptin receptor in GFAP positive cells in mice decreased the number and length of astrocyte projections in hypothalamic neurons involved in feeding control, such as POMC and AGRP neurons of the arcuate nucleus. In addition, leptin-regulated feeding was diminished in mice with astrocyte-specific leptin receptor deficiency (Kim et al., 2014).

Regarding the contribution of astrocytes in BBB development, they do not appear to participate in this process at early embryonic stages (see development section) (Daneman et al., 2010b). Indeed, mature astrocytes produce factors that regulate BBB function and integrity. Astrocytes also secrete angiopoietin-1 and angiotensin that restrict BBB permeability by supporting efficient organization of TJs (Lee et al., 2003; Wosik et al., 2007; Siegenthaler et al., 2013). Thus, astrocytes are critical in sustaining BBB functionality and integrity as well as in the regulation of neuronal and synaptic activity.

Microglia

In addition to pericytes and astrocytes, the brain endothelium at the NUV is in close contact with immune cells. The two main immune cell populations within the CNS are perivascular macrophages and microglia.

Perivascular macrophages are monocytic lineage cells located outside of the CNS parenchyma. In fact, these cells reside in and circulate through the Virchow–Robin spaces, which lie between the BM around pericytes and at the surface of the glia interface of the brain vessels. The perivascular macrophage number is continuously maintained by replacement from blood-borne cells macrophages. They provide a first line of innate immunity due to their ability to quickly phagocytose particles from the cerebrospinal fluid (Daneman and Prat, 2015).

The brain parenchyma is populated by microglia, the most abundant CNS innate immune cells. Microglial cells, also referred as resident macrophages of the brain, are derived from progenitors in the yolk sac, which migrate into the CNS parenchyma during neonatal development. Microglia colonization comes first during BECs invasion into the brain (da Fonseca et al., 2014) and are shown to be involved in CNS vasculogenesis, promoting endothelial cell fusion to increase vascular complexity (Fantin et al., 2010), as well as decreasing paracellular permeability in cultured BECs (Zenker et al., 2003). Accordingly, these data suggest that the interactions between microglia and the brain endothelium could participate in the BBB formation and regulation (Correale and Villa, 2009; da Fonseca et al., 2014).

Generally, microglia displays two distinct morphological patterns. The steady-state population of microglia in the healthy brain exhibits a 'resting' phenotype, which is characterized by a small, and circular cell body with extensively ramified processes. As a part of their homeostatic functions, microglial cell bodies remain stationary, but their processes continuously scan the surrounding extracellular space and communicate directly with neurons, astrocytes, and blood vessels (Nayak et al., 2014). Microglia rapidly respond to injury signals or infection through an activated phenotype characterized by a morphological change into an amoeboid shape and alterations in signaling and gene expression in order to perform inflammatory functions (Lull and Block, 2010; Saijo and Glass, 2011).

Prolonged microglia activation and consequent chronic neuroinflammatory state in CNS might induce impairments in BBB integrity that, in turn, contribute to the progression of neurodegenerative diseases (reviewed in de Vries et al., 2012). Evidence from *in vitro* studies has shown that microglia activation may be related to BBB disruption. Sumi et al. (2010) demonstrated that the treatment of a rat brain microvascular endothelial cell/microglia co-culture system with lipopolysaccharide, a microglial activator, induced an increase in endothelial cell permeability and changes in the expression pattern of tight junction proteins. Another study using a similar *in vitro* co-culture system found that the tumoral necrosis factor α (TNF-α) released from activated microglia also increased the permeability of BECs, which could be blocked by a neutralizing antibody against TNF-α (Nishioku et al., 2010).

Although, these *in vitro* BBB models are important for unraveling the mechanisms involved in the crosstalk between microglia activation and BBB integrity, more studies are needed to improve our understanding on how these cell types interact *in vivo*.

BBB DEVELOPMENT

The development and differentiation of the BBB can be subdivided into three phases: i, angiogenesis; ii, differentiation; and iii, maturation (summarized in **Figure 2**).

The angiogenic phase begins early during neural tube development (as early as E9.0-E10.5 in mice). Endothelial cells from the perineural vascular plexus penetrate the neuroectoderm according to a vascular endothelial growth factor (VEGF) concentration gradient giving rise to immature brain vessels (Raab et al., 2004; Potente et al., 2011). VEGF is expressed by the neural progenitors of the ventricular neuroepithelium and serves, together with angiopoietin, as a major driving force for the migrating endothelial cells (EC) (Risau et al., 1986). VEGF deficiency is lethal (Shalaby et al., 1995; Carmeliet et al., 1996).

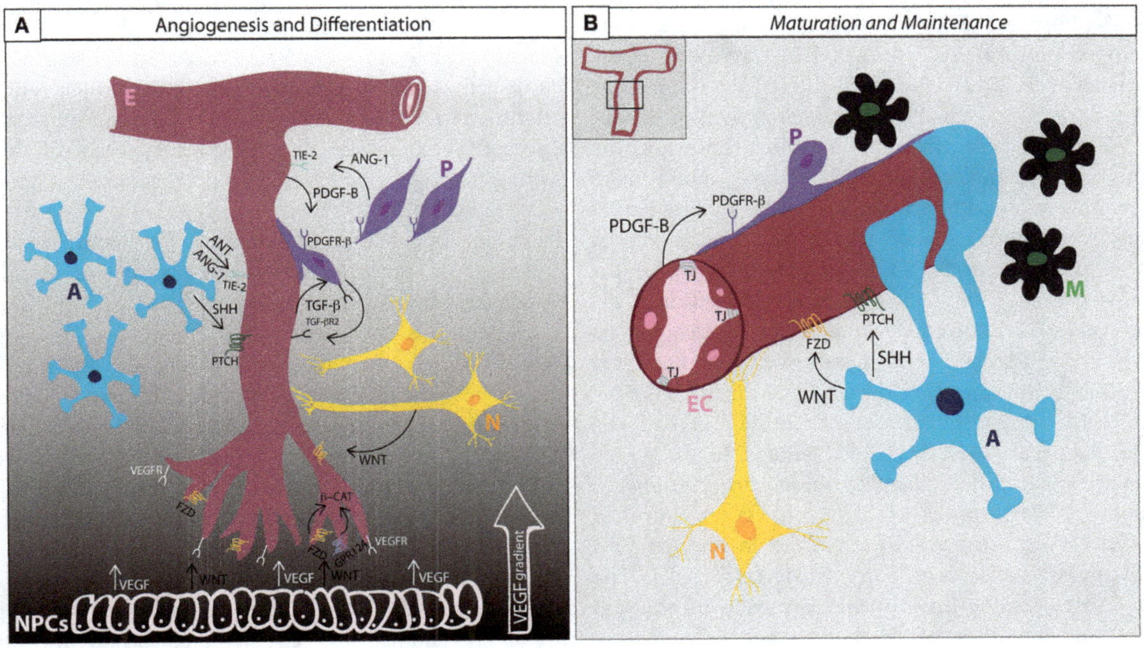

FIGURE 2 | BBB development and maintenance. (A) Angiogenesis and differentiation. VEGF secretion from neural progenitor cells induces endothelial cells penetration into the brain parenchyma according to a VEGF concentration gradient. Wnt ligands also secreted from the NPCs induces the migration of the endothelial cells and activate β-catenin signaling through the binding to Frizzled receptors, inducing the expression of BBB specific genes. GPR124, together with WNT, co-activates β-catenin signaling. Endothelial cells secrete PDGF-B and attract pericytes expressing PDGFR-β. The interaction between ECs and Ps induce the mutual expression of TGF-β and TGF-βR2. The activation of TGF-β signaling regulates basement membrane formation and the induction of Ang-1 expression in pericytes, that acting through the endothelial receptor Tie-2, enhance tight junction expression. Astrocytes release SHH, that when bound to PTCH receptor induces Shh signaling activation in ECs and contributes to BBB formation. Astrocytes also express ANT and ANG-1, which by limiting BBB permeability contributes to the maturation of BBB function. **(B)** Maturation and Maintenance. Pericytes and astrocytic end-feet cover the endothelium and secrete matrix proteins that will constitute the basement membrane. Astrocytes continue secreting SHH and WNT in order to maintain BBB functionality throughout life. A, astrocytes; E, endothelium; EC, endothelial cell; M, microglia; N, neuron; NPC, neural progenitor cell; P, pericyte; TJ, tight junction; Ang-1, angiopoietin-1; ANT, angiotensin; β-cat, beta-catenin; VEGF, vascular endothelial growth factor; VEGFR, vascular endothelial growth factor receptor; FZD, frizzled; GPR124, adhesion G protein coupled receptor A2; Shh, sonic hedgehog; Ptch, Patched 1; PDGF-B, platelet derived growth factor B; PDGFR-β, platelet derived growth factor receptor beta; TGF-β, transforming growth factor-beta; TGF-βR2, transforming growth factor beta receptor type-2.

Downstream VEGF signaling supports angiogenesis through endothelial cell proliferation, migration and survival (Olsson et al., 2006). Together with VEGF, neural Wnt signaling plays an important role in the development of the BBB (Daneman et al., 2009). Different Wnt ligands, including Wnt7a, Wnt7b, and Wnt3a are secreted by the neuroepithelium (Wang et al., 2012) and induce further ingression of ECs into the neural tissue, activating Wnt/B-catenin signaling in the newborn endothelial cells (Liebner et al., 2008; Daneman et al., 2009; Zhou and Nathans, 2014) that leads to induction of genes critical for the BBB formation and vascular patterning, such as glucose transporter Glut-1 (Stenman et al., 2008), death receptors DR6 and TROY (Tam et al., 2012) and tight junction proteins. Defects in Wnt/β-catenin signaling result in major vascular malformations and BBB breakdown (Stenman et al., 2008; Daneman et al., 2009; Wang et al., 2012). Retinoic acid, Notch signaling receptor tyrosine kinase, cadherins and ephrins also contribute to angiogenesis in the CNS (Adams and Alitalo, 2007; Dejana and Vestweber, 2013).

At about E15.5, the newly formed vessels continue to differentiate and mature as a complete NVU forming the basis for the BBB. During the differentiation phase (between E15.5 and E18.5 in mice), the brain barrier is structured properly by the induction of anti-angiogenic signals and the recruitment of pericytes and astrocytes to the newly formed vessels. Pericytes express the platelet-derived growth factor receptor- β (Pdgfr-β) and are directed to the endothelial developing capillaries that secrete Pdgf-B (Lindahl et al., 1997; Hellstrom et al., 1999). Pdgfr-β mouse mutants completely lack brain pericytes, and die as consequence of brain microhemorrhages (Lindahl et al., 1997; Lindblom et al., 2003; Tallquist et al., 2003); thus, pericyte recruitment to the developing endothelial capillaries is critical for the formation and maintenance of the BBB (Armulik et al., 2010; Bell et al., 2010; Daneman et al., 2010a). The lack of Pdgf-β or Pdgfr-β leads to erroneous TJ distribution and increased vascular permeability (Hellstrom et al., 2001).

Interactions between pericytes and the brain endothelial cells lead to the expression of transforming growth factor-β (Tgf-β) and its receptor (Tgf-βR2) by both cell types. TGF secretion induces cell adhesion through the production of cadherin-2 by the endothelial cells and the secretion of different extracellular matrix components that contribute to basement membrane (BM) formation by the pericytes (Winkler et al., 2011). Notch and sphingosine-1-phosphate (S1P) signaling also contribute to the regulation of cadherin-2 expression in BECs (Winkler et al., 2011; Obermeier et al., 2013). Upon activation of Tgf-β signaling, pericytes produce Ang-1 that, by enhancing tight junctions formation, limit BBB permeability, and reduce the expression of leukocyte adhesion molecules (LAMs). Pdgf-β and Wnt/β-catenin signaling is also important during the differentiation of the BBB by the induction of transporters and increased expression of tight junctions. This provides integrity to the barrier (Liebner et al., 2008; Daneman et al., 2009; Tam et al., 2012; Wang et al., 2012; Zhou and Nathans, 2014; Andreone et al., 2015). In the BBB, Gpr124 has been described as a necessary endothelial receptor specifically in the CNS and function as a co-activator of Wnt/b-catenin signaling to mature the BBB (Kuhnert et al., 2010; Cullen et al., 2011; Zhou and Nathans, 2014).

Pericytes are apparently required to guide astrocytes toward the developing BBB (Armulik et al., 2010). Once recruited to the forming NVU, astrocytes are involved in limiting BBB permeability by the release of Sonic Hedgehog (Shh). The activation of Shh signaling leads to the expression of occludin and claudin5 and inhibition of chemokines and cell adhesion molecules in the endothelial cells, suggesting a role for astrocytes and Shh in maintenance of BBB functionality and immune surveillance (Alvarez et al., 2011; Obermeier et al., 2013; Siegenthaler et al., 2013). Recent studies have uncovered yet another important role for astrocytes in the production of retinoic acid, which is also necessary for the correct development of BBB vessels (Halilagic et al., 2007; Mizee et al., 2013).

Maturation and maintenance of the BBB is achieved by the persistence of tight junction proteins expression and their redistribution throughout the whole BBB structure. The production of TJs is regulated by Wnt signaling between astrocytes and BECs. Close contact between the endothelial cells, pericytes, astrocytes, and possibly neurons and microglia sustain BBB integrity and function as a stabilized neurovascular unit (reviewed in Obermeier et al., 2013; reviewed in Engelhardt and Liebner, 2014; reviewed in Zhao et al., 2015). The BBB is already formed and completely functional during late gestation in rodents and in the third trimester in humans (Bauer et al., 1995; Daneman et al., 2010a; Ben-Zvi et al., 2014). In the rat embryo, the BBB is already functional at E16 (Saunders et al., 2012). The exact time window remains elusive and is likely species dependent (Saunders et al., 2013; Hagan and Ben-Zvi, 2015).

There has been intense debate on the BBB features that provide its correct function. To date, it is believed that tight junctions are functional in sealing the space between BBB endothelial cells very early in development (Dziegielewska et al., 1979; Bondjers et al., 2006; Tam et al., 2012; Ben-Zvi et al., 2014) but only when the intracellular pathway of transcytosis is partially downregulated will the complete restrictive properties of the barrier become fully matured (Hagan and Ben-Zvi, 2015). Little is known about the functionality of transporters at the embryonic BBB, although some transporters, like Glut-1, are known to be expressed very early (Boado and Pardridge, 1990; Farrell and Pardridge, 1991; Bauer et al., 1995; Hagan and Ben-Zvi, 2015). A role of Mfsd2a in participating in the inhibition of vesicular trafficking and inducing a more sealed barrier during development was suggested recently (Ben-Zvi et al., 2014; reviewed in Hagan and Ben-Zvi, 2015). Mfsd2a mutants have a defective BBB even though presenting proper and functional tight junctions (Ben-Zvi et al., 2014). Thus, barrier transporting properties would be determined very early in development while the sealing function would be acquired gradually across development, first with the suppression of fenestrations, then with the appearance of functional TJs, and finally with the decrease of transcytosis by the expression of Mfsd2 (Ben-Zvi et al., 2014; Hagan and Ben-Zvi, 2015).

Alterations in barrier development and in TJ expression could lead to anomalies later in life as well as to increased predisposition to develop metabolic diseases. Maternal obesity increases BBB permeability in the offspring (Kim et al., 2016), leading to higher exposure to leptin and ghrelin. In consistence with that, overnutrition during early postnatal life alters brain sensitivity to ghrelin (Collden et al., 2014), suggesting that nutrient sensing control alterations during specific hypothalamic developmental time-points could contribute to metabolic defects in the adult life. These alterations can affect the programming of energy homeostasis circuits predisposing the offspring to the development of metabolic syndrome at early life and/or adulthood.

BBB IN THE HYPOTHALAMIC AREA

In some areas of the brain, the BBB is modified in order to allow the access of certain substances from systemic circulation into the central nervous system. This occurs particularly in periventricular areas creating a blood/spinal fluid interface (Bennett et al., 2009). In these regions, the BBB capillaries are highly fenestrated with less tight junctions between endothelial cells creating a more permeable barrier (Bennett et al., 2009). Seven periventricular regions display differential barrier properties and are collectively known as the circumventricular organs: i, sub-fornical organ; ii, organum vasculosum of the lamina terminalis; iii, pituitary; iv, area postrema; v, median eminence (ME); vi, subcomissural organ; and vii, pineal (Bennett et al., 2009; Szathmari et al., 2013). In these regions, in addition to the cells that classically form the BBB vessels, a differential type of radial glial cell, termed tanycytes are also found in the interface between the spinal fluid and the capillaries (Rodríguez et al., 2010). Because of its physical proximity with the hypothalamus, the BBB at the ME is of particular interest regarding whole-body energy homeostasis and metabolism.

The median eminence is adjacent to the arcuate nucleus (ARC) of the hypothalamus. This region harbors neurons that play important roles in the control of whole body metabolism (Velloso and Schwartz, 2011; Cavadas et al., 2016). Classically, two main neuronal populations control energy homeostasis in the ARC: i, NPY/AgRP neurons, which are active during fasting and provide orexigenic and anti-thermogenic signals; ii, POMC/CART neurons, which are active following food intake and provide anorexigenic and pro-thermogenic signals (Velloso and Schwartz, 2011; Cavadas et al., 2016). In addition,

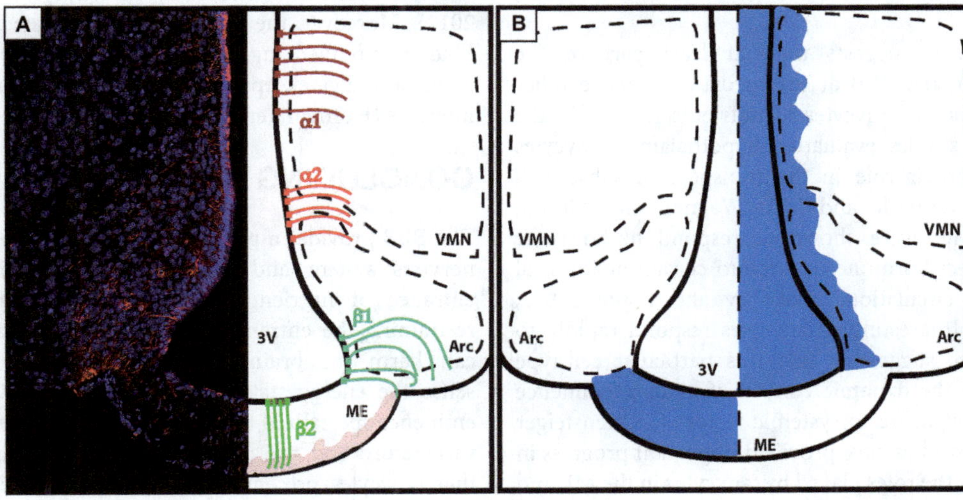

FIGURE 3 | Organization of the BBB in the energy-sensing hypothalamus. (A) Coronal section of the tuberal hypothalamus showing the distribution of tanycytes along the third ventricle wall. Left: vimentin staining (red) shows the projections of tanycytes to the brain parenchyma. Right: tanycytes line the third ventricle and can be classified according to location and function. α tanycytes don't possess barrier properties. α1 tanycytes (dark red) lye in the dorsal ventro-medial nucleus of the hypothalamus, while α2 tanycytes (light red) are found in between the ARC and the VMH. β tanycytes are located ventrally and function as gatekeeper cells controlling the passage of substances from the leaky ME to the ARC. β1 tanycytes (turquose) divide the ME from the ARC, while β2 tanycytes (green) are located in the ME, and characterized by processes with direct access to the blood capillaries. Blood capillaries are displayed in light pink. **(B)** Diagram showing how the diffusion of dyes injected peripherally do not penetrate the brain (exemplified here by the action of tanycytes lining the ME and the ARC) (left). On the other hand, dyes that are infused inside of the brain ventricles diffuse trhough the CSF and penetrate the brain parenchyma but do not pass the ME in the direction of the portal capillaries (right). VMN, ventro-medial nucleus; ARC, arcuate nucleus; ME, median eminence; 3V, third ventricle.

other distinct hypothalamic neuronal subpopulations have been described recently (Zhang and van den Pol, 2016; Campbell et al., 2017; Fenselau et al., 2017; Lam et al., 2017). Of note, a recent study has identified ARC neurons that express the dopamine-synthesizing enzyme, tyrosine hydroxylase (TH). These cells are involved in the integration of homeostatic and hedonic feeding signals and are potential targets for the treatment of obesity (Zhang and van den Pol, 2016).

Because ARC neurons are involved in the sensing of the nutritional status of the body, it would be expected that they were located in an anatomical area where the access to nutrients and energy-status signaling substances would be facilitated. In fact, studies have shown that the interface between the median eminence and the ARC is somewhat leaky to hormones and nutrients (Obici and Rossetti, 2003; Lam et al., 2005). For example, fatty acids present in the systemic circulation are not freely diffusible to most areas of the CNS (Mitchell and Hatch, 2011). In general, they rely on particular transport systems present in the structures of the BBB (Betsholtz, 2014). The proper function and distribution of these transport systems is of major importance in the development and physiology of the brain throughout life because most fatty acids that comprise the central nervous system phospholipids cannot be synthesized *de novo* in the brain, and thus, must be obtained from the systemic circulation (Mitchell and Hatch, 2011). However, in the ME specific conditions make circulating fatty acids more available to ARC neurons (Obici and Rossetti, 2003; Lam et al., 2005).

As early as the 1970's, studies have revealed that hormones involved in energy homeostasis and nutrients have particular properties to cross the BBB at the ME/ARC interface. Systemic insulin crosses the BBB by a saturable system (Woods and Porte, 1977) and concentrates mostly in the olfactory bulb and hypothalamus (Havrankova et al., 1981). Similarly, leptin reaches the brain by a saturable system, which is independent of insulin and is highly detectable in the choroid plexus, the ME and the ARC (Banks et al., 1996). A major advance in understanding how hypothalamic neurons are exposed to hormones and nutrients to respond to systemic variations in whole body energy status was obtained by the characterization of the presence of nutrient transporters in BBB endothelial cells. Beginning in the 1990's a series of studies have explored the particularities of how peptides can cross the BBB (Cashion et al., 1996; Pam et al., 1996; Banks et al., 1997). The BBB endothelial cells are also provided with transport systems for glucose (Pardridge et al., 1990); fatty acids (Obici and Rossetti, 2003; Lam et al., 2005) and aminoacids (Hawkins et al., 2006), and the variations in whole body energy status, such as in fasting/feeding or metabolic diseases can affect function of such transport systems (Kastin and Akerstrom, 2000; Kastin et al., 2001). This implies that the BBB at the ME/ARC interface plays a major role in controlling the way hypothalamic neurons are exposed to systemic factors involved in metabolism and nutrition. In this context, important advance in the field by exploring the mechanism involved in the regulation of the ME tanycytes has been provided over the last few years.

Tanycytes are originated from the radial bipolar glia around E17.5 in mice and have a morphology that is somewhere in between the aspects of an ependymal cell and an astrocyte; differing from the last by having a single basal projection directed toward the parenchyma of the brain (Rodríguez et al., 2010; **Figure 3A**).

Mounting evidence suggests that, at least part of the selective leakiness of the BBB at the median eminence relies on the responsiveness of tanycytes to nutrients present in the bloodstream. Early studies evaluating hypothalamic tanycytes have demonstrated their role in the transport of substances between the third ventricle and ME (Wagner and Pilgrim, 1974). Also, tanycytes were shown to respond to hormone production and direct hormone delivery to certain anatomical sites and systemic circulation (Akmayev and Popov, 1977; Vallet et al., 1991). Interestingly, tanycytes respond rapidly to systemic stimulation, suggesting that this particular cell-type could play a role in the dynamic control of median eminence and adjacent areas exposure to systemic factors (Lichtensteiger et al., 1978). Recent studies have provided important progress in the understanding of the roles played by tanycytes in the ME and ARC (Langlet et al., 2013a,b).

The identification of leptin in the mid 1990's placed the ARC in the center of a complex system that controls body energy status (Zhang et al., 1994). With this concept in mind, researchers looked for a potential involvement of ME tanycytes as gatekeepers controlling the access of substances (particularly nutrients and hormones) that could modulate ARC-neuron function. However, it was only in 2011 that first evidence was provided showing that tanycytes are responsive to glucose fluctuations promoted by feeding (Frayling et al., 2011). Glucose leads to a powerful ATP-mediated Ca^{2+} release into the tanycytes, which in turn release ATP to adjacent cells. Therefore, it was proposed that by responding to glucose and releasing ATP, ME tanycytes could modulate the activity of ARC neurons (Frayling et al., 2011). Furthermore, ME tanycytes can transport leptin into the mediobasal hypothalamus (Balland et al., 2014). When leptin present in the bloodstream reaches the median eminence it activates leptin receptors expressed in the tanycytes. This in turn, activates the protein ERK that transduces the signals required for an appropriate transport of leptin through the cerebrospinal fluid into the ARC (Balland et al., 2014).

Interestingly, in order to respond to the constant changes in nutrient and hormone availability in the circulation, the plasticity of the median eminence tanycytes has proven remarkable. During the physiological cycles of fasting and feeding these cells undergo both morphological and functional changes (Langlet et al., 2013a). The decreased blood levels of glucose during fasting are capable of inducing changes in the structure of the interface between the blood and the ARC. At least in part, these morphological and functional changes are dependent of the expression of VEGF-A by the tanycytes (Langlet et al., 2013a).

In addition to glucose and leptin, fatty acids can also affect ME tanycytes. In diet-induced obesity, the amount of lipid droplets increase considerably in tanycytes (Hofmann et al., 2017). Moreover, the ratio between saturated and unsaturated lipids is modified suggesting that this cell type may also act as a sensor and gatekeeper for lipids in the median eminence/ARC interface (Hofmann et al., 2017).

CONCLUDING REMARKS

The BBB provides a physiological interface between the central nervous system and the systemic circulation allowing the entrance of nutrients and certain signaling molecules and restraining the entrance of microorganisms and particles that can harm the brain. Because hypothalamic neurons must sense the energy status of the body, the BBB at the median eminence specialized to a more permeable interface between the vasculature and the brain. Recent studies have demonstrated that tanycytes present in the interface between the ARC and the median eminence are very sensitive to nutrients. They can be rapidly modified in response to fast and fed states and also, can be disturbed by abnormal consumption of nutrients derived from the diet. In obesity and in metabolic conditions associated with the obese phenotype, hypothalamic neurons are affected by a local inflammatory response that is triggered by the excessive amount of fatty acids in the diet. Mounting evidence suggest that, at least in part, the anomalous activity of the hypothalamic tanycytes can play a role in the defective neuronal activity in obesity and associated conditions. Future studies should focus on the identification of mechanisms that may protect the tanycytes from diet-induced abnormalities and the impact of such protection in the progression of metabolic diseases.

AUTHOR CONTRIBUTIONS

RHT, NRVD, and LAV discussed the structure of the manuscript. NRVD wrote the aspects of the BBB structure and function and RHT wrote the developmental topic. LAV and AFSR wrote BBB specialization in the hypothalamus. RHT, NRVD, and LAV wrote the introduction, abstract, and conclusion remarks. RHT made the figures and figure legends.

ACKNOWLEDGMENTS

The writing of this article was supported by São Paulo Research Foundation (2013/07607-8 and 2015/50278-0). Funding was provided by São Paulo Research Foundation as postdoctoral fellowships to RHT (2015/02913-9 and 2016/01868-2) and NRVD (2014/26942-5). The Laboratory of Cell Signaling belongs to the Obesity and Comorbidities Research Center and the National Institute of Science and Technology—Diabetes and Obesity.

REFERENCES

Abbott, N. J., Patabendige, A. A., Dolman, D. E., Yusof, S. R., and Begley, D. J. (2010). Structure and function of the blood-brain barrier. *Neurobiol. Dis.* 37, 13–25. doi: 10.1016/j.nbd.2009.07.030

Adams, R. H., and Alitalo, K. (2007). Molecular regulation of angiogenesis and lymphangiogenesis. *Nat. Rev. Mol. Cell Biol.* 8, 464–478. doi: 10.1038/nrm2183

Akmayev, I. G., and Popov, A. P. (1977). Morphological aspects of the hypothalamic-hypophyseal system, VII The tanycytes: their relation to the hypophyseal adrenocorticotrophic function, An ultrastructural study. *Cell Tissue Res.* 180, 263–282. doi: 10.1007/bf00231958

Alvarez, J. I., Dodelet-Devillers, A., Kebir, H., Ifergan, I., Fabre, P. J., Terouz, S., Sabbagh, M., et al. (2011). The Hedgehog pathway promotes blood–brain barrier integrity and CNS immune quiescence. *Science* 334, 1727–1731. doi: 10.1126/science.1206936

Alvarez, J. I., Katayama, T., and Prat, A. (2013). Glial influence on the blood brain barrier. *Glia* 61, 1939–1958. doi: 10.1002/glia.22575

Andreone, B. J., Lacoste, B., and Gu, C. (2015). Neuronal and vascular interactions. *Annu. Rev. Neurosci.* 38, 25–46. doi: 10.1146/annurev-neuro-071714-033835

Argente-Arizón, P., Freire-Regatillo, A., Argente, J., and Chowen, J. A. (2015). Role of non-neuronal cells in body weight and appetite control. *Front. Endocrinol.* 6:42. doi: 10.3389/fendo.2015.00042

Armulik, A., Genové, G., and Betsholtz, C. (2011). Pericytes: developmental, physiological, and pathological perspectives, problems, and promises. *Dev. Cell.* 21, 193–215. doi: 10.1016/j.devcel.2011.07.001

Armulik, A., Genové, G., Mäe, M., Nisancioglu, M. H., Wallgard, E., Niaudet, C., et al. (2010). Pericytes regulate the blood-brain barrier. *Nature* 468, 557–556. doi: 10.1038/nature09522

Bady, I., Marty, N., Dallaporta, M., Emery, M., Gyger, J., Tarussio, D., et al. (2006). Evidence from glut2-null mice that glucose is a criticalphysiological regulator of feeding. *Diabetes* 55, 988–995. doi: 10.2337/diabetes.55.04.06.db05-1386

Balland, E., Dam, J., Langlet, F., Caron, E., Steculorum, S., Messina, A. et al. (2014). Hypothalamic tanycytes are an ERK-gated conduit for leptin into the brain. *Cell Metab.* 19, 293–301. doi: 10.1016/j.cmet.2013.12.015

Banks, W. A. (2016). From blood–brain barrier to blood–brain interface: new opportunities for CNS drug delivery. *Nat. Ver. Drug Discov.* 15, 275–292. doi: 10.1038/nrd.2015.21

Banks, W. A., Jaspan, J. B., and Kastin, A. J. (1997). Effect of diabetes mellitus on the permeability of the blood-brain barrier to insulin. *Peptides* 18, 1577–1584. doi: 10.1016/S0196-9781(97)00238-6

Banks, W. A., Kastin, A. J., Huang, W., Jaspan, J. B., and Maness, L. M. (1996). Leptin enters the brain by a saturable system independent of insulin. *Peptides* 17, 305–311. doi: 10.1016/0196-9781(96)00025-3

Bauer, H., Sonnleitner, U., Lametschwandtner, A., Steiner, M., Adam, H., and Bauer, H. C. (1995). Ontogenic expression of the erythroid-type glucose transporter (Glut 1) in the telencephalon of the mouse: correlation to the tightening of the blood-brain barrier. *Brain Res. Dev. Brain Res.* 86, 317–325. doi: 10.1016/0165-3806(95)00044-E

Bell, R. D., Winkler, E. A., Sagare, A. P., Singh, I., LaRue, B., Deane, R., et al. (2010). Pericytes control key neurovascular functions and neuronal phenotype in the adult brain and during brain aging. *Neuron* 68, 409–427. doi: 10.1016/j.neuron.2010.09.043

Bennett, L., Yang, M., Enikolopov, G., and Iacovitti, L. (2009). Circumventricular organs: a novel site of neural stem cells in the adult brain. *Mol. Cell. Neurosci.* 41, 337–347. doi: 10.1016/j.mcn.2009.04.007

Ben-Zvi, A., Lacoste, B., Kur, E., Andreone, B. J., Mayshar, Y., and Yan, H. (2014). Mfsd2ais critical for the formation and function of the blood–brain barrier. *Nature* 22, 507–511. doi: 10.1038/nature13324

Berger, M., Bergers, G., Arnold, B., Hämmerling, G. J., and Ganss, R. (2005). Regulator of G-protein signaling-5 induction in pericytes coincides with active vessel remodeling during neovascularization. *Blood* 105, 1094–1101. doi: 10.1182/blood-2004-06-2315

Betsholtz, C. (2014). Physiology: double function at the blood-brain barrier. *Nature* 509, 432–433. doi: 10.1038/nature13339

Blanchette, M., and Daneman, R. (2015). Formation and maintenance of the BBB. *Mech. Dev.* 138, 8–16. doi: 10.1016/j.mod.2015.07.007

Boado, R. J., and Pardridge, W. M. (1990). The brain-type glucose transporter mRNA is specifically expressed at the blood-brain barrier. *Biochem. Biophys. Res. Commun.* 166, 174–179. doi: 10.1016/0006-291X(90)91927-K

Bondjers, C., He, L., Takemoto, M., Norlin, J., Asker, N., Hellström, M., et al. (2006). Microarray analysis of blood microvessels from PDGF-B and PDGF-Rbeta mutant mice identifies novel markers for brain pericytes. *FASEB J.* 20, 1703–1705. doi: 10.1096/fj.05-4944fje

Bribair, A., Zhang, T., Wang, Z. M., Messi, M. L., Enikolopov, G. N., Mintz, A., et al. (2013). Skeletal muscle pericyte subtypes differ in their differentiation potential. *Stem Cell Res.* 10, 67–84. doi: 10.1016/j.scr.2012.09.003

Cabezas, R., Ávila, M., Gonzalez, J., El-Bachá, S., and Báez, E., García-Segura, L. M. (2014). Astrocytic modulation of blood brain barrier: perspectives on Parkinson's disease. *Front. Cell. Neurosci.* 8:211. doi: 10.3389/fncel.2014.00211

Campbell, J. N., Macosko, E. Z., Fenselau, H., Pers, T. H., Lyubetskaya, A., Tenen, D., et al. (2017). A molecular census of arcuate hypothalamus and median eminence cell types. *Nat. Neurosci.* 20, 484–496. doi: 10.1038/nn.4495

Carmeliet, P., Ferreira, V., Breier, G., Pollefeyt, S., Kieckens, L., Gersenstein, M., et al. (1996). Abnormal blood vessel development and lethality in embryos lacking a single VEGF allele. *Nature* 380, 435–439. doi: 10.1038/380435a0

Cashion, M. F., Banks, W. A., and Kastin, A. J. (1996). Sequestration of centrally administered insulin by the brain: effects of starvation, aluminum, and TNF-alpha. *Horm. Behav.* 30, 280–286. doi: 10.1006/hbeh.1996.0034

Cavadas, C., Aveleira, C. A., Souza, G. F., and Velloso, L. A. (2016). The pathophysiology of defective proteostasis in the hypothalamus - from obesity to ageing. *Nat. Rev. Endocrinol.* 12, 723–733. doi: 10.1038/nrendo.2016.107

Chow, B. W., and Gu, C. (2015). The molecular constituents of the blood-brain barrier. *Trends Neurosci.* 38, 598–608. doi: 10.1016/j.tins.2015.08.003

Chowen, J. A., Argente-Arizón, P., Freire-Regatillo, A., Frago, L. M., Horvath, T. L., and Argente, J. (2016). The role of astrocytes in the hypothalamic response and adaptation to metabolic signals. *Prog Neurobiol.* 144, 68–87. doi: 10.1016/j.pneurobio.2016.03.001

Collden, G., Balland, E., Parkash, J., Caron, E., Langlet, F., Prevot, V., et al. (2014). Neonatal overnutrition causes early alterations in the central response to peripheral ghrelin. *Mol. Metab.* 4, 15–24. doi: 10.1016/j.molmet.2014.10.003

Correale, J., and Villa, A. (2009). Cellular elements of the blood-brain barrier. *Neurochem. Res.* 34, 2067–2077. doi: 10.1007/s11064-009-0081-y

Cullen, M., Elzarrad, M. K., Seaman, S., Zudaire, E., Stevens, J., Yang, M. Y., et al. (2011). GPR124, an orphan G protein-coupled receptor, is required for CNS-specific vascularization and establishment of the blood-brain-barrier. *Proc. Natl. Acad. Sci. U.S.A.* 108, 5759–5764. doi: 10.1073/pnas.1017192108

da Fonseca, A. C., Matias, D., Garcia, C., Amaral, R., Geraldo, L. H., Freitas, C., et al. (2014). The impact of microglial activation on blood-brain barrier in brain diseases. *Front. Cell. Neurosci.* 8:362. doi: 10.3389/fncel.2014.00362

Daneman, R., Agalliu, D., Zhou, L., Kuhnert, F., Kuo, C. J., and Barres, B. A. (2009). Wnt/beta-catenin signaling is required for CNS, but not non-CNS, angiogenesis. *Proc. Natl. Acad. Sci. U.S.A.* 106, 641–646. doi: 10.1073/pnas.0805165106

Daneman, R., and Prat, A. (2015). The blood–brain barrier. *Cold Spring Harb. Perspect. Biol.* 7:a020412. doi: 10.1101/cshperspect.a020412

Daneman, R., Zhou, L., Agalliu, D., Cahoy, J. D., Kaushal, A., and Barres, B. A. (2010a). The mouse blood–brain barrier transcriptome: A new resource for understanding the development and function of brain endothelial cells. *PLoS ONE* 5:e13741. doi: 10.1371/journal.pone.0013741

Daneman, R., Zhou, L., Kebede, A. A., and Barres, B. A. (2010b). Pericytes are required for blood–brain barrier integrity during embryogenesis. *Nature* 468, 562–566. doi: 10.1038/nature09513

Dejana, E., and Vestweber, D. (2013). The role of VE-cadherin in vascular morphogenesis and permeability control. *Prog. Mol. Biol. Transl. Sci.*116, 119–144. doi: 10.1016/B978-0-12-394311-8.00006-6

de Vries, H. E., Kooij, G., Frenkel, D., Georgopoulos, S., Monsonego, A., and Janigro, D. (2012). Inflammatory events at blood-brain barrier in neuroinflammatory and neurodegenerative disorders: implications for clinical disease. *Epilepsia* 6, 45–52. doi: 10.1111/j.1528-1167.2012.03702.x

Dore-Duffy, P., and Cleary, K. (2011). Morphology and properties of pericytes. *Methods Mol. Biol.* 686, 49–68. doi: 10.1007/978-1-60761-938-3_2

Dziegielewska, K. M., Evans, C. A., Malinowska, D. H., Møllgård, K., Reynolds, J. M., Reynolds, M. L., et al. (1979). Studies of the development of brain barrier systems to lipid insoluble molecules in fetal sheep. *J. Physiol.* 292, 207–231. doi: 10.1113/jphysiol.1979.sp012847

Eberth, C. J. (1871). *Handbuch der Lehre von der Gewegen des Menschen und der Tiere, Vol. 1.* Leipzig: Engelmann.

Ehrlich, P. (1885). *Das Sauerstoff-Bedürfniss des Organismus: eine Farbenanalytische Studie.* Berlin: Hirschwald.

Engelhardt, B., and Liebner, S. (2014). Novel insights into the development and maintenance of the blood-brain barrier. *Cell Tissue Res.* 355, 687–699. doi: 10.1007/s00441-014-1811-2

Fantin, A., Vieira, J. M., Gestri, G., Denti, L., Schwarz, Q., Prykhozhij, S., et al. (2010). Tissue macrophages act as cellular chaperones for vascular anastomosis downstream of VEGF-mediated endothelial tip cell induction. *Blood* 116, 829–840. doi: 10.1182/blood-2009-12-257832

Farrell, C. L., and Pardridge, W. M. (1991). Blood–brain barrier glucose transporter is asym-metrically distributed on brain capillary endothelial lumenal and ablumenalmembranes: an electron microscopic immunogold study. *Proc. Natl. Acad. Sci. U.S.A.* 88, 5779–5783. doi: 10.1073/pnas.88.13.5779

Fenselau, H., Campbell, J. N., Verstegen, A. M., Madara, J. C., Xu, J., Shah, B. P., et al. (2017). A rapidly acting glutamatergic ARC→PVH satiety circuit postsynaptically regulated by α-MSH. *Nat. Neurosci.* 20, 42–51. doi: 10.1038/nn.4442

Fernández-Klett, F., Offenhauser, N., Dirnagl, U., Priller, J., and Lindauer, U. (2010). Pericytes in capillaries are contractile *in vivo*, but arterioles mediate functional hyperemia in the mouse brain. *Proc. Natl. Acad. Sci. USA,* 107, 22290–22295. doi: 10.1073/pnas.1011321108

Frayling, C., Britton, R., and Dale, N. (2011). ATP-mediated glucosensing by hypothalamic tanycytes. *J. Physiol.* 589(Pt 9), 2275–2286. doi: 10.1113/jphysiol.2010.202051

Ganong, W. F. (2000). Circumventricular organs: definition and role in the regulation of endocrine and autonomic function. *Clin. Exp. Pharmacol. Physiol.* 27, 422–427. doi: 10.1046/j.1440-1681.2000.03259.x

Goldmann, E. E. (1909). Dieäussere und innere Sekretion des gesunden und kranken Organismus im Lichte der 'vitalen Färbung.' *Beiträg Klinische Chirurgie* 64, 192–265.

Goldmann, E. E. (1913). Vitalfärbung am Zentralnervensyatem. Beitrag zur Physio-Pathologie dês plexus chorioideus und der Hirnhäute. *Abh preuss, Akad Wiss Phys-Math Kl* 1, 1–60.

Haan, N., Goodman, T., Najdi-Samiei, A., Stratford, C. M., Rice, R., El Agha, E., et al. (2013). Fgf10-expressing tanycytes add new neurons to the appetite/energy-balance regulating centers of the postnatal and adult hypothalamus. *J. Neurosci.* 33, 6170–6180. doi: 10.1523/JNEUROSCI.2437-12.2013

Hagan, N., and Ben-Zvi, A. (2015). The molecular, cellular, and morphological components of blood–brain barrier development during embryogenesis. *Semin. Cell Biol.* 38, 7–15. doi: 10.1016/j.semcdb.2014.12.006

Halilagic, A., Ribes, V., Ghyselinck, N. B., Zile, M. H., Dollé, P., and Studer, M. (2007). Retinoids control anterior and dorsal properties in the developing forebrain. *Dev Biol.* 303, 362–375. doi: 10.1016/j.ydbio.2006.11.021

Hall, C. N., Reynell, C., Gesslein, B., Hamilton, N. B., Mishra, A., Sutherland, B. A., et al. (2014). Capillary pericytes regulate cerebral blood flow in health and disease. *Nature* 508, 55–60. doi: 10.1038/nature13165

Havrankova, J., Brownstein, M., and Roth, J. (1981). Insulin and insulin receptors in rodent brain. *Diabetologia* 20, 268–273. doi: 10.1007/BF00254492

Hawkins, R. A., O'Kane, R. L., Simpson, I. A., and Viña, J. R. (2006). Structure of the blood-brain barrier and its role in the transport of amino acids. *J. Nutr.* 36, 218S–226S.

Hellstrom, M., Gerhardt, H., Kalén, M., Li, X., Eriksson, U., Wolburg, H., et al. (2001). Lack of pericytes leads to endothelial hyperplasia and abnormal vascular morphogenesis. *J. Cell Biol.* 153, 543–553. doi: 10.1083/jcb.153.3.543

Hellstrom, M., Kalen, M., Lindahl, P., Abramsson, A., and Betsholtz, C. (1999). Role of PDGF-B and PDGFR-β in recruitment of vascular smooth muscle cells and pericytes during embryonic blood vessel formation in the mouse. *Development* 126, 3047–3055.

Hill, R. A., Tong, L., Yuan, P., Murikinati, S., Gupta, S., and Grutzendler, J. (2015). Regional blood flow in the normal and ischemic brain is controlled by arteriolar smooth muscle cell contractility and not by capillary pericytes. *Neuron* 87, 95–110. doi: 10.1016/j.neuron.2015.06.001

Hofmann, K., Lamberz, C., Piotrowitz, K., Offermann, N., But, D., Scheller, A., et al. (2017). Tanycytes and a differential fatty acid metabolism in the hypothalamus. *Glia* 65, 231–249. doi: 10.1002/glia.23088

Holly, J., and Perks, C. (2006). The role of insulin-like growth factor binding proteins. *Neuroendocrin* 83, 154–160. doi: 10.1159/000095523

Janzer, R. C., and Raff, M. C. (1987). Astrocytes induce blood–brain barrier properties in endothelial cells. *Nature* 325, 253–257. doi: 10.1038/325253a0

Kastin, A. J., and Akerstrom, V. (2000). Fasting, but not adrenalectomy, reduces transport of leptin into the brain. *Peptides* 21, 679–682. doi: 10.1016/S0196-9781(00)00195-9

Kastin, A. J., Akerstrom, V., and Hackler, L. (2001). Food deprivation decreases blood galanin-like peptide and its rapid entry into the brain. *Neuroendocrinology* 74, 423–432. doi: 10.1159/000054708

Keaney, J., and Campbell, M. (2015). The dynamic blood–brain barrier. *FEBS J.* 282, 4067–4079. doi: 10.1111/febs.13412

Keller, A. (2013). Breaking and building the wall: the biology of the blood-brain barrier in health and disease. *Swiss Med.* Wkly. 143, 1–9. doi: 10.4414/smw.2013.13892

Kim, D. W., Glendining, K. A., Grattan, D. R., and Jasoni, C. L. (2016). Maternal obesity in the mouse compromises the blood-brain barrier in the arcuate nucleus of offspring. *Endocrinology* 157, 2229–2242. doi: 10.1210/en.2016-1014

Kim, J. G., Suyama, S., Koch, M., Jin, S., Argente-Arizon, P., Argente, J., et al. (2014). Leptin signaling in astrocytes regulates hypothalamic neuronal circuits and feeding. *Nat. Neurosci.* 17, 908–910. doi: 10.1038/nn.3725

Kuhnert, F., Mancuso, M. R., Shamloo, A., Wang, H. T., Choksi, V., Florek, M., et al. (2010). Essential regulation of CNS angiogenesis by the orphan G protein-coupled receptor GPR124. *Science* 330, 985–989. doi: 10.1126/science.1196554

Lam, B. Y. H., Cimino, I., Polex-Wolf, J., Kohnke, S. N., Rimmington, D., Iyemere, V., et al. (2017). Heterogeneity of hypothalamic Pro-opiomelanocortin-expressing neurons revealed by single-cell RNA sequencing. *Mol. Met.* 6, 1–10. doi: 10.1016/j.molmet.2017.02.007

Lam, T. K., Schwartz, G. J., and Rossetti, L. (2005). Hypothalamic sensing of fatty acids. *Nat. Neurosci.* 8, 579–584. doi: 10.1038/nn1456

Langlet, F., Levin, B. E., Luquet, S., Mazzone, M., Messina, A., et al. (2013a). Tanycytic VEGF-A boosts blood-hypothalamus barrier plasticity and access of metabolic signals to the arcuate nucleus in response to fasting. *Cell Metab.* 17, 607–617. doi: 10.1016/j.cmet.2013.03.004

Langlet, F., Mullier, A., Bouret, S. G., Prevot, V., and Dehouck, B. (2013b). Tanycyte-like cells form a blood-cerebrospinal fluid barrier in the circumventricular organs of the mouse brain. *J. Comp. Neurol.* 21, 3389–3405. doi: 10.1002/cne.23355

Lee, D. A., Bedont, J. L., Pak, T., Wang, H., Song, J., Miranda-Angulo, A., et al. (2012). Tanycytes of the hypothalamic median eminence form a diet-responsive neurogenic niche. *Nat. Neurosci.* 15, 700–702. doi: 10.1038/nn.3079

Lee, S. W., Kim, W. J., Choi, Y. K., Song, H. S., Son, M. J., et al. (2003). SSeCKS regulates angiogenesis and tight junction formation in blood-brain barrier. *Nat. Med.* 9, 900–906. doi: 10.1038/nm889

Lewandowsky, M. (1900). Zur Lehre von der Cerebrospinalflüssgkeit. Z. *Clin. Med.* 40, 480–494.

Lichtensteiger, W., Richards, J. G., and Kopp, H. G. (1978). Changes in the distribution of non-neuronal elements in rat median eminence and in anterior pituitary hormone secretion after activation of tuberoinfundibular dopamine neurones by brain stimulation or nicotine. *Brain Res.* 157, 73–88. doi: 10.1016/0006-8993(78)90997-6

Liebner, S., Corada, M., Bangsow, T., Babbage, J., Taddei, A., Czupalla, C. J., et al. (2008). Wnt/beta-catenin signaling controls development of the blood-brain barrier. *J. Cell Biol.* 183, 409–417. doi: 10.1083/jcb.200806024

Lindahl, P., Johansson, B. R., Levéen, P., and Betsholtz, C. (1997). Pericyte loss and microaneurysm formation in PDGF-B-deficient mice. *Science* 277, 242–245. doi: 10.1126/science.277.5323.242

Lindblom, P., Gerhardt, H., Liebner, S., Abramsson, A., Hellström, M., Bäckström, G., et al. (2003). Endothelial PDGF-B retention is required for proper investment of pericytes in the microvessel wall. *Genes Dev.* 17, 1835–1840. doi: 10.1101/gad.266803

Luissint, A. C., Artus, C., Glacial, F., Ganeshamoorthy, K., and Couraud, P. O. (2012). Tight junctions at the blood brain barrier: physiological architecture and disease-associated dysregulation. *Fluids Barriers CNS* 9:23. doi: 10.1186/2045-8118-9-23

Lull, M. E., and Block, M. L. (2010). Microglial activation and chronic neurodegeneration. *Neurotherapeutics* 4, 354–365. doi: 10.1016/j.nurt.2010.05.014

Marty, N., Dallaporta, M., Foretz, M., Emery, M., Tarussio, D., Bady, I., et al. (2005). Regulation of glucagon secretion by glucose transporter type 2 (glut2) and astrocytedependent glucose sensors. *J Clin. Invest.* 115, 3545–3553. doi: 10.1172/JCI26309

Millis, S. J., Cowin, A. J., and Kaur, P. (2013). Pericytes, mesenchymal stem cells and the wound healing process. *Cells.* 2, 621–634 doi: 10.3390/cells2030621

Mitchell, R. W., and Hatch, G. M. (2011). Fatty acid transport into the brain: of fatty acid fables and lipid tails. *Prostaglandins Leukot. Essent. Fatty Acids.* 85, 293–302. doi: 10.1016/j.plefa.2011.04.007

Mizee, M. R., Wooldrik, D., Lakeman, K. A., van het Hof, B., Drexhage, J. A., Geerts, D., et al. (2013). Retinoic acid induces blood-brain barrier development. *J. Neurosci* 33, 1660–1671. doi: 10.1523/JNEUROSCI.1338-12.2013

Mullier, A., Bouret, S. G., Prevot, V., and Dehouck, B. (2010). Differential distribution of tight junction proteins suggests a role for tanycytes in blood-hypothalamus barrier regulation in the adult mouse brain. *J. Comp. Neurol.* 518, 943–962. doi: 10.1002/cne.22273

Nayak, D., Roth, T. L., and McGavern, D. B. (2014). Microglia development and function. *Annu. Rev. Immunol.* 32, 367–402. doi: 10.1146/annurev-immunol-032713-120240

Nishioku, T., Matsumoto, J., Dohgu, S., Sumi, N., Miyao, K., Takata, F., et al. (2010). Tumor necrosis factor-alpha mediates the blood-brain barrier dysfunction induced by activated microglia in mouse brain microvascular endothelial cells. *J. Pharmacol. Sci.* 112, 251–254. doi: 10.1254/jphs.09292SC

Obermeier, B., Daneman, R., and Ransohoff, R. M. (2013). Development, maintenance and disruption of the blood-brain barrier. *Nat. Med.* 19, 1584–1596. doi: 10.1038/nm.3407

Obici, S., and Rossetti, L. (2003). Minireview: nutrient sensing and the regulation of insulin action and energy balance. *Endocrinology*144, 5172–5178. doi: 10.1210/en.2003-0999

Olsson, A. K., Dimberg, A., Kreuger, J., and Claesson-Welsh, L. (2006). VEGF receptor signalling–in control of vascular function. *Nat. Rev. Mol. Cell Biol.* 7, 359–371. doi: 10.1038/nrm1911

Pam, W., Banks, W. A., Kennedy, M. K., Guiterrez, E. G., and Kastin, A. J. (1996). Differential permeability of the BBB in acute EAE: enhanced transport of TNT-alpha. *Am. J. Physiol.* 271, E636–E642.

Pardridge, W. M., Boado, R. J., and Farrell, C. R. (1990). Brain-type glucose transporter (GLUT-1) is selectively localized to the blood-brain barrier. Studies with quantitative western blotting and in situ hybridization. *J. Biol Chem.* 265, 18035–18040.

Peppiatt, C. M., Howarth, C., Mobbs, P., and Attwell, D. (2006). Bidirectional control of CNS capillary diameter by pericytes. *Nature* 443, 700–704. doi: 10.1038/nature05193

Potente, M., Gerhardt, H., and Carmeliet, P. (2011). Basic and therapeutic aspects of angiogenesis. *Cell* 146, 873–887. doi: 10.1016/j.cell.2011.08.039

Raab, S., Beck, H., Gaumann, A., Yüce, A., Gerber, H. B., Plate, K., et al. (2004). Impaired brain angiogenesis and neuronal apoptosis induced by conditional homozygous inactivation of vascular endothelial growth factor. *Thromb. Haemost.* 91, 595–605. doi: 10.1160/th03-09-0582

Reese, T. S., and Karnovsky, M. J. (1967). Fine structural localization of a blood-brain barrier to exogenous peroxidase. *J. Cell Biol.* 34, 207–217. doi: 10.1083/jcb.34.1.207

Ribatti, D., Nico, B., Crivellato, E., and Artico, M. (2006).Development of the blood-brain barrier: a historical point of view. *Anat. Rec. B New Anat.* 289B, 3–8. doi: 10.1002/ar.b.20087

Risau, W., Hallmann, R., and Albrecht, U. (1986). Differentiation dependent expression of proteins in brain endothelium during development of the blood-brain barrier. *Dev. Biol.* 117, 537–545. doi: 10.1016/0012-1606(86)90321-0

Rodríguez, E. M., Blázquez, J. L., and Guerra, M. (2010). The design of barriers in the hypothalamus allows the median eminence and the arcuate nucleus to enjoy private milieus: the former opens to the portal blood and the latter to the cerebrospinal fluid. *Peptides* 31, 757–776. doi: 10.1016/j.peptides.2010.01.003

Rouget, C. (1873). Memoire sur le developpement, la structures et les proprietes des capillaires sanguins et lymphatiques. *Archs. Physiol. Norm. Pathol.* 5, 603–633.

Rustenhoven, J., Jansson, D., Smyth, L. C., and Dragunow, M. (2016). Brain pericytes as mediators of neuroinflammation. *Trends Pharmacol. Sci.* 38, 291–304. doi: 10.1016/j.tips.2016.12.001

Saijo, K., and Glass, C. K. (2011). Microglial cell origin and phenotypes in health and disease. *Nat. Rev. Immunol.* 11, 775–787. doi: 10.1038/nri3086

Saunders, N. R., Daneman, R., Dziegielewska, K. M., and Liddelow, S. A. (2013). Transporters of the blood–brain and blood–CSF interfaces in development and in the adult. *Mol. Aspects Med.* 34, 742–752. doi: 10.1016/j.mam.2012.11.006

Saunders, N. R., Liddelow, S. A., and Dziegielewska, K. M. (2012). Barrier mechanisms in the developing brain. *Front. Pharmacol.* 3:46. doi: 10.3389/fphar.2012.00046

Shalaby, F., Rossant, J., Yamaguchi, T. P., Gersenstein, M., Wu, X. F., Breitman, M. L., et al. (1995). Failure of blood-island formation and vasculogenesis in Flk-1-deficient mice. *Nature* 376, 62–66. doi: 10.1038/376062a0

Shepro, D., and Morel, N. M. (1993). Pericyte physiology. *FASEB J.* 7, 1031–1038.

Siegenthaler, J. A., Sohet, F., and Daneman, R. (2013). 'Sealing off the CNS': cellular and molecular regulation of blood–brain barriergenesis. *Curr. Opin. Neurobiol.* 23, 1057–1064. doi: 10.1016/j.conb.2013.06.006

Sofroniew, M. V., and Vinters, H. V. (2010). Astrocytes: biology and pathology *Acta Neuropathol.* 119, 7–35. doi: 10.1007/s00401-009-0619-8

Stenman, J. M., Rajagopal, J., Carroll, T. J., Ishibashi, M., McMahon, J., and McMahon, A. P. (2008). Canonical Wnt signaling regulates organ-specific assembly and differentiation of CNS vasculature. *Science* 322, 1247–1250. doi: 10.1126/science.1164594

Stolarczyk, E., Guissard, C., Michau, A., Even, P. C., Grosfeld, A., Serradas, P., et al. (2010). Detection of extracellular glucose by GLUT2 contributes to hypothalamic control of food intake. *Am J Physiol Endocrinol. Metab.* 298, E1078–E1087.doi: 10.1152/ajpendo.00737.2009

Sumi, N., Nishioku, T., Takata, F., Matsumoto, J., Watanabe, T., Shuto, H., et al. (2010). Lipopolysaccharide-activated microglia induce dysfunction of the blood-brain barrier in rat microvascular endothelial cells co-cultured with microglia. *Cell. Mol. Neurobiol.* 30, 247–253. doi: 10.1007/s10571-009-9446-7

Szathmari, A., Champier, J., Ghersi-Egea, J. F., Jouvet, A., Watrin, C., Wierinckx, A., et al (2013). Molecular characterization of circumventricular organs and third ventricle ependyma in the rat: potential markers for periventricular tumors. *Neuropathology* 33, 17–29. doi: 10.1111/j.1440-1789.2012.01321.x

Tallquist, M. D., French, W. J., and Soriano, P. (2003). Additive effects of PDGF receptor beta signaling pathways in vascular smooth muscle cell development. *PLoS Biol.* 1:E52. doi: 10.1371/journal.pbio.0000052

Tam, S. J., Richmond, D. L., Kaminker, J. S., Modrusan, Z., Martin-McNulty, B., Cao, T. C., et al. (2012). Death receptors DR6 and TROY regulate brain vascular development. *Dev. Cell* 22, 403–417. doi: 10.1016/j.devcel.2011.11.018

Theis, M., Sohl, G., Eiberger, J., and Willecke, K. (2005). Emerging complexities in identity and function of glial connexins. *Trends Neurosci.* 28, 188–195. doi: 10.1016/j.tins.2005.02.006

Tietz, S., and Engelhardt, B. (2015). Brain barriers: crosstalk between complex tight junctions and adherens junctions. *J. Cell Biol.* 209, 493–506. doi: 10.1083/jcb.201412147

Trost, A., Lange, S., Schroedl, F., Bruckner, D., Motloch, A. K., Bogner, B. et al. (2016). Brain and retinal pericytes: origin, function and role. *Front. Cell. Neurosci.* 4:20. doi: 10.3389/fncel.2016.00020

Vallet, P. G., Charnay, Y., Boura, C., and Kiss, J. Z. (1991). Colocalization of delta sleep inducing peptide and luteinizing hormone releasing hormone in neurosecretory vesicles in rat median eminence. *Neuroendocrinology* 53, 103–106. doi: 10.1159/000125705

Velloso, L. A., and Schwartz, M. W. (2011). Altered hypothalamic function in diet-induced obesity. *Int. J. Obes.* 35, 1455–1465. doi: 10.1038/ijo.2011.56

Wagner, H. J., and Pilgrim, C. (1974). Extracellular and transcellular transport of horseradish peroxidase (HRP) through the hypothalamic tanycyte ependyma. *Cell Tissue Res.* 152, 477–491. doi: 10.1007/BF00218933

Wang, Y., Rattner, A., Zhou, Y., Williams, J., Smallwood, P. M., and Nathans, J. (2012). Norrin/Frizzled4 signaling in retinal vascular development and blood-brain barrier plasticity. *Cell* 151, 1332–1344. doi: 10.1016/j.cell.2012.10.042

Weindl, A., and Joynt, R. J. (1973). Barrier properties of the subcommissural organ. *Arch. Neurol.* 29, 16–22.

Winkler, E. A., Bell, R., and Zlokovic, B. V. (2011). Central nervous system pericytes in health and disease. *Nat. Neurosci.* 14, 1398–1405. doi: 10.1038/nn.2946

Woods, S. C., and Porte, D. Jr. (1977). Relationship between plasma and cerebrospinal fluid insulin levels of dogs. *Am J. Physiol.* 233, E331–E334.

Wosik, K., Cayrol, R., Dodelet-Devillers, A., Berthelet, F., Bernard, M., Moumdjian, R., et al. (2007). Angiotensin II controls occludin function and is required for blood–brain barrier maintenance: relevance to multiple sclerosis. *J. Neurosci.* 27, 9032–9042. doi: 10.1523/JNEUROSCI.2088-07.2007

Xiao, G., and Gan, L. S. (2013). Receptor-mediated endocytosis and brain delivery of therapeutic biologics. *Int. J. Cell Biol.* 2013:703545. doi: 10.1155/2013/703545

Zenker, D., Begley, D., Bratzke, H., Rübsamen-Waigmann, H., and von Briesen, H. (2003). Human blood-derived macrophages enhance barrier function of cultured primary bovine and human brain capillary endothelial cells. *J. Physiol.* 551(Pt 3), 1023–1032. doi: 10.1113/jphysiol.2003.045880

Zhang, X., and van den Pol, N. A. (2016). Hypothalamic arcuate nucleus tyrosine hydroxylase neurons play orexigenic role in energy homeostasis. *Nat. Neurosci.* 19, 1341–1347. doi: 10.1038/nn.4372

Zhang, Y., Proenca, R., Maffei, M., Barone, M., Leopold, L., and Friedman, J. M. (1994). Positional cloning of the mouse obese gene and its human homologue. *Nature* 372, 425–432.

Zhao, Z., Nelson, A. R., Betsholtz, C., and Zlokovic, B. V. (2015). Establishment and dysfunction of the blood-brain barrier. *Cell* 163, 1064–1078. doi: 10.1016/j.cell.2015.10.067

Zhou, Y., and Nathans, J. (2014). Gpr124 controls CNS angiogenesis and blood-brain barrier integrity by promoting ligand-specific canonical Wnt signaling. *Dev. Cell* 31, 248–256. doi: 10.1016/j.devcel.2014.08.018

Zimmermann, K. W. (1923). Der feinere bau der blutcapillares. *Z. Anat. Entwicklungsgesch.* 68, 3–109. doi: 10.1007/978-3-642-92456-9

Zlokovic, B. V. (2008). The blood-brain barrier in health and chronic neurodegenerative disorders. *Neuron* 57, 178–201. doi: 10.1016/j.neuron.2008.01.003

15

Effects of Fat and Sugar, Either Consumed or Infused toward the Brain, on Hypothalamic ER Stress Markers

Evita Belegri[1], Merel Rijnsburger[1], Leslie Eggels[1], Unga Unmehopa[1], Wiep Scheper[2], Anita Boelen[1†] and Susanne E. la Fleur[1,3†]*

[1] Laboratory of Endocrinology, Department of Clinical Chemistry and Department of Endocrinology and Metabolism, Academic Medical Center, University of Amsterdam, Amsterdam, Netherlands, [2] Clincal Genetics, VU Medical Center, Amsterdam, Netherlands, [3] Metabolism and Reward Group, Netherlands Institute for Neuroscience, Amsterdam, Netherlands

***Correspondence:**
Susanne E. la Fleur
s.e.lafleur@amc.uva.nl

[†] These authors have contributed equally to this work.

Protein-folding stress at the Endoplasmic Reticulum (ER) occurs in the hypothalamus during diet-induced obesity (DIO) and is linked to metabolic disease development. ER stress is buffered by the activation of the unfolded protein response (UPR), a controlled network of pathways inducing a set of genes that recovers ER function. However, it is unclear whether hypothalamic ER stress during DIO results from obesity related changes or from direct nutrient effects in the brain. We here investigated mRNA expression of UPR markers in the hypothalamus of rats that were exposed to a free choice high-fat high-sugar (fcHFHS) diet for 1 week and then overnight fed *ad libitum*, or fasted, or fat/sugar deprived (i.e., switched from obesogenic diet to chow). In addition, we determined the direct effects of fat/sugar on mRNA expression of hypothalamus UPR markers by intracarotic infusions of intralipids and/or glucose in chow-fed rats that were fasted overnight. Short term (1 week) exposure to fcHFHS diet increased adiposity compared to chow-feeding. Short term exposure to a fcHFHS diet, followed by mild food restriction overnight, induced hypothalamic ER stress in rats as characterized by an increase in spliced to unspliced X-box binding protein 1 mRNA ratio in hypothalamus of fcHFHS fed rats compared to chow fed rats. Moreover, infused lipids toward the brain of overnight fasted rats, were able to induce a similar response. Non-restricted *ad libitum* fcHFHS-diet fed or totally fasted rats did not show altered ratios. We also observed a clear increase in hypothalamic activating transcription factor 4 mRNA in rats on the fcHFHS diet while being *ad libitum* fed or when infused with intralipid via the carotic artery compared to vehicle infusions. However, we did not observe induction of downstream targets implying that this effect is a more general stress response and not related to ER stress. Overall, we conclude that the hypothalamic stress response might be a sensitive sensor of fat and energy status.

Keywords: ER stress response, hypothalamus, food restriction, fatty acids, sugar

INTRODUCTION

Obesity is the result of a mismatch between energy intake and energy expenditure. Although a sedentary lifestyle can contribute to obesity development, the consumption of sugar-sweetened beverages and high amounts of saturated fat in foods has been linked to the risk to become obese and develop metabolic disorders (Hall et al., 2012). Over the last decades, the intake of sugar-based beverages has clearly increased worldwide, and from recent surveys it has become clear that consumption of both sugar-sweetened beverages and saturated fats (especially from snack foods) exceeds recommended daily levels (Popkin et al., 2012). It is, therefore, of utmost importance to understand how fat and sugar affect energy balance.

The hypothalamus is an important brain area in regulating energy balance (Elmquist and Flier, 2004; Schwartz and Porte, 2005). Under normal conditions the hypothalamus senses whole body energy demands via nutrient, neuronal and hormonal signaling and adjusts feeding behavior and energy expenditure via the production of orexigenic and anorexigenic peptides. For example leptin, the hormone secreted by adipose tissue in proportion to fat mass, activates the release of α-melanocyte stimulating hormone [α-MSH; derived from pro-opiomelanocortin (POMC)] and inhibits the release of the orexigenic neuropeptide Y (NPY) and agouti related peptide (AgRP) (Sahu, 2011). During obesity, however, the function of intracellular organelles in AGRP/NPY or POMC neurons like the endoplasmic reticulum (ER) was shown to be impaired leading to disturbed leptin signaling and energy imbalance (Hosoi et al., 2008; Zhang et al., 2008; Ozcan et al., 2009; Cakir et al., 2013; Ramírez and Claret, 2015).

The ER is a complex membrane network responsible for the synthesis and folding of various transmembrane and secreted proteins (Westrate et al., 2015). Accumulation of toxic, misfolded proteins in the ER leads to ER stress and activation of the unfolded protein response (UPR). The UPR is a network of pathways controlled by three sensors; PKR-like ER kinase (PERK), the activating transcription factor 6 (ATF6) and the inositol-requiring protein-1 alpha (IREα). Activation of these pathways induces the expression of genes that lead to the expansion of the ER, reduction of protein translation and increase of protein folding capacity promoting cell survival or induces apoptosis (Walter and Ron, 2011; Lee and Ozcan, 2014). Upon PERK activation, activating transcription factor 4 (ATF4) mRNA is translated which increases the transcription of specific UPR target genes, including C/EBP homologous protein (CHOP) (Harding et al., 2000; Han et al., 2013). Immunoglobulin-heavy-chain-binding protein (BiP) mRNA is increased upon ATF6 activation and splicing of unspliced X box binding protein 1 to spliced XBP1 (sXBP1/usXBP1) occurs upon IREα activation (Yoshida et al., 2001). Both usXBP1 and sXBP1 were related to cell viability under ER stress conditions. Under severe ER stress, IREα activation can also lead to degradation of mRNAs and miRNAs and cell apoptosis via the c-Jun N-terminal kinase (JNK) pathway (Todd et al., 2008). DP5 (Death protein 5/harakiri) and FasL (Fas ligand) are genes expressed downstream of JNK indicating activation of the IREα—apoptotic pathway (Schenkel, 2004; Guan et al., 2006; Ma et al., 2007).

Long term high fat diet (HFD) feeding, resulting in profound body weight gain, induces hypothalamic ER stress characterized by increased protein levels of UPR markers like p-PERK, p-IREα, and phospho-eukaryotic initiation factor 2 alpha (p-eIF2α) (Ozcan et al., 2009; Cakir et al., 2013). Activation of UPR pathways was also reported when fatty acids (FA) [arachidic acid, palmitic acid, or ceramide] were directly supplied to the brain via intracerebroventricular (ICV) infusion in rodents (Milanski et al., 2009; Contreras et al., 2014) or when administered to murine neuronal cell lines (Choi et al., 2010) implying a more direct role for FA in hypothalamic ER stress induction. Although many of the HFD used also contain considerable amounts of sugar, the effects of sugar alone on the ER stress induction has not been studied so far.

The fact that long term HFD feeding, but also ICV infusions of FA, induce hypothalamic ER stress marker expression points to the idea that nutrients like FA can induce hypothalamic ER stress. However, it is not clear whether other nutrients or the increased adiposity reflecting a positive energy status or a combination of nutrients and energy status affects hypothalamic ER stress. We therefore determined whether overfeeding/fasting status and its interaction with diet-induced obesity affected genetic markers for ER stress in the hypothalamus. We exposed male Wistar rats to a free choice high-fat high-sugar (fcHFHS) diet or chow for 1 week followed by overnight *ad libitum* feeding, fat/sugar deprivation or fasting. In addition, we investigated if fat and sugar have a direct effect on the ER stress markers in the hypothalamus by intracarotic infusions of Intralipids (IL), IL and glucose, or glucose to the brain of overnight fasted lean rats. For both experiments, mRNA of different UPR markers was measured using RT-PCR as an indication for the induction of hypothalamic ER stress.

MATERIALS AND METHODS

Animals

Adult male Wistar rats (250–280 g, Charles River, Germany) were individually housed in a temperature controlled room (19 ± 1°C) on a 12 h light/ 12 h dark cycle (lights on at 7:00 a.m.). During the experiments animals had *ad libitum* access to water and standard laboratory chow (SDS, UK) unless stated differently. All the studies were approved by and performed according to the regulations of the Committee for Animal Experimentation of the Academic Medical Centre of the University of Amsterdam, Netherlands.

fcHFHS Diet Experiments

Three experiments were performed to study the effect of nutrient availability on the hypothalamic ER stress response and its interaction with obesity. In all experiments rats were on a fcHFHS diet or chow for 1 week. The fcHFHS diet consisted of *ad libitum* access to chow, tap water, 30% sugar water (1.0 M sucrose mixed from commercial grade sugar and water) and a dish of pure animal fat (beef tallow; Ossewit/Blanc de Boeuf, Vandermoortele, Belgium) (composition: 34% oleic acid, 25% plamitc, and 22%

stearic acid and 4% linoleic acid). After this period the three experiments differed in feeding regime the night before the end of the experiment (4:00 p.m. day 7–9:00 a.m. day 8).

- *experiment 1*: rats had *ad libitum* access to the control chow diet or to the fcHFHS diet.
- *experiment 2*: all rats received 10 g chow overnight (fat/sugar deprivation for rats on fcHFHS).
- *experiment 3*: all rats were fasted overnight.

Fat/sugar deprivation in our diet model is characterized by removing the fat/sugar components of the diet (i.e., saturated fat and sugar water) overnight. We previously showed that removing fat and sugar from the fcHFHS diet results in consumption of 10–15 g chow spontaneously without caloric compensation for the fat/sugar components of the diet (Pandit, 2015). To ensure equal intake overnight between fcHFHS and chow-fed rats we provided all animals with 10 g of chow. Food components of the diet were weighed 5 times a week and the amounts of components eaten were multiplied with the caloric value of each component to determine energy intake in kcals.

At the end of the experiment, rats were anesthetized via 30% CO_2/70% O_2 and decapitated between 9:00 a.m. and 11:00 a.m. Epididymal, mesenteric, subcutaneous and peritoneal fat were dissected and weighed, trunk blood collected and brains were removed and stored at −80°C until further analysis. Plasma leptin concentrations were determined by radioimmunoassay (Linco Research, Inc., St. Charles, MO, USA). Samples were assayed in duplicate. Amounts of sample, standards, label, antibody and precipitating reagent as described in the procedures of the assay were divided by 4. The detection limit was 0.5 ng/ml and the inter- and intra-assay coefficients were 8% or less.

TABLE 1 | Content of intralipid 20%.

Fatty acid	Amount (%)
Linoleic acid	52
Oleic acid	22
Palmitic acid	13
Linolenic acid	8
Stearic acid	4
Myristic acid	<1
Others	1

Source; Fresenius Kabi.

Intracarotic Infusion Experiment

Rats ($n = 6$–9 per group) underwent surgery under anesthesia induced with an i.p. injection of 80 mg/kg Ketamin (Eurovet Animal Health, Netherlands), 8 mg/kg Xylazin (Bayer Health Care) and 0.1 mg/kg Atropin (Pharmachemie, Netherlands). A silicon catheter was inserted in the carotid artery and directed toward the brain (according to the method of Steffens, 1969). The catheter was externalized at the vertex of the head and the animals were allowed to recover for 7 days.

To study the direct effect of fat and/or glucose on hypothalamic ER stress markers, NaCl (control), 20% IL [(Fresenuis Kabi); composition of IL is displayed in **Table 1**] or IL + 1% glucose (G) were infused via the carotid artery toward the brain (*experiment 4*). Another infusion experiment was performed to study the effect of glucose on hypothalamic ER stress response using glucose (1% in NaCl) or NaCl (*experiment 5*). All solutions were heparinized (0.04%) and Infusion rate was 5 μl/min for 2 h. One hour after the end of infusion the animals received a single shot of pentobarbital via the carotid artery (100–150 mg/kg BW) and were decapitated. Brains were removed and stored at −80°C for further analysis.

Brain Harvesting—Isolation of the Hypothalamus

Coronal brain slices of 250 μm were obtained from −0.96 to −4.36 mm Bregma (Rat brain atlas; Paxinos and Watson, 2007) and directly put in RNAlater solution (Ambion Life Technologies). The hypothalamic part in each section was isolated using syringe needles (0.4 × 19 mm, BD Microlance) and used for RT-PCR.

RNA Isolation—RT-PCR

One half of the hypothalamus was homogenized in lysis buffer provided with the "High Pure RNA isolation kit" (Roche

TABLE 2 | Primer sequences used for RT-PCR.

Primers	Forward 5′–3′	Reverse 5′–3′
ATF4	CTGAACAGCGAAGTGTTGGC	TCTGTCCCGGAAAAGGCATC
us-XBP1	GTCCGCAGCACTCAGACTAC	ATGAGGTCCCCACTGACAGA
s-XBP1	CTGAGTCCGAATCAGGTGCAG	ATCCATGGGAAGATGTTCTGG
DP5	ATGAAGCTGTGTTGCCGAGA	GCTTCAGTCCCACAGACTCC
FasL	TATCCTGGGGATCTGGTGCTA	TGCAGGCATTAAGGACCACT
Ddit3 (CHOP)	AGAGTGGTCAGTGCGCAGC	CTCATTCTCCTGCTCCTTCTCG*
Hspa (Bip)	TGGGTACATTTGATCTGACTGGA	CTCAAAGGTGACTTCAATCTGGG*
β-actin	CATGTACGTAGCCATCCAGGC	CTCTTTAATGTCACGCACGAT
Cyclophilin	ATGTGGTCTTTGGGAAGGTG	GAAGGAATGGTTTGATGGGT
HPRT	GCAGTACAGCCCCAAAATGG	AACAAAGTCTGGCCTGTATCCAA

*Oslowski and Urano (2011).

Molecular Biochemicals, Manheim, Germany) and total RNA was isolated according to the manufacturer's instructions. RNA was quantified by spectrophotometry at 260 nm (Nanodrop 1000, Willmington, Delaware, USA) and cDNA synthesis was performed using the "Transcriptor First Strand cDNA synthesis kit" for RT PCR with oligo(dT) primers (Roche Molecular Biochemicals, Manheim, Germany). The mRNA levels of ER stress markers as well as Hypoxanthine-guanine phosphoribosyltransferase (Hprt), Cyclophilin A and β-actin were determined by RT-PCR using SensiFAST SYBR No-Rox mix (Bioline, Luckenwalde, Germany) at the Lightcycler 480 apparatus (Roche Molecular Biochemicals, Manheim, Germany). The primers were designed using "Primer Blast" (**Table 2**). Samples were baseline corrected and individually checked for their PCR efficiency using the "LC480 Conversion" and "LinRegPCR" software. Median efficiency was calculated for each assay and samples that differed more than 0.05 from the mean efficiency were excluded from statistical analysis. Specific gene expression was normalized to the geometric mean of three housekeeping genes; $(\text{Hprt} \times \beta\text{-actin} \times \text{Cyclophilin A})^{1/3}$.

Statistical Analysis

Data are presented as Mean ± SEM. Outliers were detected using "Dixon's *Q* test" and excluded. Differences between diet groups were evaluated using *Student's t-test* [experiments 1–4, 5 (NaCl vs. G)] or ANOVA followed by *post-hoc* Tukey test (experiment 5, NaCl vs. IL vs. IL+G). Difference between groups was considered significant when $p < 0.05$. In order to determine the effects of low vs. high fat intake and low vs. high sugar intake a median split was performed whereby the median was calculated for fat or for sugar intake and the animals that consumed more than the median were depicted as high consumers and those that consumed lower as low consumers. All tests were performed using Graphpad Prism 6 (Graphpad software Inc., la Jolla, CA, USA).

RESULTS

One Week of fcHFHS Diet Does Not Induce Hypothalamic ER Stress Markers

Rats exposed to the fcHFHS diet for 1 week were hyperphagic as shown by increased caloric intake compared to those on chow (**Table 3**). As a result, % WAT/BW and plasma leptin levels were significantly higher in rats on the fcHFHS diet compared to rats on chow whereas ΔBW did not differ between the groups (**Table 3**).

One week of fcHFHS diet exposure significantly increased ATF4 mRNA expression (**Figure 1A**). However, mRNA expression of CHOP, a target gene of ATF4, and BiP, a target gene of ATF6, was not significantly changed in hypothalami of fcHFHS-fed rats compared to chow-fed controls (**Figures 1B,C**). Splicing of usXBP1 to sXBP1 as shown by the ratio sXBP1/usXBP1 (**Figure 1D**), as well as DP5 and FasL mRNA expression did not differ between the groups.

Overnight Fat/Sugar Deprivation Induces ER Stress in Animals Exposed to the fcHFHS Diet for 1 Week

ΔBW, % WAT/BW and leptin were still increased in fcHFHS-fed rats compared to chow-fed rats when overnight deprived of fat and sugar (**Table 3**), but no changes were observed in hypothalamic ATF4, CHOP, and BiP mRNA expression between the groups (**Figures 2A–C**; left column). However, sXBP1/usXBP1 mRNA was higher and DP5 mRNA was lower in the fcHFHS-fed group compared to the chow controls (**Figures 2D,E**; left column).

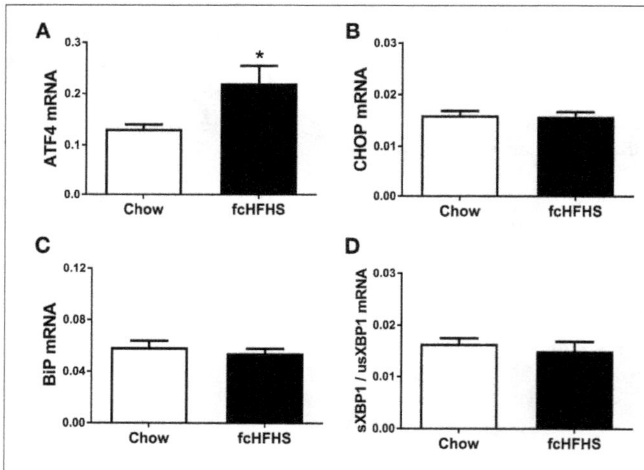

FIGURE 1 | ER stress markers in rat hypothalamus after 1 week *ad libitum* fcHFHS diet or chow. (A) ATF4 and **(B)** CHOP **(C)** BiP, and **(D)** sXBP1/usXBP1 mRNA expression. mRNA expression of specific genes was normalized to the geometric mean of three housekeeping genes. Significant differences between the fcHFHS and control group: $^*p < 0.05$.

TABLE 3 | Characteristics of chow and fcHFHS animals.

Exp.	ΔBW (gr)		% WAT/BW		Leptin (ng/ml)		Average intake/day (Kcal)	
	Chow	fcHFHS	Chow	fcHFHS	Chow	fcHFHS	Chow	fcHFHS
1	34 ± 2.2	37 ± 2.3	2.58 ± 0.09	3.41 ± 0.05****	4.9 ± 0.8	7.6 ± 0.6**	76.0 ± 1.5	100 ± 2.5***
2	41 ± 3.4	52 ± 5.1	1.94 ± 0.13	2.81 ± 0.12***	2.01 ± 0.2	2.73 ± 0.3***	81.6 ± 4.4	122.1 ± 3.7****
3	51 ± 4.8	54 ± 3.7	2.20 ± 0.16	2.72 ± 0.16*	2.34 ± 0.3	3.24 ± 0.4**	88.0 ± 3.8	121.2 ± 5.5***

Delta body weight, average food intake per day, % total white adipose tissue (WAT) relative to final body weight of animals and leptin plasma concentrations in experiment 1 (ad lib fed o/n), 2 (10 g chow fed o/n) and experiment 3 (fasted o/n) are shown as mean (n = 8) ± SEM. Total WAT represents the sum of mesenteric, peritoneal, subcutaneous and epididymal fat. Significant differences between the fcHFHS and chow control group: $^*p < 0.05$, $^{**}p < 0.01$, $^{***}p < 0.001$, $^{****}p < 0.0001$.

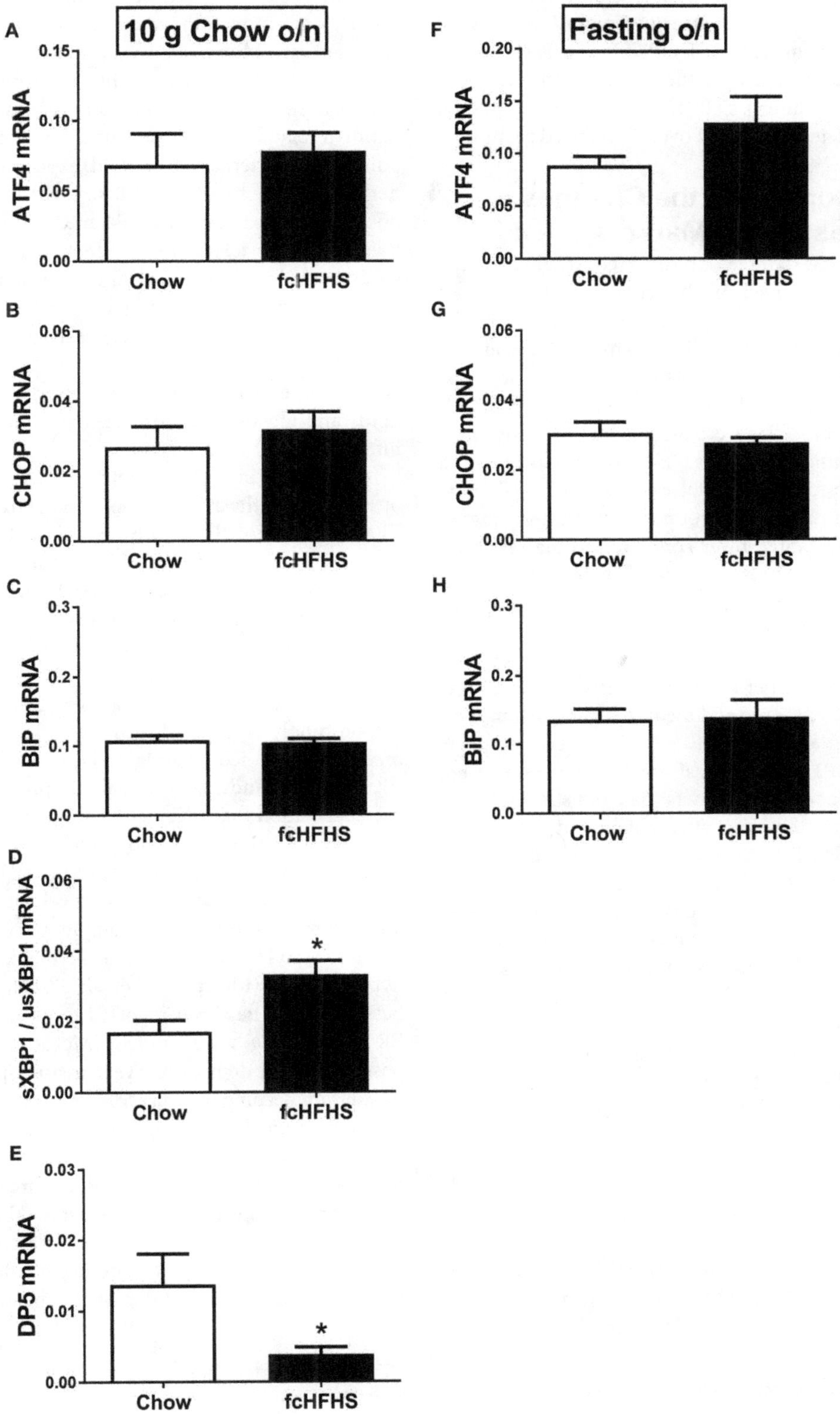

FIGURE 2 | The effect of overnight fat/sugar deprivation (10 g chow; left column) or fasting (right column) after 1 week fcHFHS diet or chow on the mRNA expression of hypothalamic (A,F) ATF4, **(B,G)** CHOP, **(C,H)** BiP, **(D)** sXBP1/usXBP1, and **(E)** DP5. mRNA expression of specific genes was normalized to the geometric mean of three housekeeping genes. Significant cifferences between the fcHFHS and control groups: *$p < 0.05$.

No change in FasL mRNA expression was observed between the groups after removing fat and sugar overnight (not shown). Similarly, no differences in ATF4, CHOP, BiP, and FasL mRNA expression were observed between the groups after overnight fasting (**Figure 2**, right column). sXBP1/usXBP1 and DP5 mRNA expression were not detectable in the overnight fasted groups.

Fat Consumption Leads the Changes Induced in Stress Gene Markers

To determine to what extent fat or sugar contributed to the observed differences observed in hypothalamic mRNA, we divided the fcHFHS group according to fat and sugar intake using a median split forming either low or high fat consumers (LF or HF) or low or high sugar consumers (LS or HS). The median fat consumption was 10% out of total caloric intake. Rats that consumed <10% fat were assigned as LF consumers and those that consumed >10% as HF consumers. LF and HF consumers had similar BW, total caloric intake and chow intake, but fat consumption in HF group was significantly higher and sugar intake significantly lower compared to the LF group (**Table 4**). ATF4 mRNA expression tended to be higher ($p = 0.07$), in the hypothalamus of the HF consumers compared to the LF consumers, whereas sXBP1/usXBP1, DP5 and FasL mRNA expression was not different between the groups (data not shown). Similar analysis was performed for consumption of sugar over a week of fcHFHS exposure and median sugar consumption out of total caloric intake was 38%. No differences in ATF4, usXBP1, sXBP1/usXBP1, DP5, or FasL mRNA expression were observed between HS and LS consumers (data not shown).

To further investigate the direct effects of fat and sugar in the brain on hypothalamic ER stress markers, we infused IL, IL + glucose (ILG), glucose or saline (control) via the carotid artery directly to the brain of overnight fasted rats. IL and ILG increased hypothalamic ATF4 mRNA expression compared to saline but did not affect CHOP, DP5, and FasL mRNA (**Figures 3A–D**). In addition, IL infusion resulted in increased sXBP1/usXBP1 mRNA expression, and tended to increase BiP mRNA expression (**Figures 3E,F**). Glucose infusion did not have an effect on AFT4, sXBP1/usXBP1, and DP5 mRNA expression (**Figures 3G–I,K**), but reduced BiP and FasL mRNA levels compared to saline infusion (**Figures 3J,L**).

DISCUSSION

We showed that short term exposure to a fcHFHS diet, followed by mild food restriction overnight induces hypothalamic ER stress in rats as characterized by an increase in sXPB1/usXBP1 mRNA ratio in hypothalamus of fcHFHS fed rats compared to chow fed rats. Moreover, we showed that lipids, directly infused towards the brain of overnight fasted rats, are able to induce a similar response. As non-restricted *ad libitum* fcHFHS-diet fed or totally fasted rats do not show altered ratios, these data point to an interaction of lipid exposure to the brain and a negative energy balance in ER stress induction. In addition, we observed an increase in ATF4 mRNA when animals were *ad libitum* fed the fcHFHS diet which is abolished when rats are either provided with 10 g of chow overnight or totally fasted. In addition, high fat consumers on the fcHFHS diet have higher ATF4 mRNA, pointing to a direct role for fat intake in the increase in hypothalamic ATF4 mRNA. Indeed, ATF4 mRNA is also increased when animals are directly infused with lipids or lipids and glucose towards the brain, but not when glucose is infused alone.

An increase in sXPB1/usXBP1mRNA ratio implies activation of the IREα pathway (Yoshida et al., 2001; Calfon et al., 2002). The activation of IREα pathway due to HFD-feeding has been reported earlier. However, this was after long-term (8 or 20 weeks) exposure (Ozcan et al., 2009; Won et al., 2009). Here we showed for the first time that short term exposure to a fcHFHS diet is enough to induce activation of this pathway, but only under mild food restriction.

It is unclear why animals on a fcHFHS diet display this response only when food restricted while absent when animals are *ad libitum* fed overnight. One possibility might be that ER stress was induced via anabolic processes as illustrated by the observation that overnight fasting and subsequent refeeding increases sXBP1 mRNA and protein in the liver (Deng et al., 2013) and in the hypothalamus of mice (Williams et al., 2014). It is also possible that protective mechanisms play a role under *ad libitum* conditions. For example, we observed recently that 1 week fcHFHS diet increases beta- oxidation genes in the hypothalamus (Rijnsburger et al., 2016), and since enhanced beta-oxidation has been reported to counter palmitate-induced ER stress in *in vitro* models (McFadden et al., 2014), it is possible that we do not observe increased splicing of XPB1 under *ad libitum* feeding because of counter-active regulatory fatty acid oxidation. In line, we observed no changes in fatty acid oxidation genes after lipid infusion directly to the brain while it does induce XBP1 splicing (M. Rijnsburger, unpublished data). Further research is needed to determine the exact role of energy status and nutrient sensing on hypothalamic ER stress induction.

We observed a clear increase in hypothalamic ATF4 mRNA in rats on the fcHFHS diet while being *ad libitum* fed or

TABLE 4 | Characteristics of low fat and high fat consumers over 1 week of fcHFHS diet.

	Total (Kcal)	Chow (Kcal)	Fat (Kcal)	Sugar (Kcal)	BW (g)	% FAT/BW
HF	105 ± 2.3	50 ± 1.9	19 ± 1.40	36 ± 0.8	331 ± 1.8	3.26 ± 0.06
LF	98 ± 2.6	47 ± 3.0	6.9 ± 0.44**	49 ± 1.4**	331 ± 5.2	3.07 ± 0.08

Average Total, Chow, Fat, or Sugar caloric intake as well as body weight and % Fat/BW of animals over 1 week on fcHFHS diet. High fat (HF) and low fat (LF) animals were determined using median split. The median of fat intake was 10% out of total caloric intake. Significant differences between the HF and LF group: $^{**}p < 0.01$.

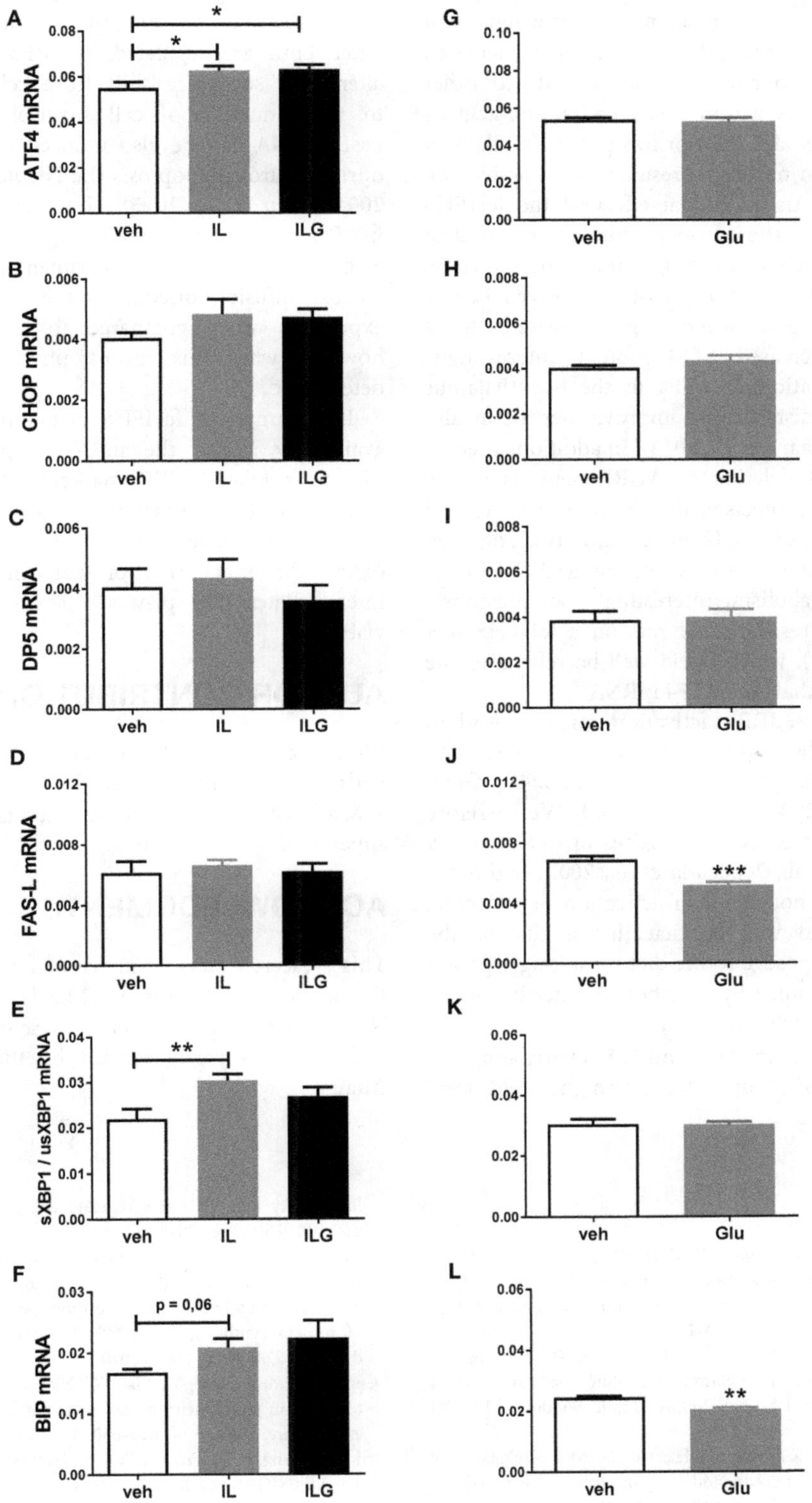

FIGURE 3 | The effect of central infusion of Intralipid (IL), Intralipid and Glucose (ILG) or Glucose on hypothalamic (A,G) ATF4, **(B,H)** CHOP **(C)**, **(C,I)** DP5, **(D,J)** FasL, **(E,K)** sXBP1/usXBP1, **(F,L)** Bip **mRNA expression in chow rats.** mRNA expression of specific genes was normalized to the geometric mean of three housekeeping genes. Significant differences between groups: $^{*}p < 0.05$, $^{**}p \leq 0.01$; $^{***}p < 0.001$.

when infused with intralipids via the carotic artery compared to vehicle infusions. However, we did not observe induction of downstream targets. It might be possible that increased ATF4 mRNA expression in our models is associated with other general stress related events within a cell i.e., amino-acid or glucose deprivation (Siu et al., 2002) or less protein availability (which has been shown in muscle to result in UPR activation; Deldicque et al., 2010). An additional effect of the fcHFHS diet is reduced chow—and thus protein—intake compared to chow controls, it is well possible that this might be the cause for the changes in ATF4 mRNA expression observed in our study. It is unclear at this point whether this increase in ATF4 mRNA will result in increased ATF4 protein. Interestingly, overexpression and inhibition of ATF4 in the hypothalamus induces hepatic insulin resistance and improves hepatic insulin sensitivity, respectively (Zhang et al., 2013). In addition, a recent study showed that ATF4 deletion in AGRP neurons of the hypothalamus specifically protects against high fat diet induced weight gain and insulin resistance (Deng et al., 2016). Together, this suggests an important role for hypothalamic ATF4 in the regulation of energy metabolism. Interestingly, we previously reported hepatic insulin resistance in rats on a fcHFHS diet (Diepenbroek et al., 2017), which could well be related to the observed increase in hypothalamic ATF4 mRNA.

Under severe ER stress, IREα activation can also lead to cell apoptosis via the JNK pathway (Todd et al., 2008) and to activation of apoptotic genes (Urano et al., 2000; Guan et al., 2006; Kim et al., 2006; Ma et al., 2007). We therefore measured DP5 and FasL mRNA, target genes of JNK pathway (Schenkel, 2004; Guan et al., 2006; Ma et al., 2007). However, 1 week fcHFHS diet did not result in activation of apoptotic gene expression. It could well be that this is due to the duration of the diet, as exposure to the diet for a longer period induces apoptosis accompanied by obesity and other metabolic disturbances (Ozcan et al., 2009; Won et al., 2009).

Interestingly a decrease in DP5 mRNA expression was observed in the fcHFHS group after overnight mild food restriction (10 g chow intake). That might be related to the increase in sXBP1 mRNA under the same conditions. Since both are regulated by IREα activation, the observed alterations suggest a shift from cell death related pathways to the induction of cell survival mechanisms. Like DP5, FasL mRNA can be also induced upon IREα/JNK activation during neuronal apoptosis (Le-Niculescu et al., 1999; Schenkel, 2004; Chen et al., 2015). However, no change was observed in FasL expression indicating that FasL does not play a major role in our experimental setting. In addition, a glucose infusion directly to the brain lowered FasL mRNA expression when compared to a vehicle control infusion, however what this means physiologically remains to be determined.

In summary, a fcHFHS diet and overnight fat and sugar availability affects the mRNA expression of hypothalamic ER stress related UPR markers. Overall, the UPR markers seemed to be a sensitive sensor of fatty acid availability as well as nutrient load. More studies are necessary to define the exact role of nutrients in induction of UPR intermediates that play a role in cellular metabolism and viability.

AUTHOR CONTRIBUTIONS

EB, AB, and Sl designed experiments. EB, MR, LE, UU, and Sl performed experiments. EB, AB, and Sl prepared the manuscript. WS, MR, LE, and UU edited the manuscript. The entire study was supervised by AB and Sl.

ACKNOWLEDGMENTS

This research was supported by the Dutch Technology Foundation STW (grant 12264), which is part of the Netherlands Organization for Scientific Research (NWO), and which is partly funded by the Ministry of Economic Affairs.

REFERENCES

Cakir, I., Cyr, N. E., Perello, M., Litvinov, B. P., Romero, A., Stuart, R. C., et al. (2013). Obesity induces hypothalamic endoplasmic reticulum stress and impairs proopiomelanocortin (POMC) post-translational processing. *J. Biol. Chem.* 288, 17675–17688. doi: 10.1074/jbc.M113.475343

Calfon, M., Zeng, H., Urano, F., Till, J. H., Hubbard, S. R., Harding, H. P., et al. (2002). IRE1 couples endoplasmic reticulum load to secretory capacity by processing the XBP-1 mRNA. *Nature* 415, 92–96. doi: 10.1038/415092a

Chen, X., Shen, J., Wang, Y., Chen, X., Yu, S., Shi, H., et al. (2015). Up-regulation of c-Fos associated with neuronal apoptosis following intracerebral hemorrhage. *Cell. Mol. Neurobiol.* 35, 363–376. doi: 10.1007/s10571-014-0132-z

Choi, S. J., Kim, F., Schwartz, M. W., and Wisse, B. E. (2010). Cultured hypothalamic neurons are resistant to inflammation and insulin resistance induced by saturated fatty acids. *Am. J. Physiol. Endocrinol. Metab.* 298, E1122–E1130. doi: 10.1152/ajpendo.00006.2010

Contreras, C., González-García, I., Martínez-Sánchez, N., Seoane-Collazo, P., Jacas, J., Morgan, D. A., et al. (2014). Central ceramide-induced hypothalamic lipotoxicity and ER stress regulate energy balance. *Cell Rep.* 9, 366–377. doi: 10.1016/j.celrep.2014.08.057

Deldicque, L., Cani, P. D., Philp, A., Raymackers, J. M., Meakin, P. J., Ashford, M. L., et al. (2010). The unfolded protein response is activated in skeletal muscle by high-fat feeding: potential role in the downregulation of protein synthesis. *Am. J. Physiol. Endocrinol. Metab.* 299, E695–E705. doi: 10.1152/ajpendo.00038.2010

Deng, J., Yuan, F., Guo, Y., Xiao, Y., Niu, Y., Deng, Y., et al. (2016). Deletion of ATF4 in AgRP neurons promotes fat loss mainly via increasing energy expenditure. *Diabetes* 66, 640–650. doi: 10.2337/db16-0954

Deng, Y., Wang, Z. V., Tao, C., Gao, N., Holland, W. L., Ferdous, A., et al. (2013). The Xbp1s/GalE axis links ER stress to postprandial hepatic metabolism. *J. Clin. Invest.* 123, 455–468. doi: 10.1172/JCI62819

Diepenbroek, C., Eggels, L., Ackermans, M. T., Fliers, E., Kalsbeek, A., Serlie, M. J., et al. (2017). Differential effects of hypercaloric choice diets on insulin sensitivity in rats. *J. Endocrinol.* 232, 49–57. doi: 10.1530/JOE-16-0265

Elmquist, J. K., and Flier, J. S. (2004). Neuroscience. The fat-brain axis enters a new dimension. *Science* 304, 63–64. doi: 10.1126/science.1096746

Guan, Q. H., Pei, D. S., Xu, T. L., and Zhang, G. Y. (2006). Brain ischemia/reperfusion-induced expression of DP5 and its interaction with Bcl-2, thus freeing Bax from Bcl-2/Bax dimmers are mediated by c-Jun N-terminal kinase (JNK) pathway. *Neurosci. Lett.* 393, 226–230. doi: 10.1016/j.neulet.2005.09.075

Hall, K. D., Heymsfield, S. B., Kemnitz, J. W., Klein, S., Schoeller, D. A., and Speakman, J. R. (2012). Energy balance and its components: implications for body weight regulation. *Am. J. Clin. Nutr.* 95, 989–994. doi: 10.3945/ajcn.112.036350

Han, J., Back, S. H., Hur, J., Lin, Y. H., Gildersleeve, R., Shan, J., et al. (2013). ER-stress-induced transcriptional regulation increases protein synthesis leading to cell death. *Nat. Cell Biol.* 15, 481–490. doi: 10.1038/ncb2738

Harding, H. P., Novoa, I., Zhang, Y., Zeng, H., Wek, R., Schapira, M., et al. (2000). Regulated translation initiation controls stress-induced gene expression in mammalian cells. *Mol. Cell* 6, 1099–1108. doi: 10.1016/S1097-2765(00)00108-8

Hosoi, T., Sasaki, M., Miyahara, T., Hashimoto, C., Matsuo, S., Yoshii, M., et al. (2008). Endoplasmic reticulum stress induces leptin resistance. *Mol. Pharmacol.* 74, 1610–1619. doi: 10.1124/mol.108.050070

Kim, B. J., Ryu, S. W., and Song, B. J. (2006). JNK- and p38 kinase-mediated phosphorylation of Bax leads to its activation and mitochondrial translocation and to apoptosis of human hepatoma HepG2 cells. *J. Biol. Chem.* 281, 21256–21265. doi: 10.1074/jbc.M510644200

Lee, J., and Ozcan, U. (2014). Unfolded protein response signaling and metabolic diseases. *J. Biol. Chem.* 289, 1203–1211. doi: 10.1074/jbc.R113.534743

Le-Niculescu, H., Bonfoco, E., Kasuya, Y., Claret, F. X., Green, D. R., and Karin, M. (1999). Withdrawal of survival factors results in activation of the JNK pathway in neuronal cells leading to Fas ligand induction and cell death. *Mol. Cell. Biol.* 19, 751–763. doi: 10.1128/MCB.19.1.751

Ma, C., Ying, C., Yuan, Z., Song, B., Li, D., Liu, Y., et al. (2007). dp5/HRK is a c-Jun target gene and required for apoptosis induced by potassium deprivation in cerebellar granule neurons. *J. Biol. Chem.* 282, 30901–30909. doi: 10.1074/jbc.M608694200

McFadden, J. W., Aja, S., Li, Q., Bandaru, V. V., Kim, E. K., Haughey, N. J., et al. (2014). Increasing fatty acid oxidation remodels the hypothalamic neurometabolome to mitigate stress and inflammation. *PLoS ONE* 9:e115642. doi: 10.1371/journal.pone.0115642

Milanski, M., Degasperi, G., Coope, A., Morari, J., Denis, R., Cintra, D. E., et al. (2009). Saturated fatty acids produce an inflammatory response predominantly through the activation of TLR4 signaling in hypothalamus: implications for the pathogenesis of obesity. *J. Neurosci.* 29, 359–370. doi: 10.1523/JNEUROSCI.2760-08.2009

Oslowski, C. M., and Urano, F. (2011). Measuring ER stress and the unfolded protein response using mammalian tissue culture system. *Meth. Enzymol.* 490, 71–92. doi: 10.1016/B978-0-12-385114-7.00004-0

Ozcan, L., Ergin, A. S., Lu, A., Chung, J., Sarkar, S., Nie, D., et al. (2009). Endoplasmic reticulum stress plays a central role in development of leptin resistance. *Cell Metab.* 9, 35–51. doi: 10.1016/j.cmet.2008.12.004

Pandit, R. (2015). *Of Diet and Leptin.* Thesis, Utrecht University.

Paxinos, G., and Watson, C. (2007). *The Rat Brain in Stereotaxic Coordinates, 6th Edn.* San Diego, CA: Academic Press; Elsevier.

Popkin, B. M., Adair, L. S., and Ng, S. W. (2012). Global nutrition transition and the pandemic of obesity in developing countries. *Nutr. Rev.* 70, 3–21. doi: 10.1111/j.1753-4887.2011.00456.x

Ramírez, S., and Claret, M. (2015). Hypothalamic ER stress: a bridge between leptin resistance and obesity. *FEBS Lett.* 589, 1678–1687. doi: 10.1016/j.febslet.2015.04.025

Rijnsburger, M., Belegri, E., Eggels, L., Unmehopa, U. A., Boelen, A., Serlie, M. J., et al. (2016). The effect of diet interventions on hypothalamic nutrient sensing pathways in rodents. *Physiol. Behav.* 162, 61–68. doi: 10.1016/j.physbeh.2016.04.011

Sahu, A. (2011). Intracellular leptin-signaling pathways in hypothalamic neurons: the emerging role of phosphatidylinositol-3 kinase-phosphodiesterase-3B-cAMP pathway. *Neuroendocrinology* 93, 201–210. doi: 10.1159/000326785

Schenkel, J. (2004). Activation of the c-Jun transcription factor following neurodegeneration *in vivo. Neurosci. Lett.* 361, 36–39. doi: 10.1016/j.neulet.2003.12.011

Schwartz, M. W., and Porte, D. Jr. (2005). Diabetes, obesity, and the brain. *Science* 307, 375–379. doi: 10.1126/science.1104344

Siu, F., Bain, P. J., LeBlanc-Chaffin, R., Chen, H., and Kilberg, M. S. (2002). ATF4 is a mediator of the nutrient-sensing response pathway that activates the human asparagine synthetase gene. *J. Biol. Chem.* 277, 24120–24127. doi: 10.1074/jbc.M201959200

Steffens, A. B. (1969). Blood glucose and FFA levels in relation to the meal pattern in the normal rat and the ventromedial hypothalamic lesioned rat. *Physiol. Behav.* 4, 215–216, IN11–IN12, 217–225. doi: 10.1016/0031-9384(69)90083-3

Todd, D. J., Lee, A. H., and Glimcher, L. H. (2008). The endoplasmic reticulum stress response in immunity and autoimmunity. *Nat. Rev. Immunol.* 8, 663–674. doi: 10.1038/nri2359

Urano, F., Wang, X., Bertolotti, A., Zhang, Y., Chung, P., Harding, H. P., et al. (2000). Coupling of stress in the ER to activation of JNK protein kinases by transmembrane protein kinase IRE1. *Science* 287, 664–666. doi: 10.1126/science.287.5453.664

Walter, P., and Ron, D. (2011). The unfolded protein response: from stress pathway to homeostatic regulation. *Science* 334, 1081–1086. doi: 10.1126/science.1209038

Westrate, L. M., Lee, J. E., Prinz, W. A., and Voeltz, G. K. (2015). Form follows function: the importance of endoplasmic reticulum shape. *Annu. Rev. Biochem.* 84, 791–811. doi: 10.1146/annurev-biochem-072711-163501

Williams, K. W., Liu, T., Kong, X., Fukuda, M., Deng, Y., Berglund, E. D., et al. (2014). Xbp1s in Pomc neurons connects ER stress with energy balance and glucose homeostasis. *Cell Metab.* 20, 471–482. doi: 10.1016/j.cmet.2014.06.002

Won, J. C., Jang, P. G., Namkoong, C., Koh, E. H., Kim, S. K., Park, J. Y., et al. (2009). Central administration of an endoplasmic reticulum stress inducer inhibits the anorexigenic effects of leptin and insulin. *Obesity (Silver. Spring).* 17, 1861–1865. doi: 10.1038/oby.2009.194

Yoshida, H., Matsui, T., Yamamoto, A., Okada, T., and Mori, K. (2001). XBP1 mRNA is induced by ATF6 and spliced by IRE1 in response to ER stress to produce a highly active transcription factor. *Cell* 107, 881–891. doi: 10.1016/S0092-8674(01)00611-0

Zhang, Q., Yu, J., Liu, B., Lv, Z., Xia, T., Xiao, F., et al. (2013). Central activating transcription factor 4 (ATF4) regulates hepatic insulin resistance in mice via S6K1 signaling and the vagus nerve. *Diabetes* 62, 2230–2239. doi: 10.2337/db12-1050

Zhang, X., Zhang, G., Zhang, H., Karin, M., Bai, H., and Cai, D. (2008). Hypothalamic IKKbeta/NF-kappaB and ER stress link overnutrition to energy imbalance and obesity. *Cell* 135, 61–73. doi: 10.1016/j.cell.2008.07.043

16

Prebiotics Supplementation Impact on the Reinforcing and Motivational Aspect of Feeding

*Anne-Sophie Delbès[1], Julien Castel[1], Raphaël G. P. Denis[1], Chloé Morel[1], Mar Quiñones[1], Amandine Everard[2], Patrice D. Cani[2], Florence Massiera[3] and Serge H. Luquet[1]**

[1] Université Paris Diderot, Sorbonne Paris Cité, Unité de Biologie Fonctionnelle et Adaptative, CNRS UMR 8251, Paris, France, [2] Walloon Excellence in Life Sciences and Biotechnology (WELBIO), Metabolism and Nutrition Research Group, Louvain Drug Research Institute, Université catholique de Louvain, Brussels, Belgium, [3] Laboratoire de Recherche Nutritionnelle KOT CEPRODI SA, Paris, France

Correspondence:
Serge H. Luquet
serge.luquet@univ-paris-diderot.fr

Energy homeostasis is tightly regulated by the central nervous system which responds to nervous and circulating inputs to adapt food intake and energy expenditure. However, the rewarding and motivational aspect of food is tightly dependent of dopamine (DA) release in mesocorticolimbic (MCL) system and could be operant in uncontrolled caloric intake and obesity. Accumulating evidence indicate that manipulating the microbiota–gut–brain axis through prebiotic supplementation can have beneficial impact of the host appetite and body weight. However, the consequences of manipulating the implication of the microbiota–gut–brain axis in the control motivational and hedonic/reinforcing aspects of food are still underexplored. In this study, we investigate whether and how dietary prebiotic fructo-oligosaccharides (FOS) could oppose, or revert, the change in hedonic and homeostatic control of feeding occurring after a 2-months exposure to high-fat high-sugar (HFHS) diet. The reinforcing and motivational components of food reward were assessed using a two-food choice paradigm and a food operant behavioral test in mice exposed to FOS either during or after HFHS exposure. We also performed mRNA expression analysis for key genes involved in limbic and hypothalamic control of feeding. We show in a preventive-like approach, FOS addition of HFHS diet had beneficial impact of hypothalamic neuropeptides, and decreased the operant performance for food but only after an overnight fast while it did not prevent the imbalance in mesolimbic markers for DA signaling induced by palatable diet exposure nor the spontaneous tropism for palatable food when given the choice. However, when FOS was added to control diet after chronic HFHS exposure, although it did not significantly alter body weight loss, it greatly decreased palatable food tropism and consumption and was associated with normalization of MCL markers for DA signaling. We conclude that the nature of the diet (regular chow or HFHS) as well as the timing at which prebiotic supplementation is introduced (preventive or curative) greatly influence the efficacy of the gut–microbiota–brain axis. This crosstalk selectively alters the hedonic or motivational drive to eat and triggers molecular changes in neural substrates involved in the homeostatic and non-homeostatic control of body weight.

Keywords: food intake, hedonic and motivational component, dopaminergic system, prebiotic, reward

INTRODUCTION

Obesity and corollary pathologies, such as dyslipidemia, diabetes, and cardiovascular diseases are spreading in both developed and developing countries as a result of increased accessibility to energy-dense food associated with a general decrease in physical activity and energy expenditure (1). Whereas some genetic loci were clearly identified and extensively studied as monogenic causes for obesity, it is widely accepted that the metabolic syndrome is in essence a multifactorial disease that encloses a complex network of molecular, cellular, and physiologic alterations (1, 2). Understanding the complex pathology of the metabolic syndrome will be critical in shaping effective preventive and therapeutic strategies. However, despite the encouraging results obtained through pharmacological and surgical interventions, no effective anti-obesity treatment with long-lasting effects on body weight is nowadays available.

Proper energy balance is insured by the ability of the central nervous system to integrate nervous and circulating signals that reflect nutritional status to produce adaptive metabolic and behavioral responses aiming at maintaining body weight within a physiological narrow range (3). In addition, the rewarding aspects of energy-dense food largely depends on dopamine (DA) release from dopaminergic neurons in the ventral tegmental area that project to limbic regions, notably the prefrontal cortex and the nucleus accumbens (NAcc) (4, 5). This neural substrate referred as to mesolimbic "reward" circuit is instrumental in the encoding of both the volume of desire, i.e., "motivation" and the hedonic aspect, i.e., "liking" in food rewards (6).

Hence, the complex behavioral sequence leading to food intake results from the integration of metabolic needs but also reinforcing aspects of food. Multiple lines of evidence suggest that high-fat feeding and obesity *per se* can promote long-lasting adaptations in both hypothalamic and limbic regions thus leading to increased vulnerability to over-consume energy-dense food. In turn, such vulnerability can promote aberrant behaviors (7, 8) in which the reward becomes the primary driving force to consume energy-dense food (9–12). For instance, emerging theories suggest that chronic exposure to palatable food might impair the proper encoding of reward and, similar to drug of abuse, lead to desensitization of the DA mesolimbic system, and ultimately promote craving and addictive-like consummatory behavior (4, 6).

However, despite similar exposure to palatable and hypercaloric food, the development of eating-habits dissociated from actual homeostatic needs does not occur in every individual, suggesting differential degrees of vulnerability. In that regard, the microbiota–gut–brain axis has recently emerged as a key regulator of brain structures involved in stress-like responses (13, 14) together with resilience to high-fat-induced body weight gain (15). Dietary prebiotic such as the soluble fibers fructo-oligosaccharides (FOS) represents selectively fermented compounds that promote changes in the activity and composition of the gut microbiota, that are associated with a wide spectrum of beneficial effects including reduced appetite (16–20), decreased body weight (15), improved glucose metabolism (15), dampened susceptibility to stress (21, 22), and improved learning discrimination in rodents (23).

These observations suggest that prebiotic manipulation of the microbiota–gut–brain axis could directly impact both homeostatic and non-homeostatic control of food intake. However, the behavioral and molecular consequences of prebiotic supplementation onto the reinforcing and motivational components of food seeking have hitherto been largely unexplored.

In the current study, we investigated how administration of FOS could oppose-in a preventive-like approach or reverse-in a curative approach the behavioral and molecular adaptations induced by high-fat high-sucrose exposure and their consequences on food preference and motivation for food seeking.

MATERIALS AND METHODS

Animals and Diets

Ten-weeks-old male mice C57Bl/6J (25–30 g, Janvier, Le Genest Saint Isle, France) were housed in stainless steel cages in a room maintained at 22 ± 1°C with light from 7:00 a.m. to 7:00 p.m. Food (Safe, Augy, France) and water were given *ad libitum* unless otherwise stated. C57Bl/6J were split in six groups (n = 12/group). The first four groups were exposed, respectively, during 2-months to a control diet (Ctrl, 3,438 kcal/kg, protein 19%, lipid 5%, carbohydrates 55%, reference #U8959 version 63 Safe, Augy, France), a control diet enriched in fructo-oligosaccharide (Ctrl-FOS, 3,438 kcal/kg, protein 17%, lipid 8%, carbohydrates 49%, oligofructose 10%), a high-fat high-sugar diet (HFHS, 4,362 kcal/kg, proteins 20%, lipid 23%, carbohydrate 37%, reference #U8954 version 14 Safe, Augy, France), and an HFHS diet enriched in fructo-oligosaccharide (HFHS-FOS, 4,362 kcal/kg, proteins 18%, lipid 20%, carbohydrate 34%, oligofructose 10%). The last two groups were subjected to a 2-months HFHS diet and split in two groups (n = 12) that received during the following 2-months a "control" diet (HFHS/Ctrl) and a control diet enriched in fructo-oligosaccharide (HFHS/Ctrl-FOS). Groups supplemented with FOS will also be referred in the text by preventive (Ctrl-FOS, HFHS-FOS) or corrective (HFHS/Ctrl-FOS) effects of FOS. All animal experiments were performed with approval of the Animal Care Committee of the University Paris Diderot-Paris 7 and according to European directives.

Body Composition Analysis

Mice were monitored for body weight and composition at the beginning and the end of the experiment. Body mass composition (lean tissue mass, fat mass, free water, and total water content) was analyzed using an Echo Medical systems' EchoMRI (Whole Body Composition Analyzers, EchoMRI, Houston, TX, USA), according to manufacturer's instructions.

Measurement of Food Intake and Food Preference

Analyses were performed in an automated online measurement system using high sensitivity feeding and drinking sensors and an infrared beam-based activity monitoring system (Phenomaster, TSE Systems GmbH, Bad Homburg, Germany).

Mice were evaluated for food preference when exposed to HFHS and control chow diet (CTRL). Food preference was measured during six short sessions of 2 h (days 1–6) using animals as their own controls.

Operant Conditioning System

Operant responding performance was performed as previously described (24). Computer-controlled operant conditioning was conducted in 12 identical conditioning chambers equipped with a swiveling infusion device (Phenomaster, TSE Systems GmbH, Bad Homburg, Germany). Each chamber contains an operant wall with a food cup, two levers located 3 cm lateral to the food cup, with the left lever designated the active lever (for food pellet delivery). Mice are maintained at 90% of initial body weight to facilitate initial learning and performance of a fixed ratio (FR1) operant learning task. The reinforcer was a single 20-mg peanut butter flavored sucrose tablet (TestDiet, Richmond, VA, USA).

Operant training was carried out over six consecutive days with two overnight fix ratio of 1 (FR) and then four consecutive days with one 2-h trial of FR1 per day. At the conclusion of the 6-days operant training period, animals were given four trials to lever press for sucrose under a progressive ratio of 3 (PR), lever press requirement for each subsequent reinforcer increased by 3 with an initial requirement of 3 lever press ($r = 3N + 3$; N = reinforcer number).

The PR schedule requires the mouse to perform an increasing number of lever presses for each consecutive reward, the number of rewards received (also called breakpoint) was used to assess motivation or effort to work for a food reward.

At the end of the experiment, animals were sacrificed, brain, liver, cecum tissues, and plasma collected.

Gut Microbiota Analysis

At the end of the experiment, the total cecum content was collected and weighed before storage at −80°C. Metagenomic DNA was extracted from the cecal content using the QIAamp DNA stool mini kit (Qiagen, Hilden, Germany) according to the manufacturer's instructions. Quantitative PCR (qPCR) for total bacteria, *Bifidobacterium* spp., *Lactobacillus* spp., *Akkermansia muciniphila*, *Roseburia* spp., and *Bacteroides-Prevotella* spp. were performed by using Mesa Fast qPCR™ (Eurogentec, Seraing, Belgium). Real-time PCRs were performed with the StepOnePlus™ real-time PCR system and software (Applied Biosystems, Den Ijssel, The Netherlands). The primers sequences were described previously (15, 25). Cycle threshold of each sample was then compared with a standard curve (performed in triplicate) made by diluting genomic DNA obtained from BCCM/LMG (Ghent, Belgium) or DSMZ (Braunshweig, Germany). Prior to isolating the DNA, the cell counts were determined by BCCM/LMG or DSMZ, respectively; fivefold serial dilution of *Bifidobacterium animalis* BCCM/LMG 18900 for *Bifidobacterium* spp., *Bacteroides fragilis* BCCM/LMG 10263 for *Bacteroides-Prevotella* spp., *Lactobacillus acidophilus* DSM 20079 for *Lactobacillus* spp., *A. muciniphila MucT* (ATTC BAA-835, DSMZ22959) for *A. muciniphila*, *Roseburia intestinalis* (DSMZ 14610) for *Roseburia* spp., and *Lactobacillus acidophilus* DSM 20079 for total bacteria.

Isolation of Total RNA and Quantitative RT-PCR

From all groups, total hypothalamic RNA was extracted and analyzed by qRT-PCR for agouti-related protein (AgRP), neuropeptide Y (NPY), pro-opiomelanocortin (POMC), and cocaine and amphetamine-regulated transcript (CART), and total nucleus accumbens (NAcc) RNA was extracted and analyzed by qRT-PCR for dopamine transporter (DAT), dopamine receptor D1 (DR1), dopamine receptor D2 (DR2), dopamine beta hydroxylase (DBH), and tyrosine hydroxylase (TH).

Total RNA was isolated as described previously (9). We retro transcribed 1 µg RNA using Superscript II (Invitrogen). Real-time quantitative (qRT-PCR) analyses were performed with 25 ng cDNA and 250 nM sense and antisense primers (Eurogentec) in a final reaction volume of 25 µl by using qPCR Core Kit (Eurogentec) and the MyiQ real-time PCR detection system (Bio-Rad). Specific primers were designed using Primer Express software (version 1.0, Applied Biosystems) and primers sequences and house-keeping gene (HKG) are listed below. Relative quantification of hypothalamic and NAcc RNA for each gene was calculated after normalization to HKG by using the comparative Ct method.

Primers	Sequences
POMC	Forward: 5′-AGTGCCAGGACCTCACCA-3′ Reverse: 5′-CAGCGAGAGGTCGAGTTTG-3′
NPY	Forward: 5′-CCGCTCTGCGACACTACAT-3′ Reverse: 5′-TGTCTCAGGGCTGGATCTCT-3′
AgRP	Forward: 5′-CGGAGGTGCTAGATCCACAGA-3′ Reverse: 5′-AGGACTCGTGCAGCCTTACAC-3′
CART	Forward: 5′-CGAGAAGAAGTACGGCCAAG-3′ Reverse: 5′-CTGGCCCCTTTCCTCACT-3′
DAT	Forward: 5′-GCCCTACCTGCTCTTCATGC-3′ Reverse: 5′-GGATGACAGTGAAGCCCACA-3′
DR1	Forward: 5′-TCTGGTTTACCTGATCCCTCA-3′ Reverse: 5′-GCCTCCTCCCTCTTCAGGT-3′
DR2	forward: 5′-TGAACAGGCGGAGAATGG-3′ Reverse: 5′-CTGGTGCTTGACAGCATCTC-3′
DBH	Forward: 5′-ATCTCCATGCATTGCAACAA-3′ Reverse: 5′-AGGCTGCAGATTCCACTCAC-3′
TH	Forward: 5′-GGTATACGCCACGCTGAAGG-3′ Reverse: 5′-TAGCCACAGTACCGTTCCAGA-3′
RPL19 HKG	Forward: 5′-GGGCAGGCATATGGGCATA-3′ Reverse: 5′-GGCGGTCAATCTTCTTGGATT-3′
H1A HKG	Forward: 5′-AGAAGAACAACAGCCGCATC-3′ Reverse: 5′-TGCACCAGTGTGCCTTTATT-3′
HPRT HKG	Forward: 5′-GTTGGATACAGGCCAGACTTTGTTG-3′ Reverse: 5′-GATTCAACTTGCGCTCATCTTAGGC-3′
CYCLOA HKG	Forward: 5′-ACGCCACTGTCGCTTTTC-3′ Reverse: 5′-GCAAACAGCTCGAAGGAGAC-3′

Statistical Analysis

Displayed values are mean ± SEM. Variance equality was analyzed by a paired t-test (GraphPad Prism 6®). Unless otherwise stated, comparisons between groups were carried out using analysis of variance (ANOVA, GraphPad Prism 6®). A P-value of less than 0.05 was considered statistically significant.

RESULTS

Preventive vs Corrective Prebiotic Supplementation Differentially Impact Body Weight and Gut Microbiota Composition

Four groups were subjected to a 2-months long preventing-like approach of prebiotic supplementation in which two groups received regular chow diet with or without soluble fibers FOS (Ctrl or Ctrl-FOS groups) while two last groups received a similar treatment but were raised on palatable high-fat high-sucrose diet with or without FOS (HFHS or HFHS-FOS groups) (**Figure 1A**). An additional two animal cohorts were dedicated to explore the corrective potency of prebiotic supplementation onto metabolic and behavioral changes induced by a 2 months exposure to HFHS diet. In this setting, 12 weeks-old C57Bl/6J male mice were first raised on HFHS diet for 2-months then shifted onto Ctrl or Ctrl-FOS diet and will be referred as to HFHS/Ctrl or HFHS/Ctrl-FOS, respectively (**Figure 1A**). Based on the extensive literature in the field, we chose a 10% FOS enrichment since it was described to promote metabolic benefits (26–28) together with improvement in learning discrimination and improved cognitive performances (23, 29).

While average body weight did not differ among groups before the treatment, a significant increase in body weight was reached after HFHS but not HFHS-FOS exposure (**Figures 1B,E,H**). Body weight gain was mostly attributable to adipose tissue as revealed by body composition analysis (**Figures 1C,D,F,G**; Figures S1A–D in Supplementary Material). In HFHS/Ctrl and HFHS/Ctrl-FOS groups, the switch of HFHS to control diet stopped diet-induced body weight gain (**Figure 1H**) in similar way between FOS and non-FOS-treated group (**Figure 1H**; Figure S1E in Supplementary Material).

Prebiotic supplementation is known to change the composition and activity of specific gastrointestinal microbiota (30, 31). Therefore, we decided to investigate if specific bacteria were modified following our diets. qPCR analysis of the cecum bacterial content revealed that the prevalence of *Bifidobacterium* spp., *A. muciniphila*, and to a lesser extent *Lactobacillus* spp. was significantly increased but only in condition in which both prebiotics and HFHS were combined either simultaneously or when FOS supplementation followed HFHS exposure. It is worth to mention that other bacterial families, such as *Roseburia* spp. and *Bacteroides* spp., were not affected by dietary regimens (**Figures 1I,J**). However, when mice were exposed to Ctrl or Ctrl-FOS diets, we could not identify significant changes in the microbiota ecosystem (**Figures 1I,J**).

Timing in Prebiotic Supplementation Is Instrumental in the Beneficial Impact on Hedonic and Motivational Component Feeding

Previous data suggest that modifications in the microbial diversity may influence food choice and tropism in the host and participate to satiety responses by regulating the gut–brain axis (16, 30, 32). After nutritional manipulation aimed at either preventing or correcting any metabolic and behavioral changes induced by HFHS exposure, the six groups were subjected to a two-food choice paradigm consisting in a seven daily consecutive 2 h-limited access to both Ctrl and HFHS diet followed by an overnight exposure to food choice (**Figure 2A**). Short-term access to two-food choice aimed at deciphering the preference to select and consume palatable over chow pellets in a non-fasted condition. While Ctrl-fed animals displayed a tropism for HFHS over control chow diet (CTRL), Ctrl-FOS maximized their consumption of HFHS starting from the first session (**Figures 2B–D**). During the overnight exposure to food choice, a similar pattern was observed with increased HFHS consumption in Ctrl and Ctrl-FOS animals with an overall 90% preference for the palatable diet (**Figure 2E**).

Interestingly both cohorts exposed to HFHS diet (HFHS and HFHS-FOS) displayed minimal consumption of palatable diet when given the choice on a short period of time (**Figures 2B–D**), in agreement with the reduction in palatable food preference observed in animal fed with high-fat diet (33). This result contrasted, however, with a large preference for HFHS over CTRL in the overnight access in both HFHS and HFHS-FOS groups (**Figure 2E**). In addition, FOS supplementation in HFHS-FOS led to increased tropism for palatable diet compared to HFHS group (**Figure 2E**). These results indicate that mice exposed to diets supplemented with FOS (Ctrl or HFHS) show increased preference for palatable food (**Figures 2B–E**).

In sharp contrast with the lack of preventive action, when prebiotics were added in the diet after a 2 months HFHS exposure (HFHS/Ctrl-FOS), we observed a strong corrective action of FOS on both 2-h time-restricted and overnight palatable diet intake (**Figures 2F–I**).

Food preference and seeking strongly rely on dopamine whose release within the mesocorticolimbic (MCL) system participate in driving the motivational and reinforcing values of food reward (6, 34–36). Hence, we next sought to behaviorally dissect the consequences of FOS supplementation on the motivational drive to obtain food rewards. After nutritional manipulation, the different cohorts underwent through an operant conditioning task to obtain food rewards. Animals were first subjected to fixed ratio (FR) reinforcement schedule in which a single lever press triggers the delivery of a palatable food pellet. Once mice have reached their discriminatory ability between active and inactive lever, they are shifted to a progressive ratio (PR) in which the number of lever presses required to obtain a reward increases progressively (**Figure 3A**). If a subject abnormally inflates the reinforcing aspect of a reward it will be more likely to exert effort to obtain it. Alternatively, if the perceived value of the reward is abnormally diminished, the willingness to engage in effortful behavior to obtain it will be reduced. In all conditions, operant responding for sucrose pellets reward was evaluated on mice gradually food restricted to 90% of body weight or following acute overnight in fed or fasting condition (**Figure 3A**).

Here again, the behavioral output of prebiotic supplementation was different according to the timing (preventive or corrective) of FOS addition in the diet. Ctrl and Ctrl-FOS groups had a similar profile with enhanced operant responding for food reward compared to both HFHS and HFHS-FOS group

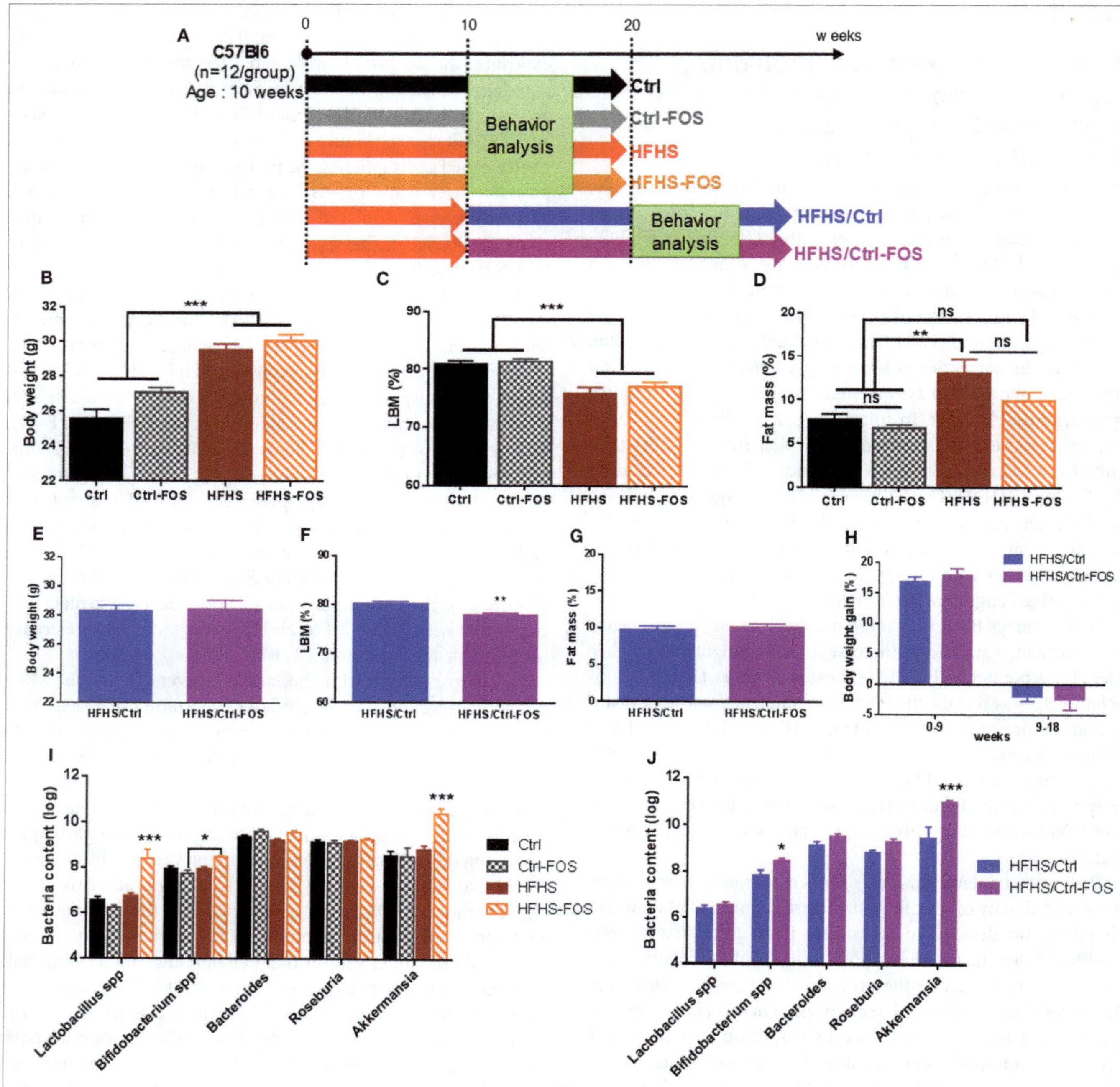

FIGURE 1 | **(A).** Experimental design of diet manipulation in which mice were fed, respectively, regular chow (Ctrl, black), high-fat high-sucrose diet (HFHS, red), or diet enriched in fructo-oligosaccharides (FOS) (Ctrl-FOS, gray and HFHS-FOS, orange) in a protective approach. Two additional groups were fed an HFHS and switched onto either regular chow diet (HFHS/Ctrl, blue) or regular chow enriched in FOS (HFHS/Ctrl-FOS, purple). **(B–H)** Body weight and body composition evolution during diet manipulation in the six different groups. **(B,E)** Body weight evolution, **(C,D,F,G)** body composition in **(C,F)** lean body mass (LBM) and **(D,G)** fat body mass in Ctrl (black), Ctrl-FOS (gray), HFHS (red), HFHS-FOS (orange), HFHS/Ctrl (blue), and HFHS/Ctrl-FOS (purple). **(I,J)** Targeted metagenomics analysis of cecum bacterial content in animal fed Ctrl (black), Ctrl-FOS (gray), HFHS (red), and HFHS-FOS (orange) and **(J)** after switch on Ctrl or Ctrl-FOS diet in HFHS/Ctrl (blue) and HFHS/Ctrl-FOS (purple). Data are expressed as mean ± SEM of 12 mice in each group. Significant differences from a one-way ANOVA **(B–D)**, paired *t*-test **(F)** and a two-way ANOVA **(I,J)**, *Bonferroni Post hoc* test are shown (*$P < 0.005$, **$P < 0.001$, ***$P < 0.0005$).

(**Figure 3B**). These results are consistent with the previous studies showing attenuated operant performance in high-fat fed animals (37). Surprisingly, FOS addition did not alter the number of collected rewards (**Figure 3B**), active lever press (**Figure 3C**), and discriminatory capacity between active and inactive lever (**Figures 3D,J**) in animal exposed to Ctrl diet (Ctrl and Ctrl-FOS) under both chronic and acute fasting-induced body weight loss (**Figures 3E,F,H**). However, FOS supplementation on HFHS diet decreased the motivational drive to collect food reward under conditions of drastic energy deprivation (**Figures 3G,I**).

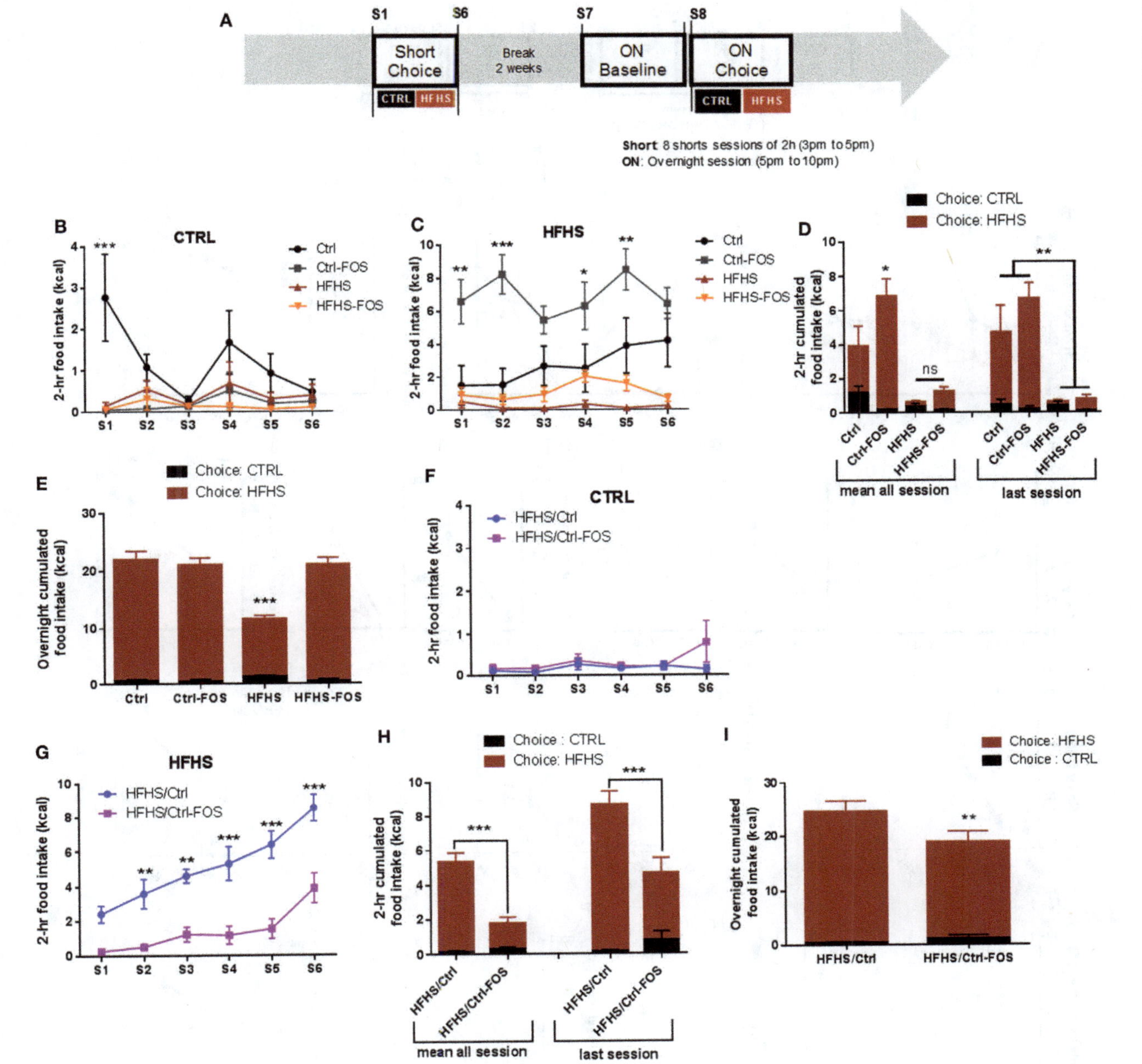

FIGURE 2 | **(A)** Experimental design for food tropism analysis using short or overnight access to a two-food choice protocol using regular chow diet or palatable HFHS diet for six mice per group. Regular chow diet [CTRL **(B,D,F,H)**] or HFHS intake **(C,D,G,H)** during seven sessions consisting of a 2-h two-food choice access, **(D,H)** representative tropism for CTRL *vs* HFHS as average cumulated intake through all session or during the last session, **(E,I)** representative tropism for CTRL vs HFHS as average cumulated intake overnight in Ctrl (black), Ctrl-fructo-oligosaccharides (FOS) (gray), HFHS (red), HFHS-FOS (orange), HFHS/Ctrl (blue), and HFHS/Ctrl-FOS (purple). Data are expressed as mean ± SEM of six mice in each group. Significant differences from a two-way ANOVA, *Bonferroni Post hoc* test (*$P < 0.005$, **$P < 0.001$, ***$P < 0.0005$) **(B–I)**.

A similar experimental design was carried out to evaluate operant conditioning in animals previously fed with an HFHS diet and shifted under Ctrl or Ctrl-FOS diets (HFHS/Crtl, HFHS/Ctrl-FOS).

While a corrective property of FOS supplementation was evident in palatable diet intake and preference (**Figures 2F–I**), HFHS/Crtl and HFHS/Ctrl-FOS exhibited identical performance in every aspect of operant response for food reward in both tested conditions (chronic or acute food deprivation) (**Figures 3K–Q**).

These results highlight that prebiotics might exert a distinct and specific action onto the hedonic "liking," and motivational "wanting" drive to consume palatable food as well as feeding response to energy deprivation. Furthermore, our data support the notion that time-dependent exposure to prebiotics may be instrumental in their action onto reward-seeking behavior.

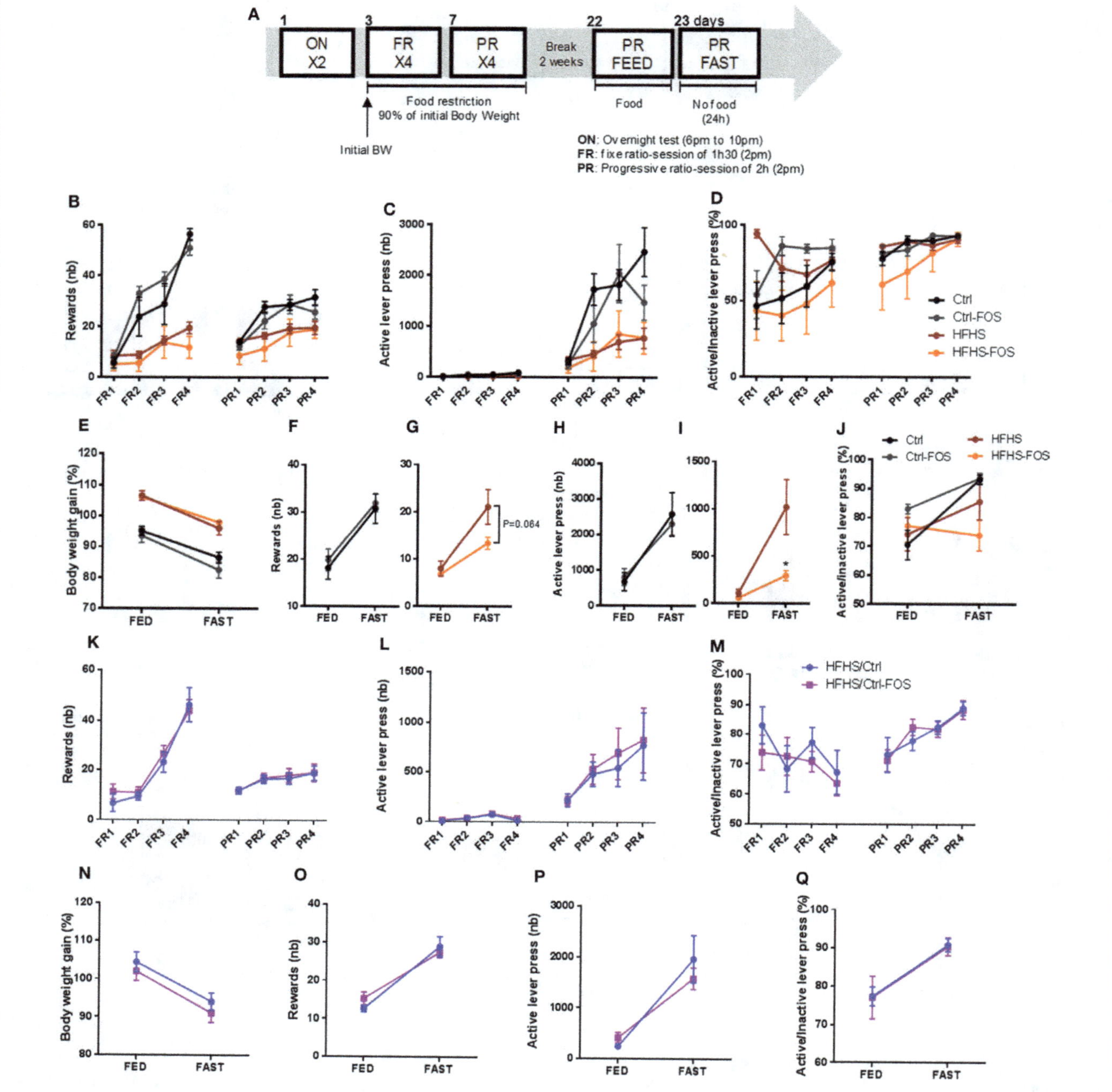

FIGURE 3 | **(A)** Experimental design for the operant responding performance assessment for six mice per group. **(B,K)** Reward number, **(C,L)** active lever press, **(D,M)** ratio between the active and inactive lever presses in **(B–D)** Ctrl (black), Ctrl-fructo-oligosaccharides (FOS) (gray), HFHS (red), **(K–M)** HFHS-FOS (orange), HFHS/Ctrl (blue), and HFHS/Ctrl-FOS (purple) during a 90% body weight reduction. **(E,N)** body weight change, reward number **(F,G,O)**, active lever press **(H,I,P)** or active vs inactive lever press ratio **(J,Q)** in response to an overnight fast in Ctrl (black), Ctrl-FOS (gray), HFHS (red), HFHS-FOS (orange), HFHS/Ctrl (blue), and HFHS/Ctrl-FOS (purple). Data are expressed as mean ± SEM of six mice per group. Significant differences from a two-way ANOVA, *Bonferroni Post hoc* test are shown (**P* < 0.005) **(I)**.

Timing in Prebiotic Supplementation Is Instrumental in Molecular Adaptation in Mesolimbic and Hypothalamic Structures

The action of feeding results from the ability of the brain to properly integrate circulating signals of hunger and satiety together with food-related cues coding for palatable and rewarding values (38). The hypothalamus–brainstem axis, by primarily encoding metabolic needs, is regarded as the key neural network in the homeostatic control of body weight whereas the dopaminergic system is mainly involved in encoding the rewarding and reinforcing values of food seeking. Hence, hypothalamic–brainstem circuit is typically referred as to homeostatic while mesolimbic circuit are referred as to non-homeostatic regulation of feeding (38, 39). Interestingly, obesity and high-fat feeding have been shown to provoke various adaptive changes in both MCL and hypothalamic structures which could account for the toxic effect of energy-dense food (8, 10, 40–43).

We therefore explored how time-dependent prebiotic manipulation modulated the molecular adaptations of dopaminoceptive and hypothalamic structures in response to high-fat feeding. mRNA were extracted from the NAcc and hypothalamus and analyzed for expression of genes involved in dopamine synthesis and signaling, i.e., DAT, DBH, DR1, DR2, and TH in the NAcc, while genes encoding neuropeptides involved in melanocortin signaling and body weight regulation i.e., NPY, agouti-related protein (AgRP), POMC, and cocaine and amphetamine-regulated transcript (CART) in the hypothalamus (**Figures 4A,B**).

In a preventive approach, the effect of FOS addition to Ctrl or HFHS diets was evident in hypothalamic expression of energy-related neuropeptides but failed to alter expression of dopamine-associated genes in the NAcc. Both Ctrl and Ctrl-FOS displayed similar levels of mRNA encoding DAT and DR2 that were significantly higher than those observed in either HFHS or HFHS-FOS (**Figure 4A**). In the hypothalamus, however, while exposure to energy-dense food led to increased mRNA contents for NPY and AgRP in HFHS group, prebiotic supplementation induced a significant decrease in NPY expression (**Figure 4B**). These results are in agreement with published observations showing that high-fat diet and/or obesity result in decreased expression of DR2 and DAT (7, 8) and, on the one hand, increased expression of hypothalamic orexigenic peptides (44, 45). Our results show that, in a preventive-like approach, FOS supplementation partially restores hypothalamic expression of orexigenic peptides but fails to correct the modifications induced by energy-dense food in the NAcc (**Figures 4A,B**).

Surprisingly, FOS enrichment had an opposite consequence onto hypothalamic peptides on mice exposed to Ctrl or HFHS

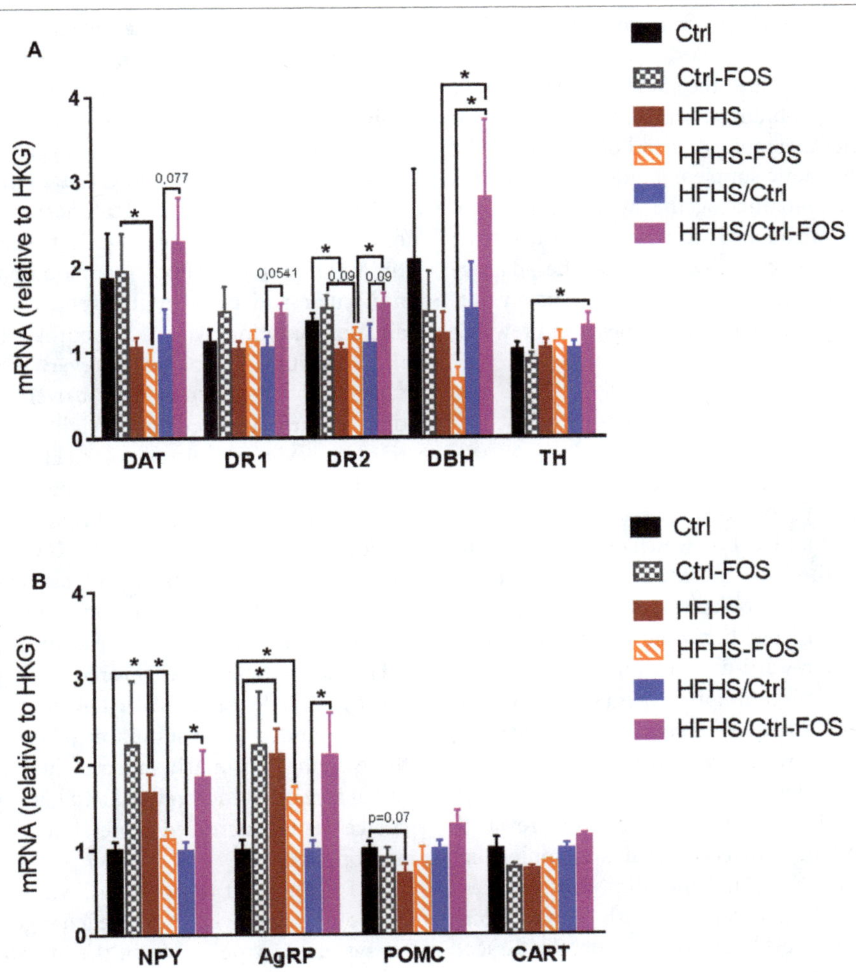

FIGURE 4 | Real-time PCR analysis of mRNA content **(A)** in the nucleus accumbens, for gene encoding for dopamine transporter (DAT), dopamine receptor 1 (DR1), dopamine receptor 2 (DR2), dopamine beta hydroxylase (DBH), and tyrosine hydroxylase (TH) and **(B)** in the hypothalamus for neuropeptide Y (NPY), Agouti-related protein (AgRP), Pro-opiomelanocortin (POMC), and cocaine and amphetamine-regulated transcript (CART) in Ctrl (black), Ctrl-fructo-oligosaccharides (FOS) (gray), HFHS (red), HFHS-FOS (orange), HFHS/Ctrl (blue), and HFHS/Ctrl-FOS (purple). Expression level corresponds to a ratio relative to housekeeping gene (HKG). Data are expressed as mean ± SEM of eight mice in each group. Significant differences from a two-way ANOVA, *Bonferroni Post hoc* test (*$P < 0.005$) **(A,B)**.

diets. Ctrl-FOS diet led to increases in both orexigenic peptides NPY and AgRP compared to Ctrl group while the same nutritional manipulation operated onto HFHS diet led to a decrease of these peptides (**Figure 4B**). In both conditions, the modulation of NPY and AgRP were not counterbalanced by a change in the expression of the anorectic transcripts for POMC or CART (**Figure 4B**).

This result provides a molecular underpinning supporting the relative hyperphagia observed in Ctrl-FOS compared to Ctrl animals in food choice condition (**Figures 2C,D**). In the same food choice paradigm, FOS enrichment in HFHS diet led to increased consumption of palatable diet in an overnight session (**Figure 2E**) which point toward a decorrelation between hypothalamic decrease in NPY, AgRP and food reward seeking.

In a corrective-like approach, however, prebiotic supplementation to Ctrl diet in animal previously exposed to HFHS diet for 2 months fully restored Nacc level of DAT, DR2, and DBH (**Figure 4A**). However, while the shift onto Ctrl diet was *per se* sufficient to restore normal hypothalamic levels for NPY and AgRP, this benefic action was counterbalanced by FOS addition which was associated to sustained level of both orexigenic peptides (**Figure 4B**).

Altogether our results show that the molecular adaptations induced by high-fat feeding in brain structures that govern food intake in response to either metabolic demand or reward can be restored or opposed by prebiotic supplementation. Importantly, the timing in FOS supplementation together with the nature of the diet in which FOS is introduced with have critical impact on the direction by which prebiotic will operate the adaptive changes in MCL or hypothalamic structures and ultimately predict the ability of prebiotic to change food tropism and reward-seeking behavior.

DISCUSSION

While metabolic needs are primarily encoded in the hypothalamus, the reinforcing value of food encompasses a multisensory component including flavors and texture which ultimately modulates the release of DA in the MCL system. In modern society, calorie-dense foods are widely available and were associated with the progression of obesity together with the development of compulsive eating in which reward-driven eating behaviors are bypassing homeostatic regulation of nutrients intake (4, 46, 47). The microbiota–gut–brain axis has emerged as a pivotal player in appetite control as well as reward-driven behavior (48).

In the present study, we described the impact of prebiotic supplementation onto various components of food reward-seeking behavior, gut microbiota ecosystem and molecular adaptation in both hypothalamic and mesolimbic structures. We used food choice paradigm associated with operant conditioning to lever press for food reward in order to dissect out how FOS supplementation could prevent or correct the consequence of chronic exposure to palatable, energy-rich diet onto the hedonic and motivational component of food seeking behavior. We manipulated the timing of FOS introduction in the diet using, first, a preventive-like approach in which animals were exposed to CTRL diet or HFHS diet with or without FOS supplementation and second, a corrective-like approach in which animal were first raised on HFHS diet and then switched onto CTRL diet with or without FOS. In both cases, the consequences onto gut microbiota, hedonic and motivational aspect of food reward together with brain expression of genes involved homeostatic and non-homeostatic control of feeding.

We found that prebiotics act in synergy with the diet supplied to operate change in microbiota composition, tropism for palatable food, and hypothalamic and MCL response. Using targeted metagenomics approach, we could only identify selected changes in the gut–microbiota ecosystem, especially modifying the contents of *Bifidobacterium* spp., *A. muciniphila*- and *Lactobacillus* spp., but only in animals that were either raised or had been exposed chronically to HFHS diet (**Figures 1I,J**). In the same line we found that, while FOS addition to CTRL diet increased both the drive for palatable diet (**Figures 2C–E**) and hypothalamic expression of orexigenic neuropeptides NPY and AgRP (**Figure 4B**), prebiotic addition decreased the motivation to collect food rewards after a fast and decreased hypothalamic NPY content in HFHS fed animals (**Figures 3G,I** and **4B**).

Surprisingly enough, in our hands FOS introduction to the diet only modestly affected HFHS-induced fat mass gain (**Figure 1D**; Figure S1B in Supplementary Material) but had no significantly impact of body weight gain or body weight loss after the transition from HFS to CTRL diet (**Figures 1E–H**; Figures S1C–E in Supplementary Material). However, despite the lack of effect on body weight, we could clearly demonstrate that the timing of prebiotic supplementation had a pivotal role in both molecular and behavioral responses in food reward seeking and consumption. After a 2-months HFHS exposure, we tested the capacity of prebiotic to revert molecular and behavioral dysfunctions induced by caloric overload. The shift onto CTRL diet similarly surfeited body weight gain regardless of FOS addition, however, in contrast to the chronic preventive approach, prebiotic supplementation resulted in decreased palatable food tropism and consumption (**Figures 2F–I**) without affecting operant performance (**Figures 3K–Q**) and was associated with concomitant increase in hypothalamic orexigenic markers and NAcc expression of gene involved in DA signaling. This latter result suggests that, unlike the preventive addition of FOS, prebiotic treatment after chronic HFHS exposure helped restoring the imbalance in MCL DA signaling and reward-driven tropism and overconsumption of palatable diet. Importantly, these changes primarily affected hedonic rather than motivational aspects of food reward and had a positive impact on food choice despite increased expression of hypothalamic orexigenic neuropeptides.

It is important to note that, while 10% FOS supplementation correlated with positive change in the gut microbiota ecosystem as expected from the literature, we did not observe a clear benefit on body weight. FOS introduction did mitigate fat mass gain in animal raised onto HFHS diet (**Figure 1D**) but on overall did not significantly modify body weight. Of note, however, while a decrease in body weight could be expected from prebiotic treatment it is important to highlight that while FOS supplementation has been shown to increase post-meal satiety and hunger, change in body weight were not always consistently observed. Indeed it when compared to other dietary fibers FOS supplementation was associated with body weight gain in lean rodents (28) and obese mice (49) while other report clearly show a preventive action of FOS on high-fat-mediated body weight gain (50). A genetic model of metabolic syndrome FOS supplementation was shown to drastically alleviate excessive feeding but had no impact on body weight (29). This study comes in addition with several report that clearly established the benefits of FOS onto glucose control and insulin sensitivity (51) and in that regards it is tempting to speculate that enhanced insulin sensitivity (29), while promoting a more healthy adipose development, could mitigate the overall body weight loss.

Despite overall similar body weight in within cohort, we found very different outcomes at the behavioral and molecular level when FOS supplementation was added during or after HFHS diet exposure. We first described a paradoxical action of FOS when assessed onto CTRL diet that increased the tropism for palatable diet when assessed on a two-food choice paradigm (**Figures 2B–D**) and while this result is in good agreement with the increase in hypothalamic orexigenic peptides (**Figure 4B**) it could also potentially be the consequence of anxiolytic-like properties of prebiotic (21) which might alleviate food neophobia classically observed in C57BL6 mice (29, 52) and result in faster maximization of palatable diet intake when given the choice. Importantly, however, it should be noted that our behavioral assay was designed to address how animals spontaneously prefer, or are willing to work for food reward and although alteration on reward feeding might lead to overconsumption (46), our protocol does not provide a measure on the long-term consequence onto body weight.

Chronic palatable diet exposure has been shown to promote changes in the reward system at both molecular and behavioral levels (8, 10, 46). One possible explanation for this timing effect of prebiotic action that we observed might be encapsulated in the fact that pre exposure to energy-dense food might initiate both peripheral and central adaptive changes among which some could be selectively corrected by FOS addition. Indeed, once rodent have been exposed to reinforcing stimulus such as palatable diet or drug of abuse they are typically more prone to develop addictive-like behavior (8, 46). These adaptive changes can involve one or many components of the DA system (7, 8, 46, 53) in association with alteration of the gut microbial ecosystem (54). For instance, energy-dense food exposure leads to diet-induced central inflammation (55), neuropeptide signaling alteration (29, 44), and decrease in dopamine receptor abundance (8, 10, 46), which would presumably participate in the development of addictive/compulsive eating behavior. Aside of a direct action onto the brain, energy-dense food also target the gut to control reward acquisition. Gut detection of dietary lipids have been shown to directly control DA release and action by route of the vagal nerves (56). These regulatory processes are probably part of larger integrative aspects by which the combination of diet and microbiota can influence host appetite through change in gut-derived metabolite, intestinal barrier, immune system (48).

Hence, the combination of HFHS exposure followed by prebiotic addition might overall change the microbia–gut–brain axis resulting in the fine-tuning or resetting of DA signaling and reward-driven behavior. Indeed, when FOS was added after HFHS exposure, we could observe a restoration of mesolimbic markers of DA signaling (**Figures 4A,B**) and, despite the increase in orexigenic NPY and AgRP observed the HFHS/CTRL-FOS group displayed strong reduction in food reward tropism (**Figures 2F–H**). This points at a rather dominant function of the reward system in the control of feeding in animals pre-exposed to palatable diet. Interestingly, the study from de Cossio and colleagues also described a beneficial action of prebiotic onto hyperphagia in obese animals that was independent of any changes in NPY, POMC was blunted by prebiotic addition, hypothalamic neuropeptide related (29).

Our results suggest that manipulating of the gut–brain axis can, in specific condition, exert a satietogenic effect primarily by modulating hedonic and motivational drive for food reward. This is in good agreement with the emerging concept that microbiota–gut–brain axis is a potential avenue to modulate reward and in general addictive behavior (57, 58). Notwithstanding, a great limitation of our study lies in the use of targeted metagenomics approach that only accounted for specific bacterial strain changes. It is clear that prebiotic treatment will have consequences on gut flora that extend far beyond the changes that we described here (**Figures 1I,J**) and it is formally possible that one or multiple changes in the gut ecosystem that were not addressed here might reveal potential molecular underpinning by which bacterial–host interaction alters food reward.

In conclusion, our study depicts how timely controlled prebiotic manipulation can differentially and selectively affect positive reinforcement and motivational aspects of food reward-seeking behavior and demonstrate the efficacy of the gut–microbiota–brain axis to operate molecular adaptations in neural substrates involved in both homeostatic and non-homeostatic control of body weight. However, further studies will be warrant to precisely describe the molecular underpinning of the bacterial–host interaction in the control of food reward.

AUTHOR CONTRIBUTIONS

A-SD performed all the studies. JC, RD, CM, and MQ provided technical and conceptual support for behavioral and metabolic analysis and PCR analysis. AE and PC provide analysis of microbiota composition and conceptual support. FM and SL designed the study, secured the funding, and wrote the manuscript.

ACKNOWLEDGMENTS

This work was supported by a collaborative research grant from Laboratoire de Recherche Nutritionnelle KOT CEPRODI SA, Paris, the Centre National la Recherche Scientifique (CNRS), and the University Paris Diderot-Paris 7. RD received a postdoctoral grant from the Région Île-de-France and a fellowship from the Région Ile de France and merit grant from the Société Francophone de Nutrition (SFN-LU). AE is research associate from the FRS-FNRS (Fonds de la Recherche Scientifique), PC is senior research associate from the FRS-FNRS. PC was the recipient of grants from FNRS. This work was supported by the FRFS-WELBIO under grant WELBIO-CGR-2017-C02 and the Funds Baillet Latour (Grant for Medical Research 2015). PC was a recipient of an ERC Starting Grant in 2013 (European Research Council, Starting grant 336452-ENIGMO). MQ is recipient of a Postdoctoral fellowship from Galician Government (Xunta de Galicia ED481B2014/039-0). We acknowledge the technical platform Functional and Physiological Exploration platform (FPE) of the Unit "Biologie Fonctionnelle et Adaptative," (University Paris Diderot, Sorbonne Paris Cité, BFA, UMR 8251 CNRS, F-75205 Paris, France) for metabolic and behavioral analysis. We also acknowledge the animal core facility "Buffon" of the University Paris Diderot-Paris 7/Institut Jacques Monod, Paris for animal husbandry and breeding. We thank Olja Kacanski for administrative support; Isabelle Le Parco, Ludovic Maingault, and Daniel Quintas for care of animals; Giuseppe Gangarossa, Claire Martin, and Chloé Berland for helpful comments on the manuscript; and Dr. Reginald Allouche for help in the experimental design.

REFERENCES

Kahn BB, Flier JS. Obesity and insulin resistance. *J Clin Invest* (2000) 106:473–81. doi:10.1172/JCI10842

Kopelman PG, Hitman GA. Diabetes. Exploding type II. *Lancet* (1998) 352(Suppl 4):SIV5. doi:10.1016/S0140-6736(98)90267-7

Schwartz MW, Woods SC, Porte D Jr, Seeley RJ, Baskin DG. Central ner- vous system control of food intake. *Nature* (2000) 404:661–71. doi:10.1038/35007534

DiLeone RJ, Taylor JR, Picciotto MR. The drive to eat: comparisons and distinctions between mechanisms of food reward and drug addiction. *Nat Neurosci* (2012) 15:1330–5. doi:10.1038/nn.3202

Narayanan NS, Guarnieri DJ, DiLeone RJ. Metabolic hormones, dopamine circuits, and feeding. *Front Neuroendocrinol* (2010) 31:104–12. doi:10.1016/j.yfrne.2009.10.004

Berridge KC. 'Liking' and 'wanting' food rewards: brain substrates and roles in eating disorders. *Physiol Behav* (2009) 97:537–50. doi:10.1016/j.physbeh.2009.02.044

Wu C, Garamszegi SP, Xie X, Mash DC. Altered dopamine synaptic markers in postmortem brain of obese subjects. *Front Hum Neurosci* (2017) 11:386. doi:10.3389/fnhum.2017.00386

Johnson PM, Kenny PJ. Dopamine D2 receptors in addiction-like reward dysfunction and compulsive eating in obese rats. *Nat Neurosci* (2010) 13:635–41. doi:10.1038/nn.2519

Denis RG, Joly-Amado A, Webber E, Langlet F, Schaeffer M, Padilla SL, et al. Palatability can drive feeding independent of AgRP neurons. *Cell Metab* (2015) 22:646–57. doi:10.1016/j.cmet.2015.07.011

Kenny PJ, Voren G, Johnson PM. Dopamine D2 receptors and striatopallidal transmission in addiction and obesity. *Curr Opin Neurobiol* (2013) 23:535–8. doi:10.1016/j.conb.2013.04.012

Berthoud HR. Mind versus metabolism in the control of food intake and energy balance. *Physiol Behav* (2004) 81:781–93. doi:10.1016/j.physbeh.2004.04.034

Kelley AE, Baldo BA, Pratt WE. A proposed hypothalamic-thalamic-striatal axis for the integration of energy balance, arousal, and food reward. *J Comp Neurol* (2005) 493:72–85. doi:10.1002/cne.20769

Burokas A, Moloney RD, Dinan TG, Cryan JF. Microbiota regulation of the mammalian gut-brain axis. *Adv Appl Microbiol* (2015) 91:1–62. doi:10.1016/bs.aambs.2015.02.001

Dinan TG, Cryan JF. Regulation of the stress response by the gut microbiota: implications for psychoneuroendocrinology. *Psychoneuroendocrinology* (2012) 37:1369–78. doi:10.1016/j.psyneuen.2012.03.007

Everard A, Belzer C, Geurts L, Ouwerkerk JP, Druart C, Bindels LB, et al. Cross-talk between *Akkermansia muciniphila* and intestinal epithelium controls diet-induced obesity. *Proc Natl Acad Sci U S A* (2013) 110:9066–71. doi:10.1073/pnas.1219451110

Cani PD, Joly E, Horsmans Y, Delzenne NM. Oligofructose promotes satiety in healthy human: a pilot study. *Eur J Clin Nutr* (2006) 60:567–72. doi:10.1038/sj.ejcn.1602350

Cani PD, Neyrinck AM, Maton N, Delzenne NM. Oligofructose promotes satiety in rats fed a high-fat diet: involvement of glucagon-like Peptide-1. *Obes Res* (2005) 13:1000–7. doi:10.1038/oby.2005.117

Bindels LB, Neyrinck AM, Salazar N, Taminiau B, Druart C, Muccioli GG, et al. Non digestible oligosaccharides modulate the gut microbiota to control the development of leukemia and associated cachexia in mice. *PLoS One* (2015) 10:e0131009. doi:10.1371/journal.pone.0131009

Hadri Z, Chaumontet C, Fromentin G, Even PC, Darcel N, Bouras AD, et al. Long term ingestion of a preload containing fructo-oligosaccharide or guar gum decreases fat mass but not food intake in mice. *Physiol Behav* (2015) 147:198–204. doi:10.1016/j.physbeh.2015.04.039

Gibson GR, Hutkins R, Sanders ME, Prescott SL, Reimer RA, Salminen SJ, et al. Expert consensus document: The International Scientific Association for Probiotics and Prebiotics (ISAPP) consensus statement on the definition and scope of prebiotics. *Nat Rev Gastroenterol Hepatol* (2017) 14:491–502. doi:10.1038/nrgastro.2017.75

Burokas A, Arboleya S, Moloney RD, Peterson VL, Murphy K, Clarke G, et al. Targeting the microbiota-gut-brain axis: prebiotics have anxiolytic and antidepressant-like effects and reverse the impact of chronic stress in mice. *Biol Psychiatry* (2017) 82:472–87. doi:10.1016/j.biopsych.2016. 12.031

McLean PG, Bergonzelli GE, Collins SM, Bercik P. Targeting the microbiota-gut-brain axis to modulate behavior: which bacterial strain will translate best to humans? *Proc Natl Acad Sci U S A* (2012) 109:E174; author reply E176. doi:10.1073/pnas.1118626109

Messaoudi M, Rozan P, Nejdi A, Hidalgo S, Desor D. Behavioural and cognitive effects of oligofructose-enriched inulin in rats. *Br J Nutr* (2005) 93(Suppl 1): S27–30. doi:10.1079/BJN20041348

Cansell C, Castel J, Denis RG, Rouch C, Delbes AS, Martinez S, et al. Dietary triglycerides act on mesolimbic structures to regulate the rewarding and motivational aspects of feeding. *Mol Psychiatry* (2014) 1095–105. doi:10.1038/mp.2014.31

Muccioli GG, Naslain D, Backhed F, Reigstad CS, Lambert DM, Delzenne NM, et al. The endocannabinoid system links gut microbiota to adipogenesis. *Mol Syst Biol* (2010) 6:392. doi:10.1038/msb.2010.46

Daubioul CA, Taper HS, De Wispelaere LD, Delzenne NM. Dietary oligofructose lessens hepatic steatosis, but does not prevent hypertriglyceridemia in obese zucker rats. *J Nutr* (2000) 130:1314–9. doi:10.1093/jn/130.5.1314

Cani PD, Possemiers S, Van de Wiele T, Guiot Y, Everard A, Rottier O, et al. Changes in gut microbiota control inflammation in obese mice through a mechanism involving GLP-2-driven improvement of gut permeability. *Gut* (2009) 58:1091–103. doi:10.1136/gut.2008.165886

Li S, Yingyi G, Chen L, Lijuan G, Ou S, Peng X. Lean rats gained more body weight from a high-fructooligosaccharide diet. *Food Funct* (2015) 6:2315–21. doi:10.1039/c5fo00376h

de Cossio LF, Fourrier C, Sauvant J, Everard A, Capuron L, Cani PD, et al. Impact of prebiotics on metabolic and behavioral alterations in a mouse model of metabolic syndrome. *Brain Behav Immun* (2017) 64:33–49. doi:10.1016/j.bbi.2016.12.022

Cani PD, Lecourt E, Dewulf EM, Sohet FM, Pachikian BD, Naslain D, et al. Gut microbiota fermentation of prebiotics increases satietogenic and incretin gut peptide production with consequences for appetite sensation and glucose response after a meal. *Am J Clin Nutr* (2009) 90:1236–43. doi:10.3945/ ajcn.2009.28095

Wang J, Tang H, Zhang C, Zhao Y, Derrien M, Rocher E, et al. Modulation of gut microbiota during probiotic-mediated attenuation of metabolic syndrome in high fat diet-fed mice. *ISME J* (2015) 9:1–15. doi:10.1038/ismej.2014.99

Alcock J, Maley CC, Aktipis CA. Is eating behavior manipulated by the gastrointestinal microbiota? Evolutionary pressures and potential mechanisms. *Bioessays* (2014) 36:940–9. doi:10.1002/bies.201400071

Vucetic Z, Carlin JL, Totoki K, Reyes TM. Epigenetic dysregulation of the dopamine system in diet-induced obesity. *J Neurochem* (2012) 120:891–8. doi:10.1111/j.1471-4159.2012.07649.x

Kelley AE, Baldo BA, Pratt WE, Will MJ. Corticostriatal-hypothalamic circuitry and food motivation: integration of energy, action and reward. *Physiol Behav* (2005) 86:773–95. doi:10.1016/j.physbeh.2005.08.066

DiLeone RJ. The influence of leptin on the dopamine system and implications for ingestive behavior. *Int J Obes (Lond)* (2009) 33(Suppl 2):S25–9. doi:10.1038/ijo.2009.68

Berridge KC, Robinson TE. What is the role of dopamine in reward: hedonic impact, reward learning, or incentive salience? *Brain Res Brain Res Rev* (1998) 28:309–69. doi:10.1016/S0165-0173(98)00019-8

Davis JF, Tracy AL, Schurdak JD, Tschop MH, Lipton JW, Clegg DJ, et al. Exposure to elevated levels of dietary fat attenuates psychostimulant reward and mesolimbic dopamine turnover in the rat. *Behav Neurosci* (2008) 122: 1257–63. doi:10.1037/a0013111

Morton GJ, Cummings DE, Baskin DG, Barsh GS, Schwartz MW. Central nervous system control of food intake and body weight. *Nature* (2006) 443:289–95. doi:10.1038/nature05026

Wise RA. Role of brain dopamine in food reward and reinforcement. *Philos Trans R Soc Lond B Biol Sci* (2006) 361:1149–58. doi:10.1098/rstb. 2006.1854

Blouet C, Schwartz GJ. Hypothalamic nutrient sensing in the control of energy homeostasis. *Behav Brain Res* (2010) 209:1–12. doi:10.1016/j.bbr.2009.12.024

Dorfman MD, Thaler JP. Hypothalamic inflammation and gliosis in obesity. *Curr Opin Endocrinol Diabetes Obes* (2015) 22:325–30. doi:10.1097/MED.0000000000000182

Thaler JP, Yi CX, Schur EA, Guyenet SJ, Hwang BH, Dietrich MO, et al. Obesity is associated with hypothalamic injury in rodents and humans. *J Clin Invest* (2012) 122:153–62. doi:10.1172/JCI59660

Alsio J, Olszewski PK, Norback AH, Gunnarsson ZE, Levine AS, Pickering C, et al. Dopamine D1 receptor gene expression decreases in the nucleus accumbens upon long-term exposure to palatable food and differs depending on diet-induced obesity phenotype in rats. *Neuroscience* (2010) 171:779–87. doi:10.1016/j.neuroscience.2010.09.046

la Fleur SE, van Rozen AJ, Luijendijk MC, Groeneweg F, Adan RA. A free-choice high-fat high-sugar diet induces changes in arcuate neuropeptide expression that support hyperphagia. *Int J Obes (Lond)* (2010) 34:537–46. doi:10.1038/ijo.2009.257

van de Giessen E, la Fleur SE, de Bruin K, van den Brink W, Booij J. Free-choice and no-choice high-fat diets affect striatal dopamine D2/3 receptor availability, caloric intake, and adiposity. *Obesity (Silver Spring)* (2012) 20: 1738–40. doi:10.1038/oby.2012.17

Kenny PJ. Reward mechanisms in obesity: new insights and future directions. *Neuron* (2011) 69:664–79. doi:10.1016/j.neuron.2011.02.016

Saper CB, Chou TC, Elmquist JK. The need to feed: homeostatic and hedonic control of eating. *Neuron* (2002) 36:199–211. doi:10.1016/ S0896-6273(02)00969-8

van de Wouw M, Schellekens H, Dinan TG, Cryan JF. Microbiota-gut-brain axis: modulator of host metabolism and appetite. *J Nutr* (2017) 147:727–45. doi:10.3945/jn.116.240481

Liu TW, Cephas KD, Holscher HD, Kerr KR, Mangian HF, Tappenden KA, et al. Nondigestible fructans alter gastrointestinal barrier function, gene expression, histomorphology, and the microbiota profiles of diet-induced obese C57BL/6J mice. *J Nutr* (2016) 146:949–56. doi:10.3945/jn.115.227504

Nakamura Y, Natsume M, Yasuda A, Ishizaka M, Kawahata K, Koga J. Fructooligosaccharides suppress high-fat diet-induced fat accumulation in C57BL/6J mice. *Biofactors* (2017) 43:145–51. doi:10.1002/biof.147

Schneeberger M, Everard A, Gomez-Valades AG, Matamoros S, Ramirez S, Delzenne NM, et al. *Akkermansia muciniphila* inversely correlates with the onset of inflammation, altered adipose tissue metabolism and metabolic disorders during obesity in mice. *Sci Rep* (2015) 5:16643. doi:10.1038/ srep16643

Kronenberger JP, Medioni J. Food neophobia in wild and laboratory mice (*Mus musculus* domesticus). *Behav Processes* (1985) 11:53–9. doi:10.1016/ 0376-6357(85)90102-0

Wang GJ, Volkow ND, Logan J, Pappas NR, Wong CT, Zhu W, et al. Brain dopamine and obesity. *Lancet* (2001) 357:354–7. doi:10.1016/S0140-6736(00)03643-6

Everard A, Geurts L, Caesar R, Van Hul M, Matamoros S, Duparc T, et al. Intestinal epithelial MyD88 is a sensor switching host metabolism towards obe- sity according to nutritional status. *Nat Commun* (2014) 5:5648. doi:10.1038/ ncomms6648

Velloso LA, Araujo EP, de Souza CT. Diet-induced inflammation of the hypo- thalamus in obesity. *Neuroimmunomodulation* (2008) 15:189–93. doi:10.1159/ 000153423

Tellez LA, Medina S, Han W, Ferreira JG, Licona-Limon P, Ren X, et al. A gut lipid messenger links excess dietary fat to dopamine deficiency. *Science* (2013) 341:800–2. doi:10.1126/science.1239275

Skosnik PD, Cortes-Briones JA. Targeting the ecology within: the role of the gut-brain axis and human microbiota in drug addiction. *Med Hypotheses* (2016) 93:77–80. doi:10.1016/j.mehy.2016.05.021

Kiraly DD, Walker DM, Calipari ES, Labonte B, Issler O, Pena CJ, et al. Alterations of the host microbiome affect behavioral responses to cocaine. *Sci Rep* (2016) 6:35455. doi:10.1038/srep35455

17

Lipoprotein Lipase Expression in Hypothalamus is Involved in the Central Regulation of Thermogenesis and the Response to Cold Exposure

Elise Laperrousaz[1], Raphaël G. Denis[1], Nadim Kassis[1], Cristina Contreras[2,3], Miguel López[2,3], Serge Luquet[1], Céline Cruciani-Guglielmacci[1] and Christophe Magnan[1]*

[1] Unité de Biologie Fonctionnelle et Adaptative, CNRS UMR 8251, Sorbonne Paris Cité, Université Denis Diderot, Paris, France, [2] NeurObesity Group, Department of Physiology, Centro de Investigación en Medicina Molecular y Enfermedades Crónicas (CiMUS), University of Santiago de Compostela-Instituto de Investigación Sanitaria, Santiago de Compostela, Spain, [3] CIBER Fisiopatología de la Obesidad y Nutrición (CIBERobn), Santiago de Compostela, Spain

***Correspondence:**
Céline Cruciani-Guglielmacci
cruciani@univ-paris-diderot.fr

Lipoprotein lipase (LPL) is expressed in different areas of the brain, including the hypothalamus and plays an important role in neural control of the energy balance, including feeding behavior and metabolic fluxes. This study tested the hypothesis that hypothalamic LPL participates in the control of body temperature. We first showed that cold exposure induces decreased activity and expression of LPL in the mouse hypothalamus. We then selectively deleted LPL in the mediobasal hypothalamus (MBH) through an adeno-associated virus approach in LPL-floxed mice and generated MBHΔ^{Lpl} mice with 30–35% decrease in hypothalamic LPL activity. Results showed a decrease in body temperature in MBHΔ^{Lpl} mice when compared with controls at 22°C. Exposure to cold (4°C for 4 h) decreased the body temperature of the control mice while that of the MBHΔ^{Lpl} mice remained similar to that observed at 22°C. MBHΔ^{Lpl} mice also showed increased energy expenditure during cold exposure, when compared to controls. Finally, the selective MBH deletion of LPL also increased the expression of the thermogenic PRMD16 and Dio2 in subcutaneous and perigonadal adipose tissues. Thus, the MBH LPL deletion seems to favor thermogenesis. These data demonstrate that for the first time hypothalamic LPL appears to function as a regulator of body temperature and cold-induced thermogenesis.

Keywords: lipoprotein lipase, cold exposure, hypothalamus, brown adipose tissue, browning of white adipose tissue

INTRODUCTION

Adaptation to change in ambient temperature, especially cold exposure, is one of the mechanisms essential to the survival of mammals. This adaptation involves numerous signals of neural or hormonal origin and acute responses or acclimatization to prolonged cold exposures (1). Acute responses include vasoconstriction or shivering. The hypothalamus is a key area of central nervous system (CNS) involved in the adaptation to cold exposure. Indeed, afferent signals from the skin are sensed by the preoptic area of the anterior hypothalamus. The measurement of c-fos expression also suggests a role for the dorsomedial, medial, and the ventromedial hypothalamus after cold exposure in rats (2). In addition, several studies have also highlighted a role for arcuate (ARC) or ventromedial (VMH) nuclei in this adaptation (3, 4). Peripheral adaptation to cold exposure involves the activation of the sympathetic nervous system (SNS) and hypothalamic–pituitary–thyroid axis (5, 6), including an increase in type 2 iodothyronine deiodinase (Dio2) expression that activates thyroxine (T4) to 3,3′,5-triiodothyronine (T3) (7). These signals combine to activate catabolic pathways with release of energy substrates such as free fatty acids (FFA) into the bloodstream from white adipose tissue (WAT). FFA can then serve to fuel shivering thermogenesis in muscle (8). In contrast, triglycerides (TG) stored in the brown adipose tissue (BAT) are also mobilized as FFA *via* activation of the SNS, however, these FFA are used primarily within the BAT itself as a fuel to generate heat through uncoupling of oxidative phosphorylation (8). Furthermore, browning of WAT during cold exposure can also be an adaptive mechanism to produce thermogenesis accompanied by increased expression of beige adipocyte markers such as Dio2, PR domain containing 16 (PRDM16), cell death-inducing DNA fragmentation factor α-subunit effector 1 (Cidea), and carnitine palmitoyl transferase-1b (Cpt1b) (9–11). In Humans, short-term cooling increases serum FFA, TG, and total cholesterol concentration (12). Short-term cooling also enhances large very low-density lipoprotein, small low-density lipoprotein, and small high-density lipoprotein particle number (12). Hydrolysis of TG during cold exposure is mainly due to lipoprotein lipase (LPL) that supplies FFA for nonshivering thermogenesis. Short-term cold exposure (i.e., 4–8 h) increased LPL activity in BAT in rats (13), Djungarian hamsters (14), and mice (15). Of note, other lipases such as patatin like phospholipase domain containing 2 [Pnpla2, also known as adipose triglyceride lipase (ATGL)] and hormone-sensitive lipase (HSL) are also affected by cold exposure (16). Interestingly, this cold-induced rise of LPL activity is specific to BAT, while cold exposure decreases epididymal WAT LPL activity in rats (17). Finally, LPL is strongly expressed in the CNS especially in regions involved in the control of the energy balance (18). We have previously shown that a decrease in the expression of LPL in hippocampus (19) or hypothalamus (20) led to the development of obesity and dysregulation of energy homeostasis. Thus, it was tempting to investigate whether hypothalamic LPL was involved in regulation of body temperature depending on different ambient conditions, such as moderate hypothermia relative to thermoneutrality (22°C) or cold (4°C). The passage from 22 to 4°C represents an adaptive challenge requiring increased thermogenic needs (21). To that end, mice deficient for LPL in mediobasal (ARC + VMH) hypothalamus (MBHΔ^{Lpl}) were generated by bilateral injections of adeno-associated virus (AAV)-cre in the mediobasal hypothalamus (MBH) of Lpl$^{lox/lox}$ male mice, leading to a 30–35% decrease in hypothalamic LPL activity as previously published (20). The results obtained from these mice suggest that MBH LPL dampens cold-induced thermogenesis and its deletion promotes cold adaptation.

MATERIALS AND METHODS

The experimental protocol was approved by the institutional animal care and use committee of the Paris Diderot University (CEEA40) and the agreement # 03752.02 was given to the project.

Animal Models

Ten-week-old Lpl$^{lox/lox}$ male mice (Jackson laboratory, strain B6.129S4-Lpltm1Ijg/J, no. 006503) and wild-type littermates were used as controls. They were housed individually in stainless steel cages in a room maintained at 22 ± 1°C with lights on from 07:00 a.m. to 07:00 p.m. They were given a standard laboratory diet (proteins 19.4%, carbohydrates 59.5%, lipids 4.6%, vitamins, and minerals 16.5%) and water *ad libitum*.

Viral Production

An AAV Cre-GFP was used in order to induce genetic recombination within the hypothalamus in Lpl$^{lox/lox}$ mice. The plasmid CBA.nls myc Cre.eGFP expressing the myc-nls-Cre-GFP fusion protein was kindly provided by Richard Palmiter (University of Washington, Seattle, WA, USA). Adeno-associated viruses of the serotype 2/9 (AAV2/9) (6×10^{11} vg/ml and 1.7×10^{8} pi/μl) known to have a neuronal tropism (22) were produced by the viral production facility of the UMR INSERM 1089 (Nantes, France).

Surgical and Stereotactic Procedures

At 10 weeks of age, mice were anesthetized with isoflurane and received an i.p. injection of 180 μg/kg buprenorphine hydrochloride (Axiance, Pantin, France) analgesic before being placed on a stereotaxic frame. AAVs were injected bilaterally into the MBH (stereotactic coordinates are relative to bregma: $x \pm 0.5$ mm; y −1.64 mm; z −5.7 mm) at a rate of 0.20 μl/min for a total of 0.5 μl per side, in Lpl$^{lox/lox}$ mice (MBHΔ^{Lpl} mice) and in wild-type C57Bl6/J used as controls (MBH^{Lpl} mice). At the end of surgical procedures, mice received an i.p. injection of 50 μg/kg ketoprofen (Mérial, Lyon, France). Intraperitoneal probes (Anipill, Caen, France) were placed in animals during a laparotomy, to measure their body temperature. Animals had 7 days postsurgery to recover.

Indirect Calorimetry

Animals were individually housed in a cage with lights on from 7 a.m. to 7 p.m. and an ambient temperature of 22 ± 0.5 or 7°C (see Cold Exposure). All animals were acclimated to their cages for 48 h before experimental measurements. Data were collected every 15 min. Animals were analyzed for total energy expenditure (kcal/h), oxygen consumption and carbon dioxide production (VO_2 and VCO_2, where V is the volume), respiratory exchange rate (RER = VCO_2/VO_2), food intake (g), and locomotor activity (beam breaks/h) using calorimetric cages with bedding, food and water *ad libitum* (Labmaster, TSE Systems GmbH, Bad Homburg, Germany). The instrument combined a set of highly sensitive feeding and drinking sensors for automated online measurement. To allow measurement of ambulatory movements, each cage was embedded in a frame with an infrared light beam-based activity monitoring system with online measurement at 100 Hz; the detection of movement operated efficiently in both light and dark phases, allowing continuous recording. Gas ratio was determined using an indirect open-circuit calorimeter (23), which monitored O_2 and CO_2 concentrations by volume at the inlet ports of a tide cage with an airflow of 0.4 l/min, with regular comparisons to an empty reference cage. Total energy expenditure was calculated according to the Weir equation, using respiratory gas exchange measurements (24). The flow was previously calibrated with O_2 and CO_2 mixture of known concentrations (Air Liquide, S.A. France). Fatty acid oxidation was calculated from the following equation: fat ox (kcal/h) = energy expenditure × (1 − RER/0.3) according to Bruss et al. (25). Animals were monitored for body weight and composition at the beginning and end of the experiment. Data analysis was carried out with Excel XP using extracted raw values of VO_2 consumption, VCO_2 production (ml/h), and energy expenditure (kcal/h). Subsequently, each value was expressed either as a function of total body weight or total lean tissue mass extracted from the EchoMRI analysis.

Cold Exposure

Mice were exposed to cold at 10 days postsurgery. For the acute cold exposure, animals were exposed to 4°C for 4 h in a refrigerated bench, closed by a Plexiglas plate. Additional mice were exposed to 7°C for 24 h in the calorimetric cages described above.

Body Temperature Measurement

Body temperature was measured every 15 min by telemetry with intraperitoneal probes (Anipill, Caen, France). Data were collected by an electronic monitor and transferred to a computer with Anipill Software (Anipill, Caen, France) and were then extracted to an Excel XP file (Microsoft France, Issy-les-Moulineaux, France) before analysis.

BAT Temperature Measurement

Skin temperature surrounding BAT was recorded with an infrared camera (B335: Compact-Infrared-Thermal-Imaging-Camera; FLIR; West Malling, Kent, UK) and analyzed with a FLIR-Tools-Software (FLIR; West Malling, Kent, UK) as previously described (26, 27). For each image, the area surrounding BAT was delimited and the average temperature of the skin area was calculated as the average of two pictures/animal.

Tissue Collection

Brain tissues were dissected following the Glowinski and Iversen technique (28); hypothalamus, hippocampus, striatum, and cerebral cortex were immediately frozen. In addition, subcutaneous (WATsc) and gonadal white adipose tissue (WATgon) and intrascapular BAT were also collected and immediately frozen for further measurement of mRNA of gene of interest.

LPL Activity Assay

Heparin-releasable LPL activity was assayed in brain regions using a Roar LPL activity assay kit (RB-LPL, Roar Biomedical, Inc.). Briefly, tissues were lysed in 500 μl of assay buffer (150 mM NaCl, 10 mM Tris, 2 mM EDTA, pH 7.4) and incubated for 45 min at 37°C with an equivalent volume of heparin (100 U/ml). After incubation, samples were centrifuged for 10 min at 3,000 *g*, and aliquots (10 μl for mice) of the aqueous phase deposited on LPL substrate emulsion in 96-well black microplates (VWR International, # 25227-304) and incubated for 1 h at 37°C. Finally, fluorescence was read using a fluorimeter (370 nm excitation/450 nm emission), and compared to a standard curve made using known concentrations of prehydrolyzed LPL substrate. LPL activity was expressed as μmoles of FFA produced per minute per gram of tissue.

Real-Time Quantitative PCR

Total RNA was isolated from the hippocampus dissected at day 28 at the end of the experimentation using RNeasy Lipid Tissue mini kit (Qiagen, Courtaboeuf, France). Real-time quantitative PCR was carried out in a LightCycler 480 detection system (Roche, Meylan, France) using the Light-Cycler FastStart DNA Master plus SYBR Green I kit (Roche). The mRNA transcript level for each gene was normalized against the mean of 2 HKG: rpL19 and TBP, which we have previously shown to be unaffected by LPL inhibition (**Table 1**: primers sequences).

Statistical Analysis

Data are expressed as mean ± SEM. Statistical analysis were performed using Student's test or ANOVA followed by two-by-two Bonferroni *post hoc* test (GraphPad software). $p < 0.05$ was considered significant. Representative bar graph is expressed as mean ± SEM.

RESULTS

Cold Exposure Decreases Hypothalamic LPL Activity in Control Mice

There was no effect of nutritional status (i.e., fed or fasted) on hypothalamic LPL activity at either ambient temperatures of 22 or 4°C (**Figure 1A**). In contrast, in fed and fasted mice, exposure

TABLE 1 | Primers used for RT-qPCR.

Gene	Forward primers	Reverse primers
Rpl19	gggcaggcatatgggcata	ggcggtcaatcttcttggatt
Tbp	ggggagctgtgatgtgaagt	ccaggaaataattctggctca
Abhd5	atctttggagcccgatcct	cttctggctgatctgcatacac
Pnpla2	tgaccatctgccttccaga	tgtaggtggcgcaagaca
Plin5	Agctggagcccgtgtcta	gggcatccactgcattct
Lipe HSL	gcctggcaaaatctgagg	gcctccgtggatgtgaac
Lpl	tttgtgaaatgccatgacaag	cagatgctttcttctcttgtttgt
CerS1	ggagctactgcgcttacctg	ccatgcctgacctccagt
Clock	ccagtcagttggtccatcatt	tggctcctaactgagctgaaa
Bmal1	cgactcattgatgccaagac	tgcacttcattctacagaacagaga
Cidea	ttcaaggccgtgttaagga	cctttggtgctaggcttgg
Cpt1b	Ctcctttcctggctgaggt	gatctggaactgggggatct
Prdm16	Cctaaggtgtgcccagca	caccttccgcttttctaccc
Dio2	tggcatgccctgtaggtt	tgagaagtctggtacatcagcaa
Ucp1	ggctctgcaggagtccgaagt	ggcgtgagtgcaagaacaaaa
Ucp2	tttgggtttggttgtttttga	ggaggcagatgcaggtagat
Ucp3	ctgcctgtccatcagttcaa	ccagtcctaacaattccctaaaga
AdRβ3	cagccagccctgttgaag	ccttcatagccatcaaacctg

Rpl19, ribosomal protein L19; Tbp, TATA-box binding protein; Abhd5, α/β hydrolase domain containing 5; Pnpla2, patatin-like phospholipase domain containing 2 (ATGL); Plin5, perilipin5; Lipe HSL, lipase hormone sensitive; Lpl, lipoprotein lipase; CerS1, ceramide synthase1; Clock, clock circadian regulator; Bmal1, brain and muscle Arnt-like protein-1; CIDEA, cell death-inducing DNA fragmentation factor alpha subunit-like effector A; Cpt1b, carnitine palmitoyltransferase 1B; PRDM16, PR/SET domain 16; Dio2, type 2 iodothyronine deiodinase; UCP, uncoupling protein; AdRβ3, β3-adrenergic receptor.

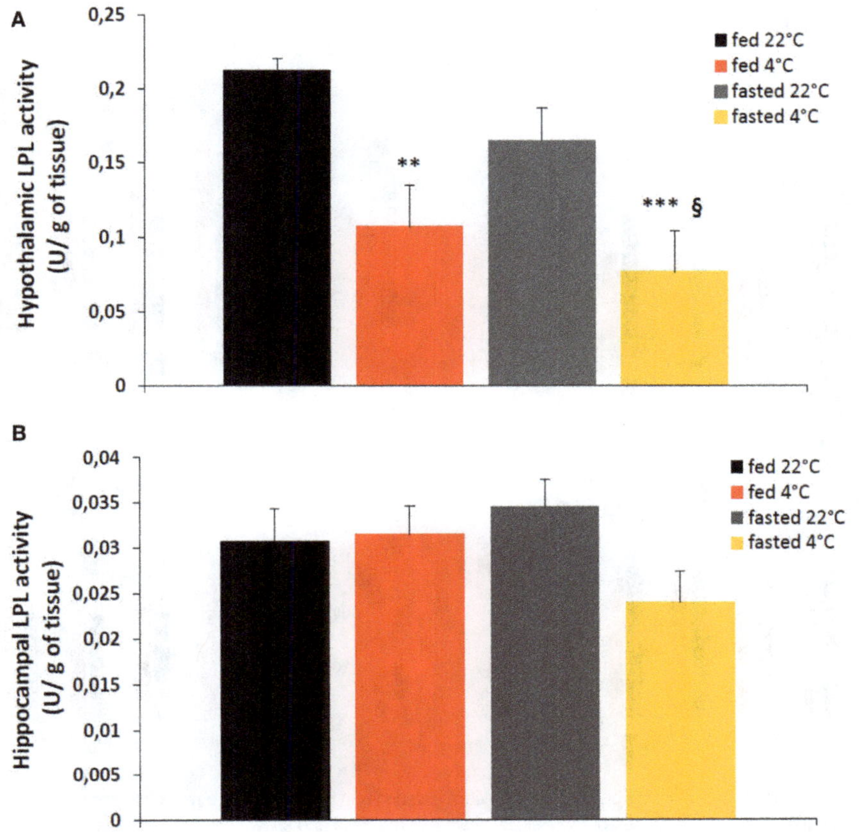

FIGURE 1 | An acute cold exposure (4 h at 4°C) decreases significantly enzymatic activity of lipoprotein lipase (LPL) in hypothalamus **(A)** but not in hippocampus **(B)**. LPL activity is expressed in enzymatic units (U, μmol/min) per g of tissue. Data are mean ± SEM, $n = 6$–8 for each group. *$p < 0.05$ and ***$p < 0.001$ vs. mice "fed 22°C", §$p < 0.05$ vs. "fasted 22°C" mice.

after 4 h at 4°C, there was a significant decrease of ~50% in hypothalamic LPL activity when compared with LPL activity at 22°C (**Figure 1A**). Of note, neither nutritional status nor ambient temperature exposure affected hippocampal LPL activity (**Figure 1B**).

Cold Exposure-Induced Changes in Brain Gene Expression in Control Mice

Cold exposure induced changes in the expression of genes involved in lipid metabolism in several brains areas (**Figure 2**). LPL mRNA expression was decreased in response to cold exposure in the hypothalamus, as well as hormone sensitive lipase (Lipe HSL) and abhydrolase domain containing 5 (Abhd5) mRNA. Conversely, acute cold exposure significantly increased the expression of hypothalamic perilipin 5 (Plin 5). Abdh5 and Plin5 are cofactors of the Pnpla2 (also known as ATGL) which catalyzes the first step of intracellular TG hydrolysis (16). No change was observed in the expression of other hypothalamic genes involved in lipid metabolism. In the hippocampus and in the cerebral cortex, cold exposure significantly increased the expression of the perilipin 5 gene, as in the hypothalamus, but also of Pnpla2 (ATGL). No change in expression of mRNAs for lipases or their cofactors was seen in the striatum. For clock genes, the expression of hypothalamic Bmal1 and Clock and striatal Bmal1 mRNA was decreased, while hippocampal Bmal1 expression was increased after cold exposure.

MBH LPL Depletion Dysregulates Body Temperature and Energy Metabolism

As shown in **Table 2** and **Figure 3A**, MBHΔ^{Lpl} mice had a significantly lower basal temperature at 22°C when compared with controls mice. However, after 4 h of exposure to 4°C, MBHΔ^{Lpl} mice maintained their body temperature, whereas body temperature fell by 1.2°C during the first hour of cold exposure in control MBH^{Lpl} mice and remained lower than that in MBHΔ^{Lpl} mice for the remainder of the 4 h exposure period. Figure S1 in Supplementary Material shows the temperature time courses for MBH^{Lpl} and MBHΔ^{Lpl} mice with their respective controls maintained at 22°C during 4 h. The thermogenic images over intrascapular BAT pads (**Figures 3B–E**) and their quantification (**Figure 3F**) appear to correlate with comparable changes in core body temperature measured with the intraperitoneal probes: MBHΔ^{Lpl} mice maintained their BAT temperature after 4 h at 4°C, whereas BAT temperature significantly dropped in controls. The expression of uncoupling protein 1 (UCP1) mRNA was upregulated by 4 h of cold exposure in both MBH^{Lpl} and MBHΔ^{Lpl} mice (**Figure 3G**), and there was no difference

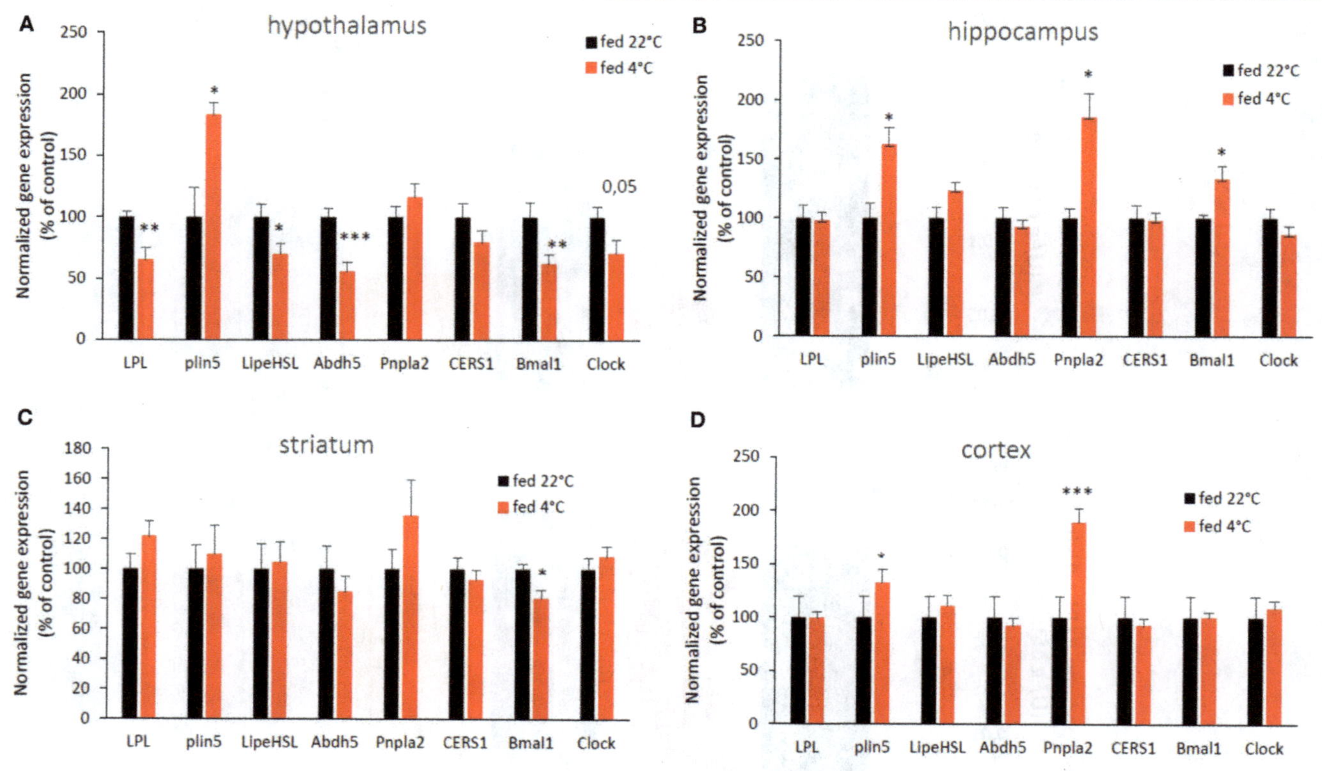

FIGURE 2 | An acute cold exposure modifies the expression of several genes involved in lipid metabolism and circadian clock. mRNA expression in **(A)** hypothalamus, **(B)** hippocampus, **(C)** striatum, and **(D)** cerebral cortex. Data are mean ± SEM and show change of expression rate relative to mRNA for mice at 22°C. $n = 8–10$ for each group. *$p < 0.05$, **$p < 0.01$, and ***$p < 0.001$ vs. "fed 22°C" group.

TABLE 2 | Comparison of physiological parameters of MBH^{Lpl} vs. MBHΔ^{Lpl}.

	MBH^{Lpl}	MBHΔ^{Lpl}
Body weight (g)	33.07 ± 0.63	31.45 ± 0.88
Body temperature before cold exposure (°C)	37.02 ± 0.12	36.26 ± 0.10***
Body temperature after cold exposure (°C)	35.58 ± 0.21	36.34 ± 0.15*
Temperature change (°C)	−1.31 ± 0.14	+0.02 ± 0.11***
Weight of BAT at 22°C (g)	0.11 ± 0.026	0.15 ± 0.025
Weight of BAT at 4°C (g)	0.094 ± 0.015	0.16 ± 0.021*

Data are mean ± SEM, n ≥ 6 for each group.
**p < 0.05 vs. MBH^{Lpl}.*
****p < 0.001 vs. MBH^{Lpl}.*

in UCP2 and UCP3 expressions in MBHΔ^{Lpl} mice compared to controls. In MBH^{Lpl} mice, expression of β3-adrenoreceptor mRNA was significantly downregulated by the cold exposure, whereas it remained higher in MBHΔ^{Lpl} mice than their 4°C controls (**Figure 3G**).

During 24 h cold exposure in metabolic cages, food intake was similar in the two groups (Figure S2 in Supplementary Material), and the locomotor activity was decreased during the daylight (cf. **Figure 4A**) whereas energy expenditure normalized to lean mass was significantly increased in MBHΔ^{Lpl} mice (**Figure 4B**). A shown in **Figure 4C**, these mice presented a trend toward carbohydrate-oriented metabolism before the nighttime, as demonstrated by the increased RER, and consequently a lower rate of fatty acid oxidation (**Figure 4D**).

The Expression of "Beige" Genes Is Increased in WAT of MBHΔ^{Lpl} Mice

Beige adipocytes share some common characteristics with brown adipocytes and have a thermogenic potential. In the subcutaneous adipose tissue, some genes involved in WAT thermogenic function ("beige" markers; CPT1b and PRDM16) were significantly increased in basal conditions (22°C) and remained higher compared than controls after a cold exposure. Moreover, Dio2 gene expression was higher at 22°C in MBHΔ^{Lpl} mice (**Figure 5A**). In gonadal WAT, PRDM6 trended to be more expressed in MBHΔ^{Lpl} mice compared to controls at 22°C, and DiO2 expression showed a ninefold increase following cold exposure (cf. **Figure 5B**).

DISCUSSION

In the present study, we first demonstrated that hypothalamic LPL mRNA expression and activity were regulated as a function of ambient temperatures between 22 and 4°C. Indeed, cold exposure induced a selective decrease in both LPL activity and gene expression in hypothalamus with no change in mRNA expression in the hippocampus, striatum, or cerebral cortex when temperature dropped from 22 to 4°C. It has already been reported that the expression of the brain LPL was regulated by the 72 h fasted or fed states (29), but to our knowledge it is the first time that a regulation as a function of the ambient temperature is described. We and others previously reported that brain LPL

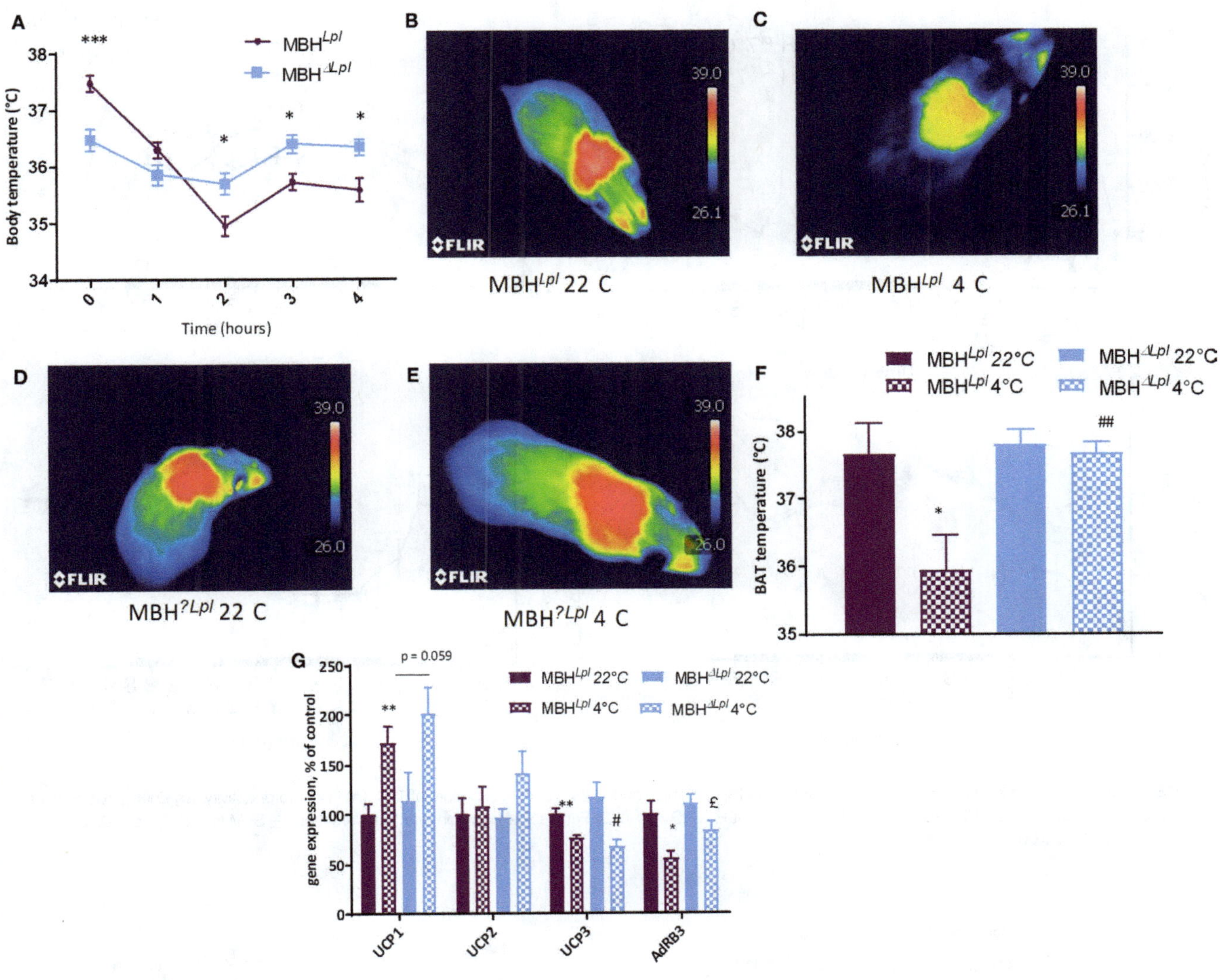

FIGURE 3 | An acute exposure to cold decreases body and skin temperature of MBH^{Lpl} mice but not of MBHΔ^{Lp} **(A)**. Thermic images of brown adipose tissue (BAT) temperature of MBH^{Lpl} at 22°C **(B)** and at 4°C **(C)** shows a decrease during the acute cold exposure whereas BAT temperature of MBHΔ^{Lpl} at 22°C **(D)**, is maintained at 4°C **(E)**. The value of BAT temperature for MBH^{Lpl} and MBHΔ^{LPL} mice at 22°C and at 4°C is presented in a global histogram, showing a decrease of BAT temperature at 4°C for MBH^{Lpl} whereas MBHΔ^{Lpl} mice present no difference at 4°C **(F)**. Measurement of mRNA expression in BAT **(G)** for uncoupling proteins (UCPs) show no difference between MBH^{Lpl} and MBHΔ^{Lpl} at 22 or at 4°C. mRNA expression of AdRβ3 is increased at 4°C in MBHΔ^{LPL} group compared to MBH^{Lpl}. Data are mean ± SEM (*n* = 6). $^{*}p < 0.05$, $^{**}p < 0.01$ vs. MBH^{Lpl} mice at 22°C, $^{£}p < 0.05$ vs. MBH^{Lpl} mice at 4°C.

regulated energy balance. Wang et al. showed that neuronal LPL deficiency promoted obesity and maladaptive responses to environmental challenges (30–32). In addition, we reported that specific deletion of hypothalamic LPL induced body weight gain without hyperphagia, but with increased food efficiency in mice (20). Such increased body weight gain was partly explained by an early decrease in locomotor activity, a trend toward lower energy expenditure at night, and a preferential use of carbohydrate rather than lipid metabolism (20).

In the present study, after having shown that LPL in the hypothalamus was regulated by ambient temperature, it seemed important to investigate whether partial invalidation of LPL in the hypothalamus could therefore influence cold adaptation in mice in order to establish a cause-and-effect relationship between the expression of the enzyme and body temperature. It is well known that the control of BAT thermogenesis is regulated by the CNS (33, 34), and numerous studies have highlighted the role of the hypothalamus and the SNS in such control (4, 27, 35, 36). Besides the preoptic area of the hypothalamus, which is considered as a major coordinator of thermoregulation since it receives inputs from skin and visceral thermoreceptors, other nuclei participate in thermoregulation such as the paraventricular, the ARC and the VMH [review by Labbe et al. (4)]. Although the characterization of the neurons controlling thermogenesis remains unsolved, data pointed toward a role for the melanocortin system in stimulating BAT thermogenesis (3). In the ARC, NPY/AgRP neurons inhibit this system while POMC neurons activate it. In the VMH, steroidogenic factor 1 (SF1) neurons are known to affect BAT thermogenesis (37), by integrating both AMPK and mTOR signaling (27, 38, 39). We showed here that

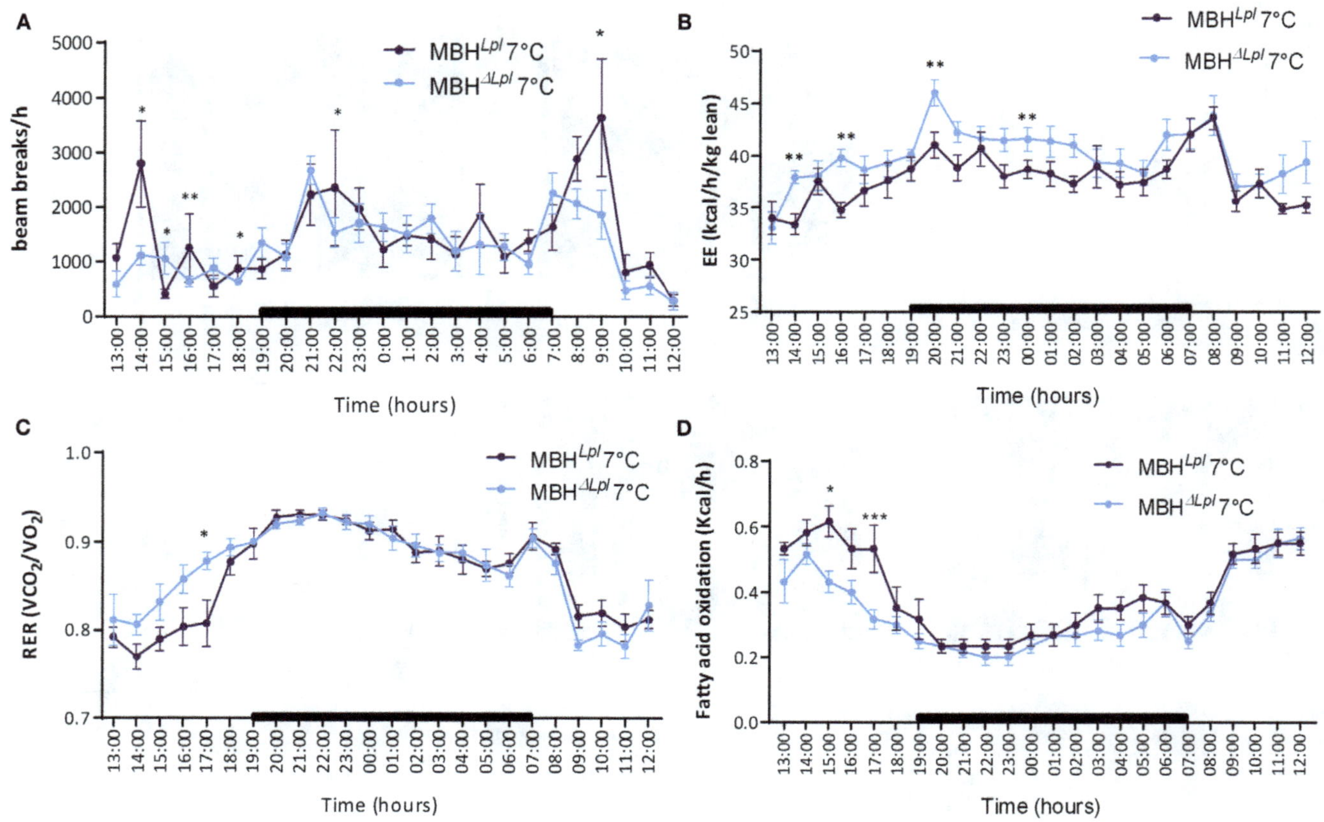

FIGURE 4 | Calorimetry and locomotor activity for MBH^{LPL} and $MBH\Delta^{LPL}$ mice during 24 h of cold exposure at 7°C. **(A)** Locomotor activity. **(B)** Energy expenditure normalized per lean body mass. **(C)** Respiratory exchange rate (RER, VCO_2/VO_2). **(D)** Fatty acids oxidation rate. Data are mean ± SEM (n = 5–6). $^{*}p < 0.05$, $^{**}p < 0.01$, and $^{***}p < 0.001$ vs. MBH^{Lpl} mice.

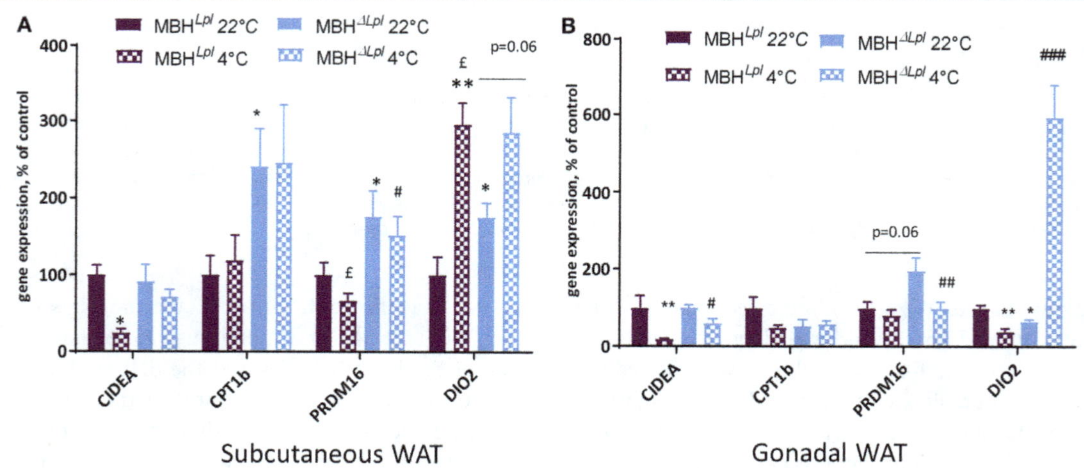

FIGURE 5 | Depletion of lipoprotein lipase in the mediobasal hypothalamus (MBH) increases mRNA expression of genes responsible for "beigeing" in white adipose tissues (WATs). **(A)** mRNA expression in subcutaneous WAT. **(B)** mRNA expression in gonadal WAT. Data are mean ± SEM and show change of expression rate relative to mRNA for mice at 22°C. n = 4–6 for each group. $^{*}p < 0.05$, $^{**}p < 0.01$ vs. MBH^{Lpl} mice at 22°C, $^{\#}p < 0.05$, $^{\#\#}p < 0.01$, and $^{\#\#\#}p < 0.001$ vs. MBH^{Lpl} mice at 4°C, $^{£}p < 0.05$ vs. $MBH\Delta^{Lpl}$ mice at 22°C.

LPL deficiency in the hypothalamus induced a dysregulation of thermogenesis in mice at both normal vivarium temperature of 22 and at 4°C. Specifically, $MBH\Delta^{Lpl}$ mice had a significant lower core body temperature compared to controls when the ambient temperature was 22°C. This result seemed to be consistent with our previous observations (i.e., sparing fatty acids and decrease of locomotor activity) (20). As mentioned above, we observed a decrease in both LPL expression and activity in the hypothalamus in normal mice during cold exposure. This result could suggest that the physiological decrease of LPL activity in the hypothalamus, in response to decreased ambient temperature plays a role in adaptive thermogenesis. In accordance with this hypothesis, when the hypothalamic LPL was permanently depleted, the animals presented higher energy expenditure and were able to defend their body temperature more successfully than controls when exposed at 4°C for 4 h. At mild temperature corresponding to their basal housing conditions (22°C), LPL depleted animals displayed a significantly lower body temperature (0.76°C), which could be interpreted as an attempt of saving energy for the long-term. The subsequent question might be to understand how a drop in hypothalamic LPL activity could induce this change in energy flow and control body temperature. It can be hypothesized that a decrease in hypothalamic LPL activity and thus a consequent local decrease in TG hydrolysis and FFA availability could be sensed by specialized neurons (18, 40) as a "thrifty" signal and a need for metabolic adaption. By specifically decreasing LPL in MBH, we therefore mimicked such a "thrifty behavior" that was observed during cold exposure (41). Because $MBH\Delta^{Lpl}$ mice had already displayed some metabolic features of cold exposure, the actual exposure to cold (at least during a short period) did not induce a greater decrease in their body temperature, whereas this occurred in the control mice (decreased body temperature from 37 to 35°C). This adaption could be explained by a modulation of the circadian clock, as it has been shown that transcription of genes involved in the metabolism can be regulated by the circadian clock. For example, Clock and Bmal1 genes favor transcription of Lpl (42). Interestingly, we showed that exposure to cold decreased the expression of Bmal1 and Clock. The downregulation of Bmal1 and Clock mRNA could partly explain the decrease observed for LPL mRNA. Furthermore, a recent study suggested the existence of an independent circadian clock in the VMH (43). Exposure to cold could have an impact on hypothalamic circadian clock and thus on LPL expression. Finally, this study by Orozco-Solis et al. showed that a mouse model KO for Bmal1 in Sf1 neurons of the VMH was associated with increased BAT temperature throughout the diurnal cycle. Therefore, a decrease of Bmal1 expression during cold exposure in $MBH\Delta^{Lpl}$ compared to MBH^{Lpl} could contribute to explain the preservation of BAT temperature.

Partial deletion of hypothalamic LPL also resulted in changes in mRNA expression of some marker genes of adipocyte function as well as thermogenesis-related genes. We measured some of these genes of interest in subcutaneous and gonadal adipose tissues. Interestingly, $MBH\Delta^{Lpl}$ mice that were exposed to mild temperature showed a significant increase in PRDM16 expression in WATsc and a tendency in WATgon when compared with controls. PRDM16 is a critical transcriptional regulator of thermogenesis and the increase of PRDM16 in WATsc of $MBH\Delta^{Lpl}$ mice could be interpreted as an attempt to adapt to their decreased body temperature at an ambient temperature of 22°C. It has been reported that adipocyte-specific deletion of PRDM16 markedly inhibited beige adipocyte function in subcutaneous fat following cold exposure or β3-agonist treatment (44). Thus, browning may occur in WATsc of $MBH\Delta^{Lpl}$ mice as an adaptation to chronically lowered body temperature. However, it must be pointed out that such adaptation was not sufficient to bring the body temperature back to that observed in the control mice. This can be explained by the fact that other parameters were also affected by the hypothalamic deletion of LPL (20).

Interestingly, mRNA expression of Dio2, the enzyme that activates T4 to 3,3′,5-triiodothyronine (T3) was also significantly elevated in WATsc of $MBH\Delta^{Lpl}$ mice compared to controls exposed to 22°C. Dio2 is also known as being a thermogenesis-related gene (9). As for PRDM16, the local increase in Dio2 mRNA could be interpreted as an adaptation to the decrease in body temperature through increased local production of T3. During cold exposure, mRNA expression of Dio2 in WATsc was significantly increased in controls to reach a value similar to $MBH\Delta^{Lp}$ mice. As mentioned, exposure to cold induced a decrease in the body temperature of control mice (from 37 to 35°C) while that of $MBH\Delta^{LPL}$ mice remained constant compared to exposure to mild. During cold exposure, PRDM16 expression remained significantly higher in WATsc of $MBH\Delta^{LPL}$ mice compared to controls. In WATgon, Dio2 was significantly upregulated in $MBH\Delta^{Lp}$ mice exposed to 4°C as compared with their controls. This could be related to the fact that they managed to maintain their body temperature: the upregulation of browning markers, already present at 22°C, may in part explain the absence of significant fluctuation in body temperature during exposure to cold. In particular, de Jesus et al. showed that increased Dio2 expression in BAT played a key role for local production of T3, even in a situation where serum concentrations of both T3 and T4 remained constant during cold stress (24 h at 4°C) (7). Such a result highlighted a key role for local production of T3 through activation of Dio2.

Finally, skin temperature surrounding BAT was recorded as an indirect index of thermogenesis and BAT function. In control mice, skin temperature decreased when mice were exposed to cold whereas it remained unchanged compared to mild temperature exposure for $MBH\Delta^{Lpl}$. This could be related to the decrease in body temperature that we also observed. However, in both groups UCP1 mRNA expression was increased during cold temperature when compared to mild exposure. Again, this difference in response between the two groups in the face of cold exposure suggests that the deficiency of LPL in the hypothalamus regulated energy homeostasis and especially thermogenesis.

In conclusion, we demonstrate here for the first time, that LPL in hypothalamus is a negative regulator of thermogenesis. Normal adaptation to a drop-in temperature involves a decrease in hypothalamic LPL activity that promotes cold-induced thermogenesis. A chronic decreased in LPL activity in hypothalamus could impair the regulation of body temperature in response to changes in ambient temperature. More generally, a defect in the central sensing of lipids could compromise the survival of individuals during winter and more particularly when a lack of food also occurred.

AUTHOR CONTRIBUTIONS

ML, SL, CC-G, and CM designed experiments. EL, RD, NK, CC, and CC-G performed experiments. EL, CC-G, and CM prepared the manuscript. RD, CC, and ML edited the manuscript. The entire study was supervised by CC-G and CM.

ACKNOWLEDGMENTS

This study was supported by grants from National Research Agency (ANR SVSE 1 2011: "lipobrain") and ANR-16-CE14-0026 "Fat4Brain," from the European Foundation for Study of Diabetes (EFSD/Lilly Research Fellowship Programme 2014), from Ministerio de Economía y Competitividad (MINECO cofunded by the FEDER Program of EU (ML: SAF2015-71026-R and from Xunta de Galicia (ML: 2015-CP079 and 2016-PG068. CC was recipient of Sara Borrell Contract from ISCIII. We want to warmly thank Pr Barry E. Levin for reading and editing the manuscript.

REFERENCES

Castellani JW, Young AJ. Human physiological responses to cold exposure: Acute responses and acclimatization to prolonged exposure. *Auton Neurosci* (2016) 196:63–74. doi:10.1016/j.autneu.2016.02.009

McKitrick DJ. Expression of fos in the hypothalamus of rats exposed to warm and cold temperatures. *Brain Res Bull* (2000) 53(3):307–15. doi:10.1016/S0361-9230(00)00346-4

De Jonghe BC, Hayes MR, Banno R, Skibicka KP, Zimmer DJ, Bowen KA, et al. Deficiency of PTP1B in POMC neurons leads to alterations in energy balance and homeostatic response to cold exposure. *Am J Physiol Endocrinol Metab* (2011) 300(6):E1002–11. doi:10.1152/ajpendo.00639.2010

Labbe SM, Caron A, Lanfray D, Monge-Rofarello B, Bartness TJ, Richard D. Hypothalamic control of brown adipose tissue thermogenesis. *Front Syst Neurosci* (2015) 9:150. doi:10.3389/fnsys.2015.00150

Fregly MJ. Activity of the hypothalamic-pituitary-thyroid axis during exposure to cold. *Pharmacol Ther* (1989) 41(1–2):85–142. doi:10.1016/0163-7258 (89)90103-4

Lopez M, Alvarez CV, Nogueiras R, Dieguez C. Energy balance regulation by thyroid hormones at central level. *Trends Mol Med* (2013) 19(7):418–27. doi:10.1016/j.molmed.2013.04.004

de Jesus LA, Carvalho SD, Ribeiro MO, Schneider M, Kim SW, Harney JW, et al. The type 2 iodothyronine deiodinase is essential for adaptive thermogenesis in brown adipose tissue. *J Clin Invest* (2001) 108(9):1379–85. doi:10.1172/JCI13803

Himms-Hagen J. Lipid metabolism during cold-exposure and during cold-acclimation. *Lipids* (1972) 7(5):310–23. doi:10.1007/BF02532649

Kurylowicz A, Jonas M, Lisik W, Jonas M, Wicik ZA, Wierzbicki Z, et al. Obesity is associated with a decrease in expression but not with the hypermethylation of thermogenesis-related genes in adipose tissues. *J Transl Med* (2015) 13:31. doi:10.1186/s12967-015-0395-2

Lau P, Tuong ZK, Wang SC, Fitzsimmons RL, Goode JM, Thomas GP, et al. Roralpha deficiency and decreased adiposity are associated with induction of thermogenic gene expression in subcutaneous white adipose and brown adipose tissue. *Am J Physiol Endocrinol Metab* (2015) 308(2):E159–71. doi:10.1152/ajpendo.00056.2014

Velazquez-Villegas LA, Perino A, Lemos V, Zietak M, Nomura M, Pols TWH, et al. TGR5 signalling promotes mitochondrial fission and beige remodelling of white adipose tissue. *Nat Commun* (2018) 9(1):245. doi:10.1038/s41467-017-02068-0

Hoeke G, Nahon K, Bartelt A, Dinnes D, Drettwan D, Pagel P, et al. Cold exposure beneficially modulates HDL metabolism in mice and humans. *Atherosclerosis* (2017) 263:e95. doi:10.1016/j.atherosclerosis.2017.06.308

Carneheim C, Nedergaard J, Cannon B. Beta-adrenergic stimulation of lipoprotein lipase in rat brown adipose tissue during acclimation to cold. *Am J Physiol* (1984) 246(4 Pt 1):E327–33. doi:10.1152/ajpendo.1984.246.4.E327

Klingenspor M, Ebbinghaus C, Hulshorst G, Stohr S, Spiegelhalter F, Haas K, et al. Multiple regulatory steps are involved in the control of lipoprotein lipase activity in brown adipose tissue. *J Lipid Res* (1996) 37(8):1685–95.

Kuusela P, Jacobsson A, Klingenspor M, Rehnmark S, Heldmaier G, Cannon B, et al. Contrasting adrenergic effects on lipoprotein lipase gene expression in the brown adipose tissue of intact mice and in cultured brown adipocytes from mice. *Biochim Biophys Acta* (1997) 1345(3):327–37. doi:10.1016/S0005-2760(97)00008-8

Caimari A, Oliver P, Palou A. Adipose triglyceride lipase expression and fasting regulation are differently affected by cold exposure in adipose tissues of lean and obese Zucker rats. *J Nutr Biochem* (2012) 23(9):1041–50. doi:10.1016/j.jnutbio.2011.05.008

Radomski MW. Effect of cold exposure on serum lipids and lipoproteins in the rat. *Can J Physiol Pharmacol* (1966) 44(5):711–9. doi:10.1139/y66-091

Cruciani-Guglielmacci C, Magnan C. Brain lipoprotein lipase as a regulator of energy balance. *Biochimie* (2017) 143:51–5. doi:10.1016/j.biochi.2017.07.012

PicardA,RouchC,KassisN,MoulleVS,CroizierS,DenisRG,etal.Hippocampal lipoprotein lipase regulates energy balance in rodents. *Mol Metab* (2014) 3(2):167–76. doi:10.1016/j.molmet.2013.11.002S2212-8778(13)00120-8

Laperrousaz E, Moulle VS, Denis RG, Kassis N, Berland C, Colsch B, et al. Lipoprotein lipase in hypothalamus is a key regulator of body weight gain and glucose homeostasis in mice. *Diabetologia* (2017) 60:1314–24. doi:10.1007/ s00125-017-4282-7

Abreu-Vieira G, Xiao C, Gavrilova O, Reitman ML. Integration of body temperature into the analysis of energy expenditure in the mouse. *Mol Metab* (2015) 4(6):461–70. doi:10.1016/j.molmet.2015.03.001

Chakrabarty P, Rosario A, Cruz P, Siemienski Z, Ceballos-Diaz C, Crosby K, et al. Capsid serotype and timing of injection determines AAV transduction in the neonatal mice brain. *PLoS One* (2013) 8(6):e67680. doi:10.1371/journal.pone.0067680

Arch JR, Hislop D, Wang SJ, Speakman JR. Some mathematical and tech- nical issues in the measurement and interpretation of open-circuit indirect calorimetry in small animals. *Int J Obes (Lond)* (2006) 30(9):1322–31. doi:10.1038/sj.ijo.0803280

Weir JB. New methods for calculating metabolic rate with special reference to protein metabolism. *J Physiol* (1949) 109(1–2):1–9. doi:10.1113/jphysiol.1949. sp004363

Bruss MD, Khambatta CF, Ruby MA, Aggarwal I, Hellerstein MK. Calorie restriction increases fatty acid synthesis and whole body fat oxidation rates. *Am J Physiol Endocrinol Metab* (2010) 298(1):E108–16. doi:10.1152/ajpendo.00524.2009

Contreras C, Nogueiras R, Dieguez C, Rahmouni K, Lopez M. Traveling from the hypothalamus to the adipose tissue: the thermogenic pathway. *Redox Biol* (2017) 12:854–63. doi:10.1016/j.redox.2017.04.019

Martinez-Sanchez N, Seoane-Collazo P, Contreras C, Varela L, Villarroya J, Rial-Pensado E, et al. Hypothalamic AMPK-ER stress-JNK1 axis mediates the central actions of thyroid hormones on energy balance. *Cell Metab* (2017) 26(1):212–29.e212. doi:10.1016/j.cmet.2017.06.014

Glowinski J, Iversen LL. Regional studies of catecholamines in the rat brain.

The disposition of [3H]norepinephrine, [3H]dopamine and [3H]dopa in various regions of the brain. *J Neurochem* (1966) 13(8):655–69. doi:10.1111/j.1471-4159.1966.tb09873.x

Gavin LA, Cavalieri RR, Moeller M, McMahon FA, Castle JN, Gulli R. Brain lipoprotein lipase is responsive to nutritional and hormonal mod- ulation. *Metabolism* (1987) 36(10):919–24. doi:10.1016/0026-0495(87) 90124-7

Wang H, Astarita G, Taussig MD, Bharadwaj KG, DiPatrizio NV, Nave KA, et al. Deficiency of lipoprotein lipase in neurons modifies the regulation of energy balance and leads to obesity. *Cell Metab* (2011) 13(1):105–13. doi:10.1016/j.cmet.2010.12.006

Wang H, Eckel RH. Lipoprotein lipase in the brain and nervous system. *Annu Rev Nutr* (2012) 32:147–60. doi:10.1146/annurev-nutr-071811-150703

Pellinen J, Wang H, Eckel RH. Mice with altered brain lipoprotein metabolism display maladaptive responses to environmental challenges that may predispose to weight gain. *Metab Syndr Relat Disord* (2014) 12(6):339–46. doi:10.1089/met.2013.0141

Cannon B, Nedergaard J. Brown adipose tissue: function and physiological sig- nificance. *Physiol Rev* (2004) 84(1):277–359. doi:10.1152/physrev.00015.2003

Morrison SF, Madden CJ, Tupone D. Central neural regulation of brown adipose tissue thermogenesis and energy expenditure. *Cell Metab* (2014) 19(5):741–56. doi:10.1016/j.cmet.2014.02.007

Contreras C, Gonzalez-Garcia I, Martinez-Sanchez N, Seoane-Collazo P, Jacas J, Morgan DA, et al. Central ceramide-induced hypothalamic lipotox-icity and ER stress regulate energy balance. *Cell Rep* (2014) 9(1):366–77. doi:10.1016/j.celrep.2014.08.057

Richard D. Cognitive and autonomic determinants of energy homeostasis in obesity. *Nat Rev Endocrinol* (2015) 11(8):489–501. doi:10.1038/nrendo.2015.103

Choi YH, Fujikawa T, Lee J, Reuter A, Kim KW. Revisiting the ventral medial nucleus of the hypothalamus: the roles of SF-1 neurons in energy homeostasis. *Front Neurosci* (2013) 7:71. doi:10.3389/fnins.2013.00071

Martinez de Morentin PB, Gonzalez-Garcia I, Martins L, Lage R, Fernandez-Mallo D, Martinez-Sanchez N, et al. Estradiol regulates brown adipose tissue thermogenesis via hypothalamic AMPK. *Cell Metab* (2014) 20(1):41–53. doi:10.1016/j.cmet.2014.03.031

Martinez de Morentin PB, Martinez-Sanchez N, Roa J, Ferno J, Nogueiras R, Tena-Sempere M, et al. Hypothalamic mTOR: the rookie energy sensor. *Curr Mol Med* (2014) 14(1):3–21. doi:10.2174/1566524013666131118103706

Magnan C, Levin BE, Luquet S. Brain lipid sensing and the neural control of energy balance. *Mol Cell Endocrinol* (2015) 418(Pt 1):3–8. doi:10.1016/j.mce.2015.09.019

Zhao ZJ, Chi QS, Cao J, Han YD. The energy budget, thermogenic capacity and behavior in Swiss mice exposed to a consecutive decrease in tempera-tures. *J Exp Biol* (2010) 213(Pt 23):3988–97. doi:10.1242/jeb.046821

Delezie J, Dumont S, Dardente H, Oudart H, Grechez-Cassiau A, Klosen P, et al. The nuclear receptor REV-ERBalpha is required for the daily balance of carbohydrate and lipid metabolism. *FASEB J* (2012) 26(8):3321–35. doi:10.1096/fj.12-208751

Orozco-Solis R, Aguilar-Arnal L, Murakami M, Peruquetti R, Ramadori G, Coppari R, et al. The circadian clock in the ventromedial hypothalamus con-trols cyclic energy expenditure. *Cell Metab* (2016) 23(3):467–78. doi:10.1016/j. cmet.2016.02.003

Cohen P, Levy JD, Zhang Y, Frontini A, Kolodin DP, Svensson KJ, et al.

Ablation of PRDM16 and beige adipose causes metabolic dysfunction and a subcutaneous to visceral fat switch. *Cell* (2014) 156(1–2):304–16. doi:10.1016/j.cell.2013.12.021

18

Overlapping Neural Endophenotypes in Addiction and Obesity

*Andréanne Michaud[1], Uku Vainik[1,2], Isabel Garcia-Garcia[1] and Alain Dagher[1]**

[1] *Department of Neurology and Neurosurgery, Montreal Neurological Institute, McGill University, Montreal, QC, Canada,*
[2] *Faculty of Social Sciences, Institute of Psychology, University of Tartu, Tartu, Estonia*

Correspondence:
Alain Dagher
alain.dagher@mcgill.ca

Impulsivity refers to a tendency to act rapidly without full consideration of consequences. The trait is thought to result from the interaction between high arousal responses to potential rewards and poor self-control. Studies have suggested that impulsivity confers vulnerability to both addiction and obesity. However, results in this area are unclear, perhaps due to the high phenotypic complexity of addictions and obesity. Focusing on impulsivity, the aim of this review is to tackle the putative overlaps between addiction and obesity in four domains: (1) personality research, (2) neurocognitive tasks, (3) brain imaging, and (4) clinical evidence. We suggest that three impulsivity-related domains are particularly relevant for our understanding of similarities between addiction and obesity: lower self-control (high Disinhibition/low Conscientiousness), reward sensitivity (high Extraversion/Positive Emotionality), and negative affect (high Neuroticism/Negative Emotionality). Neurocognitive studies have shown that obesity and addiction are both associated with increased impulsive decision-making and attention bias in response to drug or food cues, respectively. Mirroring this, obesity and different forms of addiction seem to exhibit similar alterations in functional MRI brain activity in response to reward processing and during self-control tasks. Overall, our review provides an integrative approach to understand those facets of obesity that present similarities to addictive behaviors. In addition, we suggest that therapeutic interventions targeting inhibitory control may represent a promising approach for the prevention and/or treatment of obesity.

Keywords: obesity, addiction, impulsivity, brain, personality and neurocognitive characteristics

INTRODUCTION

Obesity and addiction are complex and heterogeneous conditions at the intersection of biology and mental health. A bulk of scientific literature has highlighted the importance of neurobiological and neuropsychological factors in the pathophysiology of obesity (**Figure 1**) (1, 2). More importantly, growing evidence suggests that obesity shares common mechanisms with addiction in terms of neurobiological systems that underlie reward and self-regulation processes (3–5). The goal of this review is to critically assess the putative overlaps between addiction and obesity in four domains: (1) personality research, (2) neurocognitive task, (3) brain imaging, and (4) clinical evidence.

BRAIN MECHANISMS OF APPETITE CONTROL AND UNDER CONTROL

Three interconnected brain systems control food intake and eating behavior: (1) the hypothalamus, which responds to internal energy-balance signals, (2) the limbic system [amygdala/hippocampus, insula, orbitofrontal cortex (OFC), and striatum], which is involved in learning and memory and

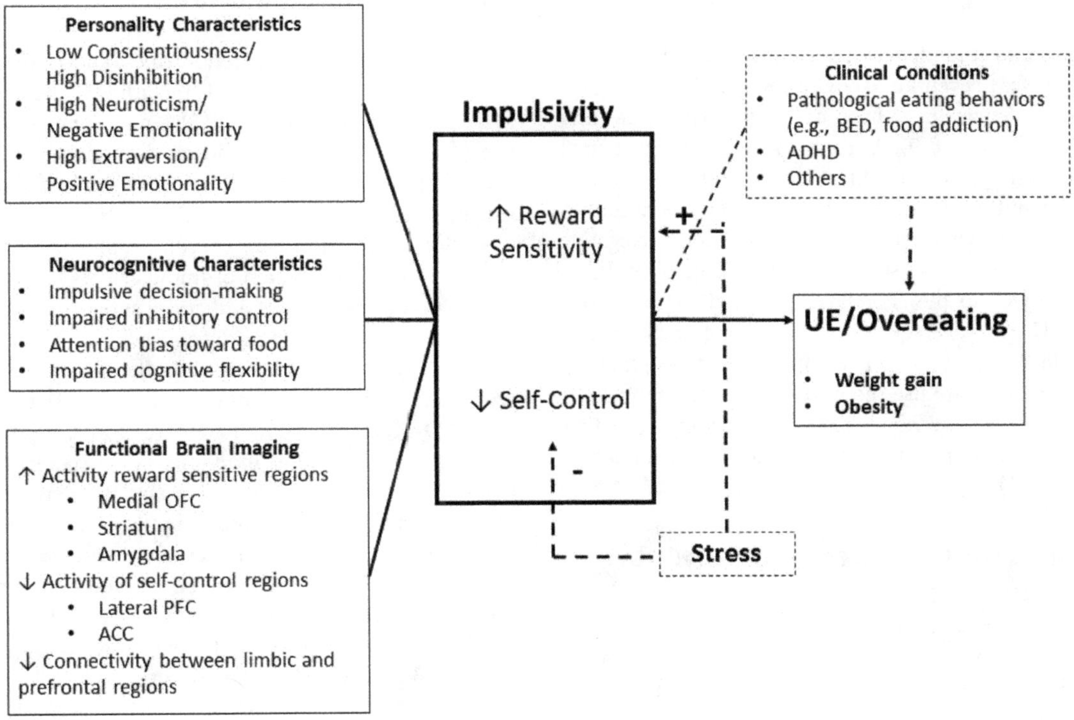

FIGURE 1 | Brain endophenotype of obesity vulnerability. Personality, cognitive, and functional brain imaging characteristics that increase obesity vulnerability. Uncontrolled eating (UE) results from an interaction of elevated reward sensitivity and poor self-control. OFC, orbitofrontal cortex; PFC, prefrontal cortex; ACC, anterior cingulate cortex; BED, binge-eating disorder; ADHD, attention deficit/hyperactivity disorder; BMI, body mass index.

encodes the value or incentive salience of foods, and (3) the cortical (mostly prefrontal) cognitive control system, which enables behavioral self-regulation (6, 7). The normal function of these systems maintains energy homeostasis, enables learning about the nutrient content of foods, and promotes motivation to seek and consume foods as appropriate.

However, individual differences in neurobiological mechanisms involved in the control of food choices and food intake likely explain why some individuals are more susceptible to weight gain than others (8). Indeed, obese individuals may have neurocognitive characteristics that predispose them to overeating upon exposure to favorable environmental or endogenous conditions. One such characteristic is impulsivity. Although many definitions exist (9–14), impulsivity is generally considered as the tendency to act rapidly without full consideration of consequences (15). Sharma et al. (16) recently conducted a meta-analytic principal-components analysis and proposed that impulsivity is a multidimensional construct that includes various distinct psychological components such as disinhibition, neuroticism, extraversion, sensation seeking, inattention, impulsive decision-making, insufficient inhibitory control, and lack of cognitive flexibility (16–19).

Impulsivity is a key component of several neuropsychiatric disorders such as attention deficit/hyperactivity disorder (ADHD), mania, and personality disorders (20, 21). Numerous studies have reported that impulsivity, a personality trait generally observed in individuals with addiction (22–26), may also be associated with high-calorie dietary choices, undercontrolled eating, and the development of obesity (27–31). For instance, individuals characterized by frequent disinhibited behavior and elevated response to potential rewards may be more vulnerable to develop unhealthy weight gain when exposed to the so-called "obesogenic" food-abundant environment (8, 28, 32). Neurobehavioral processes that lead to impulsivity result from the interaction of high arousal response to potential rewards (i.e., reward sensitivity) and poor self-control (i.e., rash spontaneous impulsivity) (14, 28). The reward system is generally thought to encompass projection sites of mesolimbic dopamine neurons, while self-control is dependent on the prefrontal cortex (PFC), especially the lateral PFC, and dorsal anterior cingulate cortex (ACC). Individual differences in impulsivity might constitute a common denominator across obesity and drug addiction. In this regard, several studies have suggested the existence of similarities between addiction and obesity in reward processing (4, 5, 33, 34). In fact, addictive drugs are thought to be addictive by virtue of their actions on neural systems that primarily control appetitive responses to natural rewards such as food (4, 34–36). Dopamine circuitry plays an important role in encoding the reinforcing values of addictive substances (37, 38).

Considering that some neurobehavioral characteristics that confer vulnerability to addiction may also represent risk factors for obesity, this review is aimed at tackling the following question: is the impulsive and poor self-control phenotype identified in drug addiction also present in obesity? The next sections review the evidence in terms of personality, neurocognitive tasks, neuroimaging, and clinical evidence.

PERSONALITY CHARACTERISTICS

Personality traits reflect tendencies for cognitive, emotional, and behavioral responses to events and environments. Traits that capture impulsive tendencies have been associated with unhealthy weight gain and addiction (39). A recent meta-analytic principal component analysis of personality questionnaires identified three distinct impulsivity subdomains (16): (1) Disinhibition versus Constraint/Conscientiousness, (2) Neuroticism/Negative Emotionality, and (3) Extraversion/Positive Emotionality. These dimensions map well to the "Big Five" personality framework (40), the UPPS (Urgency, Perseverance, Premeditation, Sensation Seeking) scale (19), and many other impulsivity conceptualizations (9, 11). Therefore, we use this three-factor decomposition of impulsivity (16) as a base framework to organize evidence that personality-measured impulsivity is associated with addiction and obesity (**Table 1**).

High Disinhibition and Low Constraint/ Conscientiousness

The Disinhibition versus Constraint/Conscientiousness factor is comprised of two subfactors associated with behavioral dyscontrol: lack of planning, leading to an inability to refrain from hasty actions, and a lack or perseverance, leading to an inability to maintain self-control in the face of adversity (16). This factor relates to the following measures from commonly used personality scales: lack of perseverance and lack of premeditation from the UPPS, low Conscientiousness from the NEO-Personality Inventory-Revised NEO-PI-R, and motor impulsivity and non-planning impulsivity from the Barratt Impulsiveness Scale (BIS) (16).

TABLE 1 | Summary of the main associations between addiction or obesity and impulsivity measurements.

	Addiction	Obesity
Personality characteristics		
High Disinhibition and low Constraint or Conscientiousness	+	+
High Neuroticism/Negative Emotionality	+	+, NS
High Extraversion/Positive Emotionality	+	+, NS
Neurocognitive characteristics		
Impulsive decision-making	+	+
Impaired inhibition	+, NS	+
Inattention	+	+, NS
Impaired set-shifting	+, NS	+
Functional brain imaging		
Reward/motivation system		
Medial OFC/VMPFC	↑ Activity	↑ Activity
Striatum	↑ Activity	↑ Activity
Amygdala	↑ Activity	↑ Activity
Self-regulation system		
Lateral PFC	↓ Activity	↓ Activity ↓ OFC–PCF connectivity
ACC	↓ Activity ↓ ACC–striatum connectivity	↓ Activity

+, positive associations; NS, association not significant; ↑, increase; ↓, decrease; OFC, orbitofrontal cortex; VMPFC, ventromedial prefrontal cortex; PFC, prefrontal cortex; ACC, anterior cingulate cortex.

Low scores on Conscientiousness have been related to various addictive behaviors (41) including illegal substance abuse (42–44), gambling problems (45), smoking (46–48), and alcohol use (49, 50). Furthermore, lower Conscientiousness increases the risk of relapse after treatment (51). Lack of planning or premeditation assessed using the UPPS scale is also an independent predictor of addiction (52). Thus, the high Disinhibition and low Conscientiousness domain of impulsivity is consistently associated with a higher risk of addiction, supporting the importance of self-control in resisting drug abuse.

Similarly, obesity has consistently been associated with a reduced level of Conscientiousness (28, 53) as measured by the NEO-PI, an association confirmed in a large meta-analysis involving close to 50,000 individuals (54). In a large heterogeneous sample using the BIS, Meule and Blechert (31) found that higher attentional and motor impulsivities were predictive of higher body mass index (BMI) after statistical adjustment for age and sex. However, the effect was small, and non-planning impulsivity was not significantly associated with BMI (31). Finally, studies using the UPPS have also found an association between BMI and lack of perseverance, which is the inability to persist with challenging tasks (55, 56). Furthermore, higher levels of habitual disinhibition, as measured by the Three-Factor Eating Questionnaire, have been associated with body weight gain over time (57). Disinhibition here refers to a tendency to overeat upon exposure to palatable foods or stressful situations, a trait related to consciousness and self-control. In light of these studies, obesity seems to be associated with high Disinhibition and low Conscientiousness. These traits may increase the tendency of an individual to overeat in certain situations and may complicate the maintenance of behaviors associated with body weight reduction in obese individuals (58).

Neuroticism/Negative Emotionality

The factor Neuroticism/Negative Emotionality reflects a tendency to act rashly in response to negative emotions and to experience cravings when in negative mood states (16). It is reflected in neuroticism in the NEO-PI-R, negative urgency in the UPPS, and attentional impulsivity in the BIS (16).

Neuroticism (NEO-PI-R) has been related to various addiction syndromes, including substance abuse (42–44), problem gambling (45), smoking (46–48), and alcohol use (49, 50), and also with increased risk of relapse after treatment (51). Other studies have also reported an association between negative urgency (UPPS) and substance addiction (59–62). In sum, individuals with addictive behavior may engage in drug use as a way of coping with stress and negative emotion.

The relationship between obesity and neuroticism is less evident. While previous reviews have reported a link between the two (28, 53), a recent meta-analysis found no association (54). A possibility for this lack of significant relationship is that body weight is specifically linked only to some facets of negative emotionality. For example, it has been consistently shown that only the impulsiveness subfactor ("N5:Impulsiveness") of the NEO-PI-R correlates with adiposity (39, 63). Findings from the UPPS support this notion, as negative urgency, a tendency to experience strong impulses during negative affect, has been linked to greater BMI (55, 56). Other factors that could obscure the link between obesity and Neuroticism/Negative Emotionality include the fact that the association may be present only in women and that neuroticism may also predispose to underweight, *via* a link to eating disorders (64). This could obscure a linear relationship between obesity and neuroticism in population studies. Finally, the link between neuroticism and obesity could be driven by two questions in the Neuroticism scale of the NEO PI-R that specifically target uncontrolled eating (UE) behavior (65, 66).

In summary, the association between the Neuroticism/Negative Emotionality domain and obesity is somewhat less consistent than that with Conscientiousness and Disinhibition. Nonetheless, this personality trait may predispose an individual to overeating in conditions of emotional distress (67), which may lead to adiposity in the long term.

Extraversion/Positive Emotionality

The Extraversion/Positive Emotionality factor refers to sensation seeking and sensitivity to appetitive or rewarding cues (16). Individuals with high Extraversion/Positive Emotionality are sensitive to positive environmental stimuli and more likely to engage in impulsive or reward-seeking behaviors when they experience positive emotions. They are said to seek novel and exciting experiences. Extraversion/Positive Emotionality correlates with the Extraversion domain in the Five-Factor Model of personality and with Sensation Seeking of the UPPS (16). The Sensitivity to Reward portion of the Sensitivity to Punishment and Sensitivity to Reward Questionnaire (SPSR) is a self-report questionnaire that also assesses this dimension (28, 68).

Numerous studies suggest that reward-driven impulsivity represents a risk factor for both drug addiction and overeating by enhancing the motivation to obtain drugs or palatable foods (69, 70). Higher scores in Extraversion have been related to drug addiction (47). A related trait, positive urgency, the tendency to act rapidly in response to positive emotions, was also correlated to substance addiction (59–62). In addition, Sensation Seeking is commonly associated with substance-use disorders and alcohol problems (62). In sum, the literature is consistent in associating the Extraversion/Positive Emotionality domain of impulsivity to addictive disorders.

Some studies have proposed that high BMI is associated with increased levels of Extraversion (28, 53). Higher scores in Extraversion also seem to predict prospective weight gain (after 2 years) (71). However, contradictory findings do exist, with a meta-analysis (54) failing to show a consistent relationship between obesity and Extraversion in longitudinal studies. However, Davis et al. (72) found that reward sensitivity, as assessed by the SPSR, was associated with maladaptive eating behaviors such as preference for high-calorie foods and overeating (72). They suggested that some individuals may have greater reactivity to food cues and that weight management, in these individuals, may represent a continuous struggle in the modern obesity-promoting food environment. Using the SPSR, this group also demonstrated an inverted U-shaped relationship between reward sensitivity and BMI in a sample of subjects covering a large spectrum of adiposity values, suggesting that lean and severely obese subjects were less sensitive to reward than overweight and obese subjects (73). By using the Behavioral Activation Scale, other groups have also provided evidence of a quadratic relationship between BMI and reward sensitivity (74, 75). To explain this curvilinear relationship, Davis and Fox (73) proposed that both hyper- and hyposensitivity to reward could predispose to obesity. The possibility of an inverted U-shape relationship between BMI and Extraversion suggests that differences in the range of sampled BMI across studies might account for the discrepancies in the literature. In addition to this, gender might modulate the correlation between Extraversion and BMI. For women, lower scores in Extraversion seem to relate to higher adiposity (76, 77), while the opposite has been reported in males (76, 78).

Overall, although contradictory findings do exist, the current evidence points in the direction of similar impulsivity profiles in obesity and addictive disorders. Specifically, these two disorders seem to share lower cognitive control (high Disinhibition/low Conscientiousness), and a tendency toward making impulsive decisions in response to positive (high Extraversion/Positive Emotionality) and negative (high Neuroticism/Negative Emotionality) mood states. **Figure 2** displays a comprehensive overview of personality differences in obesity and addiction as derived from Ref. (39, 42, 79). This shows that while, on a broad level, obesity seems to be similar to addictive behaviors, there are also differences at the finer level of personality subscales.

NEUROCOGNITIVE TASKS

Laboratory-based neurocognitive tasks can be used to measure inhibitory control or self-regulation. Commonly used examples are the delay discounting task, the stop-signal task (SST), the Go/No-Go task, the Stroop task, and the Wisconsin card sorting task (WCST) (80). These neurocognitive tests assess various dissociable dimensions of impulsivity, including impulsive choice, impulsive responding, and inattention (15, 81). Sharma et al. (16) also performed a meta-analytic principal-components factor analysis of the most commonly used behavioral task measures of impulsivity and they identified four major domains: (1) impulsive decision-making, (2) inattention, (3) inhibition, and (4) shifting. The next sections describe how these four domains of impulsivity are associated with addiction and obesity (**Table 1**).

Impulsive Decision-Making

Impulsive decision-making (or impulsive choice) refers to a tendency not to delay gratification and to prefer immediately available rewards (16). It is typically tested with the delay discounting task, in which participants must choose between an immediate, smaller monetary sum and a larger, delayed amount (82). A steeper delay discounting rate is associated with a greater preference for immediate rewards, which reflects impulsive decision-making.

Kirby and Petry (83) have demonstrated using a questionnaire version of this task that substance-addicted individuals have higher discounting rates for delayed rewards than controls. Two meta-analyses also provided strong evidence that steeper impulsive discounting rate is associated with the severity and the frequency of addictive behaviors (84, 85). The magnitude of the

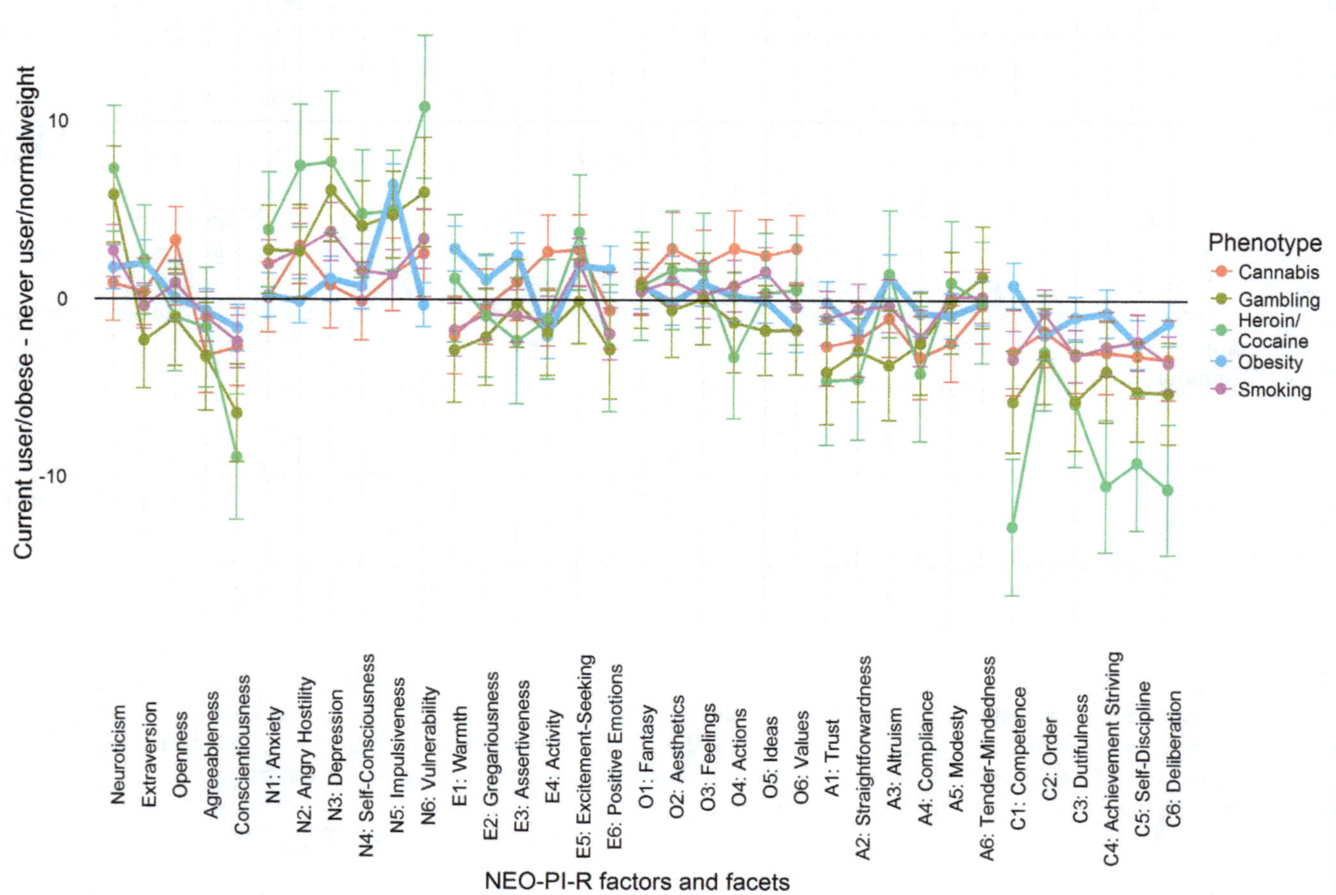

FIGURE 2 | Personality profiles of obesity and addictive phenotypes according to NEO-personality inventory revised. We present the difference in T-score units between obese minus normal weight group and addiction phenotype group minus control group. On a broad factor level, all phenotypes share higher Neuroticism (high Negative Emotionality) and lower Agreeableness and Conscientiousness (high Disinhibition). However, on a finer facet level, the profiles become less similar. For instance, obesity sets apart from other addictions only peaking at one facet of Neuroticism, and not on all facets of Conscientiousness. Therefore, while there are broad similarities, obesity and addictive phenotypes are not fully similar to each other. Mean scores were obtained from these papers (39, 42, 79).

association was similar between various types of addictive problems (alcohol, gambling, tobacco, cannabis, opiates, and stimulants) (85). The same group also reported a similar relationship in obesity: although results vary, their meta-analysis concluded that obesity is associated with steeper delay discounting of future monetary and food rewards (86). Interestingly, Weygandt et al. (87) recently found that less functional MRI (fMRI) activation of inhibitory-control areas during a delay discounting task is associated with poor weight loss maintenance in the long term. More specifically, obese subjects seem to have greater delay discounting for food compared to other type of rewards. Similarly, substance-addicted subjects have greater delay discounting for drugs compared to other type of rewards (28, 85, 86). Impulsive decision-making in addiction and obesity may explain why some individuals engage in maladaptive behaviors that are immediately rewarding but detrimental in the long run.

Another perspective in impulsive decision-making revolves around the concept of risk sensitivity. Risk sensitivity refers to the individual degree of attraction or aversion to uncertain outcomes (88). A moderate risk-seeking behavior may confer advantages in the discovery of new environments and resources and might lead to experiencing exciting adventures. However, an excessive attraction toward risk may also be associated with adverse consequences and might have a role in the development of drug addiction. In recent years, the concept of risk sensitivity has been used to describe impulsive behavior in addiction and obesity (89, 90). Both addiction and obesity might involve to some extent an approach tendency toward short-term pleasure despite the risk of long-term negative consequences (89, 91). Several studies have suggested the existence of addiction-related alterations in risky choices. For example, compared with healthy controls, participants who binge drink exhibited increased risk-seeking when anticipating large unlikely monetary losses (92). Risky decision-making and higher delay discounting also appear to hamper the maintenance of abstinence following treatment (93).

Relatively few studies have directly examined risk-taking similarities or differences between addiction and obesity to date. One study found that obese individuals with and without binge-eating disorder (BED) made as many risky choices in a monetary task as drug addicts (94).

Inhibition

The inhibition domain refers to the ability to suppress prepotent motor responses (16). Tasks that test inhibition include the Go/No-Go and the SST (80, 82). In the Go/No-Go task, individuals are asked to answer as quickly as possible when a repeated visual stimulus appears (Go signal) but to inhibit their response when a rare stop signal appears (No-Go signal). In the SST task, the stop signal is presented after the Go signal to measure the ability of an individual to stop an already initiated response (95).

Considerable evidence links drug addiction to impaired inhibitory control (96–98). A meta-analysis of 97 studies using the SST or Go/No-Go tasks reported that impaired inhibitory control is generally observed in subjects with heavy substance-use disorders and pathological gambling (99). However, there was lack of evidence for inhibitory deficit in subjects diagnosed with cannabis, opioid, or Internet addiction (99).

Similarly, obesity has been linked to poor inhibitory control. A comprehensive literature review found that obese and overweight individuals have lower inhibitory-control performance in food-specific versions of the SST (100). The authors proposed that the SST may be a good marker to identify individuals at high risk of weight gain or less responsive to weight loss interventions (100). Poor inhibitory control is also associated with higher prospective weight gain (101, 102) and food intake (103). Furthermore, a recent meta-analysis confirmed that obese adults display inhibitory-control deficits compared to lean controls (104). Similar findings have been reported in children and adolescents (104–108). However, Loeber et al. (109) found no significant differences between lean and obese participants in performance during a food-related Go/No-Go task. Furthermore, others did not find an effect of BMI *per se* on SST performance in response to food, but rather a complex interaction between BMI and impulsivity (110).

Furthermore, Voon et al. (111) used a serial reaction time task adapted from rodent experiments to assess a somewhat different form of motor impulsivity: waiting impulsivity or premature responding. They found that premature responses were significantly higher in addicted individuals (alcohol, smoking, and drugs) but not in obese or BED subjects. Thus, certain forms of motor impulsivity seen in addiction are not present in obesity.

Inattention

The third impulsivity domain considered here refers to the ability to focus attention on specific activities while suppressing the response to distracting stimuli (16). The Stroop task is typically used to measure the inattention domain of impulsivity (16). This task requires participants to identify (usually verbally) the color of a written color word, without reading the word itself. When the word is printed in a color that is incongruent with the word (for example, the word blue printed in green), there is a conflict between word reading and color naming. PFC has been implicated in the performance of the Stroop task (112).

A refinement of this task, the "addiction-Stroop," in which the distractor stimuli represent the addictive substance of interest, has also been used to assess altered attentional processes associated with addictive behaviors (113). Indeed, there is considerable evidence that individuals with addiction have an attentional bias toward drug-related cues, which may play an important role in drug craving, consumption, and relapse (114). Similarly, some studies have reported that obese individuals may have attentional biases toward food-related cues, which may increase food consumption and weight gain over time (115). Hall et al. (116) found that elevated levels of inattention were predictors of high-calorie snack consumption. Furthermore, a recent study demonstrated that obese individuals are characterized by lower scores on the traditional Stroop task (117). Even though some reviews reported inconsistent associations between attentional bias for food-related cues and obesity (28, 115, 118, 119), we previously concluded in a comprehensive review that the Stroop task seems to be one of the most consistent cognitive control tasks demonstrating replicated associations with obesity and weight-related eating behaviors (28).

Shifting

Behavioral flexibility, or the ability to switch attentional or task set in response to changing rules, has also been linked to impulsivity (16). It is typically evaluated with the WCST (16). During this task, participants are asked to match a response card to one of four category cards based on specific rules (e.g., color, shape, or number) (120). The rules change over time and subjects need to modify their response accordingly. A tendency to fail to switch is called perseveration, and it may reflect a form of impulsivity. Poor cognitive flexibility has been associated with compulsive behaviors (121, 122).

A recent review by Morris and Voon (122) argued that the links between cognitive flexibility assessed using the WCST and addiction are inconsistent. Indeed, some studies reported impaired cognitive flexibility in substance-addicted (123) and non-substance-addicted (gambling, bulimia) individuals (124). However, others found no significant association between performance on the WCST and addiction (125–127). With respect to obesity, a recent study reported impaired performance on the WCST in obese individuals compared to individuals with other eating disorders (128). In addition, a meta-analysis (121) and systematic review (118) both reported impaired WCST performance in obese individuals compared to controls. However, overweight rather than obese individuals were not characterized by set-shifting impairment (121).

Overall, current evidence from neurocognitive tasks is that obese and addicted individuals are both generally characterized by higher impulsive decision-making and attentional bias in response to drug or food cues. In addition, obesity is usually associated with altered cognitive flexibility (set-shifting) assessed with the WCST and poor inhibitory control assessed with the SST.

NEUROIMAGING

Neuroimaging has been used to investigate functional and anatomical neural correlates of the vulnerability to drug abuse and overeating. Vulnerability to addiction can be considered as resulting from the interaction of increased incentive response to drug cues, propensity for habit formation, poor self-control, and heightened negative emotionality (129, 130). These processes are related to different but interconnected brain systems: (1) the mesolimbic dopamine system, implicated in reward, motivation, and habit formation, which includes the ventral tegmental area, ventral striatum, anterior insula, OFC, amygdala, and hippocampus and (2) cognitive control circuits, implicated in self-regulation, including middle and inferior lateral PFC, ACC, and insula (131). Previous neuroimaging studies have shed light on the role of the mesolimbic system in the pathophysiology of addiction (132–139). Participants with addiction seem to exhibit increased fMRI activation in ventral striatum, amygdala, and medial regions of OFC in response to drug cues (133). In general, these results are consistent with the observation that participants with drug addictions exhibit a heightened attentional or motivational focus toward drug-related stimuli (130).

With regards to cognitive control circuits, adolescents who initiate substance use seem to exhibit reduced blood oxygen level dependent (BOLD) activity in the dorsolateral prefrontal cortex (DLPFC), putamen, and inferior parietal cortex during a Go/No-Go task, suggesting that baseline dysfunction in these areas could predict the initiation of drug use (140, 141). In this vein, theoretical work has highlighted the key role of PFC areas in the endophenotype of addiction vulnerability (112). For instance, participants with addiction seem to exhibit prefrontal dysfunction, implicating the dorsal PFC (dACC and DLPFC) involved in self-control, the ventromedial prefrontal cortex (VMPFC) involved in emotional regulation and salience attribution, as well as the ventrolateral prefrontal cortex and lateral OFC involved in inhibitory or automatic responses (112). It has been proposed that the PFC is involved in addictive behaviors through its capacity to regulate subcortical regions implicated in reward processes (112, 142). For example, the strength of the connectivity between dACC and striatum has been negatively associated with the severity of nicotine addiction (143). PFC dysfunction might be implicated in an endophenotype named *impaired response inhibition and salience attribution* (112). This endophenotype both increases sensitivity to drug cues and reduces the capacity to inhibit maladaptive behaviors (144). Consistent with these findings, drug craving seems to involve the amygdala, ACC, OFC, and DLPFC (145), suggesting the involvement of both reward-related and inhibitory-control resources.

Numerous brain imaging studies also support the notion that vulnerability to weight gain and overeating may result from the interaction between elevated food reward sensitivity (incentive salience of the cue) and poor inhibitory control. In response to visual food stimuli, participants with obesity exhibit increased activation in the dorsomedial PFC, the ventral striatum, the parahippocampal gyrus, the precentral gyrus, the superior/inferior frontal gyrus (IFG), and the ACC relative to lean subjects (119–121). These brain regions are thought to encode reward responses, incentive salience, motor coordination, and memory. Longitudinal study designs have shown that increased BOLD activity in reward-related areas (i.e., ventral striatum and OFC) predicts weight gain, suggesting a link between heightened reward responsivity and the development of obesity (146, 147). With regards to inhibitory-control circuits, participants with obesity seem to show consistent blunted activity in the DLPFC and insula in response to visual food cues (148), suggesting a reduced engagement of neural resources associated with inhibition, executive control, and interoceptive awareness. Of note, longitudinal studies have reported that increased activation in the DLPFC in response to high-calorie food images is associated with successful voluntary weight loss (149, 150). An interesting possibility is that self-control processes in the DLPFC may downregulate the activity of the VMPFC and thus, modulate eating choices (151). Supporting this model, stronger functional coupling between the DLPFC and the VMPFC has been associated with successful dietary weight loss (102) and healthier dietary decisions (151). Furthermore, other fMRI studies have reported that the regulation of food craving was associated with increased activity in the DLPFC, IFG, and dorsal ACC (152–154).

A few neuroimaging studies in obesity have specifically addressed cognitive control processes by using cued inhibitory-control paradigms. Here, fMRI studies have found negative associations between brain activation in executive-control regions (lateral PFC) and BMI (155–157). Longitudinal studies have reported that activity in the DLPFC during cognitive control tasks seems to predict successful weight loss after treatment (87, 102). Conversely, impairment of cognitive control over appetitive regions may (1) decrease the acquisition of behaviors leading to successful weight loss and (2) enhance the motivation to consume palatable foods, even in the absence of energy requirements (6, 158).

Together, the aforementioned studies suggest that participants with obesity and patients with addictions present similar functional alterations in frontal regions and in mesocorticolimbic circuits. However, to date few neuroimaging studies have directly compared the impact of obesity and various types of addictions on brain activation. This last point is especially relevant, since food and drug cues seem to activate similar brain regions involved in reward processes, such as striatum, amygdala, OFC, and insula (135). A previous meta-analysis observed that participants with obesity and subjects with different forms of substance addiction exhibited similar heightened BOLD activity in the amygdala and ventral striatum in response to the relevant cues (food in obesity and drugs in addiction) (159).

Overall, current fMRI studies provide evidence for the existence of shared neural mechanisms associated with obesity and different forms of addiction. Poor inhibitory control in combination with increased reward sensitivity and attention to cues (foods or drugs) may be relevant for both obesity and addictive disorders.

CLINICAL EVIDENCE

Binge-Eating Disorder

Binge-eating disorder (BED) is an eating disorder characterized by recurrent episodes of consumption of larger than normal amounts of food in short periods of time (160). These binges are associated with a sense of loss of control and subsequent distress and culpability. Many studies report that individuals with BED display increased impulsivity, altered reward sensitivity, and altered attentional and memory biases to food-related stimuli (161, 162). For example, individuals with BED have steeper delay discounting of rewards (163) and lower activation in the PFC regions during inhibitory-control tasks (164, 165), suggesting that impulsivity may be importantly related to BED. BED presents phenotypic similarities with substance-use disorders (166). Indeed, substance-use disorders and BED are both characterized by loss of control over consumption, and chronic overconsumption despite negative consequences (167).

The observation that BED shares behavioral and neural underpinnings with substance-use disorders has led to the use of the expression "food addiction," specifically with respect to individuals who meet BED diagnostic criteria, but also more generally as an explanation for obesity. The model hypothesizes that hyper-palatable foods may lead to an addictive response in vulnerable and high-risk individuals (168, 169). Individual variations in "food addiction" can be operationalized by means of scales such as the Yale Food Addiction Scale (YFAS) (166, 170, 171) or the YFAS 2.0 (a revised version adapted for the DSM-5 criteria for substance-related and addictive disorders) (172). However, the model of "food addiction" in humans remains controversial (173–177). The main criticism is that the model is based mostly on animal studies and that the type and quantity of food that characterize "food addiction" are imprecise (173, 174, 177). Furthermore, animals rarely exhibit addition-like behaviors toward sugar; these behaviors only occur when access to sugar is intermittent, and not because of some neurochemical effect of sugar (177). This failure in characterizing what constitutes an addictive agent in foods has led to some theorists to advocate in favor of referring to the phenomenon as "eating addiction" instead (178). We have proposed the term "UE" (65). In addition, even though "food addiction" scores are positively correlated with several measures of adiposity (179), not all individuals with obesity or BED exhibit "food addiction," and conversely, some individuals displaying "food addiction" are not obese (174, 180). Davis (171) suggests that "food addiction" constitutes the last stage of an overeating spectrum (65) and may represent an extreme subtype of BED. In a similar vein, BED has been strongly associated with obesity; however, BED can also occur in individuals with a wide spectrum of body weight (181). As suggested by previous studies, obese individuals with BED seem to represent a specific and possibly rare subtype of obesity (166, 182). Nonetheless, while the lines between BED, "food addiction," and obesity are ill-defined, these conditions seem to share common characteristics including impulsivity and reward dysfunction.

Attention Deficit/Hyperactivity Disorder

Attention deficit/hyperactivity disorder is a neurodevelopmental disorder characterized by inattention, hyperactivity, and impulsivity (160). Neuroimaging studies have suggested a link between ADHD and dysfunction in frontostriatal circuits. For instance, anatomical studies have observed that participants with ADHD exhibit cortical thinning in the PFC, associated with inhibitory-control deficits (183, 184). A frequent comorbidity of ADHD is substance-use disorders (185–187). For example, a longitudinal study found that children and adolescents with ADHD are at higher risk of substance-use disorders and tobacco smoking after a 10-year follow-up period (188).

There is also growing evidence of a link between ADHD and obesity. However, this relationship remains controversial (189, 190). A recent meta-analytic report found a significant association between obesity and ADHD in both children and adults after controlling for possible confounding factors (e.g., gender, study design, country, and study quality) (190). Conversely, another recent meta-analysis reported that the strength of the association between ADHD and obesity was weak. Nevertheless, the effect size increases with age suggesting that the association is stronger in adults than children (189). Two longitudinal studies found that individuals with ADHD are at higher risk of obesity than controls (191, 192). A recent systematic review found that the strength of the association between ADHD and disordered-eating behavior was moderate (193). Furthermore, genetic correlations were found between ADHD, BMI, and smoking (194). To explain the link between ADHD and obesity, researchers have hypothesized that these two disorders exhibit common neurocognitive features, such as impulsivity and inattention (195). Davis et al. (196) also suggested that individuals with ADHD may be more inattentive to their internal signals of hunger and satiety, which may lead to subsequent overeating. Interestingly, the pharmacological treatment of ADHD with dopaminomimetics may facilitate weight control by modulating satiety signals and eating behaviors (197). Overall, ADHD appears to be associated with both addiction and obesity and with the neural endophenotypes that predispose to both, namely, self-control deficits and impulsivity.

Stress or Emotion Dysregulation

Stress is a ubiquitous risk factor across several psychiatric disorders, and it has important implications for our current understanding of addiction and obesity (198, 199). Studies have shown associations between stress and drug craving (200, 201). Chronic exposure to life stressors also predisposes to the transition from casual drug use to substance abuse (202), and it seems to increase the risk of relapse among abstinent users (202). Stress is one of the central elements of the model of addiction proposed by Koob and Le Moal (203). According to this framework, addiction can be conceived as a continuous process of hedonic and homeostasis dysregulation (204). The *spiraling distress* cycle describes how continued drug use along with failures in self-regulation can cause chronic dysregulation of the reward system. As the drug use escalates, patients reach a pathological state that is characterized by increased negative affect and distress, which are particularly pronounced after drug withdrawal. The model hypothesizes that this aversive emotional state constitutes a powerful motivator for drug-seeking, since patients at severe stages of drug addiction will consume drugs to find relief from distress (203).

With regards to obesity, mounting evidence suggests that stress can modify eating patterns (198, 205). Negative mood states or chronic stress increase subjective appetite or food cravings, selective attention toward food, and individual preferences for high-calorie snacks (e.g., sweets and chocolate) (206–209). Increments in food seeking and food consumption during emotionally demanding situations might relate to the fact that eating a so-called "comfort food" promotes improvements in negative affect (210, 211), in line with the model of Koob and Le Moal. The relationship between stress and food intake, however, presents remarkable interindividual variations. Indeed, stress can be associated with both augmented and diminished appetite (205), with around 30% of the population experiencing increases in appetite, 48% appetite suppression, and the rest no change (212). Studies have suggested that obesity constitutes a crucial predictor of increases in food intake during stress. For instance, while work stress has been associated with weight gain in male participants with elevated BMI, the same psychological stressor leads to weight loss in lean participants (213). Finally, individuals with obesity seem to suffer a higher numbers of adverse life events and chronic stressors compared to lean individuals (198).

Stress acts on brain areas involved in both sides of appetite regulation: the reward/motivation system and the inhibitory-control pathways. For example, Tryon et al. (214) found that in response to high-calorie food pictures, women characterized by higher chronic stress have increased activation in brain regions involved in reward and motivation as well as reduced activation in prefrontal regions. These women also demonstrated greater consumption of high-calorie foods after the scanning session. In a similar vein, Maier et al. (215) compared the neural responses between participants assigned to a laboratory stressor versus those assigned to a neutral condition during a food choice task. Subjects assigned to the stressor put greater value on the taste of the food items presented. Paralleling this, bilateral amygdala and right nucleus accumbens reflected the relative taste value of chosen options more strongly in stressed compared to control participants. The authors interpreted these findings as suggesting that acute stress may increase the rewarding attributes of food stimuli (215). Furthermore, Jastreboff et al. (216) observed that obese individuals exhibit increased activation in striatal, insular, and hypothalamic regions in response to stress and favorite-palatable food cues compared to lean individuals. These increased corticolimbic-striatal activations in response to food cues and stress were also positively associated with food craving ratings, suggesting that some individuals may be at higher risk to consume high-calorie foods during stressful periods (216). On the basis of the theoretical model proposed by Sinha and Jastreboff (198), highly palatable food cues in combination with chronic stress exposure could modulate emotions, metabolic responses (e.g., glucose and energy-balance hormones), and stress-responsive hormones (e.g., adrenocorticotrophin cortisol) that influence brain regions involved in reward, motivation, self-control, and decision-making. Thus, stress sensitivity likely interacts with reward systems to promote either drug use or overeating (or both) in vulnerable individuals (217).

CONCLUSION

Evidence of Non-Overlap

Despite the similarities exposed here there is also evidence that obesity and other addictive behaviors differ and may only overlap partially (218). While some studies have observed higher rates of addictive disorders in obese populations (219, 220), others have reported a lack of significant relationships between addiction and obesity (221–224). Methodological aspects (224) as well as the remarkable intrinsic complexity and heterogeneity associated with obesity and addiction (225) might help to explain the discrepancies observed between studies. Multiple factors (e.g., impulsivity and depressive symptoms) might interact with obesity/eating behavior in complex ways that are difficult to account for in studies with relatively small sample sizes. These factors may explain conflicting studies in the literature. Furthermore, an interesting possibility is that some subtypes of obesity might be at higher risk for developing addictive behavior (33). For instance, some post-bariatric surgery patients seem to exhibit increased rates of addictive problems (226–228). This phenomenon is commonly referred to as "cross addiction" or "addiction transfer."

Limitations of the present review should be acknowledged. Obesity results from a chronic positive imbalance between energy intake and energy expenditure. Almost all studies in obesity and impulsivity presented here describe obese participants in terms of the BMI (kg/m^2). While the BMI is an indicator of total adiposity, an important disadvantage is that it might not necessarily be associated with addictive-like eating patterns. In this vein, it is thus crucial to include a description of the participants in terms of their eating behavior or their UE patterns. Furthermore, clinical conditions that often present in comorbidity with obesity, such as BED or ADHD are not systematically evaluated and excluded in all the studies included in the present review. This point constitutes an important limitation that might obscure or inflate the overlap between addiction and obesity.

Concluding Sentences

Addiction and obesity are health problems with high phenotypic complexity. Growing evidence from personality, cognitive neuroscience, and brain imaging studies suggest that the combination of reduced cognitive control and, to a lesser extent, increased reward sensitivity is a risk factor for the development and maintenance of both syndromes. This is especially true in the domain of cognitive control (**Figure 2**) as measured by the Conscientiousness versus Disinhibition factors on personality questionnaires, by cognitive tasks of executive function, or by diminished recruitment of areas associated with cognitive control, such as the lateral PFC, in fMRI studies. Individuals characterized by high food drive and high cognitive control might better control their body weight in an environment rich in palatable foods.

The present review provides a comprehensive view of impulsivity-related alterations in obesity and addiction, covering results from the personality, neurocognitive, neuroimaging, and clinical fields. The conclusions of the review have the potential to inform clinical approaches aimed at the prevention or treatment of obesity. Diminished self-control is a predictor of poorer treatment outcomes in substance abuse disorders (51) and might also be one in obesity treatment. The findings of the present review might, as such, be of interest to cognitive behavioral therapists aiming to foster impulse control strategies in participants with obesity. Specific inhibitory-control interventions may also represent a promising approach for the prevention of obesity in individuals with poor self-control and high reward sensitivity.

AUTHOR CONTRIBUTIONS

AM: design and conception of the manuscript; wrote the manuscript; and gave final approval. UV and IG: wrote and critically revised the manuscript; gave final approval. AD: design and conception of the manuscript; wrote and critically revised the manuscript; study supervision and responsible for funding; and gave final approval.

FUNDING

This work was supported by operating funds from the Canadian Institutes of Health Research to AD. AM is the recipient of a post-doctoral fellowship from Canadian Institutes of Health Research.

REFERENCES

O'Rahilly S, Farooqi IS. Human obesity: a heritable neurobehavioral disorder that is highly sensitive to environmental conditions. *Diabetes* (2008) 57(11):2905–10. doi:10.2337/db08-0210

Volkow ND, O'Brien CP. Issues for DSM-V: should obesity be included as a brain disorder? *Am J Psychiatry* (2007) 164(5):708–10. doi:10.1176/ajp.2007.164.5.708

Frascella J, Potenza MN, Brown LL, Childress AR. Carving addiction at a new joint? Shared brain vulnerabilities open the way for non-substance addictions. *Ann NYAcad Sci*(2010) 1187:294–315. doi:10.1111/j.1749-6632.2009.05420.x

Volkow ND, Wise RA. How can drug addiction help us understand obesity? *Nat Neurosci* (2005) 8(5):555–60. doi:10.1038/nn1452

Volkow ND, Baler RD. NOW vs LATER brain circuits: implications for obesity and addiction. *Trends Neurosci* (2015) 38(6):345–52. doi:10.1016/j.tins.2015.04.002

Dagher A. Functional brain imaging of appetite. *Trends Endocrinol Metab* (2012) 23(5):250–60. doi:10.1016/j.tem.2012.02.009

Rangel A. Regulation of dietary choice by the decision-making circuitry. *Nat Neurosci* (2013) 16(12):1717–24. doi:10.1038/nn.3561

Boswell RG, Kober H. Food cue reactivity and craving predict eating and weight gain: a meta-analytic review. *Obes Rev* (2016) 17(2):159–77. doi:10.1111/obr.12354

Gray JA. The psychophysiological basis of introversion-extraversion. *Behav Res Ther* (1970) 8(3):249–66. doi:10.1016/0005-7967(70)90069-0

Eysenck SB, Eysenck HJ. The place of impulsiveness in a dimensional system of personality description. *Br J Soc Clin Psychol* (1977) 16(1):57–68. doi:10.1111/j.2044-8260.1977.tb01003.x

Patton JH, Stanford MS, Barratt ES. Factor structure of the Barratt impulsiveness scale. *J Clin Psychol* (1995) 51(6):768–74. doi:10.1002/1097-4679(199511)51:6<768::AID-JCLP2270510607>3.0.CO;2-1

Zuckerman M. *Behavioral Expressions and Biosocial Bases of Sensation Seeking.* New York: Cambridge University Press (1994).

Cloninger CR. A systematic method for clinical description and classification of personality variants. A proposal. *Arch Gen Psychiatry* (1987) 44(6):573–88. doi:10.1001/archpsyc.1987.01800180093014

Dawe S, Loxton NJ. Theroleofimpulsivityinthedevelopmentofsubstanceuse andeatingdisorders.*NeurosciBiobehavRev*(2004)28(3):343–51.doi:10.1016/j.neubiorev.2004.03.007

Dalley JW, Everitt BJ, Robbins TW. Impulsivity, compulsivity, and top-down cognitive control. *Neuron* (2011) 69(4):680–94. doi:10.1016/j.neuron.2011.01.020

Sharma L, Markon KE, Clark LA. Toward a theory of distinct types of "impulsive" behaviors: a meta-analysis of self-report and behavioral measures. *Psychol Bull* (2014) 140(2):374–408. doi:10.1037/a0034418

Robbins TW, Gillan CM, Smith DG, de Wit S, Ersche KD. Neurocognitive endophenotypes of impulsivity and compulsivity: towards dimensional psychiatry. *Trends Cogn Sci* (2012) 16(1):81–91. doi:10.1016/j.tics.2011.11.009

Franken IHA, van Strien JW, Nijs I, Muris P. Impulsivity is associated with behavioral decision-making deficits. *Psychiatry Res* (2008) 158(2):155–63. doi:10.1016/j.psychres.2007.06.002

Whiteside S, Lynam D. The Five Factor Model and impulsivity: using a structural model of personality to understand impulsivity. *Pers Individ Dif* (2001) 4:669–89. doi:10.1016/S0191-8869(00)00064-7

Grant JE, Potenza MN, editors. *The Oxford Handbook of Impulse Control Disorders.* 1st ed. Oxford University Press (2011). Available from: http://www.oxfordhandbooks.com/view/10.1093/oxfordhb/9780195389715.001.0001/oxfordhb-9780195389715

Chamberlain SR, Sahakian BJ. The neuropsychiatry of impulsivity. *Curr Opin Psychiatry* (2007) 20(3):255–61. doi:10.1097/YCO.0b013e3280ba4989

Perry JL, Carroll ME. The role of impulsive behavior in drug abuse. *Psychopharmacology(Berl)*(2008)200(1):1–26.doi:10.1007/s00213-008-1173-0

Potenza MN, Taylor JR. Found in translation: understanding impulsivity and related constructs through integrative preclinical and clinical research. *Biol Psychiatry* (2009) 66(8):714–6. doi:10.1016/j.biopsych.2009.08.004

Verdejo-García A, Bechara A. A somatic marker theory of addiction. *Neuropharmacology* (2009) 56(Suppl 1):48–62. doi:10.1016/j.neuropharm.2008.07.035

Belin D, Mar AC, Dalley JW, Robbins TW, Everitt BJ. High impulsivity predicts the switch to compulsive cocaine taking. *Science* (2008) 320(5881):1352–5. doi:10.1126/science.1158136

Brewer JA, Potenza MN. The neurobiology and genetics of impulse control disorders: relationships to drug addictions. *Biochem Pharmacol* (2008) 75(1):63–75. doi:10.1016/j.bcp.2007.06.043

Davis C. Psychobiological traits in the risk profile for overeating and weight gain. *Int J Obes* (2005) 2009(33 Suppl 2):S49–53. doi:10.1038/ijo.2009.72

Vainik U, Dagher A, Dubé L, Fellows LK. Neurobehavioural correlates of body mass index and eating behaviours in adults: a systematic review. *Neurosci Biobehav Rev* (2013) 37(3):279–99. doi:10.1016/j.neubiorev.2012.11.008

Guerrieri R, Nederkoorn C, Jansen A. The interaction between impulsivity and a varied food environment: its influence on food intake and overweight. *Int J Obes (Lond)* (2008) 32(4):708–14. doi:10.1038/sj.ijo.0803770

Guerrieri R, Nederkoorn C, Stankiewicz K, Alberts H, Geschwind N, Martijn C, et al. The influence of trait and induced state impulsivity on food intake in normal-weight healthy women. *Appetite* (2007) 49(1):66–73. doi:10.1016/j.appet.2006.11.008

Meule A, Blechert J. Trait impulsivity and body mass index: a cross- sectional investigation in 3073 individuals reveals positive, but very small relationships. *Health Psychol Open* (2016) 3(2):2055102916659164. doi:10.1177/2055102916659164

Bryant EJ, King NA, Blundell JE. Disinhibition: its effects on appetite and weight regulation. *Obes Rev* (2008) 9(5):409–19. doi:10.1111/j.1467-789X.2007.00426.x

Davis C, Curtis C, Levitan RD, Carter JC, Kaplan AS, Kennedy JL. Evidencethat "food addiction" is a valid phenotype of obesity. *Appetite* (2011) 57(3):711–7. doi:10.1016/j.appet.2011.08.017

Wise RA, Spindler J, deWit H, Gerberg GJ. Neuroleptic-induced "anhedonia" in rats: pimozide blocks reward quality of food. *Science* (1978) 201(4352):262–4. doi:10.1126/science.566469

Davis C, Carter JC. Compulsive overeating as an addiction disorder. A review of theory and evidence. *Appetite* (2009) 53(1):1–8. doi:10.1016/j.appet.2009.05.018

Kenny PJ. Common cellular and molecular mechanisms in obesity and drug addiction. *Nat Rev Neurosci* (2011) 12(11):638–51. doi:10.1038/ nrn3105

Wise RA. The neurobiology of craving: implications for the understanding and treatment of addiction. *J Abnorm Psychol* (1988) 97(2):118–32. doi:10.1037/0021-843X.97.2.118

Salamone JD, Correa M. Motivational views of reinforcement: impli- cations for understanding the behavioral functions of nucleus accumbens dopamine. *Behav Brain Res* (2002) 137(1–2):3–25. doi:10.1016/ S0166-4328(02)00282-6

Sutin AR, Ferrucci L, Zonderman AB, Terracciano A. Personality and obesity across the adult life span. *J Pers Soc Psychol* (2011) 101(3):579–92. doi:10.1037/a0024286

John OP, Srivastava S, editors. The big five trait taxonomy: history, measurement, and theoretical perspectives. *Handbook of Personality: Theory and Research*. 2nd ed (1999). p. 102–138.

Bogg T, Roberts BW. Conscientiousness and health-related behaviors: a meta-analysis of the leading behavioral contributors to mortality. *Psychol Bull* (2004) 130(6):887–919. doi:10.1037/0033-2909.130.6.887

Terracciano A, Löckenhoff CE, Crum RM, Bienvenu OJ, Costa PT. Five- Factor Model personality profiles of drug users. *BMC Psychiatry* (2008) 8:22. doi:10.1186/1471-244X-8-22

Kotov R, Gamez W, Schmidt F, Watson D. Linking "big" personality traits to anxiety, depressive, and substance use disorders: a meta-analysis. *Psychol Bull* (2010) 136(5):768–821. doi:10.1037/a0020327

Ruiz MA, Pincus AL, Schinka JA. Externalizing pathology and the five-factor model: a meta-analysis of personality traits associated with antisocial person- ality disorder, substance use disorder, and their co-occurrence. *J Pers Disord* (2008) 22(4):365–88. doi:10.1521/pedi.2008.22.4.365

Brunborg GS, Hanss D, Mentzoni RA, Molde H, Pallesen S. Problem gambling and the five-factor model of personality: a large population-based study. *Addiction* (2016) 111(8):1428–35. doi:10.1111/add.13388

Malouff JM, Thorsteinsson EB, Schutte NS. The five-factor model of personality and smoking: a meta-analysis. *J Drug Educ* (2006) 36(1):47–58. doi:10.2190/9EP8-17P8-EKG7-66AD

Hakulinen C, Hintsanen M, Munafò MR, Virtanen M, Kivimäki M, Batty GD, et al. Personality and smoking: individual-participant meta-analysis of nine cohort studies. *Addiction* (2015) 110(11):1844–52. doi:10.1111/add.13079

Terracciano A, Costa PT. Smoking and the five-factor model of personality. *Addiction* (2004) 99(4):472–81. doi:10.1111/j.1360-0443.2004.00687.x

Malouff JM, Thorsteinsson EB, Rooke SE, Schutte NS. Alcohol involvement and the Five-Factor model of personality: a meta-analysis. *J Drug Educ* (2007) 37(3):277–94. doi:10.2190/DE.37.3.d

Ruiz MA, Pincus AL, Dickinson KA. NEO PI-R predictors of alcohol use and alcohol-related problems. *J Pers Assess* (2003) 81(3):226–36. doi:10.1207/S15327752JPA8103_05

Bottlender M, Soyka M. Impact of different personality dimensions (NEO Five-Factor Inventory) on the outcome of alcohol-dependent patients 6 and 12 months after treatment. *Psychiatry Res* (2005) 136(1):61–7. doi:10.1016/j.psychres.2004.07.013

Torres A, Catena A, Megías A, Maldonado A, Cándido A, Verdejo-García A, et al. Emotional and non-emotional pathways to impulsive behavior and addiction. *Front Hum Neurosci* (2013) 7:43. doi:10.3389/fnhum.2013.00043

Gerlach G, Herpertz S, Loeber S. Personality traits and obesity: a systematic review. *Obes Rev* (2015) 16(1):32–63. doi:10.1111/obr.12235

Jokela M, Hintsanen M, Hakulinen C, Batty GD, Nabi H, Singh-Manoux A, et al. Association of personality with the development and persistence of obesity: a meta-analysis based on individual-participant data. *Obes Rev* (2013) 14(4):315–23. doi:10.1111/obr.12007

Murphy CM, Stojek MK, MacKillop J. Interrelationships among impulsive personality traits, food addiction, and body mass index. *Appetite* (2014) 73:45–50. doi:10.1016/j.appet.2013.10.008

Mobbs O, Crépin C, Thiéry C, Golay A, Van der Linden M. Obesity and the four facets of impulsivity. *Patient Educ Couns* (2010) 79(3):372–7. doi:10.1016/j.pec.2010.03.003

Hays NP, Roberts SB. Aspects of eating behaviors "disinhibition" and "restraint" are related to weight gain and BMI in women. *Obesity (Silver Spring)* (2008) 16(1):52–8. doi:10.1038/oby.2007.12

Sullivan S, Cloninger CR, Przybeck TR, Klein S. Personality characteristics in obesity and relationship with successful weight loss. *Int J Obes (Lond)* (2007) 31(4):669–74. doi:10.1038/sj.ijo.0803464

Smith GT, Fischer S, Cyders MA, Annus AM, Spillane NS, McCarthy DM. On the validity and utility of discriminating among impulsivity-like traits. *Assessment* (2007) 14(2):155–70. doi:10.1177/1073191106295527

Whiteside SP, Lynam DR. Understanding the role of impulsivity and externalizing psychopathology in alcohol abuse: application of the UPPS impulsive behavior scale. *Exp Clin Psychopharmacol* (2003) 11(3):210–7. doi:10.1037/1064-1297.11.3.210

Verdejo-García A, Lawrence AJ, Clark L. Impulsivity as a vulnerability marker for substance-use disorders: review of findings from high-risk research, problem gamblers and genetic association studies. *Neurosci Biobehav Rev* (2008) 32(4):777–810. doi:10.1016/j.neubiorev.2007.11.003

Mitchell MR, Potenza MN. Addictions and personality traits: impulsivity and related constructs. *Curr Behav Neurosci Rep* (2014) 1(1):1–12. doi:10.1007/s40473-013-0001-y

Terracciano A, Sutin AR, McCrae RR, Deiana B, Ferrucci L, Schlessinger D, et al. Facets of personality linked to underweight and overweight. *Psychosom Med* (2009) 71(6):682–9. doi:10.1097/PSY.0b013e3181a2925b

Sutin AR, Terracciano A. Five-Factor Model personality traits and the objective and subjective experience of body weight. *J Pers* (2016) 84(1):102–12. doi:10.1111/jopy.12143

Vainik U, Neseliler S, Konstabel K, Fellows LK, Dagher A. Eating traits questionnaires as a continuum of a single concept. Uncontrolled eating. *Appetite* (2015) 90:229–39. doi:10.1016/j.appet.2015.03.004

Vainik U, Mõttus R, Allik J, Esko T, Realo A. Are trait–outcome associations caused by scales or particular items? Example analysis of personality facets and BMI. *Eur J Pers* (2015) 29(6):622–34. doi:10.1002/per.2009

Emery RL, King KM, Fischer SF, Davis KR. The moderating role of negative urgency on the prospective association between dietary restraint and binge eating. *Appetite* (2013) 71:113–9. doi:10.1016/j.appet.2013.08.001

Torrubia R, Ávila C, Moltó J, Caseras X. The sensitivity to punishment and sensitivity to reward questionnaire (SPSRQ) as a measure of Gray's anxiety and impulsivity dimensions. *Pers Individ Dif* (2001) 31(6):837–62. doi:10.1016/S0191-8869(00)00183-5

Kreek MJ, Nielsen DA, Butelman ER, LaForge KS. Genetic influences on impulsivity, risk taking, stress responsivity and vulnerability to drug abuse and addiction. *Nat Neurosci* (2005) 8(11):1450–7. doi:10.1038/nn1583

Dagher A. The neurobiology of appetite: hunger as addiction. *Int J Obes* (2009) 33(S2):S30–3. doi:10.1038/ijo.2009.69

Magee C, Heaven P. Big five personality factors, obesity and 2-year weight gain in Australian adults. *Fac Health Behav Sci* (2011) 3:332–5. doi:10.1016/j.jrp.2011.02.009

Davis C, Patte K, Levitan R, Reid C, Tweed S, Curtis C. From motivation to behaviour: a model of reward sensitivity, overeating, and food preferences in the risk profile for obesity. *Appetite* (2007) 48(1):12–9. doi:10.1016/j.appet. 2006.05.016

Davis C, Fox J. Sensitivity to reward and body mass index (BMI): evidence for a non-linear relationship. *Appetite* (2008) 50(1):43–9. doi:10.1016/j.appet.2007.05.007

Dietrich A, Federbusch M, Grellmann C, Villringer A, Horstmann A. Body weight status, eating behavior, sensitivity to reward/punishment, and gender: relationships and interdependencies. *Front Psychol* (2014) 5:1073. doi:10.3389/fpsyg.2014.01073

Verbeken S, Braet C, Lammertyn J, Goossens L, Moens E. How is reward sensitivity related to bodyweight in children? *Appetite* (2012) 58(2):478–83. doi:10.1016/j.appet.2011.11.018

Faith MS, Flint J, Fairburn CG, Goodwin GM, Allison DB. Gender differences in the relationship between personality dimensions and relative body weight. *Obes Res* (2001) 9(10):647–50. doi:10.1038/oby.2001.86

Davis C, Cerullo D. Fat distribution in young women: associations and interactions with behavioural, physical and psychological factors. *Psychol Health Med* (1996) 1(2):159–67. doi:10.1080/13548509608400015

Brummett BH, Babyak MA, Williams RB, Barefoot JC, Costa PT, Siegler IC. NEO personality domains and gender predict levels and trends in body mass index over 14 years during midlife. *J Res Personal* (2006) 40(3):222–36. doi:10.1016/j.jrp.2004.12.002

Bagby RM, Vachon DD, Bulmash EL, Toneatto T, Quilty LC, Costa PT. Pathological gambling and the five-factor model of personality. *Pers Individ Dif* (2007) 43(4):873–80. doi:10.1016/j.paid.2007.02.011

Chambers CD, Garavan H, Bellgrove MA. Insights into the neural basis of response inhibition from cognitive and clinical neuroscience. *Neurosci Biobehav Rev* (2009) 33(5):631–46. doi:10.1016/j.neubiorev.2008. 08.016

Hamilton KR, Mitchell MR, Wing VC, Balodis IM, Bickel WK, Fillmore M, et al. Choice impulsivity: definitions, measurement issues, and clinical implications. *Personal Disord* (2015) 6(2):182–98. doi:10.1037/per0000099

MacKillop J, Weafer J, Gray JC, Oshri A, Palmer A, de Wit H. The latent structure of impulsivity: impulsive choice, impulsive action, and impulsive personality traits. *Psychopharmacology (Berl)* (2016) 233(18):3361–70. doi:10.1007/s00213-016-4372-0

Kirby KN, Petry NM. Heroin and cocaine abusers have higher discount rates for delayed rewards than alcoholics or non-drug-using controls. *Addiction* (2004) 99(4):461–71. doi:10.1111/j.1360-0443.2003.00669.x

MacKillop J, Amlung MT, Few LR, Ray LA, Sweet LH, Munafò MR. Delayed reward discounting and addictive behavior: a meta-analysis. *Psychopharmacology (Berl)* (2011) 216(3):305–21. doi:10.1007/s00213- 011-2229-0

Amlung M, Vedelago L, Acker J, Balodis I, MacKillop J. Steep delay discounting and addictive behavior: a meta-analysis of continuous associations. *Addiction* (2016). doi:10.1111/add.13535

Amlung M, Petker T, Jackson J, Balodis I, MacKillop J. Steep discounting of delayed monetary and food rewards in obesity: a meta-analysis. *Psychol Med* (2016) 46(11):2423–34. doi:10.1017/S0033291716000866

Weygandt M, Mai K, Dommes E, Ritter K, Leupelt V, Spranger J, et al. Impulse control in the dorsolateral prefrontal cortex counteracts post-diet weight regain in obesity. *Neuroimage* (2015) 109:318–27. doi:10.1016/j.neuroimage.2014.12.073

Platt ML, Watson KK, Hayden BY, Shepherd SV, Klein JT. Neuroeconomics: implications for understanding the neurobiology of addiction. 2nd ed. In: Kuhn CM, Koob GF, editors. *Advances in the Neuroscience of Addiction*. Boca Raton, FL: CRC Press/Taylor & Francis (2010). (Frontiers in Neuroscience). Available from: http://www.ncbi.nlm.nih.gov/books/NBK53362/

Weinstein SM, Mermelstein R, Shiffman S, Flay B. Mood variability and cigarette smoking escalation among adolescents. *Psychol Addict Behav* (2008) 22(4):504–13. doi:10.1037/0893-164X.22.4.504

Brogan A, Hevey D, O'Callaghan G, Yoder R, O'Shea D. Impaired decision making among morbidly obese adults. *J Psychosom Res* (2011) 70(2):189–96. doi:10.1016/j.jpsychores.2010.07.012

Leehr EJ, Krohmer K, Schag K, Dresler T, Zipfel S, Giel KE. Emotion regulation model in binge eating disorder and obesity – a systematic review. *Neurosci Biobehav Rev* (2015) 49:125–34. doi:10.1016/j.neubiorev.2014.12.008

Worbe Y, Irvine M, Lange I, Kundu P, Howell NA, Harrison NA, et al. Neuronal correlates of risk-seeking attitudes to anticipated losses in binge drinkers. *Biol Psychiatry* (2014) 76(9):717–24. doi:10.1016/j.biopsych.2013.11.028

Stevens L, Verdejo-García A, Goudriaan AE, Roeyers H, Dom G, Vanderplasschen W. Impulsivity as a vulnerability factor for poor addiction treatment outcomes: a review of neurocognitive findings among individuals with substance use disorders. *J Subst Abuse Treat* (2014) 47(1):58–72. doi:10.1016/j.jsat.2014.01.008

Voon V, Morris LS, Irvine MA, Ruck C, Worbe Y, Derbyshire K, et al. Risk-taking in disorders of natural and drug rewards: neural correlates and effects of probability, valence, and magnitude. *Neuropsychopharmacology* (2015) 40(4):804–12. doi:10.1038/npp.2014.242

Logan GD, Cowan WB, Davis KA. On the ability to inhibit simple and choice reaction time responses: a model and a method. *J Exp Psychol Hum Percept Perform* (1984) 10(2):276–91. doi:10.1037/0096-1523.10.2.276

Kaufman JN, Ross TJ, Stein EA, Garavan H. Cingulate hypoactivity in cocaine users during a GO-NOGO task as revealed by event-related functional magnetic resonance imaging. *J Neurosci* (2003) 23(21):7839–43. doi:23/21/7839 [pii]

Hester R, Garavan H. Executive dysfunction in cocaine addiction: evidence for discordant frontal, cingulate, and cerebellar activity. *J Neurosci* (2004) 24(49):11017–22. doi:10.1523/JNEUROSCI.3321-04.2004

Fu L, Bi G, Zou Z, Wang Y, Ye E, Ma L, et al. Impaired response inhibition function in abstinent heroin dependents: an fMRI study. *Neurosci Lett* (2008) 438(3):322–6. doi:10.1016/j.neulet.2008.04.033

Smith JL, Mattick RP, Jamadar SD, Iredale JM. Deficits in behavioural inhibition in substance abuse and addiction: a meta-analysis. *Drug Alcohol Depend* (2014) 145:1–33. doi:10.1016/j.drugalcdep.2014.08.009

Bartholdy S, Dalton B, O'Daly OG, Campbell IC, Schmidt U. A systematic review of the relationship between eating, weight and inhibitory control using the stop signal task. *Neurosci Biobehav Rev* (2016) 64:35–62. doi:10.1016/j. neubiorev.2016.02.010

Kulendran M, Vlaev I, Sugden C, King D, Ashrafian H, Gately P, et al. Neuropsychological assessment as a predictor of weight loss in obese adoles- cents. *Int J Obes* (2014) 38(4):507–12. doi:10.1038/ijo.2013.198

Weygandt M, Mai K, Dommes E, Leupelt V, Hackmack K, Kahnt T, et al. The role of neural impulse control mechanisms for dietary success in obesity. *Neuroimage* (2013) 83:669–78. doi:10.1016/j.neuroimage.2013. 07.028

Appelhans BM, Woolf K, Pagoto SL, Schneider KL, Whited MC, Liebman R. Inhibiting food reward: delay discounting, food reward sensitivity, and palatable food intake in overweight and obese women. *Obesity (Silver Spring)* (2011) 19(11):2175–82. doi:10.1038/oby.2011.57

Lavagnino L, Arnone D, Cao B, Soares JC, Selvaraj S. Inhibitory control in obesity and binge eating disorder: a systematic and meta-analysis of neurocognitive and neuroimaging studies. *Neurosci Biobehav Rev* (2016) 68:714–26. doi:10.1016/j.neubiorev.2016.06.041

Reinert KRS, Po'e EK, Barkin SL. The relationship between executive function and obesity in children and adolescents: a systematic literature review. *J Obes* (2013) 2013:820956. doi:10.1155/2013/820956

Miller AL, Lee HJ, Lumeng JC. Obesity-associated biomarkers and executive function in children. *Pediatr Res* (2015) 77(1–2):143–7. doi:10.1038/pr.2014.158

Liang J, Matheson BE, Kaye WH, Boutelle KN. Neurocognitive correlates of obesity and obesity-related behaviors in children and adolescents. *Int J Obes* (2014) 38(4):494–506. doi:10.1038/ijo.2013.142

Carnell S, Benson L, Pryor K, Driggin E. Appetitive traits from infancy to adolescence: using behavioral and neural measures to investigate obesity risk. *Physiol Behav* (2013) 121:79–88. doi:10.1016/j.physbeh.2013.02.015

Loeber S, Grosshans M, Korucuoglu O, Vollmert C, Vollstädt-Klein S, Schneider S, et al. Impairment of inhibitory control in response to food- associated cues and attentional bias of obese participants and normal-weight controls. *Int J Obes* (2012) 36(10):1334–9. doi:10.1038/ijo.2011.184

Mühlberg C, Mathar D, Villringer A, Horstmann A, Neumann J. Stopping at the sight of food – how gender and obesity impact on response inhibition. *Appetite* (2016) 107:663–76. doi:10.1016/j.appet.2016.08.121

Voon V, Irvine MA, Derbyshire K, Worbe Y, Lange I, Abbott S, et al. Measuring "waiting" impulsivity in substance addictions and binge eating disorder in a novel analogue of rodent serial reaction time task. *Biol Psychiatry* (2014) 75(2):148–55. doi:10.1016/j.biopsych.2013.05.013

Goldstein RZ, Volkow ND. Dysfunction of the prefrontal cortex in addiction: neuroimaging findings and clinical implications. *Nat Rev Neurosci* (2011) 12(11):652–69. doi:10.1038/nrn3119

Cox WM, Fadardi JS, Pothos EM. The addiction-Stroop test: theoretical considerations and procedural recommendations. *Psychol Bull* (2006) 132(3):443–76. doi:10.1037/0033-2909.132.3.443

Field M, Cox WM. Attentional bias in addictive behaviors: a review of its development, causes, and consequences. *Drug Alcohol Depend* (2008) 97(1–2):1–20. doi:10.1016/j.drugalcdep.2008.03.030

Nijs IMT, Franken IHA, Muris P. Food-related Stroop interference in obese and normal-weight individuals: behavioral and electrophysiological indices. *Eat Behav* (2010) 11(4):258–65. doi:10.1016/j.eatbeh.2010.07.002

Hall PA, Lowe C, Vincent C. Executive control resources and snack food consumption in the presence of restraining versus facilitating cues. *J Behav Med* (2014) 37(4):587–94. doi:10.1007/s10865-013-9528-3

Wu X, Nussbaum MA, Madigan ML. Executive function and measures of fall risk among people with obesity. *Percept Mot Skills* (2016) 122(3):825–39. doi:10.1177/0031512516646158

Fitzpatrick S, Gilbert S, Serpell L. Systematic review: are overweight and obese individuals impaired on behavioural tasks of executive functioning? *Neuropsychol Rev* (2013) 23(2):138–56. doi:10.1007/s11065-013-9224-7

Werthmann J, Jansen A, Roefs A. Worry or craving? A selective review of evidence for food-related attention biases in obese individuals, eating-disorder patients, restrained eaters and healthy samples. *Proc Nutr Soc* (2015) 74(2):99–114. doi:10.1017/S0029665114001451

Berg EA. A simple objective technique for measuring flexibility in thinking. *J Gen Psychol* (1948) 39:15–22. doi:10.1080/00221309.1948.9918159

Wu M, Brockmeyer T, Hartmann M, Skunde M, Herzog W, Friederich H-C. Set-shifting ability across the spectrum of eating disorders and in overweight and obesity: a systematic review and meta-analysis. *Psychol Med* (2014) 44(16):3365–85. doi:10.1017/S0033291714000294

Morris LS, Voon V. Dimensionality of cognitions in behavioral addiction. *Curr Behav Neurosci Rep* (2016) 3:49–57. doi:10.1007/s40473-016-0068-3

Woicik PA, Urban C, Alia-Klein N, Henry A, Maloney T, Telang F, et al. A pattern of perseveration in cocaine addiction may reveal neurocognitive processes implicit in the Wisconsin Card Sorting Test. *Neuropsychologia* (2011) 49(7):1660–9. doi:10.1016/j.neuropsychologia.2011.02.037

Alvarez-Moya EM, Jiménez-Murcia S, Moragas L, Gómez-Peña M, Aymamí MN, Ochoa C, et al. Executive functioning among female patho- logical gambling and bulimia nervosa patients: preliminary findings. *J Int Neuropsychol Soc* (2009) 15(2):302–6. doi:10.1017/S1355617709090377

Grant S, Contoreggi C, London ED. Drug abusers show impaired performance in a laboratory test of decision making. *Neuropsychologia* (2000) 38(8):1180–7. doi:10.1016/S0028-3932(99)00158-X

Nowakowska K, Jabłkowska K, Borkowska A. [Cognitive dysfunctions in patients with alcohol dependence]. *Psychiatr Pol* (2007) 41(5):693–702.

Boog M, Höppener P, Vande Wetering BJM, Goudriaan AE, Boog MC, Franken IH. Cognitive inflexibility in gamblers is primarily present in reward-related decision making. *Front Hum Neurosci* (2014) 8:569. doi:10.3389/fnhum. 2014.00569

Perpiñá C, Segura M, Sánchez-Reales S. Cognitive flexibility and decision-making in eating disorders and obesity. *Eat Weight Disord* (2016). doi:10.1007/s40519-016-0331-3

Dagher A. Alcohol and the paradox of self-control. *Biol Psychiatry* (2014) 76(9):674–5. doi:10.1016/j.biopsych.2014.08.019

Koob GF, Volkow ND. Neurobiology of addiction: a neurocircuitry analysis. *Lancet Psychiatry* (2016) 3(8):760–73. doi:10.1016/S2215-0366(16)00104-8

Garavan H, Weierstall K. The neurobiology of reward and cognitive control systems and their role in incentivizing health behavior. *Prev Med* (2012) 55(Suppl):S17–23. doi:10.1016/j.ypmed.2012.05.018

Kühn S, Gallinat J. Common biology of craving across legal and illegal drugs – a quantitative meta-analysis of cue-reactivity brain response. *Eur J Neurosci* (2011) 33(7):1318–26. doi:10.1111/j.1460-9568.2010.07590.x

Chase HW, Eickhoff SB, Laird AR, Hogarth L. The neural basis of drug stim- ulus processing and craving: an activation likelihood estimation meta-analysis. *Biol Psychiatry* (2011) 70(8):785–93. doi:10.1016/j.biopsych.2011.05.025

Schacht JP, Anton RF, Myrick H. Functional neuroimaging studies of alcohol cue reactivity: a quantitative meta-analysis and systematic review. *Addict Biol* (2013) 18(1):121–33. doi:10.1111/j.1369-1600.2012.00464.x

Tang DW, Fellows LK, Small DM, Dagher A. Food and drug cues activate similar brain regions: a meta-analysis of functional MRI studies. *Physiol Behav* (2012) 106(3):317–24. doi:10.1016/j.physbeh.2012.03.009

Hanlon CA, Dowdle LT, Naselaris T, Canterberry M, Cortese BM. Visual cortex activation to drug cues: a meta-analysis of functional neuroimaging papers in addiction and substance abuse literature. *Drug Alcohol Depend* (2014) 143:206–12. doi:10.1016/j.drugalcdep.2014.07.028

Engelmann JM, Versace F, Robinson JD, Minnix JA, Lam CY, Cui Y, et al. Neural substrates of smoking cue reactivity: a meta-analysis of fMRI studies. *Neuroimage* (2012) 60(1):252–62. doi:10.1016/j.neuroimage.2011.12.024

Noori HR, Cosa Linan A, Spanagel R. Largely overlapping neuronal substrates of reactivity to drug, gambling, food and sexual cues: a compre- hensive meta-analysis. *Eur Neuropsychopharmacol* (2016) 26(9):1419–30. doi:10.1016/j.euroneuro.2016.06.013

Meng Y, Deng W, Wang H, Guo W, Li T. The prefrontal dysfunction in individuals with Internet gaming disorder: a meta-analysis of functional magnetic resonance imaging studies. *Addict Biol* (2015) 20(4):799–808. doi:10.1111/adb.12154

Norman AL, Pulido C, Squeglia LM, Spadoni AD, Paulus MP, Tapert SF. Neural activation during inhibition predicts initiation of substance use in adolescence. *Drug Alcohol Depend* (2011) 119(3):216–23. doi:10.1016/j.drugalcdep.2011.06.019

Wetherill RR, Squeglia LM, Yang TT, Tapert SF. A longitudinal examination of adolescent response inhibition: neural differences before and after the initiation of heavy drinking. *Psychopharmacology (Berl)* (2013) 230(4):663–71. doi:10.1007/s00213-013-3198-2

Tang Y-Y, Posner MI, Rothbart MK, Volkow ND. Circuitry of self-control and its role in reducing addiction. *Trends Cogn Sci* (2015) 19(8):439–44. doi:10.1016/j.tics.2015.06.007

Hong LE, Gu H, Yang Y, Ross TJ, Salmeron BJ, Buchholz B, et al. Association of nicotine addiction and nicotine's actions with separate cingulate cortex functional circuits. *Arch Gen Psychiatry* (2009) 66(4):431–41. doi:10.1001/archgenpsychiatry.2009.2

Goldstein RZ, Volkow ND. Drug addiction and its underlying neurobi- ological basis: neuroimaging evidence for the involvement of the frontal cortex. *Am J Psychiatry* (2002) 159(10):1642–52. doi:10.1176/appi.ajp.159. 10.1642

Wilson SJ, Sayette MA, Fiez JA. Prefrontal responses to drug cues: a neurocognitive analysis. *Nat Neurosci* (2004) 7(3):211–4. doi:10.1038/nn1200

Demos KE, Heatherton TF, Kelley WM. Individual differences in nucleus accumbens activity to food and sexual images predict weight gain and sexual behavior. *J Neurosci* (2012) 32(16):5549–52. doi:10.1523/JNEUROSCI.5958-11.2012

Stice E, Burger KS, Yokum S. Reward region responsivity predicts future weight gain and moderating effects of the TaqIA allele. *J Neurosci* (2015) 35(28):10316–24. doi:10.1523/JNEUROSCI.3607-14.2015

Brooks SJ, Cedernaes J, Schiöth HB. Increased prefrontal and parahippocampal activation with reduced dorsolateral prefrontal and insular cortex activation to food images in obesity: a meta-analysis of fMRI studies. *PLoS One* (2013) 8(4):e60393. doi:10.1371/journal.pone.0060393

Goldman RL, Canterberry M, Borckardt JJ, Madan A, Byrne TK, George MS, et al. Executive control circuitry differentiates degree of success in weight loss following gastric-bypass surgery. *Obesity (Silver Spring)* (2013) 21(11):2189–96. doi:10.1002/oby.20575

Jensen CD, Kirwan CB. Functional brain response to food images in successful adolescent weight losers compared with normal-weight and overweight controls. *Obesity (Silver Spring)* (2015) 23(3):630–6. doi:10.1002/ oby.21004

Hare TA, Camerer CF, Rangel A. Self-control in decision-making involves modulation of the vmPFC valuation system. *Science* (2009) 324(5927):646–8. doi:10.1126/science.1168450

Giuliani NR, Mann T, Tomiyama AJ, Berkman ET. Neural systems underlying the reappraisal of personally craved foods. *J Cogn Neurosci* (2014) 26(7):1390–402. doi:10.1162/jocn_a_00563

Hollmann M, Hellrung L, Pleger B, Schlögl H, Kabisch S, Stumvoll M, et al. Neural correlates of the volitional regulation of the desire for food. *Int J Obes* (2012) 36(5):648–55. doi:10.1038/ijo.2011.125

Siep N, Roefs A, Roebroeck A, Havermans R, Bonte M, Jansen A. Fighting food temptations: the modulating effects of short-term cognitive reappraisal, suppression and up-regulation on mesocorticolimbic activity related to appetitive motivation. *Neuroimage* (2012) 60(1):213–20. doi:10.1016/j.neuroimage.2011.12.067

Batterink L, Yokum S, Stice E. Body mass correlates inversely with inhibitory control in response to food among adolescent girls: an fMRI study. *Neuroimage* (2010) 52(4):1696–703. doi:10.1016/j.neuroimage.2010.05.059

Hendrick OM, Luo X, Zhang S, Li C-SR. Saliency processing and obesity: a preliminary imaging study of the stop signal task. *Obesity (Silver Spring)* (2012) 20(9):1796–802. doi:10.1038/oby.2011.180

He Q, Xiao L, Xue G, Wong S, Ames SL, Schembre SM, et al. Poor ability to resist tempting calorie rich food is linked to altered balance between neural systems involved in urge and self-control. *Nutr J* (2014) 13:92. doi:10.1186/1475-2891-13-92

Appelhans BM. Neurobehavioral inhibition of reward-driven feeding: implications for dieting and obesity. *Obesity (Silver Spring)* (2009) 17(4):640– 7. doi:10.1038/oby.2008.638

García-García I, Horstmann A, Jurado MA, Garolera M, Chaudhry SJ, Margulies DS, et al. Reward processing in obesity, substance addiction and non-substance addiction. *Obes Rev* (2014) 15(11):853–69. doi:10.1111/obr.12221

American Psychiatric Association. *Diagnosticand Statistical Manualof Mental Disorders*. 5th ed. Washington, DC: DSM-5 American Psychiatric Publishing (2013).

Kessler RM, Hutson PH, Herman BK, Potenza MN. The neurobiological basis of binge-eating disorder. *Neurosci Biobehav Rev* (2016) 63:223–38. doi:10.1016/j. neubiorev.2016.01.013

Voon V. Cognitive biases in binge eating disorder: the hijacking of decision making. *CNS Spectr* (2015) 20(6):566–73. doi:10.1017/S1092852915000681

Davis C, Patte K, Curtis C, Reid C. Immediate pleasures and future consequences. A neuropsychological study of binge eating and obesity. *Appetite* (2010) 54(1):208–13. doi:10.1016/j.appet.2009.11.002

Hege MA, Stingl KT, Kullmann S, Schag K, Giel KE, Zipfel S, et al. Attentional impulsivity in binge eating disorder modulates response inhibition performance and frontal brain networks. *Int J Obes* (2015) 39(2):353–60. doi:10.1038/ijo.2014.99

Balodis IM, Molina ND, Kober H, Worhunsky PD, White MA, Sinha R, et al. Divergent neural substrates of inhibitory control in binge eating disorder relative to other manifestations of obesity. *Obesity (Silver Spring)* (2013) 21(2):367–77. doi:10.1002/oby.20068

Schulte EM, Grilo CM, Gearhardt AN. Shared and unique mechanisms underlying binge eating disorder and addictive disorders. *Clin Psychol Rev* (2016) 44:125–39. doi:10.1016/j.cpr.2016.02.001

Gearhardt AN, White MA, Potenza MN. Binge eating disorder and food addiction. *Curr Drug Abuse Rev* (2011) 4(3):201–7. doi:10.2174/18744737 11104030201

Avena NM, Rada P, Hoebel BG. Evidence for sugar addiction: behavioral and neurochemical effects of intermittent, excessive sugar intake. *Neurosci Biobehav Rev* (2008) 32(1):20–39. doi:10.1016/j.neubiorev.2007.04.019

Schulte EM, Joyner MA, Potenza MN, Grilo CM, Gearhardt AN. Current considerations regarding food addiction. *Curr Psychiatry Rep* (2015) 17(4):563. doi:10.1007/s11920-015-0563-3

Gearhardt AN, Corbin WR, Brownell KD. Preliminary validation of the Yale Food Addiction Scale. *Appetite* (2009) 52(2):430–6. doi:10.1016/j.appet.2008.12.003

Davis C. From passive overeating to "food addiction": a spectrum of compulsion and severity. *ISRN Obes* (2013) 2013:435027. doi:10.1155/2013/435027

Gearhardt AN, Corbin WR, Brownell KD. Development of the Yale Food Addiction Scale Version 2.0. *Psychol Addict Behav* (2016) 30(1):113–21. doi:10.1037/adb0000136

Ziauddeen H, Fletcher PC. Is food addiction a valid and useful concept? *Obes Rev* (2013) 14(1):19–28. doi:10.1111/j.1467-789X.2012.01046.x

Ziauddeen H, Farooqi IS, Fletcher PC. Obesity and the brain: how convincing is the addiction model? *Nat Rev Neurosci* (2012) 13(4):279–86. doi:10.1038/nrn3212

Corsica JA, Pelchat ML. Food addiction: true or false? *Curr Opin Gastroenterol* (2010) 26(2):165–9. doi:10.1097/MOG.0b013e328336528d

Avena NM, Gearhardt AN, Gold MS, Wang G-J, Potenza MN. Tossing the baby out with the bathwater after a brief rinse? The potential downside of dismissing food addiction based on limited data. *Nat Rev Neurosci* (2012) 13(7):514; author reply 514. doi:10.1038/nrn3212-c1

Westwater ML, Fletcher PC, Ziauddeen H. Sugar addiction: the state of the science. *Eur J Nutr* (2016) 55(Suppl 2):55–69. doi:10.1007/s00394-016-1229-6

Hebebrand J, Albayrak Ö, Adan R, Antel J, Dieguez C, de Jong J, et al. "Eating addiction", rather than "food addiction", better captures addictive-like eating behavior. *Neurosci Biobehav Rev* (2014) 47:295–306. doi:10.1016/j.neubiorev.2014.08.016

Pedram P, Wadden D, Amini P, Gulliver W, Randell E, Cahill F, et al. Food addiction: its prevalence and significant association with obesity in the general population. *PLoS One* (2013) 8(9):e74832. doi:10.1371/journal.pone.0074832

Long CG, Blundell JE, Finlayson G. A systematic review of the application and correlates of YFAS-diagnosed "food addiction" in humans: are eating-related "addictions" a cause for concern or empty concepts? *Obes Facts* (2015) 8(6):386–401. doi:10.1159/000442403

De Zwaan M. Binge eating disorder and obesity. *Int J Obes Relat Metab Disord* (2001) 25(Suppl 1):S51–5. doi:10.1038/sj.ijo.0801699

Schag K, Schönleber J, Teufel M, Zipfel S, Giel KE. Food-related impulsivity in obesity and binge eating disorder – a systematic review. *Obes Rev* (2013) 14(6):477–95. doi:10.1111/obr.12017

Davis C. Attention-deficit/hyperactivity disorder: associations with overeating and obesity. *Curr Psychiatry Rep* (2010) 12(5):389–95. doi:10.1007/s11920-010-0133-7

Matthews M, Nigg JT, Fair DA. Attention deficit hyperactivity disorder. In: Andersen SL, Pine DS, editors. *The Neurobiology of Childhood*. Berlin Heidelberg: Springer (2013). p. 235–66. (Current Topics in Behavioral Neurosciences). Available from: http://link.springer.com/chapter/10.1007/7854_2013_249

Ottosen C, Petersen L, Larsen JT, Dalsgaard S. Gender differences in associations between attention-deficit/hyperactivity disorder and substance use disorder. *J Am Acad Child Adolesc Psychiatry* (2016) 55(3):227.e–34.e. doi:10.1016/j.jaac.2015.12.010

Charach A, Yeung E, Climans T, Lillie E. Childhood attention-deficit/hyperactivity disorder and future substance use disorders: comparative meta-analyses. *J Am Acad Child Adolesc Psychiatry* (2011) 50(1):9–21. doi:10.1016/j.jaac.2010.09.019

Lee SS, Humphreys KL, Flory K, Liu R, Glass K. Prospective association of childhood attention-deficit/hyperactivity disorder (ADHD) and substance use and abuse/dependence: a meta-analytic review. *Clin Psychol Rev* (2011) 31(3):328–41. doi:10.1016/j.cpr.2011.01.006

Wilens TE, Martelon M, Joshi G, Bateman C, Fried R, Petty C, et al. Does ADHD predict substance-use disorders? A 10-year follow-up study of young adults with ADHD. *J Am Acad Child Adolesc Psychiatry* (2011) 50(6):543–53. doi:10.1016/j.jaac.2011.01.021

Nigg JT, Johnstone JM, Musser ED, Long HG, Willoughby MT, Shannon J. Attention-deficit/hyperactivity disorder (ADHD) and being overweight/obesity: new data and meta-analysis. *Clin Psychol Rev* (2016) 43:67–79. doi:10.1016/j.cpr.2015.11.005

Cortese S, Moreira-Maia CR, St Fleur D, Morcillo-Peñalver C, Rohde LA, Faraone SV. Association between ADHD and obesity: a systematic review and meta-analysis. *Am J Psychiatry* (2016) 173(1):34–43. doi:10.1176/appi.ajp.2015.15020266

Cortese S, Ramos Olazagasti MA, Klein RG, Castellanos FX, Proal E, Mannuzza S. Obesity in men with childhood ADHD: a 33-year controlled, prospective, follow-up study. *Pediatrics* (2013) 131(6):e1731–8. doi:10.1542/ peds.2012-0540

Khalife N, Kantomaa M, Glover V, Tammelin T, Laitinen J, Ebeling H, et al. Childhood attention-deficit/hyperactivity disorder symptoms are risk factors for obesity and physical inactivity in adolescence. *J Am Acad Child Adolesc Psychiatry* (2014) 53(4):425–36. doi:10.1016/j.jaac.2014.01.009

Kaisari P, Dourish CT, Higgs S. Attention deficit hyperactivity disorder (ADHD) and disordered eating behaviour: a systematic review and a framework for future research. *Clin Psychol Rev* (2017) 53:109–21. doi:10.1016/j.cpr.2017.03.002

Duncan L, Perry JRB, Patterson N, Robinson EB, Daly MJ, Price AL, et al. An atlas of genetic correlations across human diseases and traits. *Nat Genet* (2015) 47(11):1236–41. doi:10.1038/ng.3406

Cortese S, Isnard P, Frelut ML, Michel G, Quantin L, Guedeney A, et al. Association between symptoms of attention-deficit/hyperactivity disorder and bulimic behaviors in a clinical sample of severely obese adolescents. *Int J Obes (Lond)* (2007) 31(2):340–6. doi:10.1038/sj.ijo.0803400

Davis C, Levitan RD, Smith M, Tweed S, Curtis C. Associations among overeating, overweight, and attention deficit/hyperactivity disorder: a structural equation modelling approach. *Eat Behav* (2006) 7(3):266–74. doi:10.1016/j.eatbeh.2005.09.006

Cortese S, Castellanos FX. The relationship between ADHD and obesity: implications for therapy. *Expert Rev Neurother* (2014) 14(5):473–9. doi:10.1586/14737175.2014.904748

Sinha R, Jastreboff AM. Stress as a common risk factor for obesity and addic- tion. *Biol Psychiatry* (2013) 73(9):827–35. doi:10.1016/j.biopsych.2013.01.032

Morris MJ, Beilharz JE, Maniam J, Reichelt AC, Westbrook RF. Why is obesity such a problem in the 21st century? The intersection of palatable food, cues and reward pathways, stress, and cognition. *Neurosci Biobehav Rev* (2015) 58:36–45. doi:10.1016/j.neubiorev.2014.12.002

Epstein DH, Willner-Reid J, Vahabzadeh M, Mezghanni M, Lin J-L, Preston KL. Real-time electronic diary reports of cue exposure and mood in the hours before cocaine and heroin craving and use. *Arch Gen Psychiatry* (2009) 66(1):88–94. doi:10.1001/archgenpsychiatry.2008.509

Sinha R, Catapano D, O'Malley S. Stress-induced craving and stress response in cocaine dependent individuals. *Psychopharmacology (Berl)* (1999) 142(4):343–51. doi:10.1007/s002130050898

Sinha R. Chronic stress, drug use, and vulnerability to addiction. *Ann N Y Acad Sci* (2008) 1141:105–30. doi:10.1196/annals.1441.030

Koob GF, Le Moal M. Drug abuse: hedonic homeostatic dysregulation. *Science* (1997) 278(5335):52–8. doi:10.1126/science.278.5335.52

Koob GF, Le Moal M. Addiction and the brain antireward system. *Annu Rev Psychol* (2008) 59:29–53. doi:10.1146/annurev.psych.59.103006. 093548

Geliebter A, Aversa A. Emotional eating in overweight, normal weight, and underweight individuals. *Eat Behav* (2003) 3(4):341–7. doi:10.1016/ S1471-0153(02)00100-9

Hepworth R, Mogg K, Brignell C, Bradley BP. Negative mood increases selective attention to food cues and subjective appetite. *Appetite* (2010) 54(1):134–42. doi:10.1016/j.appet.2009.09.019

Chao A, Grilo CM, White MA, Sinha R. Food cravings mediate the relationship between chronic stress and body mass index. *J Health Psychol* (2015) 20(6):721–9. doi:10.1177/1359105315573448

Oliver G, Wardle J. Perceived effects of stress on food choice. *Physiol Behav* (1999) 66(3):511–5. doi:10.1016/S0031-9384(98)00322-9

Zellner DA, Loaiza S, Gonzalez Z, Pita J, Morales J, Pecora D, et al. Food selection changes under stress. *Physiol Behav* (2006) 87:789–93. doi:10.1016/j.physbeh.2006.01.014

Dallman MF, Pecoraro N, Akana SF, la Fleur SE, Gomez F,Houshyar H, et al. Chronic stress and obesity: a new view of "comfort food.". *Proc Natl Acad Sci U S A* (2003) 100(20):11696–701. doi:10.1073/pnas.1934666100

Macht M, Mueller J. Immediate effects of chocolate on experimentally induced mood states. *Appetite* (2007) 49:667–74. doi:10.1016/j.appet.2007. 05.004

Macht M. How emotions affect eating: a five-way model. *Appetite* (2008) 50(1):1–11. doi:10.1016/j.appet.2007.07.002

Kivimäki M, Head J, Ferrie JE, Shipley MJ, Brunner E, Vahtera J, et al. Work stress, weight gain and weight loss: evidence for bidirectional effects of job strain on body mass index in the Whitehall II study. *Int J Obes* (2006) 30(6):982–7. doi:10.1038/sj.ijo.0803229

Tryon MS, Carter CS, Decant R, Laugero KD. Chronic stress exposure may affect the brain's response to high calorie food cues and predispose to obesogenic eating habits. *Physiol Behav* (2013) 120:233–42. doi:10.1016/j.physbeh.2013.08.010

Maier SU, Makwana AB, Hare TA. Acute stress impairs self-control in goal-directed choice by altering multiple functional connections within the brain's decision circuits. *Neuron* (2015) 87(3):621–31. doi:10.1016/j.neuron.2015.07.005

Jastreboff AM, Sinha R, Lacadie C, Small DM, Sherwin RS, Potenza MN. Neural correlates of stress- and food cue-induced food craving in obesity: association with insulin levels. *Diabetes Care* (2013) 36(2):394–402. doi:10.2337/ dc12-1112

Adam TC, Epel ES. Stress, eating and the reward system. *Physiol Behav* (2007) 91(4):449–58. doi:10.1016/j.physbeh.2007.04.011

Barry D, Clarke M, Petry NM. Obesity and its relationship to addictions: is overeating a form of addictive behavior? *Am J Addict* (2009) 18(6):439–51. doi:10.3109/10550490903205579

Barry D, Petry NM. Associations between body mass index and substance use disorders differ by gender: results from the National Epidemiologic Survey on Alcohol and Related Conditions. *Addict Behav* (2009) 34(1):51–60. doi:10.1016/j.addbeh.2008.08.008

Grucza RA, Krueger RF, Racette SB, Norberg KE, Hipp PR, Bierut LJ. The emerging link between alcoholism risk and obesity in the United States. *Arch Gen Psychiatry* (2010) 67(12):1301–8. doi:10.1001/archgenpsychiatry.2010.155

Simon GE, Von Korff M, Saunders K, Miglioretti DL, Crane PK, van Belle G, et al. Association between obesity and psychiatric disorders in the US adult population. *Arch Gen Psychiatry* (2006) 63(7):824–30. doi:10.1001/archpsyc.63.7.824

Pickering RP, Grant BF, Chou SP, Compton WM. Are overweight, obesity, and extreme obesity associated with psychopathology? Results from the national epidemiologic survey on alcohol and related conditions. *J Clin Psychiatry* (2007) 68(7):998–1009. doi:10.4088/JCP.v68n0704

Scott KM, McGee MA, Wells JE, Oakley Browne MA. Obesity and mental disorders in the adult general population. *J Psychosom Res* (2008) 64(1):97–105. doi:10.1016/j.jpsychores.2007.09.006

Sansone RA, Sansone LA. Obesity and substance misuse: is there a relationship? *Innov Clin Neurosci* (2013) 10(9–10):30–5.

Green MA, Strong M, Razak F, Subramanian SV, Relton C, Bissell P. Who are the obese? A cluster analysis exploring subgroups of the obese. *J Public Health* (2015) 2:fdv040. doi:10.1093/pubmed/fdv040

King WC, Chen J-Y, Mitchell JE, Kalarchian MA, Steffen KJ, Engel SG, et al. Prevalence of alcohol use disorders before and after bariatric surgery. *JAMA* (2012) 307(23):2516–25. doi:10.1001/jama.2012.6147

Conason A, Teixeira J, Hsu C-H, Puma L, Knafo D, Geliebter A. Substance use following bariatric weight loss surgery. *JAMA Surg* (2013) 148(2):145–50. doi:10.1001/2013.jamasurg.265

Steffen KJ, Engel SG, Wonderlich JA, Pollert GA, Sondag C. Alcohol and other addictive disorders following bariatric surgery: prevalence, risk factors and possible etiologies. *Eur Eat Disord Rev* (2015) 23(6):442–50. doi:10.1002/erv.2399

Permissions

All chapters in this book were first published by Frontiers; hereby published with permission under the Creative Commons Attribution License or equivalent. Every chapter published in this book has been scrutinized by our experts. Their significance has been extensively debated. The topics covered herein carry significant findings which will fuel the growth of the discipline. They may even be implemented as practical applications or may be referred to as a beginning point for another development.

The contributors of this book come from diverse backgrounds, making this book a truly international effort. This book will bring forth new frontiers with its revolutionizing research information and detailed analysis of the nascent developments around the world.

We would like to thank all the contributing authors for lending their expertise to make the book truly unique. They have played a crucial role in the development of this book. Without their invaluable contributions this book wouldn't have been possible. They have made vital efforts to compile up to date information on the varied aspects of this subject to make this book a valuable addition to the collection of many professionals and students.

This book was conceptualized with the vision of imparting up-to-date information and advanced data in this field. To ensure the same, a matchless editorial board was set up. Every individual on the board went through rigorous rounds of assessment to prove their worth. After which they invested a large part of their time researching and compiling the most relevant data for our readers.

The editorial board has been involved in producing this book since its inception. They have spent rigorous hours researching and exploring the diverse topics which have resulted in the successful publishing of this book. They have passed on their knowledge of decades through this book. To expedite this challenging task, the publisher supported the team at every step. A small team of assistant editors was also appointed to further simplify the editing procedure and attain best results for the readers.

Apart from the editorial board, the designing team has also invested a significant amount of their time in understanding the subject and creating the most relevant covers. They scrutinized every image to scout for the most suitable representation of the subject and create an appropriate cover for the book.

The publishing team has been an ardent support to the editorial, designing and production team. Their endless efforts to recruit the best for this project, has resulted in the accomplishment of this book. They are a veteran in the field of academics and their pool of knowledge is as vast as their experience in printing. Their expertise and guidance has proved useful at every step. Their uncompromising quality standards have made this book an exceptional effort. Their encouragement from time to time has been an inspiration for everyone.

The publisher and the editorial board hope that this book will prove to be a valuable piece of knowledge for researchers, students, practitioners and scholars across the globe.

List of Contributors

Kimberley D. Bruce and Robert H. Eckel
University of Colorado School of Medicine, Division of Endocrinology, Metabolism and Diabetes, Aurora, CO, USA

Andrea Zsombok
Department of Physiology, School of Medicine, Tulane University, New Orleans, LA, USA

Dana M. Small
The John B Pierce Laboratory, New Haven, CT, USA
Department of Psychiatry, Yale University School of Medicine, New Haven, CT, USA

Sarah H. Lockie, Clare V. McAuley, Sasha Rawlinson, Natalie Guiney and Zane B. Andrews
Monash Biomedicine Discovery Institute and Department of Physiology, Monash University, Clayton, VIC, Australia

Rim Hassouna
Centre de Psychiatrie et Neurosciences, UMR-S 894 Institut National de la Santé et de la Recherche Médicale, Université Paris Descartes, Sorbonne Paris Cité, Paris, France
Department of Pediatrics, Naomi Berrie Diabetes Center, Columbia University Medical Center, New York, NY, USA

Dominique Grouselle, Virginie Tolle, Oriane Fiquet and Joanna Lipecka
Centre de Psychiatrie et Neurosciences, UMR-S 894 Institut National de la Santé et de la Recherche Médicale, Université Paris Descartes, Sorbonne Paris Cité, Paris, France

Giovanni Chiappetta and Joëlle Vinh
ESPCI Paris, PSL Research University, Spectrométrie de Masse Biologique et Protéomique (SMPB), CNRS USR 3149, Paris, France

Catherine Tomasetto
UMR-7104 Centre National de la Recherche Scientifique/U596, Institut National de la Santé et de la Recherche Médicale, Institut de génétique et de biologie moléculaire et cellulaire, Université de Strasbourg, Illkirch, France

Nicholas Heeley and Clemence Blouet
Medical Research Council Metabolic Disease Unit, Institute of Metabolic Science, University of Cambridge, Cambridge, UK

Jacques Epelbaum
Centre de Psychiatrie et Neurosciences, UMR-S 894 Institut National de la Santé et de la Recherche Médicale, Université Paris Descartes, Sorbonne Paris Cité, Paris, France
UMR 7179 Centre Nationnal de la Recherche Scientifique, MNHN, Adaptive Mechanism and Evolution (MECADEV), Brunoy, France

Ryan Michael Cassidy and Qingchun Tong
Brown Foundation of the Institute of Molecular Medicine for the Prevention of Human Diseases of McGovern Medical, USA
School, Neuroscience Program MD Anderson Cancer Center and UTHealth Graduate School of Biological Sciences, The University of Texas Health Science Center at Houston, Houston, TX, USA

João C. P. Santiago and Manfred Hallschmid
Institute of Medical Psychology and Behavioral Neurobiology, University of Tübingen, Tübingen, Germany
German Center for Diabetes Research, Tübingen, Germany
Institute for Diabetes Research and Metabolic Diseases of the Helmholtz Center Munich at the University of Tübingen, Tübingen, Germany

Ophélia Le Thuc
CNRS, Institut de Pharmacologie Moléculaire et Cellulaire, Université Côte d'Azur, Valbonne, France
Helmholtz Diabetes Center (HDC), German Center for Diabetes Research (DZD), Helmholtz Zentrum München, Neuherberg, Germany
Division of Metabolic Diseases, Technische Universität München, Munich, Germany

Katharina Stobbe, Céline Cansell, Jean-Louis Nahon, Nicolas Blondeau and Carole Rovère
CNRS, Institut de Pharmacologie Moléculaire et Cellulaire, Université Côte d'Azur, Valbonne, France

Helene Volkoff
Departments of Biology and Biochemistry, Memorial University of Newfoundland, St. John's, NL, Canada

Sergueï O. Fetissov, Nicolas Lucas and Romain Legrand
INSERM UMR1073, Nutrition, Gut and Brain Laboratory, Rouen, France
Institute for Research and Innovation in Biomedicine (IRIB), University of Rouen Normandy, Rouen, France

Daisuke Kohno
Advanced Scientific Research Leaders Development Unit, Gunma University, Maebashi, Japan
Metabolic Signal Research Center, Institute for Molecular and Cellular Regulation, Gunma University, Maebashi, Japan

Miho Koike
Advanced Scientific Research Leaders Development Unit, Gunma University, Maebashi, Japan

Yuzo Ninomiya
Division of Sensory Physiology, Research and Development Center for Taste and Odor Sensing, Kyushu University, Fukuoka, Japan
Monell Chemical Senses Center, Philadelphia, PA, USA

Itaru Kojima
Department of Cell Biology, Institute for Molecular and Cellular Regulation, Gunma University, Maebashi, Japan

Tadahiro Kitamura
Metabolic Signal Research Center, Institute for Molecular and Cellular Regulation, Gunma University, Maebashi, Japan

Toshihiko Yada
Division of Integrative Physiology, Department of Physiology, School of Medicine, Jichi Medical University, Shimotsuke, Japan

María J. Delgado
Departamento de Fisiología (Fisiología Animal II), Facultad de Biología, Universidad Complutense de Madrid, Madrid, Spain

José M. Cerdá-Reverter
Departamento de Fisiología de Peces y Biotecnología, Instituto de Acuicultura Torre de la Sal, Consejo Superior de Investigaciones Científicas, Castellón, Spain

José L. Soengas
Laboratorio de Fisioloxía Animal, Departamento de Bioloxía Funcional e Ciencias da Saúde, Facultade de Bioloxía, Universidade de Vigo, Vigo, Spain

Sophie Scharner, Philip Prinz, Peter Kobelt, Tobias Hofmann, Matthias Rose and Andreas Stengel
Division of Psychosomatic Medicine, Charité Center for Internal Medicine and Dermatology, Charité-Universitätsmedizin Berlin, Berlin, Germany

Miriam Goebel-Stengel
Department of Internal Medicine and Institute of Neurogastroenterology, Martin-Luther-Krankenhaus Berlin, Berlin, Germany

Roberta Haddad-Tóvolli, Nathalia R. V. Dragano, Albina F. S. Ramalho and Licio A. Velloso
Laboratory of Cell Signaling and Obesity and Comorbidities Research Center, Faculty of Medical Sciences, University of Campinas, Campinas, Brazil

Evita Belegri, Merel Rijnsburger, Leslie Eggels, Unga Unmehopa and Anita Boelen
Laboratory of Endocrinology, Department of Clinical Chemistry and Department of Endocrinology and Metabolism, Academic Medical Center, University of Amsterdam, Amsterdam, Netherlands

Wiep Scheper
Clincal Genetics, VU Medical Center, Amsterdam, Netherlands

Susanne E. la Fleur
Laboratory of Endocrinology, Department of Clinical Chemistry and Department of Endocrinology and Metabolism, Academic Medical Center, University of Amsterdam, Amsterdam, Netherlands
Metabolism and Reward Group, Netherlands Institute for Neuroscience, Amsterdam, Netherlands

Anne-Sophie Delbès, Julien Castel, Raphaël G. P. Denis, Chloé Morel, Mar Quiñones and Serge H. Luquet
Université Paris Diderot, Sorbonne Paris Cité, Unité de Biologie Fonctionnelle et Adaptative, CNRS UMR 8251, Paris, France

Amandine Everard and Patrice D. Cani
Walloon Excellence in Life Sciences and Biotechnology (WELBIO), Metabolism and Nutrition Research Group, Louvain Drug Research Institute, Université catholique de Louvain, Brussels, Belgium

Florence Massiera
Laboratoire de Recherche Nutritionnelle KOT CEPRODI SA, Paris, France

Elise Laperrousaz, Raphaël G. Denis, Nadim Kassis, Serge Luquet, Céline Cruciani-Guglielmacci and Christophe Magnan
Unité de Biologie Fonctionnelle et Adaptative, CNRS UMR 8251, Sorbonne Paris Cité, Université Denis Diderot, Paris, France

Cristina Contreras and Miguel López
NeurObesity Group, Department of Physiology, Centro de Investigación en Medicina Molecular y Enfermedades Crónicas (CiMUS), University of Santiago de Compostela-Instituto de Investigación Sanitaria, Santiago de Compostela, Spain
CIBER Fisiopatología de la Obesidad y Nutrición (CIBERobn), Santiago de Compostela, Spain

Andréanne Michaud, Isabel Garcia-Garcia and Alain Dagher
Department of Neurology and Neurosurgery, Montreal Neurological Institute, McGill University, Montreal, QC, Canada

Uku Vainik
Department of Neurology and Neurosurgery, Montreal Neurological Institute, McGill University, Montreal, QC, Canada
Faculty of Social Sciences, Institute of Psychology, University of Tartu, Tartu, Estonia

Index

N

O

P

S

T

U

V

Printed in the USA
CPSIA information can be obtained
at www.ICGtesting.com
LVHW080046211023
761596LV00010BA/1933

9 781639 897858